BLANCHARD & LOEB PUBLISHERS

Nurse's Choice for Better Care™

Nurse's Handbook of I.V. Drugs

D0094158

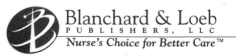

Blanchard & Loeb
PUBLISHERS, LLC
Nurse's Choice for Better Care™

San Francisco•Philadelphia•New York

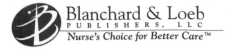

Blanchard & Loeb
PUBLISHERS, LLC
Nurse's Choice for Better Care™

Publishers: Ross Blanchard, Stanley E. Loeb
Clinical Director: Cindy Tryniszewski, RN, MSN
Clinical Project Manager: Patricia Kardish Fischer, RN, BSN
Book Editor: Doris Weinstock
Copy Editor: Dolores Connors Matthews
Indexer: Barbara Hodgson
Cover: Ray Keim
Interior Illustrations: Rolin Graphics, Inc.
Composition: Matrix Publishing Services

© 2003 Blanchard & Loeb Publishers, LLC

Printed in the United States of America

Blanchard & Loeb Publishers, LLC
865 Belfry Drive
Blue Bell, PA 19422

CONTENTS

Reviewers and Clinical Consultants iv
How to Use This Book v
Foreword xii
Overview of Pharmacology xv
Principles of I.V. Drug Administration xxiii
I.V. Drug Therapy and the Nursing Process xxxiii

INDIVIDUAL DRUGS (organized alphabetically)

A 1
B 77
C 106
D 204
E • F 272
G • H 341
I 373
K • L 410
M 442
N • O 503
P 550
Q • R • S 629
T • U • V 660
W, Z 712

APPENDICES

1 Equianalgesic Doses for Opioid Agonists 725
2 Calculating the Strength of a Solution 726
3 Calculating Parenteral Drug Dosages 728
4 Calculating I.V. Flow Rates 730
5 Selected Common Toxicity Criteria 732
6 I.V. Antineoplastic Drugs 742
7 Body Mass Index Calculation 750
8 Abbreviations 752

Index 757

Reviewers and Clinical Consultants

Karen T. Bruchak, RN, MSN, MBA
Director, Medical-Surgical Nursing
The Chester County Hospital
Chester, PA

Terri Corbo, PharmD, BCPS
Clinical Specialist, Cardiology
Christiana Care Health System
Newark, DE

Kimberly Anne Boykin Couch, PharmD
Clinical Specialist
Christiana Care Health System
Adjunct Faculty
University of Delaware School of Nursing
Newark, DE

How to Use This Book

Blanchard & Loeb Publishers Nurse's Handbook of I.V. Drugs gives you what today's nurses and nursing students need: accurate, concise, and reliable facts about I.V. drug administration. This book emphasizes the vital information you need to know before, during, and after drug administration. And the information is presented in easy-to-understand language and organized alphabetically, so you can find what you need quickly.

What's Special

In addition to the drug information you expect to find in each entry (see "Drug Entries" below for details), *Nurse's Handbook of I.V. Drugs* boasts these special features:

- **Practical trim size and good-size type** give you a book that's easy to carry, easy to read, and easy to handle. You can hold the book in one hand, see complete pages at a glance, and use your other hand to document or perform other activities.
- **Introductory material** reviews essential general information you need to know to administer I.V. drugs safely and effectively, including an overview of pharmacology and the principles of I.V. drug administration. In addition, the five steps of the nursing process are reviewed and related specifically to drug therapy.
- **Colorful illustrations** throughout the text help you visualize selected mechanisms of action by showing how drugs work at the cellular, tissue, and organ levels. In addition, the inside front cover features a chart listing all the drugs whose mechanisms of action are illustrated—along with other drugs that have similar mechanisms of action.
- **No-nonsense writing style** that uses the terms and abbreviations you typically encounter in your practice and your studies (although a few abbreviations may not be used in certain facilities). (See *Abbreviations*, pages 752 to 755.) And to avoid sexist language, we alternate male and female pronouns as we move from letter to letter throughout the book.
- **Up-to-date drug information,** including the latest FDA-approved drugs, new and changed indications, new warnings, and newly discovered adverse reactions.
- **Dosage adjustment,** highlighted in the text, alerts you to expected dosage changes for patients with a specific condition or disorder, such as advanced age or renal impairment.

- **Warning,** highlighted in the text, calls attention to important facts that you need to know before, during, and after drug administration. For example, in the alatrofloxacin entry, this feature informs you that the drug usually is reserved for hospitalized patients and is given for no longer than 2 weeks because of the high risk of severe liver damage.
- **Easy-to-use charts** for route, onset, peak, and duration provide a timesaving way to track and check this important information. (See page viii for details on route, onset, peak, and duration charts.)
- **Useful appendices** provide you with even more handy information you can use every day in your practice and studies, such as the Common Toxicity Criteria used to evaluate adverse effects of chemotherapy drugs and a chart that shows you which drugs are compatible in a syringe. (See pages 732 to 741 and the inside back cover.)

Drug Entries

Nurse's Handbook of I.V. Drugs clearly and concisely presents all the vital facts on the drugs that you'll typically administer. To help you find the information you need quickly, drug entries are organized alphabetically by generic drug name—from abciximab to zoledronic acid. For ease of use, every drug entry follows a consistent format. However, if specific details are unknown or don't apply, that heading isn't included so you can go right to the next section. (Exceptions are the headings "Adverse Reactions" and "Interactions," where "None with the usual dosages" and "None known" may be used.)

Generic and Trade Names

First, each entry identifies the drug's main generic name as well as alternate generic names. (For drugs prescribed by trade name, you can quickly check the comprehensive index, which refers you to the appropriate generic name and page.) Next, the entry lists the most common U.S. trade names for each drug. It also includes common trade names available only in Canada, marked (CAN).

Class, Category, and Schedule

Each entry lists the drug's chemical and therapeutic classes. With this information, you can compare drugs in the same chemical class but in different therapeutic classes and vice versa.

The entry also lists the FDA's pregnancy risk category, which categorizes drugs based on their potential to cause birth defects. (For details, see *FDA pregnancy risk categories*.) Where appropriate, the en-

F.D.A. PREGNANCY RISK CATEGORIES

Each drug may be placed in a pregnancy risk category based on the FDA's estimate of risk to the fetus. If the FDA hasn't provided a category, the *Nurse's Handbook of I.V. Drugs* notes that the drug is "Not rated." The categories range from A to X, signifying least to greatest fetal risk.

A Controlled studies show no risk

Adequate, well-controlled studies with pregnant women have failed to demonstrate a risk to the fetus in any trimester of pregnancy.

B No evidence of risk in humans

Adequate, well-controlled studies with pregnant women haven't shown increased risk of fetal abnormalities despite adverse findings in animals, or—in the absence of adequate human studies—animal studies show no fetal risk. The chance of fetal harm exists but is remote.

C Risk can't be ruled out

Adequate, well-controlled human studies are lacking, and animal studies are lacking as well or have demonstrated a risk to the fetus. A chance of fetal harm exists if the drug is administered during pregnancy, but the potential benefits may outweigh the potential risk.

D Positive evidence of risk

Studies in humans, or investigational or post-marketing data, have demonstrated fetal risk. Nevertheless, potential benefits from the drug's use may outweigh potential risks. For example, the drug may be acceptable if needed in a life-threatening situation or serious disease for which safer drugs can't be used or are ineffective.

X Contraindicated in pregnancy

Studies in animals or humans, or investigational or post-marketing reports, have demonstrated positive evidence of fetal abnormalities or risks; these risks clearly outweigh any possible benefit to the patient.

try also includes the drug's controlled substance schedule. (For details, see *Controlled substance schedules,* page viii.)

Indications and Dosages
This section lists FDA-approved therapeutic indications. For each indication, you'll find the applicable drug form or route, age-group

CONTROLLED SUBSTANCE SCHEDULES

The Controlled Substances Act of 1970 mandated that certain prescription drugs be categorized in schedules based on their potential for abuse. The greater their abuse potential, the greater the restrictions on their prescription. The controlled substance schedules range from I to V, signifying highest to lowest abuse potential.

I High potential for abuse

No accepted medical use exists for Schedule I drugs, which include heroin and lysergic acid diethylamide (LSD).

II High potential for abuse

Use may lead to severe physical or psychological dependence. Prescriptions must be written in ink or typewritten and must be signed by the prescriber. Oral prescriptions must be confirmed in writing within 72 hours and may be given only in a genuine emergency. No renewals are permitted.

III Some potential for abuse

Use may lead to low-to-moderate physical dependence or high psychological dependence. Prescriptions may be oral or written. Up to five renewals are permitted within 6 months.

IV Low potential for abuse

Use may lead to limited physical or psychological dependence. Prescriptions may be oral or written. Up to five renewals are permitted within 6 months.

V Subject to state and local regulation

Abuse potential is low; a prescription may not be required.

(adults, adolescents, or children), and dosage (which includes amount per dose, timing, and duration).

Route, Onset, Peak, and Duration

Quick-reference charts show the drug's onset, peak, and duration (when known) for the appropriate administration route. The *onset of action* is the time a drug takes to be absorbed, reach a therapeutic blood level, and elicit an initial therapeutic response. The *peak therapeutic effect* occurs when a drug reaches its highest blood concentration and the greatest amount of drug reaches the site of action to produce the maximum therapeutic response. The *duration of action* is the amount of time that a drug remains at a blood concentration that produces a therapeutic response.

Mechanism of Action
Set off by a box, this section concisely describes how a drug achieves its therapeutic effects at the cellular, tissue, and organ levels, as appropriate. Illustrations of selected mechanisms of action lend exceptional detail and clarity to sometimes complex processes.

Incompatibilities
This section alerts you to drugs or solutions that are incompatible with the topic drug when mixed in a syringe or solution or infused through the same I.V. line.

Contraindications
An alphabetical list details the conditions and disorders that preclude administration of the topic drug.

Interactions
This section presents the drugs, foods, and activities (such as alcohol use and smoking) that can cause important, problematic, or life-threatening interactions with the topic drug. For each interacting drug, food, or activity, you'll learn the effects of the interaction.

Adverse Reactions
Organized by body system, this section highlights common, serious, and life-threatening adverse reactions in alphabetical order.

Nursing Considerations
Warnings, general precautions, and key information that you must know before, during, and after drug administration are detailed in this section. Examples include whether or not you need to take special precautions when preparing a drug for administration and how to properly reconstitute, dilute, store, handle, or dispose of a drug.

Patient teaching information is also included here. You'll find important guidelines for patients, such as how to spot and manage adverse reactions, when to report them, which cautions to observe, and more. To save you time, however, this section doesn't repeat basic patient-teaching points. (For a summary of those, see *Teaching your patient about I.V. drug therapy,* pages x and xi.)

In short, *Nurse's Handbook of I.V. Drugs* is designed expressly to give you more of what you need in a versatile and highly useful format. It puts vital drug information at your fingertips and helps you remain ALWAYS CURRENT in this critical part of your practice or studies.

TEACHING YOUR PATIENT ABOUT I.V. DRUG THERAPY

Your teaching about I.V. drug therapy will vary with your patient's needs and your practice setting. To help guide your teaching, each drug entry provides key information that you must teach your patient about that drug. For all patients, however, you should also:

☑ Teach the generic and trade names for each prescribed drug that he'll take after discharge—even if he took the drug before admission.

☑ Clearly explain why each drug was prescribed, how it works, and what it's supposed to do. To help your patient understand the drug's therapeutic effects, relate its action to her disorder or condition.

☑ Review the I.V. administration process, and inform the patient how often the drug will be administered. If the patient will be switched from an I.V. drug to another drug form (for example, from I.V. methyldopate hydrochloride to oral methyldopa for continuing treatment of hypertension), teach him how to administer the new form correctly. Also instruct him how often to take the drug and for what length of time. Emphasize that he should take the drug exactly as prescribed.

☑ If the patient is being switched to an oral drug, describe the drug's appearance. Explain that she may break scored tablets in half for safe, accurate dosing but should *not* break unscored tablets because doing so may alter the drug dosage. If the patient has difficulty swallowing capsules, explain that she can open ones that contain sprinkles and take them with food or a drink but that she shouldn't do this with capsules that contain powder. Also, warn her not to crush or chew enteric-coated, extended-release, sustained-release, or similar drug forms.

☑ Teach the patient common adverse reactions associated with his drug therapy, and advise him to immediately report any dangerous ones, such as syncope. Also instruct the patient to report changes at the I.V. site, such as pain, redness, or leaking fluid.

☑ If the patient experiences unpleasant adverse reactions, such as a rash or mild itching, inform her that her prescriber may adjust the dosage or substitute a drug that causes fewer adverse reactions. Tell her which adverse reactions resolve with time.

☑ Caution the patient that some adverse reactions, such as dizziness and drowsiness, can impair his ability to perform activities requiring alertness, such as driving a car or operating machinery. If the drug is known to have CNS effects, advise the patient to avoid such activities until the drug's full CNS effects are known or as directed by the prescriber.

☑ If your patient will be self-administering a drug, teach her how to store the drug properly. Let her know if the drug is sensitive to light or temperature and how to protect it from these elements. Instruct the patient to store the drug in its original container, if possible, with the drug's name and dosage clearly printed on the label.

☑ Inform the patient which devices are available for drug administration and which ones to avoid. For example, advise him to ask the prescriber about using an infusion control device for administering I.V. morphine sulfate infusions.

☑ Teach your patient who will be self-administering a drug what to do if she misses a dose. Generally, she should administer a once-daily drug as soon as she remembers—provided that she remembers within the first 24 hours. If 24 hours has elapsed, she should administer the next scheduled dose, but not double the dose. If she has questions or concerns about missed doses, advise her to contact the prescriber.

☑ Provide information that is specific to the prescribed drug. For example, if your patient takes a diuretic to manage heart failure, instruct him to weigh himself daily at the same time of day, using the same scale and wearing the same amount of clothing; or if the patient takes digoxin or an antihypertensive, teach him how to measure his pulse and blood pressure and how to record the measurements. Then instruct him to bring the diary to his regular appointments so that the prescriber can monitor his response to the drug.

☑ Advise the patient to refill prescriptions promptly, unless she no longer needs the drug. Also instruct her to discard expired drugs because they may become ineffective or even dangerous over time.

☑ Warn the patient to keep all drugs out of the reach of children at all times.

FOREWORD

As you know, administering I.V. drug therapy safely and effectively is a top priority for nurses in today's health care environment. In the past, I.V. drug therapy was administered primarily in acute care settings. However, as health care has expanded to include multiple specialties, the practice settings for I.V. drug therapy have also broadened. Today, nurses care for a diverse population of patients in hospitals, outpatient clinics, extended care facilities, surgical centers, and the patient's own home.

The types of drugs that can be administered by I.V. injection or infusion are wide ranging and include antibiotics, antivirals, antineoplastics, and narcotics. New drugs are continually becoming available to manage various health problems, such as HIV infection and cancer, and to manage or prevent drug-induced complications. In addition, many patients have more than one health problem and are taking multiple medications.

Your Responsibilities in I.V. Drug Therapy

Your basic responsibilities in drug therapy—whether enteral or parenteral—include:
- administering the right drug in the right dose by the right route at the right time to the right patient
- knowing the therapeutic use, dosage, interactions, adverse effects, and warnings of each administered drug
- being aware of newly approved drugs that may be prescribed
- knowing about changes to existing drugs, such as new indications and dosages and recently discovered adverse reactions and interactions
- concentrating fully when preparing and administering drugs
- responding promptly and appropriately to serious or life-threatening adverse reactions, interactions, and other complications.

Beyond these basic responsibilities, however, you also need additional nursing knowledge and skills to meet the demands of today's I.V. drug therapy—for example, knowing when and how to observe the I.V. insertion site and surrounding area for signs and symptoms of patient complications. *Blanchard & Loeb Publishers Nurse's Handbook of I.V. Drugs* provides all this information in an accurate and easy-to-use reference that has been developed specifically for you.

Meeting Your Needs

This book offers a wealth of reliable and easy-to-understand information on virtually all of the I.V. drugs you're likely to administer. For example, you'll find:

- instructions on how to prepare a drug dose, including directions for reconstitution and further dilution when appropriate
- appropriate storage information, including specific temperatures required for storing drugs before preparation and, if indicated, after reconstitution and dilution, as well as recommended lighting conditions, if applicable
- important facts on drug stability, such as how long the drug remains stable after reconstitution and dilution, and drug compatibility
- instructions on which drugs require special equipment, such as specific filters or a diluent supplied directly by the manufacturer
- recommended administration rate, when applicable, and whether the drug is administered as a continuous infusion, an intermittent infusion, or an injection.
- appropriate guidelines for patient monitoring after drug administration—for example, for adverse reactions, such as tissue sloughing and necrosis.

You can depend on the accuracy and reliability of the information contained in *Nurse's Handbook of I.V. Drugs* because each entry has been reviewed by experts in nursing and pharmacology. What's more, every drug fact has been checked against the most respected drug references today, including the *American Hospital Formulary Service Drug Information, Drug Facts and Comparisons, The Physician's Desk Reference,* and the USP DI's *Drug Information for the Health Care Professional.*

Nurse's Handbook of I.V. Drugs is also more practical and convenient than many other drug references on the market. For example, it's organized alphabetically by generic drug name, each entry follows a consistent format, and the writing throughout is concise and clear.

Whether you work in a hospital, a clinic, or another setting, you face greater challenges than ever before: more patients who are acutely ill, tighter budgets and staffing, and more complex drug therapy. But your ultimate goal must remain to provide your patients with the best and safest care possible. That's why we highly recommend *Blanchard & Loeb Publishers Nurse's Handbook of I.V. Drugs* to help you provide that optimal care. We have found the information in this book so valuable and practical that we use it every day—in our practice and in the classroom. Just slip it in your pocket and take it with you. We're confident that you'll refer to this book again and again and that it will become one of your most essential tools.

Joseph P. Zbilut, RN,C, DNSc, PhD, ANP
Professor, Adult Health Nursing
Rush University College of Nursing
Professor, Molecular Biophysics and Physiology
Rush Medical College
Chicago, IL

Kimberly Anne Boykin Couch, PharmD
Clinical Specialist
Christiana Care Health System
Adjunct Faculty
University of Delaware School of Nursing
Newark, DE

OVERVIEW OF PHARMACOLOGY

Understanding the basics of pharmacology is an essential nursing responsibility. Pharmacology is the science that deals with the physical and chemical properties, and the biochemical and physiologic effects, of drugs. It includes the areas of pharmacokinetics, pharmacodynamics, pharmacotherapeutics, pharmacognosy, and toxicodynamics.

Blanchard & Loeb Publishers Nurse's Handbook of I.V. Drugs deals primarily with pharmacokinetics, pharmacodynamics, and pharmacotherapeutics—the information you need to administer drug therapy safely and effectively (discussed below). *Pharmacognosy* is the branch of pharmacology that deals with the biological, biochemical, and economic features of naturally occurring drugs. *Toxicodynamics* is the study of the harmful effects that excessive amounts of a drug produce in the body; in a drug overdose or drug poisoning, large drug doses may saturate or overwhelm normal mechanisms that control absorption, distribution, metabolism, and excretion.

Drug Nomenclature
Most drugs are known by several names—chemical, generic, trade, and official—each of which serves a specific function. (See *How drugs are named,* page xvi.) However, multiple drug names can also contribute to medication errors. You may find a familiar drug packaged with an unfamiliar name if your institution changes suppliers or if a familiar drug is newly approved in a different dose or for a new indication.

Drug Classification
Drugs can be classified in various ways. Most pharmacology textbooks group drugs by their functional classification, such as psychotherapeutics, which is based on common characteristics. Drugs can also be classified according to their therapeutic use, such as antibiotics and sedative-hypnotics. Drugs within a certain therapeutic class may be further divided into subgroups based on their mechanisms of action. For example, the therapeutic class antineoplastics can be further classified as alkylating agents, antibiotic antineoplastics, antimetabolites, antimitotics, biological response modifiers, and hormonal antineoplastics.

HOW DRUGS ARE NAMED

A drug's chemical, generic, trade, and official names are developed at different phases of the drug development process and serve different functions. For example, the various names of the commonly prescribed diuretic chlorothiazide sodium are:
- Chemical name: 6-chloro-*2H*–1,2,4-benzothiadiazine-7-sulfonamide 1,1-dioxide monosodium salt, or $C_7H_5ClN_3NaO_4S_2$
- Generic name: chlorothiazide sodium
- Trade name: Diuril
- Official name: Chlorothiazide Sodium for Injection, USP

A drug's *chemical name* describes its atomic and molecular structures. The chemical name of chlorothiazide sodium indicates that the drug is a substituted ring structure with a sulfonamide group as well as a sodium salt.

Once a drug successfully completes several clinical trials, it receives a *generic name*, also known as the nonproprietary name. The generic name is usually derived from, but shorter than, the chemical name. The United States Adopted Names Council is responsible for selecting generic names, which are intended for unrestricted public use.

Before submitting the drug for FDA approval, the manufacturer creates and registers a *trade name* (or brand name) when the drug appears ready to be marketed. Trade names are copyrighted and followed by the symbol ® to indicate that they're registered and that their use is restricted to the drug manufacturer. Once the original patent on a drug has expired, any manufacturer may produce the drug and market it with its own trade name.

A drug's *official name* is the name under which it's listed in the United States Pharmacopoeia (USP) and the National Formulary (NF).

Pharmacokinetics

Pharmacokinetics is the study of a drug's actions—or fate—as it passes through the body during absorption, distribution, metabolism, and excretion.

Absorption

Before a drug can begin working, it must be transformed from its pharmaceutical dosage form to a biologically available (bioavailable) substance that can pass through various biological cell membranes to reach its site of action. This process is known as absorption. A drug's absorption rate depends on its route of administration, its circulation through the tissue into which it's administered, and its solubility—that is, whether it's more water-soluble (hydrophilic) or fat-soluble (lipophilic).

Although drugs may penetrate cellular membranes either actively or passively, most drugs do so by *passive diffusion*, moving inertly from an area of higher concentration to an area of lower concentration. Passive diffusion may occur through water or fat. Passive diffusion through water—*aqueous diffusion*—occurs within large water-filled compartments, such as interstitial spaces, and across epithelial membrane tight junctions and pores in the epithelial lining of blood vessels. Aqueous diffusion is driven by concentration gradients. Drug molecules that are bound to large plasma proteins, such as albumin, are too large to pass through aqueous pores in this way. Passive diffusion through fat—*lipid diffusion*—plays an important role in drug metabolism because of the large number of lipid barriers that separate the aqueous compartments of the body. The ability of a drug to move through lipid layers between aqueous compartments often depends on the pH of the medium—that is, the ability of the water-soluble or fat-soluble drug to form weak acid or weak base.

Drugs whose molecules are too large to readily diffuse may rely on *active diffusion*, in which special carriers on molecules, including peptides, amino acids, and glucose, transport the drug through the membranes. However, some molecules with selective membrane carriers can expel foreign drug molecules; this is why many drugs can't cross the blood-brain barrier.

Drug absorption begins at the administration route. The three main administration route categories are parenteral (consisting of I.M., I.V., S.C., and intradermal routes), enteral (consisting of oral, nasogastric, and rectal routes), and transcutaneous. Depending on its nature or chemical makeup, a drug may be better absorbed from one site than from another.

I.V. drug administration allows for rapid distribution throughout the body because a drug is injected or infused directly into the blood circulation. This route usually provides the greatest bioavailability and may be used whenever other routes are contraindicated or inadequate. Drug absorption is much faster and more predictable after parenteral administration than after enteral administration.

Distribution
Distribution is the process by which a drug is transported by the circulating fluids to various sites, including its sites of action. To en-

sure maximum therapeutic effectiveness, the drug must permeate all membranes that separate it from its intended site of action. Drug distribution is influenced by blood flow, tissue availability, and protein binding.

Metabolism

Drug metabolism is the enzymatic conversion of a drug's structure into substrate molecules or polar compounds that are either less active or inactive and are readily excreted. Drugs can also be synthesized to larger molecules. Metabolism may also convert a drug to a more toxic compound. Because the primary site of drug metabolism is the liver, children, the elderly, and patients with impaired hepatic function are at risk for altered therapeutic effects.

Biotransformation is the process by which a drug changes into its active metabolite. Compounds that require metabolic biotransformation for activation are known as *prodrugs*. During phase I of biotransformation, the parent drug is converted into an inactive or partially active metabolite. Much of the original drug may be eliminated during this phase. During phase II, the inactive or partially active metabolite binds with available substrates, such as acetic acid, glucuronic acid, sulfuric acid, or water, to form its active metabolite. When biotransformation leads to synthesis, larger molecules are produced to create a pharmacologic effect.

Excretion

The body eliminates drugs by both metabolism and excretion. Drug metabolites—and, in some cases, the active drug itself—are eventually excreted from the body, usually through bile, feces, and urine. The primary organ for drug elimination is the kidney. Impaired renal function may cause excessive drug accumulation in the body, thus increasing the patient's risk of adverse drug reactions and toxicity. Other excretion routes include evaporation through the skin, exhalation from the lungs, and secretion into saliva and breast milk.

A drug's elimination *half-life* is the amount of time required for half of the drug to be eliminated from the body. The half-life roughly correlates with the drug's duration of action and is based on normal renal and hepatic function. Typically, the longer the half-life, the less often the drug has to be given and the longer it remains in the body after it's discontinued.

Pharmacodynamics

Pharmacodynamics is the study of the biochemical and physiologic effects of drugs and their mechanisms of action. A drug's actions may be structurally specific or nonspecific. Structurally specific drugs combine with cell receptors, such as proteins or glycoproteins, to enhance or inhibit cellular enzyme actions. Drug receptors are the cellular components affected at the site of action. Many drugs form chemical bonds with drug receptors, but a drug can bond with a receptor only if it has a similar shape—much the same way that a key fits into a lock. When a drug combines with a receptor, channels are either opened or closed and cellular biochemical messengers, such as cyclic adenosine monophosphate or calcium ions, are activated. Once activated, cellular functions can be turned either on or off by these messengers. Structurally nonspecific drugs, such as biological response modifiers, don't combine with cell receptors; rather, they produce changes within the cell membrane or interior.

The mechanisms by which drugs interact with the body are not always known. Drugs may work by physical action (such as the protective effects of a topical ointment) or chemical reaction (such as an antacid's effect on the gastric mucosa), or by modifying the metabolic activity of invading pathogens (such as an antibiotic) or replacing a missing biochemical substance (such as insulin).

Agonists

Agonists are drugs that interact with a receptor to stimulate a response. They alter cell physiology by binding to plasma membranes or intracellular structures. *Partial agonists* can't achieve maximal effects even though they may occupy all available receptor sites on a cell. *Strong agonists* can cause maximal effects while occupying only a small number of receptor sites on a cell. *Weak agonists* must occupy many more receptor sites than strong agonists to produce the same effect.

Antagonists

Antagonists are drugs that attach to a receptor but don't stimulate a response; instead, they inhibit or block responses that would normally be caused by agonists. *Competitive antagonists* bind to receptor sites that are also compatible with an agonist, thus preventing the agonist from binding to the site. *Noncompetitive antagonists* bind to receptor sites that aren't occupied by an agonist; this changes the receptor site so that it's no longer recognized by the agonist. *Irreversible antagonists* work in much the same way that noncompetitive ones do, except that they permanently bind with the receptor.

Antagonism plays an important role in drug interactions. When two agonists that cause opposite therapeutic effects, such as a vasodilator and a vasoconstrictor, are combined, the effects cancel each other out. When two antagonists, such as morphine and naloxone, are combined, both drugs may become inactive.

Pharmacotherapeutics

Pharmacotherapeutics is the study of how drugs are used to prevent or treat disease. Understanding why a drug is prescribed for a certain disease can assist you in prioritizing drug administration with other patient care activities. Knowing a drug's desired and unwanted effects may help you uncover problems not readily apparent from the admitting diagnosis. This information may also help you prevent such problems as adverse reactions and drug interactions.

A drug's *desired effect* is the intended or expected clinical response to the drug. This is the response you start to evaluate as soon as a drug is given. Dosage adjustments and the continuation of therapy often depend on your accurate evaluation and documentation of the patient's response.

An *adverse reaction* is any noxious and unintended response to a drug that occurs at therapeutic doses used for prophylaxis, diagnosis, or therapy. Adverse reactions associated with excessive amounts of a drug are considered drug overdoses. Be prepared to follow your institution's policy for reporting adverse drug reactions.

An *idiosyncratic response* is a genetically determined abnormal or excessive response to a drug that occurs in a particular patient. The unusual response may indicate that the drug has saturated or overwhelmed mechanisms that normally control absorption, distribution, metabolism, or excretion, thus altering the expected response. You may be unsure whether a reaction is adverse or idiosyncratic. Once you report the reaction, the pharmacist usually determines the appropriate course of action.

An *allergic reaction* is an adverse response that results from previous exposure to the same drug or to one that is chemically similar to it. The patient's immune system reacts to the drug as if it were a foreign invader and may produce a mild hypersensitivity reaction, characterized by localized dermatitis, urticaria, angioedema, or photosensitivity. Allergic reactions should be reported to the prescriber immediately and the drug should be discontinued. Follow-up care may include giving drugs, including antihistamines and corticosteroids, to counteract the allergic response.

An *anaphylactic reaction* is an immediate hypersensitivity response characterized by urticaria, pruritus, and angioedema. Left untreated, an anaphylactic reaction can lead to systemic involvement, resulting in shock. It's often associated with life-threatening hypotension and respiratory distress. Be prepared to assist with emergency life support measures, especially if the reaction occurs in response to I.V. drugs, which have the fastest rate of absorption.

A *drug interaction* occurs when one drug alters the pharmacokinetics of another drug—for example, when two or more drugs are given concurrently. Such concurrent administration can increase or decrease the therapeutic or adverse effects of either drug. Some drug interactions are beneficial. For example, when taken with penicillin G, probenecid decreases the excretion rate of penicillin G, resulting in higher blood levels of penicillin G. Drug interactions may also occur when a drug's metabolism is altered, often owing to the induction of or competition for metabolizing enzymes. For example, H_2-receptor agonists, which reduce secretion of the enzyme gastrin, may alter the breakdown of enteric coatings on other drugs. Drug interactions due to carrier protein competition typically occur when a drug inhibits the kidneys' ability to reduce excretion of other drugs. For example, probenecid is completely reabsorbed by the renal tubules and is metabolized very slowly. It competes with the same carrier protein as sulfonamides for active tubular secretion and so decreases the renal excretion of sulfonamides. This particular competition can lead to an increased risk of sulfonamide toxicity.

Special Considerations

Although every drug has a usual dosage range, certain factors—such as a patient's age, weight, culture and ethnicity, gender, pregnancy status, and renal and hepatic function—may contribute to the need for dosage adjustments. When you encounter special considerations such as these, be prepared to reassess the prescribed dosage to make sure that it's safe and effective for your patient.

Culture and Ethnicity

Certain drugs are more effective or more likely to produce adverse effects in particular ethnic groups or races. For example, blacks with hypertension respond better to thiazide diuretics than do patients of other races; on the other hand, blacks also have an increased risk of developing angioedema associated with angiotensin-converting enzyme (ACE) inhibitors. A patient's religious or cultural background may also call for special consideration. For example, a drug made from porcine products may be unacceptable to a Jewish or Muslim patient.

Elderly Patients

Because aging produces certain changes in body composition and organ function, elderly patients present unique therapeutic and dosing problems that require special attention. For example, the weight of the liver, the number of functioning hepatic cells, and hepatic blood flow all decrease as a person ages, resulting in slower drug metabolism. Renal function may also decrease with aging. These processes can lead to the accumulation of active drugs and metabolites as well as increased sensitivity to the effects of some drugs in elderly patients. Because they're also more likely to have multiple chronic illnesses, many elderly patients take multiple prescription drugs each day, thus increasing the risk of drug interactions.

Children
Because their bodily functions are not fully developed, children—particularly those under age 12—may metabolize drugs differently than adults. In infants, immature renal and hepatic function delay metabolism and excretion of drugs. As a result, pediatric drug dosages are very different from adult dosages.

The FDA has provided drug manufacturers with guidelines that define pediatric age categories. Use these categories as a guide when administering drugs, unless the manufacturer provides a specific age range:
- neonates—birth up to age 1 month
- infants—ages 1 month to 2 years
- children—ages 2 to 12
- adolescents—ages 12 to 16.

Pregnancy
The many physiologic changes that take place in the body during pregnancy may affect a drug's pharmacokinetics and alter its effectiveness. Additionally, exposure to drugs may pose risks for the developing fetus. Before administering a drug to a pregnant patient, be sure to check its assigned FDA pregnancy risk category and intervene appropriately.

Principles of I.V. Drug Administration

Because there are thousands of drugs and hundreds of facts about each one, taking responsibility for drug administration can seem overwhelming. Administering I.V. drugs requires a combination of skills—not only knowing how to administer drugs safely but also knowledge of anatomy (such as the location of veins in the body) and of assessment (for example, when and how to observe the insertion site, surrounding area, and the patient for complications).

In I.V. drug administration, a drug enters the circulatory system through a single, small-volume injection or a slow, large-volume infusion rather than through GI absorption. Because drugs injected I.V. don't encounter absorption barriers, this route produces the most rapid drug action, making it vital in emergency situations. The I.V. route is also used when the patient is uncooperative, unconscious, or unable to accept medication by the oral or I.M. route or when a drug is ineffective by other routes. Although it's the preferred route for certain situations, I.V. administration has several disadvantages: I.V. drugs are generally more expensive to administer than other dosage forms because they require strict sterility, and once the drug has been injected, it can't be removed and the dosage can't be reduced.

One way that you can enhance your understanding of the principles of I.V. drug administration is to *associate, ask,* and *predict* during the critical thinking process. For example, *associate* each drug with general information you may already know about the drug or drug class. *Ask* yourself why a drug may be given by the I.V. route or why it's given multiple times throughout the day rather than only once. Learn to *predict* a drug's actions, uses, adverse effects, and possible drug interactions based on your knowledge of the drug's mechanism of action. As you apply these principles to I.V. drug administration, you'll begin to intuitively know which facts you need to make rational clinical decisions.

Each facility or agency has its own protocols for I.V. drug administration, including care of the I.V. site. Many of them use the Intravenous Nurses Society's Standards of Practice to formulate their policies. Individual state nursing practice guidelines are another component that may be used to develop I.V. administration protocols.

"Rights" of Drug Administration

Always keep in mind the following "rights" of drug administration, which apply to all forms of drug administration, including I.V.: the right drug, right time, right dose, right patient, right route, and right preparation and administration.

Right Drug

Many drugs have similar spellings, a variety of concentrations, and several generic forms. Before administering any drug, compare the exact spelling and concentration of the prescribed drug that appears on the label with the information contained in the medication administration record or drug profile. Regardless of which drug distribution system your facility uses, you should read the drug label and compare it to the medication administration record at least three times:

- before removing the drug from the dispensing unit or unit-dose cart
- before reconstituting, diluting, or measuring the prescribed dose
- before opening a unit-dose package (just prior to administering the drug to the patient).

Right Time

Various factors can affect the time that a drug is administered, such as the timing of meals, other drugs, or scheduled diagnostic tests; standardized times used by the institution; and factors that may alter the consistency of blood levels and drug absorption. Before administering any p.r.n. drug, check the patient's chart to ensure that no one else has already administered it and that the specified time interval has passed. Also, document administration of a p.r.n. drug immediately.

Right Dose

Whenever you're dispensing an unfamiliar drug or in doubt about a dosage, check the prescribed dose against the range specified in a reliable reference. In addition, because many I.V. drugs come in different concentrations—such as urokinase, which is available in concentrations ranging from 5,000 to 250,000 IU—you must examine the label closely to ensure that you're administering the proper strength. Also make sure that you're using the appropriate concentration for the method of administration. For example, the 5,000- and 9,000-IU concentrations of urokinase are used *only* for clearing I.V. catheter occlusions, *not* for I.V. or intracoronary drug administration. Conversely, the 250,000-IU concentration is used *only* for I.V. and intracoronary drug administration.

Be sure to consider any reasons for which your patient might need a dosage adjustment, such as age, preexisting medical conditions, or response to the drug. Also, be familiar with the standard abbreviations your institution uses for writing prescriptions.

Right Patient

Always compare the name of the patient on the medication record with the name on the patient's identification bracelet. When using a unit-dose system, compare the name on the drug profile with that on the identification bracelet.

Right Route

Each prescribed drug should specify the administration route. If the administration route is missing, consult the prescribing physician. Never substitute one route for another unless you obtain a prescription for the change. Severe adverse reactions can result from administering a parenteral drug by the wrong route. For example, the antineoplastic drug vinblastine can cause potentially fatal paralysis when administered intrathecally and requires special labeling when it's being prepared.

Right Preparation and Administration

Be sure to maintain aseptic technique when handling drugs that need to be reconstituted, diluted, and measured. Follow any specific directions included in the manufacturer 's insert regarding diluent type and amount and the use of filters, if needed. Clearly label any drug that you've reconstituted with the patient's name, the strength or dose, the date and time that you prepared the drug, the amount and type of diluent that you used, the expiration date, and your initials. Be aware that certain drugs and diluents contain additives that have been known to cause adverse reactions. One example is benzyl alcohol, a preservative found in some drugs and diluents, which may cause a fatal toxic syndrome in neonates and premature infants, characterized by CNS, respiratory, circulatory, and renal impairment and metabolic acidosis. Also, determine whether your patient has an allergy to a prescribed drug or its components, to similar drugs, or to a recommended diluent; if so, report it to the prescriber. If the patient is allergic to a diluent, discuss possible alternative diluents with the pharmacist.

Become familiar with the I.V. administration method being used. For example, if you're using an I.V. administration set, find out the accurate flow rate—usually between 10 and 60 drops/ml. If you're using an infusion device, know how to use it correctly. Also, check the infusion rate periodically to ensure that the appropriate amount of drug is being administered.

Types of Venous Access

I.V. drugs can be administered through a peripheral or central venous access. The type of access depends on such factors as the patient's overall medical condition, the type of drug to be administered, and the amount of time the patient requires I.V. drug therapy.

Once I.V. access has been established, it is used for either continuous or intermittent injection or infusion. Intermittent infusion typically involves the use of a saline, or heparin, lock. This device is advantageous because it allows for immediate venous access and doesn't require continuous administration of fluids to maintain its patency.

Peripheral I.V. Drug Administration

In peripheral I.V. administration, a drug is injected or infused through a peripheral vein, usually one in the forearm. Peripheral access is used to administer various fluids and solutions, including antibiotics, chemotherapeutic drugs, blood products, and hydrating fluids. It is typically used for short-term drug administration in the hospital and in outpatient settings. For longer periods of drug administration, a midline catheter may be used. This is a longer catheter that remains in the peripheral venous system, typically in the larger veins of the arm below the axilla. A peripheral insertion site may also be used for a peripherally inserted central catheter (PICC), which delivers drugs directly into the central venous system.

Veins in the distal part of the upper extremity are typically selected first, but the choice of vein depends on the type of drug being administered, possible adverse effects, the patient's age and medical condition, which hand is dominant, and the length of time the I.V. line will be in place. These factors also influence the choice of a venipuncture device, which may range from a winged infusion set to an over-the-needle catheter made of polyethylene, silicone, or other materials. Use the shortest needle and the smallest gauge that meet the needs of the drug or solution to be infused.

Central Venous Administration

Central venous therapy is commonly used to administer long-term drug therapy to patients whose condition contraindicates the placement of a peripheral I.V. line. Central venous access may be achieved by the placement of centrally or peripherally inserted catheters or implantable ports.

If venous access is placed in the upper part of the body, the central venous catheter tip lies in the superior vena cava; if femoral venous access is used, the catheter tip lies in the inferior superior vena cava. Common sites for centrally inserted catheters are the subclavian vein and the internal or external jugular veins. Common sites for PICCs are the basilic, cephalic, and median cubital veins in the upper extremity. Surgically implanted central venous ports have a self-sealing septum with a catheter attached that leads to the superior vena cava. Ports may be accessed using noncoring needles from above or at the side of the port, depending on the type used.

The type of central catheter used varies, depending on such factors as the type and number of drugs to be administered and the amount of time the central access will be in place. Single-lumen or multi-lumen catheters may be used, depending on the patient's needs. Tunneled catheters, such as the Hickman catheter, are used when long-term use is anticipated. These catheters are radiopaque and have a cuff at the end, near the body entrance site. Part of the tunneled catheter lies within subcutaneous tissue, which over time turns into a collagenous matrix that gradually adheres to the cuff, thus helping to secure the catheter and protect against infection.

Alternative Infusion Methods

Although the focus of this book is I.V. drug therapy, you should be aware of other methods used to infuse drugs, such as subcutaneous (S.C.) and intraosseous infusion. One of the most common uses of the S.C. route is insulin administration. A programmed insulin pump administers small amounts of regular insulin throughout the day through a needle or catheter inserted into the patient's abdomen. Intraosseous infusions are administered by a needle inserted into the bone marrow. They are used in such conditions as shock, anaphylaxis, or trauma when venous access is not available.

Infusion Devices

I.V. drug therapy commonly requires the use of an infusion device to ensure that the appropriate dose is being administered—for example, when administering I.V. antiarrhythmics (such as lidocaine hydrochloride or procainamide hydrochloride) or when administering drugs to children. The type of infusion device can vary, depending on the drug used, the amount of fluid to be given, and the setting at which the drug is being administered.

Electronic infusion devices (also known as electronic infusion pumps and controllers) are powered by electricity or battery packs. These devices come in various sizes, from compact ambulatory versions designed for portable use to multidrug infusion pumps commonly used in acute care settings. Controller devices don't assist in drug delivery; rather they monitor the drop flow based on a programmed rate. Electronic infusion pumps provide a positive pressure flow to assist with drug delivery.

Electronic infusion devices may be equipped with alarms to signal increased pressure or air in the I.V. line or the completion of an infusion. Some devices prevent free flow of the solution if the I.V. line becomes disconnected from the device, which can prevent serious complications. Others contain a free-flow alarm, which can signal an uncontrolled rate of fluid administration stemming from accidental disconnection.

Patient-Controlled Analgesia

Patient-controlled analgesia (PCA) allows the patient to be actively involved in his own drug delivery. First, you administer the loading dose and program the pump to deliver additional bolus doses of the drug within predetermined limits for amount and frequency. The patient then presses a button when he wants to activate a bolus dose. You must clearly explain the drug delivery system to the patient, making sure he understands that there is a "lock-out" period during which he won't be able to administer additional doses.

Complications of I.V. Therapy

Because I.V. drug administration requires a break in the skin, it poses an increased risk of infection, ranging from local infection of surrounding tissues to sepsis. To prevent infection or detect it early, monitor the I.V. site, change dressings and tubing, and rotate the I.V. site in accordance with your facility's policy. Administration sets are typically changed every 24 to 48 hours (every 24 hours for intermittent infusion), and I.V. sites are rotated every 48 to 72 hours.

Two other potential complications of I.V. therapy are infiltration—the leakage of nonvesicant solution into surrounding tissues—and extravasation—the leakage of a vesicant solution, such as certain chemotherapeutic drugs, into surrounding tissues. To detect these complications, frequently assess the I.V. site and surrounding area. If you observe either of these conditions, restart the I.V. line at another site. Extravasation can cause tissue necrosis, gangrene, and other reactions around the injection site. If extravasation occurs, expect to use a drug such as phentolamine to antagonize vasoconstriction and minimize sloughing and tissue necrosis.

Other risks associated with I.V. drug therapy include catheter occlusion, circulatory overload, phlebitis, thrombosis, hematoma, pulmonary or air embolism, and venous spasm. Some potential complications are specific to the I.V. access route. For example, central venous catheters increase the risk of arterial puncture, pneumothorax, and hemothorax during catheter placement.

The rapid drug distribution and greater bioavailability associated with I.V. therapy mean that you must be vigilant in monitoring for adverse drug reactions. Too-rapid administration of a drug can result in a type of reaction known as speed shock. Anaphylactic reactions can occur within a few minutes of drug administration or several days afterward. Become familiar with the potential adverse effects of each drug you administer.

Safe Handling of Toxic Agents
I.V. drug administration may expose you to toxic agents, such as many antineoplastic drugs. To protect yourself from potential carcinogenic, mutagenic, and teratogenic effects of these drugs, learn how to handle them safely. Because no standard procedure exists, follow your facility's protocols for preparation and handling of antineoplastic drugs and for appropriate disposal of used equipment. In addition, before you prepare a toxic drug, consult the manufacturer's package insert for specific recommendations, such as the use of a biological containment cabinet, gloves, and gown.

Preventing Needlestick Injuries
Take steps to avoid needlestick injuries when you administer I.V. drugs and when you handle certain preparations, such as immune globulin intravenous, which is made from human plasma and therefore may contain infectious agents such as viruses. Needleless administration systems have been developed to decrease the risk of needlestick injuries and exposure to viruses such as HIV.

Other Uses for I.V. Access
In addition to drug administration, I.V. access is also used for infusions of hydrating fluids, blood and blood products, and total parenteral nutrition (TPN).

Parenteral Fluids
Parenteral fluids may be infused at a slow rate to maintain an I.V. access, to treat certain medical conditions (such as the administration of normal saline to treat hyperparathyroidism), or to restore fluid volume in patients with hypovolemic shock or burns. (See *Selected water and electrolyte solutions,* page xxx.)

SELECTED WATER AND ELECTROLYTE SOLUTIONS

The chart below provides electrolyte contents for some common solutions you may administer in your clinical practice.

I.V. Solution	Electrolyte Contents
0.5% dextrose in water	No electrolytes
Dextrose 2.5% with ½ strength lactated Ringer's injection	1.4 mEq/L of calcium 54 to 55 mEq/L of chloride 14 mEq/L of lactate 2 mEq/L of potassium 65 mEq/L of sodium
Dextrose 5% with lactated Ringer's injection	2.7 to 3 mEq/L of calcium 109 to 112 mEq/L of chloride 28 mEq/L of lactate 4 mEq/L of potassium 130 mEq/L of sodium
Lactated Ringer's injection	2.7 to 3 mEq/L of calcium 109 to 110 mEq/L of chloride 28 mEq/L of lactate 4 mEq/L of potassium 130 mEq/L of sodium
⅙ M Sodium lactate	167 mEq/L of lactate 167 mEq/L of sodium
0.45% Sodium chloride	77 mEq/L of chloride 77 mEq/L of sodium
0.9% Sodium chloride	154 mEq/L of chloride 154 mEq/L of sodium
3% Sodium chloride	513 mEq/L of chloride 513 mEq/L of sodium
5% Sodium chloride	855 mEq/L of chloride 855 mEq/L of sodium

Blood Products

I.V. access is used for transfusion of blood and blood products, including whole blood, packed red blood cells, platelets, and plasma. Learn your facility's protocols and the techniques required for administering blood products. Before you administer blood, verify the prescriber's order and that the patient has an appropriate I.V. access, typically an 18G or 20G catheter (smaller for children). Ensure that no solution other than normal saline is infusing in the I.V. line to be used. Two other critical steps are verifying the patient's ABO blood and Rh types and verifying his identity to ensure that the right product is given to the right patient. (See *Understanding blood types and Rh factor,* page xxxii.) Observe the patient continuously during the first 10 to 15 minutes because the majority of anaphylactic and ABO incompatibility reactions occur during that time. Blood infusions are generally not administered for longer than 4 hours because of the risk of septicemia.

TPN

Also referred to as I.V. hyperalimentation, TPN provides nutrition for patients who are unable to eat, digest, or absorb a sufficient amount of nutrients. TPN is typically administered by a central venous catheter, usually a subclavian catheter; however, PICC lines or tunneled catheters may also be used. Administer TPN as a continuous infusion, using an infusion pump. Monitor the patient for adverse reactions, including infection, sepsis, and venous thrombosis from the I.V. access; hyperglycemia if the patient can't metabolize the glucose in the TPN fast enough; or hypoglycemia if the infusion is stopped abruptly.

UNDERSTANDING BLOOD TYPES AND Rh FACTOR

Verification of ABO blood and Rh types is vital if you'll be administering blood products. Administering the wrong blood type or Rh factor to a patient could set off an immune response that results in the destruction of red blood cells (RBCs). Understanding the role that antigens and antibodies play in blood typing will help you understand the importance of transfusing the correct blood product.

Antigens are glycoproteins or glycolipids found on the membrane surface of RBCs. Specific antigens on the RBC designate an individual's ABO blood type. The four major blood types are A, B, AB, and O. Individuals inherit antigens and blood types from their parents. Within a few months of birth, a child develops antibodies against the antigens he doesn't have. The antigens and antibodies for the specific blood types are as follows:

Type	Antigen	Antibody
A	A	Anti-B
B	B	Anti-A
AB	A and B	None
O	None	Anti-A and Anti-B

Each patient should ideally receive his own specific blood type. However, in an emergency, type O blood can be administered to anyone because it contains no A or B antigens. For this reason, people with type O blood are called *universal donors.* Conversely, persons with type AB blood, which has both antigens, can receive any blood type and are called *universal recipients.*

Antigens are also a component of the Rh factor; one of them—the D antigen—is of particular significance. Patients who have the D antigen are considered Rh-positive, whereas patients who lack the D antigen are Rh-negative. Antibodies to the D antigen don't develop automatically; they can form if a person has received a previous transfusion or delivered a child who has the antigen. If a person with antibodies to the D antigen receives a transfusion of Rh-positive blood, he can develop a transfusion reaction that results in RBC destruction.

I.V. DRUG THERAPY AND THE NURSING PROCESS

A systematic approach to nursing care, the nursing process helps guide you as you develop, implement, and evaluate your care and ensures that you'll deliver safe, consistent, and effective I.V. drug therapy to your patients. The nursing process consists of five steps: assessment, nursing diagnosis, planning, implementation, and evaluation. Even though documentation is not a step in the nursing process, you're legally and professionally responsible for documenting all aspects of your care before, during, and after drug administration.

Assessment

The first step in the nursing process, assessment involves gathering information that is essential to guide your patient's drug therapy. This information includes the patient's drug history, present drug use, allergies, medical history, and physical examination findings. Assessment is an ongoing process that serves as a baseline against which to compare any changes in your patient's condition; it's also the basis for developing and individualizing the patient's plan of care.

Drug History

The patient's drug history is critical in your planning of drug-related care. Ask about his previous use of OTC and prescription drugs as well as herbal remedies. For each drug, determine:
• the reason the patient took it
• the prescribed dosage
• the administration route
• the frequency of administration
• the duration of the drug therapy
• any adverse reactions the patient may have experienced and how he handled them.

If the patient received previous I.V. therapy, ask him the type of vascular access that was used and how he tolerated the therapy.

Also, determine if the patient has a history of drug abuse or addiction; if he has, find out the administration route he used. Depending on his physical and emotional state, you may need to obtain the drug history from other sources, such as family members, friends, or other caregivers, and from the medical record.

Present Drug Use

Ask about the patient's current use of OTC and prescription drugs as well as herbal remedies. As you did in the drug history, find out the specific details for each drug (dosage, route, frequency, and reason for taking). Also ask the patient if he thinks the drug has been effective and when he took the last dose.

If the patient uses herbal remedies, similarly explore the use of these products because herbs may interact with certain drugs. Also ask about the patient's use of recreational drugs, such as alcohol and tobacco, as well as illegal drugs, such as marijuana and heroin. Again, be sure to ascertain the administration route he used. If the patient acknowledges use of these drugs, be alert for possible drug interactions. This information may also provide you with insight about the patient's response—or lack of response—to his current drug treatment plan.

Try to find out if the patient has any other problems that might affect his compliance with the drug treatment plan, and intervene appropriately. For instance, a patient who is unemployed and has no health insurance may fail to fill a needed prescription. In such a case, contact an appropriate individual in your facility who may be able to help the patient obtain financial assistance.

Be sure to ask the patient if his drug treatment plan requires special monitoring or follow-up laboratory tests. For example, patients who take antihypertensives need to have their blood pressure checked routinely, and those who take warfarin must have their prothrombin time tested regularly. Other patients must undergo periodic blood tests to assess their hepatic and renal function. Determine whether the patient has complied with this part of his treatment plan, and ask him if he knows the results of the latest monitoring or laboratory tests.

Allergies

Find out if the patient is allergic to any drugs or foods. If he has an allergy, explore it further by determining the type of drug or food that triggers a reaction, the first time he experienced a reaction, the characteristics of the reaction, and other related information. Keep in mind that some patients consider annoying symptoms, such as indigestion, an allergic reaction. However, be sure to document a true allergy according to your facility's policy to ensure that the patient doesn't receive that drug or any related drug that may cause a similar reaction. Also, document allergies to foods because they may lead to drug interactions or adverse drug reactions. For example, sulfite is a food additive as well as a drug additive, so a patient with a known allergy to sulfite-containing foods is likely to react to sulfite-containing drugs.

Medical History

While reviewing your patient's medical history, determine if he has any acute or chronic conditions that may interfere with his drug therapy. Certain disorders involving major body systems, such as the cardiovascular, GI, hepatic, and renal systems, may affect a drug's absorption, transport, metabolism, or excretion and interfere with its action; they may also increase the incidence of adverse reactions and lead to toxicity. For each disorder identified, try to determine when the condition was diagnosed, what drugs were prescribed, and who prescribed them. This information can help you determine whether the patient is receiving incompatible drugs and whether more than one prescriber is managing his drug therapy.

Ask a female patient if she is or may be pregnant or if she's breast-feeding. Many drugs are safe to use during pregnancy, but others may harm the fetus. Also, some drugs are distributed into breast milk. If your patient is or might be pregnant, check the FDA's pregnancy risk category for the prescribed drug and notify the prescriber if the drug may pose a risk to the fetus. If the patient is breast-feeding, find out if the drug is distributed in breast milk and intervene appropriately.

In addition, ask the patient about any preexisting conditions or procedures that may have implications for the I.V. site selection, such as a history of lymphatic or superior vena caval obstruction, lymph node dissection, mastectomy, or radiation therapy to the upper torso, or the presence of an internal arteriovenous fistula for hemodialysis.

Physical Examination Findings

As part of the physical examination, note the patient's age and weight. Be aware that age determines the dosage of certain drugs, such as sedatives and hypnotics, whereas weight determines the dosage of others, including some I.V. antibiotics and anticoagulants. As you perform the physical examination, note any abnormal findings that may point to body organ or system dysfunction. For example, if you detect liver enlargement and ascites, the patient may have impaired hepatic function, which can affect the metabolism of a drug he's taking and lead to harmful adverse or toxic effects. Also note whether a body organ or system appears to be responding to drug treatment. For example, if a patient has been taking an antibiotic to treat chronic bronchitis, thoroughly evaluate his respiratory status to measure his progress. And be sure to assess the patient for possible adverse reactions to the drugs he's taking.

Also assess the condition of potential vascular access sites, and evaluate their suitability for I.V. drug administration.

Assess the patient's neurologic function to ensure that he can understand his drug regimen and carry out required tasks, such as performing a finger stick to obtain blood for glucose measurement. If a patient can't understand essential drug information, you'll need to identify a family member or another person who is willing to become involved in the teaching process.

Nursing Diagnosis

Based on information derived from the assessment and physical examination findings, the nursing diagnoses are statements of actual or potential problems that a nurse is licensed to treat or manage alone or in collaboration with other members of the health care team. They're worded according to guidelines established by the North American Nursing Diagnosis Association.

One of the most common nursing diagnoses related to drug therapy is *knowledge deficit,* which indicates that the patient doesn't have sufficient understanding of his drug regimen. However, adverse reactions are the basis for most nursing diagnoses related to drug administration. For example, a patient receiving an opioid analgesic might have a nursing diagnosis of *constipation* related to decreased intestinal motility or *ineffective breathing pattern* related to respiratory depression. Many antiarrhythmics cause orthostatic hypotension and thus may place an elderly patient at *high risk for injury* related to possible syncope. Broad-spectrum antibiotics, such as penicillin G, may lead to the overgrowth of *Clostridium difficile,* a bacterium that is normally present in the intestines. This overgrowth, in turn, may lead to pseudomembranous enterocolitis, characterized by abdominal pain and severe diarrhea. The nursing diagnoses in such a case might include *risk for infection* related to bacterial overgrowth, *alteration in comfort* related to abdominal pain, and *fluid balance deficit* related to diarrhea.

Planning

During the planning phase, you'll establish expected outcomes—or goals—for the patient and then develop specific nursing interventions to achieve them. Expected outcomes are observable or measurable goals that should occur as a result of nursing interventions and sometimes in conjunction with medical interventions. Developed in collaboration with the patient, the outcomes should be realistic and objective and should clearly communicate to other nurses the direction of the plan of care. They should be written as behaviors or responses for the patient, not the nurse, to achieve and should include a time frame for measuring the patient's progress. An example of a typical expected outcome is: "The patient will accurately demonstrate self-administration of insulin before discharge." Based on each outcome statement that you establish, you'll then develop appropriate nursing interventions, which may include drug administration techniques, patient teaching, monitoring of vital signs, calculation of drug dosages based on weight, and recording of intake and output.

Implementation

As you implement the nursing interventions, be sure to stringently follow the classic rule of drug administration: administer the right dose of the right drug by the right route to the right patient at the right time. Also, keep in mind that you have a legal and professional responsibility to follow institutional policy regarding standing orders, prescription renewal, and the use of nursing judgment. During the implementation phase, you'll also begin to evaluate the patient's expected outcomes and nursing interventions and make necessary changes to the plan of care.

Evaluation

Evaluation is an ongoing process rather than a single step in the nursing process. During this phase, you evaluate each expected outcome to determine whether or not it has been achieved and whether the original plan of care is working or needs to be modified. In evaluating a patient's drug treatment plan, you should determine whether or not the drug is controlling the signs and symptoms for which it was prescribed. You should also evaluate the patient for psychological or physiologic responses to the drug, especially adverse reactions. This constant monitoring allows you to make appropriate and timely suggestions for changes to the plan of care, such as dosage adjustments or changes in delivery routes, until each expected outcome has been achieved.

Documentation

You're responsible for documenting all your actions related to the patient's drug therapy, from the assessment phase to evaluation. Each time you administer a drug, document the drug name, dose, time given, and your evaluation of its effect. Also document the condition of the I.V. insertion site, including the presence (be specific) or absence of any I.V.-related complications, specific interventions that were required, and the patient's response. When you administer drugs that require additional nursing judgment, such as those prescribed on an as-needed basis, document the rationale for administering the drug and follow-up assessment or interventions for each dose administered.

If you decide to withhold a prescribed drug based on your nursing judgment, document your action and the rationale for it, and notify the prescriber of your action in a timely manner. Whenever you notify a prescriber about a significant finding related to drug therapy, such as an adverse reaction, document the date and time, the person you contacted, what you discussed, and how you intervened.

A

abciximab
ReoPro

Class and Category
Chemical: Fab fragment of chimeric 7E3 antibody
Therapeutic: Platelet aggregation inhibitor
Pregnancy category: C

Indications and Dosages
▶ *To prevent acute myocardial ischemic complications after percutaneous transluminal coronary angioplasty (PTCA) in patients at high risk for abrupt closure of treated coronary artery*
I.V. INFUSION OR INJECTION
Adults. 250 mcg/kg bolus 10 to 60 min before PTCA. *Maintenance:* 0.125 mcg/kg/min by continuous infusion for 12 hr. *Maximum:* 10 mcg/min.
▶ *To treat unstable angina in patients who haven't responded to conventional therapy and are scheduled for PTCA within 24 hr*
I.V. INFUSION OR INJECTION
Adults. 250 mcg/kg bolus, then 10 mcg/min continuous infusion over 18 to 24 hr, concluding 1 hr after PTCA.

Route	Onset	Peak	Duration
I.V.	Unknown	Unknown	48 hr

Mechanism of Action
Binds to glycoprotein IIb/IIIa receptor sites on surface of activated platelets. Circulating fibrinogen can bind to these receptor sites and link platelets together, forming a clot that eventually blocks a coronary artery. By binding to receptor sites, abciximab prevents normal binding of fibrinogen and other factors and inhibits platelet aggregation.

Incompatibilities
Don't mix abciximab with other drugs. Administer it through a separate I.V. line, whenever possible.

1

Contraindications

Active internal bleeding, arteriovenous malformation or aneurysm, bleeding disorders, CVA in past 2 years or that caused significant neurologic deficit at any time, GI or GU bleeding in past 6 weeks, hypersensitivity to abciximab, intracranial neoplasm, I.V. dextran therapy before or during PTCA, oral anticoagulant therapy in past 7 days unless PT is less than 1.2 times the control, severe uncontrolled hypertension, surgery in past 6 weeks, thrombocytopenia, vasculitis

Interactions

DRUGS

cefamandole, cefoperazone, cefotetan, dipyridamole, heparin, NSAIDs, oral anticoagulants, thrombolytic drugs, ticlopidine: Increased risk of bleeding

Adverse Reactions

CNS: Confusion, dizziness, hyperesthesia
CV: Atrial fibrillation or flutter, bradycardia, embolism, hypotension, peripheral edema, pseudoaneurysm, supraventricular tachycardia, third-degree AV block, thrombophlebitis, weak pulse
GI: Dysphagia, hematemesis, nausea, vomiting
GU: Dysuria, hematuria, renal dysfunction, urinary frequency, urinary incontinence, urine retention
HEME: Anemia, bleeding, leukocytosis, thrombocytopenia
RESP: Bronchitis, bronchospasm, crackles, dyspnea, pleural effusion, pneumonia, pulmonary edema, pulmonary embolism, wheezing
SKIN: Pruritus, rash, urticaria
Other: Development of human antichimeric antibodies

Nursing Considerations

- Be aware that abciximab may be used with heparin and aspirin therapy.
- Obtain PT, APTT, and platelet count before initiating therapy.
- Inspect abciximab for particles; don't use if opaque particles are present. Don't shake container.
- Administer I.V. bolus over at least 1 minute, using a sterile, nonpyrogenic, low protein-binding 0.2- to 0.22-micron filter.
- For continuous I.V. infusion, withdraw 4.5 ml from 2-mg/ml solution and inject prescribed amount into 250-ml bag of NS or D_5W, using an in-line sterile, nonpyrogenic, low protein-binding 0.2- to 0.22-micron filter. Discard unused portion.
- Infuse prescribed amount, using a continuous infusion pump.

- Avoid I.M. injections, venipunctures, and use of indwelling urinary catheters, NG tubes, and automatic blood pressure cuffs during abciximab therapy to prevent bleeding. If appropriate, insert an intermittent I.V. access device to obtain blood samples.
- Monitor for GI, GU, and retroperitoneal bleeding and for bleeding at all puncture sites.
- **WARNING** If hemorrhage occurs, prepare to discontinue infusion immediately. Expect to treat severe thrombocytopenia with platelet transfusions if needed.
- Monitor for hypersensitivity reactions, such as rash, pruritus, wheezing, and dysphagia from laryngeal edema. If such reactions occur, discontinue infusion and notify prescriber immediately. If anaphylaxis occurs, administer epinephrine, antihistamines, and corticosteroids, as prescribed.
- Monitor PT, APTT, and activated clotting time during and after therapy.
- Obtain platelet count 2 to 4 hours after initial bolus and every 24 hours thereafter during abciximab therapy as ordered. Expect platelet function to return to normal within 48 hours of conclusion of therapy.
- Monitor vital signs and continuous ECG tracings during treatment.
- Store drug at 2° to 8° C (36° to 46° F). Protect from freezing.

PATIENT TEACHING
- Teach patient about possible adverse reactions associated with abciximab, including bleeding and hypersensitivity reactions, such as rash, urticaria, and dyspnea.
- Tell patient to prevent injury from falls by maintaining bed rest and from bleeding by keeping limb immobile while catheter sheath is in place.

acetazolamide sodium
acetazolamide
Acetazolam (CAN), Ak-Zol, Apo-Acetazolamide (CAN), Dazamide, Diamox, Diamox Sequels, Storzolamide

Class and Category
Chemical: Sulfonamide derivative
Therapeutic: Anticonvulsant, antiglaucoma agent, diuretic
Pregnancy category: C

Indications and Dosages

▶ *As short-term therapy to treat secondary glaucoma and preoperatively to treat acute congestive (angle-closure) glaucoma*

I.V. INJECTION, TABLETS

Adults. 250 mg I.V. or P.O. b.i.d. or q 4 hr; or 500 mg I.V. or P.O. initially, followed by 125 to 250 mg q 4 hr for severe acute glaucoma. To initially lower intraocular pressure rapidly, 500 mg I.V.; may repeat in 2 to 4 hours in acute cases, depending on patient response. Oral therapy usually initiated after initial I.V. dose.

S.R. CAPSULES

Adults. One S.R. capsule (500 mg) b.i.d.

I.V. INJECTION

Children. 5 to 10 mg/kg/dose q 6 hr.

S.R. CAPSULES, TABLETS

Children. 10 to 15 mg/kg/day in divided doses q 6 to 8 hr.

▶ *To treat chronic simple (open-angle) glaucoma*

I.V. INJECTION, E.R. CAPSULES, TABLETS

Adults. 250 to 1,000 mg/day (in divided doses for dosages above 250 mg).

▶ *To induce diuresis in heart failure*

I.V. INJECTION, TABLETS

Adults. *Initial:* 250 to 375 mg or 5 mg/kg q.d. in morning. *Maintenance:* 250 to 375 mg or 5 mg/kg on alternate days or for 2 days, followed by a drug-free day.

▶ *To treat drug-induced edema*

I.V. INJECTION, TABLETS

Adults. 250 to 375 mg q.d. for 1 to 2 days.

I.V. INJECTION, TABLETS

Children. 5 mg/kg/dose q.d. in morning.

▶ *To treat seizures, including generalized tonic-clonic, absence, and mixed seizures, and myoclonic jerk patterns*

I.V. INJECTION, TABLETS

Adults and children. 8 to 30 mg/kg/day in divided doses. *Optimal:* 375 to 1,000 mg/day; when used with other anticonvulsants, 250 mg q.d.

Route	Onset	Peak	Duration
I.V.*	2 min	15 min	4 to 5 hr
P.O.*	60 to 90 min	2 to 4 hr	8 to 12 hr
P.O. (S.R.)*	2 hr	8 to 12 hr	18 to 24 hr

* Effects on intraocular pressure

Mechanism of Action

Inhibits the enyzme carbonic anhydrase, which normally appears in the eyes' ciliary processes, brain's choroid plexes, and kidneys' proximal tubule cells. In the eyes, enzyme inhibition decreases aqueous humor secretion, which lowers intraocular pressure. In the brain, inhibition may delay abnormal, intermittent, and excessive discharge from neurons that cause seizures. In the kidneys, it increases bicarbonate excretion, which carries out water, potassium, and sodium, thus inducing diuresis and metabolic acidosis. This acidosis counteracts respiratory alkalosis.

Contraindications

Chronic noncongestive angle-closure glaucoma; cirrhosis; hyperchloremic acidosis; hypersensitivity to acetazolamide; hypokalemia; hyponatremia; severe pulmonary obstruction; severe renal, hepatic, or adrenocortical impairment

Interactions

DRUGS

amphetamines, methenamine, phenobarbital, procainamide, quinidine: Decreased excretion and possibly toxicity of these drugs
corticosteroids: Increased risk of hypokalemia
cyclosporine: Increased blood cyclosporine level, possibly nephrotoxicity or neurotoxicity
diflunisal: Possibly significantly decreased intraocular pressure
lithium: Increased excretion and decreased effectiveness of lithium
primidone: Decreased blood and urine primidone levels
salicylates: Increased risk of salicylate toxicity

Adverse Reactions

CNS: Ataxia, confusion, depression, disorientation, dizziness, drowsiness, fatigue, fever, flaccid paralysis, headache, lassitude, malaise, nervousness, paresthesia, seizures, tremor, weakness
EENT: Altered taste, tinnitus, transient myopia
GI: Anorexia, constipation, diarrhea, hepatic dysfunction, melena, nausea, vomiting
GU: Crystalluria, decreased libido, glycosuria, hematuria, impotence, nephrotoxicity, phosphaturia, polyuria, renal calculi, renal colic, urinary frequency
HEME: Agranulocytosis, hemolytic anemia, leukopenia, pancytopenia, thrombocytopenia, thrombocytopenic purpura

SKIN: Photosensitivity, pruritus, rash, Stevens-Johnson syndrome, urticaria
Other: Acidosis, hyperuricemia, hypokalemia, weight loss

Nursing Considerations

- Be aware that I.V. form of acetazolamide may be used if patient is unable to take oral drugs. I.V. or oral form is used to avoid painful I.M. injections.
- Be aware that acetazolamide may increase the risk of hepatic encephalopathy in patients with hepatic cirrhosis.
- Reconstitute each 500-mg vial with at least 5 ml sterile water for injection. Use within 24 hours because drug has no preservative.
- Monitor blood test results during acetazolamide therapy to detect electrolyte imbalances.
- Monitor blood and urine glucose concentrations of patients with diabetes mellitus because acetazolamide may lead to elevated levels.
- Monitor patients with a history of calcium-containing calculi for drug-induced calculi.
- Monitor patients with gout or respiratory impairment for exacerbation of these conditions.
- Monitor fluid intake and output every 8 hours and body weight daily to detect excessive fluid and weight loss.

PATIENT TEACHING

- Instruct patient to take acetazolamide exactly as prescribed. Tell him to take a missed dose as soon as he remembers but not to take a double dose.
- Inform patient that tablets may be crushed and suspended in chocolate or other sweet syrup. Alternatively, one tablet may be dissolved in 10 ml of hot water and added to 10 ml of honey or syrup.
- Advise patient to avoid potentially hazardous activities if dizziness or drowsiness occurs.
- Urge patient who takes high doses of salicylates to notify prescriber immediately if signs of salicylate toxicity, such as anorexia, tachypnea, and lethargy, occur.

acyclovir sodium
Zovirax

Class and Category
Chemical: Synthetic purine nucleoside analogue

Therapeutic: Antiviral
Pregnancy category: B

Indications and Dosages

▶ *To treat an initial episode of severe genital herpes infection*
I.V. INFUSION
Adults and children age 12 and older. 5 mg/kg q 8 hr for
5 days. *Maximum:* 20 mg/kg q 8 hr.
Infants and children up to age 12. 250 mg/m^2 q 8 hr for
5 days. *Maximum:* 20 mg/kg q 8 hr.
▶ *To treat mucocutaneous herpes simplex (HSV-1 and HSV-2) infections
in immunocompromised patients*
I.V. INFUSION
Adults and children age 12 and older. 5 mg/kg q 8 hr for
7 days. *Maximum:* 20 mg/kg q 8 hr.
Infants and children up to age 12. 10 mg/kg q 8 hr for
7 days. *Maximum:* 20 mg/kg q 8 hr.
▶ *To treat herpes simplex encephalitis*
I.V. INFUSION
Adults and children age 12 and older. 10 mg/kg q 8 hr for
10 days. *Maximum:* 20 mg/kg q 8 hr.
Children ages 3 months to 12 years. 20 mg/kg q 8 hr for 10
days. *Maximum:* 20 mg/kg q 8 hr.
▶ *To treat herpes zoster caused by varicella zoster virus in immuno-
compromised patients*
I.V. INFUSION
Adults and children age 12 and older. 10 mg/kg q 8 hr for
7 days. *Maximum:* 20 mg/kg q 8 hr.
Children up to age 12. 20 mg/kg q 8 hr for 7 days. *Maximum:*
20 mg/kg q 8 hr.
▶ *To treat neonatal herpes simplex infections*
I.V. INFUSION
Infants up to age 3 months. 10 mg/kg q 8 hr for 10 days. *Maximum:* 20 mg/kg q 8 hr.
DOSAGE ADJUSTMENT Dosing interval increased to q 12 hr
if patient's creatinine clearance is 25 to 50 ml/min/1.73 m^2 or to
q 24 hr if creatinine clearance is 10 to 25 ml/min/1.73 m^2; dosage reduced by 50% and dosing interval increased to q 24 hr if
creatinine clearance is 10 ml/min/1.73 m^2 or less. Hemodialysis
patients require an extra dose after each hemodialysis session.
Dosage for obese patients should be based on ideal body
weight.

Mechanism of Action
Prevents viral DNA replication of herpes simplex types 1 and 2 and varicella zoster virus. Infected cells selectively take up acyclovir, which is ultimately converted by virus-induced enzyme thymidine kinase to acyclovir triphosphate. Acyclovir triphosphate stops replication of viral DNA by incorporation into and termination of the growing DNA chain, and by inhibition and inactivation of the viral DNA polymerase, an enzyme used in the viral DNA replication process.

Incompatibilities
Don't mix acyclovir sodium with biological or colloidal solutions, such as blood products or protein-containing solutions. Don't mix with parabens because a precipitate may form.

Contraindications
Hypersensitivity to acyclovir or valacyclovir

Interactions
DRUGS
nephrotoxic drugs (such as aminoglycosides, penicillin, tacrolimus): Increased risk of nephrotoxicity
probenecid: Increased and prolonged blood acyclovir level
zidovudine: Increased lethargy and fatigue

Adverse Reactions
CNS: Agitation, coma, confusion, delirium, dizziness, fever, hallucinations, light-headedness, obtundation, psychosis, seizures, somnolence, tiredness, tremor, weakness
GI: Anorexia, diarrhea, elevated liver function test results, nausea, thirst, vomiting
GU: Elevated BUN and serum creatinine levels, hematuria, renal failure
HEME: Anemia, leukocytosis, leukopenia, neutropenia, neutrophilia, thrombotic thrombocytic purpura or hemolytic-uremic syndrome, thrombocytopenia, thrombocytosis
SKIN: Pruritus, rash, urticaria
Other: Injection site edema, pain, or redness

Nursing Considerations
• For initial drug reconstitution, add 10 or 20 ml of sterile water for injection to each 500-mg or 1-g vial of acyclovir, respectively, to yield a concentration of 50 mg/ml. Shake well. Don't mix with bacteriostatic water for injection containing parabens to avoid precipitation.

- **WARNING** Don't mix acyclovir with bacteriostatic water for injection containing benzyl alcohol because neonates and immature infants may develop a fatal toxic syndrome characterized by CNS, respiratory, circulatory, and renal impairment and metabolic acidosis.
- Use reconstituted acyclovir within 12 hours when stored at room temperature of 15° to 25° C (59° to 77° F). If a precipitate forms during refrigeration, allow reconstituted acyclovir to warm to room temperature to dissolve the precipitate.
- Further dilute reconstituted acyclovir with 60 to 150 ml of standard electrolyte or dextrose solution to a concentration of 7 mg/ml or less. Concentrations greater than 10 mg/ml may produce phlebitis or inflammation at injection site if extravasation occurs.
- Use final solution within 24 hours when stored at 15° to 25° C.
- Obtain baseline BUN and serum creatinine levels before and during therapy, as ordered.
- **WARNING** Administer acyclovir at a constant rate over at least 1 hour. Be aware that rapid administration may cause renal tubular damage and result in acute renal failure.
- Expect to hydrate patient during acyclovir administration to avoid precipitation of drug in renal tubules; maximum urinary concentrations are reached within 2 hours.
- Monitor BUN and serum creatinine levels and assess input and output of patients who are dehydrated, are using other nephrotoxic drugs, or have preexisting impaired renal function because acyclovir increases the risk of nephrotoxicity. Be aware that drug may precipitate in renal tubules if maximum solubility of free acyclovir (2.5 mg/ml at 37° C in water) is exceeded.
- Evaluate for altered LOC, confusion, and psychosis in patients with neurologic abnormalities or a prior neurologic reaction to cytotoxic drugs and in immunocompromised and elderly patients because of potential for neuropsychiatric toxicity.
- Be aware that immunocompromised patients receiving acyclovir may be at risk for thrombotic thrombocytopenic purpura/ hemolytic-uremic syndrome. Monitor such patients for signs and symptoms, including petechiae, fever, confusion, hematuria, and acute renal failure.
- Be aware that therapy may need to be prolonged in an immunocompromised patient because lesions take longer to heal.

- Notify prescriber if patient doesn't improve within a few days of beginning acyclovir therapy.
- Before reconstituting drug, store it at 14° to 25° C (58° to 77° F).

PATIENT TEACHING

- Inform patient that acyclovir won't prevent transmission of herpes simplex virus to sexual partners or cure the condition but that condom use may help prevent transmission. Instruct patient to avoid sexual activity if he or his partner exhibits signs or symptoms of genital herpes. However, explain that he may be contagious even before first sign of a herpetic lesion.
- To decrease irritation to genital area, encourage patient to wear loose-fitting clothes during acyclovir therapy and to keep this area clean and dry.

adenosine
Adenocard

Class and Category
Chemical: Monophosphorylated adenine riboside
Therapeutic: Antiarrhythmic
Pregnancy category: C

Indications and Dosages
▶ *To convert paroxysmal supraventricular tachycardia (PSVT) to normal sinus rhythm*

I.V. INJECTION

Adults and children who weigh 50 kg (110 lb) or more. *Initial:* 6 mg by rapid peripheral I.V. bolus over 1 to 2 sec. If PSVT continues after 1 to 2 min, 12 mg given as rapid bolus and repeated in 1 to 2 min if needed.

WARNING Don't give single doses of more than 12 mg.

Children who weigh less than 50 kg. *Initial:* 0.05 to 0.1 mg/kg as rapid central or peripheral I.V. bolus, followed by saline flush. If PSVT continues after 1 to 2 min, additional bolus injections given at doses increased incrementally by 0.05 to 0.1 mg/kg. Follow each bolus with saline flush. Injections continue until PSVT converts to normal sinus rhythm or until patient reaches maximum single dose of 0.3 mg/kg.

Route	Onset	Peak	Duration
I.V.	Immediate	Immediate	Unknown

Mechanism of Action
Slows conduction time through the AV node and can interrupt reentry pathways through the AV node to restore normal sinus rhythm.

Incompatibilities
Don't mix adenosine with other drugs.

Contraindications
Atrial fibrillation or flutter, hypersensitivity to adenosine, second- or third-degree heart block or sick sinus syndrome (unless pacemaker is present), ventricular tachycardia

Interactions
DRUGS

carbamazepine: Increased degree of heart block

digoxin, verapamil: Possibly increased depressant effect on SA or AV node

dipyridamole: Increased effects of adenosine

methylxanthines (such as theophylline): Antagonized effects of adenosine

FOODS

caffeine: Antagonized effects of adenosine

Adverse Reactions
CNS: Apprehension, dizziness, headache, heaviness in arms, light-headedness, paresthesia

CV: Chest pain or pressure, hypotension, palpitations, prolonged asystole, transient hypertension, ventricular fibrillation, ventricular tachycardia

EENT: Blurred vision, metallic taste, throat tightness

GI: Nausea

MS: Neck and back pain

RESP: Dyspnea, hyperventilation

SKIN: Diaphoresis, facial flushing

Nursing Considerations
- Before drug administration, inspect adenosine for crystals. If solution isn't clear, don't administer it. Dissolve crystals from refrigeration by warming adenosine to room temperature.
- Expect prescriber to inject adenosine directly into a vein, if appropriate, to ensure that it reaches systemic circulation. If administered into an I.V. line, it should be given as close to insertion site as possible and followed with a rapid saline flush.

- Be aware that drug will be administered by rapid I.V. bolus over 1 to 2 seconds only. Slower administration can cause systemic vasodilation and reflex tachycardia.
- Monitor heart rate and rhythm, blood pressure, and respiratory status frequently during adenosine therapy.
- Be aware that at the time of conversion to normal sinus rhythm, arrhythmias (such as PVCs, premature atrial contractions, sinus bradycardia, sinus tachycardia, and AV block) may occur for a few seconds but don't require intervention.
- **WARNING** Discontinue adenosine use and notify prescriber immediately if severe respiratory difficulties develop.
- Store drug at room temperature. Discard unused portion.

PATIENT TEACHING
- Instruct patient to report chest pain, palpitations, difficulty breathing, or severe headache that occurs during adenosine therapy.
- Inform patient that he may temporarily experience mild reactions, such as flushing, nausea, and dizziness.

alatrofloxacin mesylate
Trovan I.V.
trovafloxacin mesylate
Trovan

Class and Category
Chemical: Fluoroquinolone
Therapeutic: Antibacterial
Pregnancy category: C

Indications and Dosages
▶ *To treat life-threatening nosocomial pneumonia*
I.V. INFUSION, TABLETS
Adults. 300 mg I.V. q 24 hr, followed by 200 mg P.O. q 24 hr when patient is stabilized, for 10 to 14 days.
▶ *To treat life-threatening community-acquired pneumonia*
I.V. INFUSION, TABLETS
Adults. 200 mg I.V. q 24 hr, followed by 200 mg P.O. q 24 hr when patient is stabilized, for 7 to 14 days; or 200 mg P.O. q 24 hr for 7 to 14 days.
▶ *To treat complicated, life-threatening intra-abdominal infections, including postsurgical, gynecologic, and pelvic infections*

I.V. INFUSION, TABLETS

Adults. 300 mg I.V. q 24 hr, followed by 200 mg P.O. q 24 hr when patient is stabilized, for 7 to 14 days.

▶ *To treat complicated, life- or limb-threatening skin and soft-tissue infections, including diabetic foot infections*

I.V. INFUSION, TABLETS

Adults. 200 mg I.V. q 24 hr, followed by 200 mg P.O. q 24 hr when patient is stabilized, for 10 to 14 days; or 200 mg P.O. q 24 hr for 10 to 14 days.

DOSAGE ADJUSTMENT For patients with mild to moderate cirrhosis, 300-mg dosage reduced to 200 mg and 200-mg dosage reduced to 100 mg.

Mechanism of Action

Interferes with DNA gyrase, the enzyme necessary for DNA replication in aerobic and anaerobic bacteria. May be active against pathogens that are resistant to such antibiotics as penicillins, cephalosporins, aminoglycosides, macrolides, and tetracyclines.

Incompatibilities

Don't mix alatrofloxacin with, or infuse it simultaneously through same I.V. line as, other drugs or any solutions containing multivalent cations, such as magnesium. Don't dilute alatrofloxacin with NS or LR.

Contraindications

Hypersensitivity to alatrofloxacin, quinolone antibiotics, trovafloxacin, or their components

Interactions

DRUGS

aluminum-, citric acid–, magnesium-, or sodium citrate–containing antacids; iron; morphine sulfate; sucralfate: Decreased absorption of oral trovafloxacin

Adverse Reactions

CNS: Dizziness, headache, light-headedness, seizures
CV: Hypotension
EENT: Hoarseness, throat tightness
GI: Abdominal pain, acute hepatic failure (evidenced by anorexia, dark urine, dysphagia, fatigue, jaundice, pale stools, and vomiting)
GU: Vaginitis

RESP: Dyspnea
SKIN: Erythema, photosensitivity, pruritus, rash, urticaria
Other: Angioedema, infusion site pain

Nursing Considerations

• Using aseptic technique, withdraw appropriate amount of alatrofloxacin concentrate from vial and dilute further with appropriate I.V. solution to a final concentration of 1 to 2 mg/ml. Compatible I.V. solutions are D_5W, 0.45NS, $D_5/0.45NS$, $D_5/0.2NS$, and D_5LR.

• If you're using the same I.V. line to administer other drugs sequentially, flush line with a compatible solution before and after administering alatrofloxacin. Though it can't be used to dilute alatrofloxacin, NS can be used to flush I.V. line.

• Refrigerate diluted solution for up to 7 days or store at room temperature for 3 days in glass bottles or polyvinyl chloride I.V. containers.

• **WARNING** Infuse alatrofloxacin over 60 minutes; rapid or bolus I.V. injection may cause hypotension.

• Periodically assess liver function test results. Results may be elevated for up to 21 days after alatrofloxacin administration.

• **WARNING** Be aware that alatrofloxacin may cause severe liver damage, which may lead to death or need for liver transplantation. Expect therapy to last no longer than 2 weeks because more prolonged therapy increases the risk of liver damage. Alatrofloxacin is reserved for hospitalized patients with life- or limb-threatening infections.

• Protect vial from light before use. Store at room temperature; don't freeze.

PATIENT TEACHING

• Instruct patient who is receiving alatrofloxacin to report rash; urticaria; difficulty swallowing; swelling of lips, face, or tongue; hoarseness; throat tightness; abdominal pain; or nausea and vomiting.

• Advise patient to avoid potentially hazardous activities if he experiences dizziness or light-headedness.

• Instruct patient to avoid exposure to direct sunlight and ultraviolet light (such as tanning beds).

alglucerase
Ceredase

Class and Category
Chemical: Glucocerebrosidase-beta-glucosidase
Therapeutic: Enzyme replacement
Pregnancy category: C

Indications and Dosages
▶ *To treat chronic nonneuropathic Gaucher's disease in patients with moderate to severe anemia, thrombocytopenia with bleeding tendencies, bone disease, or significant hepatomegaly or splenomegaly*
I.V. INFUSION
Adults and children. Up to 60 U/kg infused over 1 to 2 hr, usually q 2 wk.
DOSAGE ADJUSTMENT Highly individualized dosage based on body size and disease severity. Some patients may need infusion once every other day; others may need it once q 4 wk. Maintenance dosage progressively reduced every 3 to 6 mo to as low as 1 U/kg.

Route	Onset	Peak	Duration
I.V.	Up to 60 min	Unknown	Variable

Mechanism of Action
Catalyzes the normal hydrolysis of glucocerebroside to glucose and ceramide in membrane lipids. Gaucher's disease results from deficiency of the enzyme beta-glucocerebrosidase and causes the lipid glucocerebroside to accumulate in tissue macrophages.

Contraindications
Hypersensitivity to alglucerase

Interactions
None known.

Adverse Reactions
CNS: Chills, dizziness, fatigue, fever, headache
CV: Transient peripheral edema, vasomotor irritability
EENT: Oral ulcerations
GI: Abdominal discomfort, diarrhea, nausea, vomiting
MS: Backache
Other: Infusion site burning, edema, or itching

Nursing Considerations

• Before intitiating alglucerase therapy, expect to give antihistamines to patient who is hypersensitive to drug.
• Use aseptic technique to dilute alglucerase with NS to final volume of no more than 200 ml.
• Don't shake drug; shaking could inactivate it.
• Don't use alglucerase if it's discolored or contains precipitate.
• Be aware that drug doesn't contain preservatives. Diluted product remains stable for up to 18 hr when stored at 2° to 8° C (36° to 46° F). Discard unused portion.
• Infuse alglucerase with in-line I.V. particle filter.

PATIENT TEACHING

• Explain to patient that alglucerase helps control Gaucher's disease but doesn't cure it.
• Inform patient that he may experience flulike symptoms with each dose of alglucerase.
• Instruct patient to report headache, hot flashes, nausea, and other adverse reactions.
• Inform patient that alglucerase is derived from pooled human placental tissue and poses a slight risk of viral contamination.
• Advise patient to keep appointments for scheduled infusions of alglucerase.

allopurinol sodium
Aloprim

Class and Category
Chemical: Hypoxanthine derivative, xanthine oxidase inhibitor
Therapeutic: Antihyperuricemic
Pregnancy category: C

Indications and Dosages
▶ *To treat increased serum and urine uric acid levels in patients with leukemia, lymphoma, and solid tumors whose cancer chemotherapy has increased those levels and who can't tolerate oral therapy*

I.V. INFUSION

Adults. 200 to 400 mg/m²/day as a single infusion or in equally divided infusions q 6, 8, or 12 hr. *Maximum:* 600 mg/day.
Children. 200 mg/m²/day as a single infusion or in equally divided infusions q 6, 8, or 12 hr.

DOSAGE ADJUSTMENT Dosage adjusted to 200 mg/day if creatinine clearance is 10 to 20 ml/min/1.73 m^2, to 100 mg/day if creatinine clearance is 3 to 10 ml/min/1.73 m^2, or to 100 mg q.o.d. if creatinine clearance falls below 3 ml/min/1.73 m^2.

Mechanism of Action

Inhibits uric acid production by inhibiting xanthine oxidase, the enzyme responsible for converting hypoxanthine and xanthine to uric acid. Allopurinol is metabolized to oxipurinol, which also inhibits xanthine oxidase.

Incompatibilities

Don't combine allopurinol in solution with amikacin, amphotericin B, carmustine, cefotaxime sodium, chlorpromazine hydrochloride, cimetidine hydrochloride, clindamycin phosphate, cytarabine, dacarbazine, daunorubicin hydrochloride, diphenhydramine hydrochloride, doxorubicin hydrochloride, doxycycline hyclate, droperidol, floxuridine, gentamicin sulfate, haloperidol lactate, hydroxyzine hydrochloride, idarubicin hydrochloride, imipenem and cilastatin sodium, mechlorethamine hydrochloride, meperidine hydrochloride, metoclopramide hydrochloride, methylprednisolone sodium succinate, minocycline hydrochloride, nalbuphine hydrochloride, netilmicin sulfate, ondansetron hydrochloride, prochlorperazine edisylate, promethazine hydrochloride, sodium bicarbonate, streptozocin, tobramycin sulfate, vinorelbine tartrate.

Contraindications

Hypersensitivity to allopurinol

Interactions

DRUGS

ACE inhibitors: Increased risk of hypersensitivity reactions
amoxicillin, ampicillin: Increased risk of rash
azathioprine, mercaptopurine: Inactivation of these drugs
chlorpropamide: Increased risk of hypoglycemia in patients with renal insufficiency
cyclophosphamide, other cytotoxic drugs: Enhanced bone marrow suppression
dicumarol: Increased half-life and anticoagulant action of dicumarol
thiazide diuretics: Possibly increased risk of allopurinol toxicity
uricosuric drugs: Increased urinary excretion of uric acid

vitamin C (large doses): Possibly urine acidification and increased risk of renal calculus formation

Adverse Reactions

CNS: Chills, coma, drowsiness, fever, headache, mental status changes, neuritis, paresthesia, peripheral neuropathy, seizures, somnolence

CV: Arrhythmias, cardiopulmonary arrest, hypertension, hypotension, vasculitis

EENT: Epistaxis, loss of taste

GI: Abdominal pain, diarrhea, elevated liver function test results, GI bleeding, granulomatous hepatitis, hepatic necrosis, hepatomegaly, intestinal obstruction, nausea, vomiting

GU: Exacerbation of renal calculi, hematuria, renal failure, UTI

HEME: Anemia, bone marrow depression, eosinophilia, leukocytosis, leukopenia, neutropenia, thrombocytopenia

MS: Arthralgia, exacerbation of gout, myopathy

SKIN: Alopecia; ecchymosis; jaundice; maculopapular, scaly, or exfoliative rash (sometimes fatal); pruritus; urticaria

Other: Septic shock

Nursing Considerations

- As ordered, obtain and review results of baseline CBC, uric acid levels, and renal and hepatic function studies before initiating allopurinol therapy. Continue to monitor test results during therapy.
- Reconstitute and dilute to a concentration of 6 mg/ml or less. To reconstitute, add 25 ml sterile water for injection to 30-ml vial of allopurinol powder. Dilute to desired concentration with NS or D₅W.
- Don't use if solution is discolored or contains particles.
- Store prepared solution at 20° to 25° C (68° to 77° F); don't refrigerate. Administer within 10 hours of reconstitution.
- Expect allopurinol therapy to begin 24 to 48 hours before start of chemotherapy.
- **WARNING** Discontinue allopurinol and notify prescriber immediately at first sign of a hypersensitivity reaction, such as a rash, which may precede more severe reactions.
- To decrease the risk of calculus formation, maintain fluid intake of up to 3 L/day and monitor patient for output of 2 L/day. Also, don't give patient vitamin C.

PATIENT TEACHING
- Instruct patient receiving allopurinol to drink at least 10 large glasses of water daily.

- Advise patient to report unusual bleeding or bruising, fever, chills, gout attack, numbness, and tingling.
- Inform patient that acute gout attacks may occur more frequently early in allopurinol treatment and that results may not be noticeable for 2 weeks or longer.
- Instruct patient not to drive or perform potentially hazardous tasks if allopurinol causes drowsiness.

alpha₁-proteinase inhibitor (human) (alpha₁-antitrypsin)

Prolastin

Class and Category

Chemical: Plasma protein
Therapeutic: Enzyme replacement
Pregnancy category: C

Indications and Dosages

▶ *To treat congenital alpha₁-antitrypsin deficiency in patients with signs of panacinar emphysema*

I.V. INFUSION

Adults. 60 mg/kg infused over 30 min (at rate of at least 0.08 ml/kg/min) once weekly.

Route	Onset	Peak	Duration
I.V.	In a few wk	Unknown	Unknown

Mechanism of Action

Replaces the enzyme alpha₁-antitrypsin, which normally inhibits the proteolytic enzyme elastase in patients with alpha₁-antitrypsin deficiency. Without alpha₁-proteinase inhibitor, elastase attacks and destroys alveolar membranes and causes panacinar emphysema.

Incompatibilities

Don't infuse alpha₁-proteinase inhibitor through same I.V. line as other agents or solutions.

Contraindications

Hypersensitivity to alpha₁-proteinase inhibitor, selective immunoglobulin A (IgA) deficiency in patients with anti-IgA antibodies

Interactions

ACTIVITIES

smoking: Inactivation of alpha₁-proteinase inhibitor

Adverse Reactions

CNS: Dizziness, fever (up to 12 hours after treatment)
HEME: Mild, transient leukocytosis
Other: Flulike symptoms

Nursing Considerations

- To reconstitute alpha₁-proteinase inhibitor, use sterile water for injection provided by manufacturer.
- Before administering solution, inspect it for particles and discoloration.
- Give drug up to 3 hours after reconstitution. Don't refrigerate. Discard unused reconstituted drug.
- Dilute drug with NS if necessary.
- **WARNING** Alpha₁-proteinase inhibitor is made from human plasma and may contain infectious agents, such as viruses. Ensure that patient is immunized against hepatitis B before giving drug. If time doesn't allow for antibody formation, give a single dose of hepatitis B immune globulin with hepatitis B vaccine, as prescribed.
- Seek medical attention if you experience a needle-stick injury because of possible exposure to infectious diseases.
- Monitor patient for delayed fever, which may occur up to 12 hours after therapy. Fever usually resolves within 24 hours.
- Monitor patients at risk for circulatory overload because drug is a colloidal solution that increases plasma volume.
- Before drug reconstitution, store vial at 2° to 8° C (36° to 46° F) or at a temperature not exceeding 25° C (77° F). Don't allow diluent to freeze.

PATIENT TEACHING

- Inform patient of potential risks of alpha₁-proteinase inhibitor therapy, including infection, even though drug is prescribed to reduce the risk of infectious agent transmission.
- Stress the importance of receiving weekly infusions to maintain an adequate antielastase barrier in the lungs. Explain that treatment must continue throughout the patient's lifetime.
- Caution patient not to smoke.

alteplase, recombinant
(tissue plasminogen activator, recombinant)
Activase, Activase rt-PA (CAN)

Class and Category
Chemical: Purified glycoprotein
Therapeutic: Thrombolytic
Pregnancy category: C

Indications and Dosages
▶ *To treat acute MI*
ACCELERATED I.V. INFUSION
Adults who weigh more than 67 kg (148 lb). 15-mg bolus, followed by 50 mg infused over next 30 min and then by 35 mg infused over next 60 min.
Adults who weigh 67 kg or less. 15-mg bolus, followed by 0.75 mg/kg (up to 50 mg) infused over next 30 min and then 0.5 mg/kg (up to 35 mg) infused over next 60 min.
I.V. INFUSION
Adults who weigh more than 65 kg (143 lb). 100 mg infused over 3 hr as follows: 6 to 10 mg by bolus over first 1 to 2 min, 50 to 54 mg over remainder of first hr, 20 mg over second hr, and 20 mg over third hr.
Adults who weigh 65 kg or less. 1.25 mg/kg infused over 3 hr on similar administration schedule for those weighing more than 65 kg.
▶ *To treat acute ischemic CVA*
I.V. INFUSION
Adults. 0.9 mg/kg infused over 60 min, with 10% of total dose given as bolus over first min. *Maximum:* 90 mg.
WARNING To avoid acute bleeding complications, expect to treat patient for acute ischemic CVA within 3 hr after onset of CVA symptoms and only after computed tomography or other diagnostic imaging method rules out intracranial hemorrhage.
▶ *To treat pulmonary embolism*
I.V. INFUSION
Adults. 100 mg infused over 2 hr.

Route	Onset	Peak	Duration
I.V.	Immediate	20 to 120 min	4 hr

Mechanism of Action

Binds to fibrin in a thrombus and converts trapped plasminogen to plasmin. Plasmin breaks down fibrin, fibrinogen, and other clotting factors, which dissolves the thrombus.

Incompatibilities

Don't add other drugs to solution that contains alteplase or infuse other drugs through same I.V. line.

Contraindications

For all indications: Active internal bleeding, arteriovenous malformation or aneurysm, bleeding diathesis, intracranial neoplasm, severe uncontrolled hypertension

For acute MI and pulmonary embolism only: History of CVA, intracranial or intraspinal surgery or trauma in past 2 months

For acute ischemic CVA only: Recent head trauma, recent intracranial surgery, recent previous CVA, seizure activity at onset of CVA, subarachnoid hemorrhage, suspicion or history of intracranial hemorrhage

Interactions

DRUGS

drugs that alter platelet function (such as abciximab, acetylsalicylic acid, and dipyridamole), heparin, vitamin K antagonists: Increased risk of bleeding

Adverse Reactions

CNS: Cerebral edema, cerebral herniation, CVA, fever, seizures

CV: Arrhythmias (including bradycardia and electromechanical dissociation), cardiac arrest, cardiac tamponade, cardiogenic shock, cholesterol embolism, coronary thrombolysis, heart failure, hypotension, mitral insufficiency, myocardial reinfarction or rupture, pericardial effusion, pericarditis, venous thrombosis and embolism

EENT: Epistaxis, gingival bleeding, laryngeal edema

GI: GI bleeding, nausea, retroperitoneal bleeding, vomiting

GU: GU bleeding

RESP: Pleural effusion, pulmonary edema, pulmonary reembolization

SKIN: Bleeding at puncture sites, ecchymosis, rash, urticaria

Other: Anaphylaxis

Nursing Considerations

- If possible, obtain appropriate coagulation tests, such as PT, APTT, platelet count, and fibrin-fibrinogen degradation product titer, as ordered, before initiating alteplase therapy. Monitor coagulation test results during and after therapy.
- Immediately before using alteplase, reconstitute it only with sterile water for injection provided by manufacturer. Swirl gently to dissolve powder; don't shake.
- Be aware that 50-mg vials have a vacuum and should not be used if vacuum isn't present.
- Use a large-bore (18G) needle when reconstituting 50-mg vial and the transfer device provided when reconstituting 100-mg vial to direct the flow of sterile water for injection.
- When using transfer device, hold vial of alteplase upside down while pushing down onto transfer device connected to sterile water for injection. Then invert the vials to allow the sterile water for injection to flow into the alteplase.
- Store reconstituted solution at 2° to 30° C (36° to 86° F). Use reconstituted solution within 8 hours or discard.
- Use NS or D₅W immediately before drug administration if further dilution to a concentration of 0.5 mg/ml is desired. Mix by gently swirling or slowly inverting polyvinyl chloride bag or glass vial.
- Monitor for bleeding, especially at arterial puncture sites.
- Monitor blood pressure and heart rate and rhythm frequently during and after alteplase therapy.
- **WARNING** Alteplase therapy may cause arrhythmias from sudden reperfusion of the myocardium. Monitor continuous ECG for arrhythmias during drug therapy.
- Minimize bleeding from noncompressible sites by avoiding internal jugular and subclavian venous puncture sites. Avoid I.M. injection.
- Use a small-gauge (23G or smaller) needle for venipunctures. Use a distal arm vessel for venipunctures and for arterial punctures if needed. Apply pressure for 30 minutes after an arterial puncture, then apply a pressure dressing. Evaluate site frequently for signs of bleeding.
- Discontinue alteplase infusion immediately if serious bleeding occurs.
- After administering alteplase, apply pressure for at least 30 minutes and then apply a pressure dressing.
- Protect alteplase from excessive exposure to light.

- Instruct patient beginning alteplase therapy to immediately report bleeding, including bleeding from the nose or gums.
- Advise patient to limit physical activity during alteplase administration to reduce the risk of injury and bleeding.

amikacin sulfate
Amikin

Class and Category
Chemical: Aminoglycoside
Therapeutic: Antibiotic
Pregnancy category: D

Indications and Dosages
▶ *To treat serious gram-negative bacterial infections (including septicemia; neonatal sepsis; respiratory tract, bone, joint, CNS, skin, soft-tissue, intra-abdominal, burn, and postoperative infections; and serious, complicated, and recurrent UTIs) caused by* Acinetobacter, Enterobacter, Escherichia coli, Klebsiella, Proteus, Providencia, Pseudomonas, *and* Serratia; *and staphylococcal infections when penicillin is contraindicated*

I.V. INFUSION

Adults and children. 15 mg/kg/day in equal doses at equally spaced intervals (7.5 mg/kg q 12 hr or 5 mg/kg q 8 hr) for 7 to 10 days. *Maximum:* 1,500 mg/day.

Neonates. *Loading dose:* 10 mg/kg. *Maintenance:* 7.5 mg/kg q 12 hr for 7 to 10 days.

DOSAGE ADJUSTMENT For patients with impaired renal function, loading dose of 7.5 mg/kg/day, followed by maintenance dosage based on creatinine clearance and serum creatinine level and given q 12 hr. For morbidly obese patients, dosage not to exceed 1.5 g/day.

▶ *To treat uncomplicated UTIs*

I.V. INFUSION

Adults. 250 mg b.i.d. for 7 to 10 days.

Route	Onset	Peak	Duration
I.V.	Immediate	Unknown	Unknown

Mechanism of Action

Binds to negatively charged sites on bacteria's outer cell membrane, disrupting cell integrity. Amikacin also binds to bacterial ribosomal subunits and inhibits protein synthesis. Both actions lead to cell death.

Incompatibilities

Don't mix or infuse amikacin with other drugs.

Contraindications

Hypersensitivity to amikacin or other aminoglycosides

Interactions

DRUGS

cephalosporins, enflurane, methoxyflurane, vancomycin: Increased nephrotoxic effects

general anesthetics: Increased risk of neuromuscular blockade

loop diuretics: Increased risk of *ototoxicity*

neuromuscular blockers: Possibly increased neuromuscular blockade and prolonged respiratory depression

penicillins: Possibly inactivation of or synergistic effects with amikacin

Adverse Reactions

CNS: Drowsiness, headache, loss of balance, neuromuscular blockade, tremor, vertigo

EENT: Hearing loss, ototoxicity, tinnitus

GI: Nausea, vomiting

GU: Azotemia, dysuria, nephrotoxicity, oliguria or polyuria, proteinuria

MS: Acute muscle paralysis; arthralgia; muscle fatigue, spasms, and weakness

RESP: Apnea

Other: Hyperkalemia

Nursing Considerations

- Expect to obtain results of culture and sensitivity tests before amikacin therapy begins.
- Prepare amikacin by adding contents of 500-mg vial to 100 to 200 ml of sterile diluent, such as NS or D$_5$W. Adjust amount of diluent proportionately for pediatric patients. Then infuse drug over 30 to 60 minutes.
- Don't use dark-colored solution. Solution color should range from colorless to light straw or pale yellow.

- Use 0.25- and 5-mg/ml I.V. solutions within 24 hours when stored at room temperature if they've been mixed with D_5W, D_5NS, NS, LR, or other solutions noted in manufacturer's insert. These solutions remain potent for 60 days if stored at 4° C (39° F) and for 30 days if frozen at −15° C (5° F).
- Monitor for signs of ototoxicity, such as tinnitus and vertigo, especially during high-dosage or prolonged amikacin therapy.
- **WARNING** Because amikacin may produce nephrotoxic effects, assess renal function before and daily during therapy, as ordered. To minimize renal tubule irritation, maintain patient hydration during therapy.
- Be aware that amikacin may exacerbate muscle weakness in such conditions as myasthenia gravis and Parkinson's disease.
- Measure serum amikacin concentrations as ordered, usually 30 to 90 minutes after injection (for peak concentration) and just before administering next dose (for trough concentration).
- Be aware that amikacin may be administered by I.M. injection into a large muscle mass at same dosages used for I.V. administration.

PATIENT TEACHING
- Inform patient that daily laboratory tests are necessary during amikacin treatment.
- Instruct patient to report ringing in ears, hearing changes, headache, nausea, vomiting, and changes in urination.

aminocaproic acid
Amicar

Class and Category
Chemical: Aminohexanoic acid
Therapeutic: Antifibrinolytic, antihemorrhagic
Pregnancy category: C

Indications and Dosages
▶ *To treat excessive bleeding caused by fibrinolysis*
I.V. INJECTION
Adults. 4 to 5 g in 250 ml of diluent over 1 hr, followed by continuous infusion of 1 g/hr in 50 ml of diluent. Continue for 8 hr or until bleeding stops.

Route	Onset	Peak	Duration
I.V.	Immediate	Unknown	Under 3 hr

Mechanism of Action
Inhibits the breakdown of blood clots by interfering with plasminogen activator substances and producing antiplasmin activity.

Contraindications
Hypersensitivity to aminocaproic acid; signs of active intravascular clotting, as in disseminated intravascular coagulation; upper urinary tract bleeding

Interactions
DRUGS
activated prothrombin, prothrombin complex concentrates: Increased risk of thrombosis
estrogens, oral contraceptives: Increased risk of hypercoagulation

Adverse Reactions
CNS: CVA, delirium, dizziness, hallucinations, headache, malaise, weakness
CV: Bradycardia, cardiomyopathy, edema, elevated serum CK level, hypotension, ischemia, thrombophlebitis
EENT: Nasal congestion, tinnitus
GI: Abdominal cramps and pain, diarrhea, elevated AST level, nausea, vomiting
GU: Elevated BUN level, intrarenal obstruction, renal failure
HEME: Agranulocytosis, leukopenia, thrombocytopenia
MS: Myopathy, rhabdomyolysis
RESP: Dyspnea, pulmonary embolism
SKIN: Pruritus, rash
Other: Anaphylaxis, elevated serum aldolase level

Nursing Considerations
- Mix aminocaproic acid solution with sterile water for injection, NS, D_5W, or Ringer's solution.
- **WARNING** Avoid rapid administration because of increased risks of hypotension and bradycardia.
- Monitor neurologic status for drug-induced changes. Note that increased clotting may lead to CVA.
- Be aware that dosage adjustment may be needed for patient with impaired renal function.
- Store between 15° and 30° C (59° and 86° F).

- Inform patient that he will be closely monitored during amino-caproic acid therapy and will have blood drawn for laboratory tests before, during, and after treatment.

aminophylline
(theophylline ethylenediamine)

Class and Category
Chemical: Xanthine
Therapeutic: Bronchodilator
Pregnancy category: C

Indications and Dosages
▶ *To relieve acute bronchospasm*
I.V. INFUSION

Adults (nonsmokers) who are not currently receiving theophylline products. *Initial:* 6 mg/kg (equal to 4.7 mg/kg anhydrous theophylline), not to exceed 25 mg/min. *Maintenance:* 0.7 mg/kg/hr for first 12 hr, then 0.5 mg/kg/hr.

Children ages 9 to 16 who are not currently receiving theophylline products. *Initial:* 6 mg/kg (equal to 4.7 mg/kg anhydrous theophylline), not to exceed 25 mg/min. *Maintenance:* 1 mg/kg/hr for first 12 hr, then 0.8 mg/kg/hr.

Children ages 6 months to 9 years and young adult smokers who are not currently receiving theophylline products. *Initial:* 6 mg/kg (equal to 4.7 mg/kg anhydrous theophylline), not to exceed 25 mg/min. *Maintenance:* 1.2 mg/kg/hr for first 12 hr, then 1 mg/kg/hr.

Adults and children who are currently receiving theophylline products. *Initial:* If possible, determine the time, amount, administration route, and form of last dose. Loading dose is based on principle that each 0.63 mg/kg (0.5 mg/kg anhydrous theophylline) administered as a loading dose raises serum theophylline level by 1 mcg/ml. Defer loading dose if serum theophylline level can be readily obtained. If this isn't possible and patient isn't exhibiting obvious signs of theophylline toxicity, prescriber may order 3.1 mg/kg (2.5 mg/kg anhydrous theophylline), which may increase serum theophylline level by about 5 mcg/ml. *Maintenance:* For adults (nonsmokers), 0.7 mg/kg/hr for first 12 hr, then 0.5 mg/kg/hr. For children ages 9 to 16, 1 mg/kg/hr for first 12 hr, then 0.8 mg/kg/hr. For children ages 6 months to 9 years

and young adult smokers, 1.2 mg/kg/hr for first 12 hr, then
1 mg/kg/hr.

DOSAGE ADJUSTMENT For elderly patients and those with
cor pulmonale, dosage reduced to 0.6 mg/kg for 12 hr, then to
0.3 mg/kg. For patients with heart failure and hepatic disease,
dosage reduced to 0.5 mg/kg for 12 hr, then to 0.1 to 0.2 mg/kg.

Route	Onset	Peak	Duration
I.V.	Immediate	Unknown	4 to 8 hr

Mechanism of Action

Inhibits phosphodiesterase enzymes, causing bronchodilation. Normally, these
enzymes inactivate cAMP and cGMP, which are responsible for bronchial
smooth-muscle relaxation. Other mechanisms of action may include translocation of calcium, prostaglandin antagonism, stimulation of catecholamines,
inhibition of cGMP metabolism, and adenosine receptor antagonism.

Incompatibilities

Don't add other drugs to prepared bag or bottle of aminophylline.
Don't mix aminophylline in same syringe as doxapram. Avoid administering amiodarone, ciprofloxacin, diltiazem, dobutamine, hydralazine, or ondansetron into the Y port of a continuous infusion of aminophylline.

Contraindications

Active peptic ulcer disease, hypersensitivity to aminophylline, underlying seizure disorder

Interactions

DRUGS

*activated charcoal, aminoglutethimide, barbiturates, ketoconazole, ri-
fampin, sulfinpyrazone, sympathomimetics:* Decreased blood theophylline level

*allopurinol, calcium channel blockers, cimetidine, corticosteroids, disulfi-
ram, ephedrine, influenza virus vaccine, interferon, macrolides, mexiletine, nonselective beta blockers, oral contraceptives, quinolones, thiabendazole:* Increased blood theophylline level

benzodiazepines: Antagonized sedative effects of benzodiazepines

beta agonists: Increased effects of aminophylline and beta agonist

carbamazepine, isoniazid, loop diuretics: Increased or decreased blood
theophylline level

halothane: Increased risk of cardiotoxicity

hydantoins: Decreased blood hydantoin level
ketamine: Increased risk of seizures
lithium: Decreased blood lithium level
neuromuscular blockers: Reversed neuromuscular blockade
propofol: Antagonized sedative effects of propofol
tetracyclines: Enhanced adverse effects of theophylline
FOODS
high-carbohydrate, low-protein diet: Decreased theophylline elimination and prolonged aminophylline half-life
low-carbohydrate, high-protein diet; charcoal-broiled beef: Increased theophylline elimination and shortened aminophylline half-life
ACTIVITIES
alcohol abuse: Increased effects of aminophylline
smoking (at least 1 pack/day): Decreased effects of aminophylline

Adverse Reactions
CNS: Dizziness, fever, headache, insomnia, irritability, restlessness, seizures
CV: Arrhythmias (including sinus tachycardia and life-threatening ventricular arrhythmias), hypotension, palpitations
ENDO: Hyperglycemia, syndrome of inappropriate ADH secretion
GI: Anorexia, diarrhea, epigastric pain, heavy feeling in stomach, hematemesis, indigestion, nausea, vomiting
GU: Diuresis, proteinuria, urine retention in men with prostate enlargement
MS: Muscle twitching
RESP: Respiratory arrest, tachypnea
SKIN: Alopecia, exfoliative dermatitis, flushing, rash, urticaria

Nursing Considerations
• Dilute aminophylline with D$_5$W, NS, or a dextrose and sodium chloride combination.
• **WARNING** Because aminophylline has a narrow therapeutic window (10 to 20 mcg/ml), closely monitor serum theophylline level and observe for signs of toxicity, such as tachycardia, tachypnea, nausea, vomiting, restlessness, and seizures. Keep in mind that acetaminophen, furosemide, phenylbutazone, probenecid, theobromine, coffee, tea, soft drinks, and chocolate can produce an inaccurate serum theophylline level.
• To determine peak serum theophylline level, draw blood sample 15 to 30 minutes after administering I.V. loading dose.
• Store between 15° and 30° C (59° and 86° F). Don't freeze; protect from light.

PATIENT TEACHING
- Advise patient to avoid excessive intake of caffeine (in coffee, tea, soft drinks, and chocolate), which can falsely elevate theophylline level.
- Inform patient that blood tests may be needed to monitor the effects of aminophylline.

amiodarone hydrochloride
Cordarone

Class and Category
Chemical: Iodinated benzofuran derivative
Therapeutic: Class III antiarrhythmic
Pregnancy category: D

Indications and Dosages
▶ *To treat life-threatening, recurrent ventricular fibrillation and hemodynamically unstable ventricular tachycardia when these arrhythmias don't respond to other drugs or when patient can't tolerate other drugs*
I.V. INFUSION
Adults. *Loading:* 150 mg over 10 min (15 mg/min), followed by 360 mg infused over 6 hr (1 mg/min). *Maintenance:* 540 mg infused over 18 hr (0.5 mg/min); then after the first 24 hr, 720 mg infused over 24 hr (0.5 mg/min) with dosage continued up to 96 hr or until rhythm is stable. Therapy should change to oral form as soon as possible.

Route	Onset	Peak	Duration
I.V.	Hours to 3 days	1 to 3 wk	Weeks to months

Mechanism of Action
Acts directly on cardiac cell membranes, prolonging repolarization and the refractory period and increasing ventricular fibrillation threshold. Amiodarone relaxes vascular smooth muscles, predominantly in the coronary circulation, and improves myocardial blood flow. It also relaxes peripheral vascular smooth muscles, which decreases peripheral vascular resistance and myocardial oxygen consumption.

Incompatibilities
Don't combine amiodarone mixed with D_5W to a concentration of 4 mg/ml with aminophylline, cefamandole nafate, cefazolin sodium, or mezlocillin sodium because a precipitate will form. Don't

mix amiodarone concentrations of 3 mg/ml with sodium bicarbonate because a precipitate will form. Amiodarone is incompatible with heparin.

Contraindications

Bradycardia that causes syncope (unless pacemaker is present), cardiogenic shock, children, hypersensitivity to amiodarone or its components, hypokalemia, hypomagnesemia, SA node dysfunction, second- or third-degree AV block (unless pacemaker is present)

Interactions

DRUGS

anticoagulants: Increased anticoagulant response, possibly resulting in serious bleeding

beta blockers: Increased blood levels of beta blockers and increased risk of hypotension and bradycardia

calcium channel blockers: Increased blood levels of calcium channel blockers and increased risk of AV block or hypotension

cholestyramine: Decreased blood amiodarone level

cimetidine: Increased blood amiodarone level

cyclosporine: Increased blood cyclosporine level

digoxin: Increased blood digoxin level and risk of digitalis toxicity

disopyramide: Increased blood disopyramide level with prolonged QT interval and increased risk of arrhythmias

fentanyl: Increased blood fentanyl level and increased risk of bradycardia, decreased cardiac output, and hypotension

flecainide: Increased blood flecainide level

hydantoins: Increased blood hydantoin level with long-term use, decreased blood amiodarone level

lidocaine: Increased blood lidocaine level and increased risk of seizures

methotrexate: Increased blood methotrexate level with long-term use and increased risk of methotrexate toxicity

procainamide: Increased blood procainamide or *n*-acetylprocainamide level

quinidine: Increased blood quinidine level and risk of life-threatening arrhythmias

ritonavir: Increased blood amiodarone level and risk of cardiotoxicity

theophylline: Increased blood theophylline level and risk of theophylline toxicity

Adverse Reactions

CNS: Abnormal gait, ataxia, dizziness, fatigue, headache, insomnia, involuntary movements, lack of coordination, malaise, paresthesia, peripheral neuropathy, sleep disturbances, tremor
CV: Arrhythmias (including bradycardia, electromechanical dissociation, and ventricular tachycardia), cardiac arrest, cardiogenic shock, edema, heart failure, hypotension, vasculitis
EENT: Abnormal salivation, altered smell and taste, blurred vision, corneal microdeposits, dry eyes, halo vision, lens opacities, macular degeneration, optic neuritis, optic neuropathy, papilledema, permanent blindness, photophobia, scotoma
ENDO: Hyperthyroidism, hypothyroidism
GI: Abdominal pain, anorexia, constipation, diarrhea, elevated liver function test results, hepatitis, nausea, vomiting
GU: Decreased libido, epididymitis
HEME: Coagulation abnormalities, spontaneous bruising, thrombocytopenia
RESP: Acute respiratory distress syndrome; infiltrates that lead to dyspnea, cough, pulmonary fibrosis, pulmonary intersititial pneumonitis, crackles, and wheezing; pneumonia
SKIN: Alopecia, bluish gray pigmentation, flushing, photosensitivity, rash
Other: Angioedema

Nursing Considerations

- For rapid I.V. infusion, add 3 ml (150 mg) of amiodarone (50 mg/ml) to 100 ml of D$_5$W for a concentration of 1.5 mg/ml.
- For slow I.V. infusion, add 18 ml (900 mg) of amiodarone (50 mg/ml) to 500 ml of D$_5$W for a concentration of 1.8 mg/ml.
- Use a volumetric infusion pump with polyvinyl chloride tubing and an in-line filter. Be aware that infusions lasting longer than 2 hours should be given by glass or polyolefin bottles containing D$_5$W.
- Monitor peripheral vein insertion sites for signs of inflammation. Be aware that the risk of phlebitis increases when concentrations greater than 3 mg/ml are administered. Use a central venous catheter for concentrations greater than 2 mg/ml that will be infused for longer than 1 hour.
- Monitor vital signs frequently during amiodarone treatment. Keep emergency equipment and drugs nearby.
- Monitor continuous ECG tracings and check for increased PR and QRS intervals, increased arrhythmias, and heart rate below 60 beats/minute.

- Monitor serum amiodarone level, which normally ranges from 1 to 2.5 mcg/ml.
- Monitor liver enzyme and thyroid hormone levels. Know that amiodarone inhibits conversion of T_4 to T_3.
- Be aware that amiodarone I.V. infusion may be switched to oral drug if patient's arrhythmia is suppressed.
- Store drug at 15° to 25° C (59° to 77° F). Protect from light (not necessary during administration).

PATIENT TEACHING
- Inform patient that frequent monitoring and laboratory tests will be needed during amiodarone treatment.
- Advise patient to report signs of respiratory problems, such as wheezing, dyspnea, and cough, and swollen hands and feet.
- If patient is switched to oral amiodarone, urge him to return as scheduled for follow-up appointments with prescriber and for laboratory tests.
- Instruct patient to report abnormal bleeding or bruising or changes in vision.
- Instruct patient to protect skin from sunlight by using sunscreen, covering skin, and wearing a hat when outdoors.

ammonium chloride

Class and Category
Chemical: Ammonium ion
Therapeutic: Acidifier
Pregnancy category: C

Indications and Dosages
▶ *To treat hypochloremia and metabolic alkalosis*
I.V. INFUSION
Adults. Individualized, based on serum bicarbonate level. *Usual:* 100 to 200 mEq added to 500 or 1,000 ml of NS, infused at 5 ml/min or less (about 3 hr for an infusion of 1,000 ml).

Route	Onset	Peak	Duration
I.V.	1 to 3 min	3 to 6 hr	Unknown

Mechanism of Action

Is converted to urea and hydrochloric acid in the liver. During the conversion, the drug is dissociated into ammonium and chloride ions, and hydrogen ions are released. These ions enter into the blood and extracellular fluid, where hydrogen reacts with bicarbonate ions to form water and carbon dioxide. This process decreases bicarbonate ions and increases chloride ions in the blood and extracellular fluid, which decreases blood and urine pH and corrects alkalosis.

Incompatibilities

Don't mix ammonium chloride with alkalies and their carbonates, codeine, lead or silver salts, levorphanol, methadone, or strong oxidizing agents such as potassium chlorate.

Contraindications

Hypersensitivity to ammonium chloride or its components, markedly impaired renal or hepatic function, metabolic alkalosis caused by vomiting of hydrochloric acid and accompanied by sodium loss caused by sodium bicarbonate excretion in urine

Interactions

DRUGS

amphetamines, salicylates, sulfonylureas, tricyclic antidepressants: Decreased therapeutic blood ammonium level

chlorpropamide: Increased effects of ammonium

Adverse Reactions

CNS. Fever, headache
CV: Phlebitis or thrombosis extending from injection site
GI: Indigestion, nausea, severe hepatic dysfunction, vomiting
RESP: Hyperventilation
SKIN: Extravasation
Other: Injection site infection, irritation, or pain; hypovolemia; severe metabolic acidosis (with large doses)

Nursing Considerations

• Before using ammonium chloride solution, warm it to room temperature by placing infusion in warm water to dissolve crystals.
• During I.V. administration, keep sodium bicarbonate or sodium lactate nearby to treat overdose.
• Infuse ammonium chloride slowly to avoid I.V. site pain and irritation.

- **WARNING** Monitor for signs and symptoms of ammonia tox-icity, including arrhythmias, such as bradycardia; coma; irreg-ular breathing; pallor; retching; seizures; diaphoresis; and twitching.
- Monitor for signs of metabolic acidosis, such as increased respi-rations, increased serum pH, restlessness, and diaphoresis.
- Monitor serum bicarbonate level and results of urinalysis and renal and liver function tests as appropriate.
- Store drug below 40° C (104° F). Don't freeze.

PATIENT TEACHING

- Tell patient taking ammonium chloride to consume more potas-sium-rich foods, such as bananas, oranges, cantaloupe, spinach, dried fruit, and potatoes.

amobarbital sodium
Amytal

Class, Category, and Schedule
Chemical: Barbiturate
Therapeutic: Anticonvulsant, sedative-hypnotic
Pregnancy category: D
Controlled substance: Schedule II

Indications and Dosages
▶ *To produce sedation*
I.V. INJECTION
Adults. 30 to 50 mg b.i.d. or t.i.d. and may range from 15 to 120 mg b.i.d or t.i.d. *Maximum:* 1,000 mg/dose.
Children over age 6. 65 to 500 mg/dose for preoperative seda-tion.
▶ *To induce a hypnotic state*
I.V. INJECTION
Adults. 65 to 200 mg/dose. *Maximum:* 1,000 mg/dose.
Children age 6 and older. 65 to 500 mg/dose.
▶ *To manage seizures*
I.V. INJECTION
Adults. *Usual:* 65 to 500 mg up to a maximum of 1,000 mg. Dosage for acute seizures determined by response. Doses of 200 to 500 mg are typically required to control seizures.
Children age 6 and older. 65 to 500 mg.
Children up to age 6. 3 to 5 mg/kg/dose.

WARNING Use I.V. route only when other routes aren't appropriate. Inject slowly—at a rate of 50 mg/min or less—to prevent sudden respiratory depression, apnea, laryngospasm, or hypotension.

Route	Onset	Peak	Duration
I.V.	Unknown	Unknown	10 to 12 hr

Mechanism of Action

Nonselectively acts on the CNS to depress the sensory cortex, decrease motor activity, alter cerebellar function, and produce drowsiness, sedation, and hypnosis. Appears to reduce wakefulness and alertness by acting in the thalamus, where it depresses the reticular activating system and interferes with impulse transmission from the periphery to the cortex. Produces CNS depressant effects ranging from mild sedation and anxiety reduction to anesthesia and coma.

Incompatibilities

Don't mix amobarbital in solution with other drugs.

Contraindications

Alcoholism, history of porphyria, history of sedative or barbiturate addiction, hypersensitivity to barbiturates, renal or hepatic disease, severe respiratory disease, sleep apnea, suicidal tendency, uncontrolled pain

Interactions

DRUGS

acetaminophen: Increased blood acetaminophen level and risk of hepatotoxicity

antihistamines, CNS depressants, phenothiazines, tranquilizers: Increased CNS depression

beta blockers, carbamazepine, clonazepam, corticosteroids, digitoxin, doxycycline, estrogens, griseofulvin, metronidazole, oral anticoagulants, oral contraceptives, phenylbutazones, quinidine, theophyllines, tricyclic antidepressants: Decreased blood levels and effects of these drugs

chloramphenicol: Inhibited amobarbital metabolism; enhanced chloramphenicol metabolism

MAO inhibitors: Increased blood level and sedative effects of amobarbital

methoxyflurane: Increased nephrotoxicity

phenytoin: Altered effects of phenytoin

rifampin: Decreased blood level and effects of amobarbital
valproic acid: Increased amobarbital effects
ACTIVITIES
alcohol use: Increased blood level of amobarbital and additive CNS
depressant effects

Adverse Reactions

CNS: Agitation, anxiety, ataxia, CNS depression, confusion, dizziness, hallucinations, hangover, headache, hyperkinesia, insomnia, nightmares, nervousness, paradoxical stimulation, psychiatric disturbance, somnolence, syncope, vertigo
CV: Bradycardia, hypotension, shock
EENT: Laryngospasm
GI: Constipation, diarrhea, epigastric pain, nausea, vomiting
RESP: Apnea, bronchospasm, hypoventilation, respiratory depression
SKIN: Exfoliative dermatitis, rash, Stevens-Johnson syndrome, urticaria
Other: Angioedema, gangrene of arm or leg from accidental injection into artery, injection site tissue damage and necrosis, physical and psychological dependence, potentially fatal withdrawal syndrome, tolerance

Nursing Considerations

- Be aware that amobarbital shouldn't be given during third trimester of pregnancy because repeated use can cause dependence in neonate. It also shouldn't be given to breast-feeding women because it may cause CNS depression in infants.
- Prepare amobarbital using sterile water for injection.
- Closely monitor blood pressure, pulse, and respirations during administration. Keep emergency equipment and drugs nearby in case respiratory depression or adverse hemodynamic effects occur. Be aware that patients with cardiovascular disease are at increased risk for adverse circulatory reactions, particularly when drug is administered too fast, and that those with pulmonary diseases associated with obstruction or dyspnea are at increased risk for ventilatory depression. Anticipate the risk of hypotension, even when giving drug at recommended rate.
- Monitor for hypersensitivity reactions, such as bronchospasm, difficulty breathing, facial edema, and urticaria, especially in patients with a history of asthma, angioedema, or urticaria.
- **WARNING** Don't administer solution after 30 minutes of exposure to air. Solution quickly becomes unstable because amobarbital sodium hydrolyzes in solution.

- **WARNING** To prevent tissue damage and necrosis at peripheral insertion sites, monitor closely for signs of extravasation. Be aware that accidental arterial injection may cause gangrene of arm or leg.
- Anticipate that amobarbital's CNS effects may exacerbate major depression, suicidal tendencies, or other mental disorders.
- Closely monitor debilitated or elderly patients, as appropriate, because they're more likely to experience such adverse CNS reactions as confusion, depression, and excitement. Take safety precautions.
- Be aware that amobarbital may cause paradoxical stimulation (excitement, euphoria, restlessness) in patients with acute pain and in children.
- Evaluate for signs of intensified or prolonged hypnotic effect in patients with shock or uremia.
- Assess hyperthyroid patients for exacerbated symptoms, such as increased nervousness and palpitations, due to amobarbital use.
- Be aware that barbituate-induced respiratory depression may cause complications in patients with severe anemia.
- Be aware that drug may trigger signs and symptoms in patients with acute intermittent porphyria.
- To prevent withdrawal symptoms, such as diaphoresis, insomnia, irritability, nightmares, and tremors, expect to taper amobarbital dosage gradually after long-term use, especially for epileptic patients.

PATIENT TEACHING
- Instruct patient to report severe dizziness, persistent drowsiness, rash, or skin lesions during amobarbital therapy.

amphotericin B
Amphocin, Fungizone Intravenous
amphotericin B cholesteryl sulfate complex
Amphotec
amphotericin B lipid complex
Abelcet
amphotericin B liposomal complex
AmBisome

Class and Category
Chemical: Amphoteric polyene macrolide
Therapeutic: Antifungal
Pregnancy category: B

Indications and Dosages

▶ *To treat severe fungal infections, using amphotericin B*
I.V. INFUSION

Adults and adolescents. *Initial:* 1-mg test dose in 20 ml of D_5W infused over 20 to 30 min; if test dose is tolerated, then 0.25 to 0.3 mg/kg/day prepared as a 0.1-mg/ml infusion, given over 2 to 6 hr. Increased in 5- to 10-mg increments up to 50 mg/day, based on patient tolerance and infection severity, not to exceed a total daily dose of 1.5 mg/kg. *Maximum:* 50 mg/day infused over 2 to 6 hr.

Children. *Initial:* 0.25 mg/kg/day in D_5W infused over 6 hr; then increased in 0.125- to 0.25-mg/kg increments daily or every other day as tolerated. *Maximum:* 1 mg/kg or 30 mg/m² of body surface daily.

▶ *To treat aspergillosis, using amphotericin B cholesteryl sulfate complex*
I.V. INFUSION

Adults and children. Test dose of 1.6 to 8.3 mg in 10 ml of D_5W infused over 15 to 30 min; if test dose is tolerated, then 3 to 4 mg/kg once daily infused at 1 mg/kg/hr.

▶ *To treat invasive amphotericin B–resistant fungal infections, using amphotericin B lipid complex*
I.V. INFUSION

Adults and children. 5 mg/kg/day infused at 2.5 mg/kg/hr.

▶ *To treat severe aspergillosis, candidiasis, or cryptococcosis, using amphotericin B liposomal complex*
I.V. INFUSION

Adults and children. 3 to 5 mg/kg/day infused over 2 hr. Infusion time may be decreased to 1 hr if tolerated, or increased if patient experiences discomfort.

▶ *To treat leishmaniasis, using amphotericin B liposomal complex*
I.V. INFUSION

Immunocompetent adults and children. 3 mg/kg/day infused over 2 hr on days 1 through 5 and on days 14 and 21. Infusion time may be decreased to 1 hr if tolerated, or increased if patient experiences discomfort.

Immunocompromised adults and children. 4 mg/kg/day infused over 2 hr on days 1 through 5 and on days 10, 17, 24, 31, and 38. Infusion time may be decreased to 1 hr if tolerated, or increased if patient experiences discomfort.

▶ *To treat presumed fungal infections in patients with febrile neutropenia, using amphotericin B lipid complex*

I.V. INFUSION
Adults and children. 3 mg/kg/day infused over 2 hr. Infusion time may be decreased to 1 hr if tolerated, or increased if patient experiences discomfort.

Route	Onset	Peak	Duration
I.V.	Immediate	Unknown	Unknown

Mechanism of Action
Binds to sterols in fungal cell plasma membranes, which changes membrane permeability and allows loss of potassium and small molecules from cells. This action results in cell impairment or death.

Incompatibilities
Don't reconstitute amphotericin B with diluents other than those recommended because solutions containing sodium chloride or bacteriostatic agents (such as benzyl alcohol) may cause drug precipitation.

Contraindications
Hypersensitivity to amphotericin B or its components

Interactions
DRUGS
antineoplastics: Increased risk of bronchospasm, hypotension, and nephrotoxicity
corticosteroids, corticotropin: Increased risk of hypokalemia and subsequent cardiac dysfunction
cyclosporine, nephrotoxic drugs: Increased risk of nephrotoxicity
digitalis glycosides: Possibly hypokalemia and more severe digitalis toxicity
flucytosine: Possibly increased flucytosine toxicity
leukocyte transfusion: Possibly dyspnea, hypoxemia, and pulmonary infiltrates
skeletal muscle relaxants: Possibly hypokalemia and subsequent increased muscle relaxation
zidovudine: Possibly myelotoxicity and nephrotoxicity

Adverse Reactions
CNS: Chills, fever, headache, tiredness, weakness
CV: Chest pain, hypotension, irregular heartbeat
EENT: Pharyngitis

GI: Abdominal pain, anorexia, diarrhea, dysphagia, hepatic failure, indigestion, nausea, vomiting
GU: Decreased or increased urine output, impaired renal function
HEME: Anemia, leukopenia, thrombocytopenia, unusual bleeding or bruising
MS: Arthralgia, muscle spasms, myalgia
RESP: Apnea, dyspnea, hypoxia, pulmonary edema, tachypnea
SKIN: Flushing, jaundice, maculopapular rash, pruritus and redness especially around ears, urticaria
Other: Anaphylaxis, hypocalcemia, hypokalemia, hypomagnesemia, infusion site pain and thrombophlebitis

Nursing Considerations

- To prepare amphotericin B, add 10 ml of sterile water for injection (without a bacteriostatic agent) to vial containing 50 mg of amphotericin B. For I.V. infusion, dilute the solution containing 5 mg/ml to 0.1 mg/ml by adding 1 ml (5 mg) of solution to 49 ml of D_5W with a pH above 4.2.
- Before using D_5W to dilute amphotericin B solution, aseptically determine injection's pH. If pH is below 4.2, follow manufacturer's instructions for buffering it.
- Because reconstituted amphotericin B is a colloidal suspension, avoid using an in-line membrane filter or use one with a mean pore diameter of more than 1 micron to prevent significant drug removal.
- To prepare amphotericin B cholesteryl sulfate complex, reconstitute it with sterile water for injection. Using a sterile syringe and a 20G needle, rapidly add 10 or 20 ml of sterile water for injection to a 50- or 100-mg vial, respectively, to obtain a solution containing 5 mg of amphotericin B per milliliter. Then shake gently by hand, rotating vial until all solids are dissolved. The fluid may be clear or opalescent. For infusion, further dilute reconstituted solution to about 0.6 mg/ml. Don't filter the solution. Flush existing line with D_5W or use a separate line. Don't use an in-line filter.
- To prepare amphotericin B lipid complex, shake vial gently until you see no yellow sediment. Using an 18G needle, withdraw prescribed dose from required number of vials into one or more 20-ml syringes. Replace needle with 5-micron filter needle that's supplied with each vial. Empty syringe contents into bag of D_5W so that final concentration is 1 mg/ml. Expect to use a concentration of 2 mg/ml for pediatric patients and patients

with cardiovascular disease. Before infusion, shake bag until contents are mixed thoroughly. Flush existing line with D$_5$W or use a separate line. Don't use an in-line filter. If infusion exceeds 2 hours, shake infusion bag every 2 hours.

- To prepare amphotericin B liposomal complex, add 12 ml of sterile water for injection (without a bacteriostatic agent) to each 50-mg vial to achieve a concentration of 4 mg amphotericin B per milliliter. Immediately shake vial vigorously for at least 30 seconds until all particles completely disperse. Withdraw prescribed dose of amphotericin B liposomal complex suspension. Then use a 5-micron filter to inject it into D$_5$W to provide a final concentration of 1 to 2 mg/ml. Expect to use a lower concentration (0.2 to 0.5 mg/ml) for infants and young children. Flush existing line with D$_5$W or use a separate line. You may use an in-line filter with a mean pore diameter of at least 1 micron.

- To help minimize fever and shaking chills, expect to administer an antipyretic, an antihistamine, meperidine, or a corticosteroid just before infusing amphotericin B.

- Assess I.V. insertion site regularly to detect extravasation of amphotericin B, which may cause severe local irritation. To minimize local thrombophlebitis, plan to add heparin to infusion or to administer amphotericin on alternate days, which also may help prevent anorexia. Alternate-day dose shouldn't exceed 1.5 mg/kg.

- Monitor renal function closely because of risk of renal impairment. Plan to assess serum creatinine level every other day while amphotericin B dosage is increasing and then at least twice weekly during continued therapy. If serum creatinine or BUN level increases significantly, expect to discontinue amphotericin B until renal function improves. Be aware that a cumulative dose of more than 4 g may cause irreversible renal dysfunction.

- Expect to monitor CBC and platelet count weekly throughout therapy to detect adverse hematologic effects. Also monitor serum calcium, magnesium, and potassium levels twice weekly throughout therapy to detect abnormalities.

- Before drug reconstitution, store amphotericin B at 2° to 8° C (36° to 46° F), and protect from light. Use reconstituted amphotericin B within 24 hours if stored at room temperature or within 1 week if refrigerated. Use immediately if solution was reconstituted and diluted in D$_5$W.

- Before drug reconstitution, store amphotericin B cholesteryl sulfate complex at 15° to 30° C (59° to 86° F) unless otherwise specified. After reconstitution, store at 2° to 8° C (36° to 46° F). Use reconstituted amphotericin B cholesteryl sulfate complex within 24 hours.
- Before drug dilution, store amphotericin B lipid complex at 2° to 8° C, and protect from light. Use amphotericin B lipid complex within 6 hours if stored at room temperature or within 48 hours if stored at 2° to 8° C. Don't freeze.
- Before drug reconstitution, store amphotericin B liposomal complex at 2° to 8° C. Use reconstituted amphotericin B liposomal complex within 24 hours if stored at 2° to 8° C. Begin infusion of diluted drug within 6 hours. Don't freeze.

PATIENT TEACHING

- Instruct patient to report pain or discomfort at I.V. insertion site of amphotericin.
- Advise patient to report adverse reactions immediately, especially shortness of breath, chest pain, or wheezing.

ampicillin sodium

Ampicin (CAN), Omnipen-N, Penbritin (CAN), Polycillin-N, Totacillin-N

Class and Category

Chemical: Semisynthetic aminopenicillin
Therapeutic: Broad-spectrum antibiotic
Pregnancy category: B

Indications and Dosages

▶ *To treat GI infections and genitourinary infections (other than gonorrhea) caused by susceptible strains of* **Shigella, Salmonella typhi** *and other species,* **Escherichia coli, Proteus mirabilis,** *and enterococci*
I.V. INFUSION

Adults and children who weigh 20 kg (44 lb) or more. 250 to 500 mg I.V. q 6 hr.
Children who weigh less than 20 kg. 12.5 mg/kg I.V. q 6 hr.
▶ *To treat gonorrhea caused by susceptible strains of non-penicillinase-producing* **Neisseria gonorrhoeae**
I.V. INFUSION

Adults and children who weigh 40 kg (88 lb) or more. 500 mg q 6 hr.

Children who weigh less than 40 kg. 50 mg/kg/day in divided doses q 6 to 8 hr.

▶ *To treat respiratory tract infections caused by susceptible strains of non-penicillinase-producing* Haemophilus influenzae, *staphylococci, and streptococci, including* Streptococcus pneumoniae

I.V. INFUSION

Adults and children who weigh 40 kg or more. 250 to 500 mg I.V. q 6 to 8 hr.

Children who weigh 20 to 39 kg (44 to 86 lb). 25 to 50 mg/kg/day I.V. in divided doses q 6 to 8 hr.

Children who weigh less than 20 kg. 12.5 mg/kg I.V. q 6 hr.

▶ *To treat septicemia*

I.V. INFUSION

Adults. 8 to 14 g I.V. daily in divided doses q 3 to 4 hr for at least 3 days; then may be administered I.M.

Children. 150 to 200 mg/kg/day I.V. in divided doses q 3 to 4 hr for at least 3 days; then may be administered I.M.

▶ *To prevent bacterial endocarditis from dental, oral, or upper respiratory tract procedures*

I.V. INFUSION

Adults. 2 g within 30 min of procedure.

Children. 50 mg/kg within 30 min of procedure.

▶ *To treat bacterial meningitis caused by susceptible strains of* Neisseria meningitidis

I.V. INFUSION

Adults. 8 to 14 g/day in divided doses q 3 to 4 hr for at least 3 days; then may be given I.M. at same dosage and schedule.

Children. 100 to 200 mg/kg/day in divided doses q 3 to 4 hr for at least 3 days; then may be given I.M. at same dosage and schedule.

▶ *To treat listeriosis*

I.V. INFUSION

Adults and children who weigh 20 kg or more. 50 mg/kg q 6 hr.

Children who weigh less than 20 kg. 12.5 mg/kg q 6 hr.

Route	Onset	Peak	Duration
I.V.	Immediate	Unknown	Unknown

Mechanism of Action

Inhibits bacterial cell wall synthesis. The rigid, cross-linked cell wall is assembled in several steps. Ampicillin exerts its effects on susceptible bacteria in the final stage of the cross-linking process by binding with and inactivating penicillin-binding proteins (enzymes responsible for linking the cell wall strands). This action causes bacterial cell lysis and death.

Incompatibilities

To prevent mutual inactivation, don't mix ampicillin in the same I.V. bag, bottle, or tubing with an aminoglycoside. If patient must receive both drugs, administer them in separate sites at least 1 hour apart.

Contraindications

Hypersensitivity to any penicillin, infection caused by penicillinase-producing organism

Interactions

DRUGS

allopurinol: Increased risk of rash, particularly in hyperuricemic patient

aminoglycosides: Possibly inactivation of both drugs when given together

heparin, oral anticoagulants: Increased risk of bleeding

oral contraceptives: Possibly reduced contraceptive effectiveness and breakthrough bleeding

probenecid: Possibly increased blood ampicillin level and risk of ampicillin toxicity

tetracyclines: Possibly impaired action of ampicillin

Adverse Reactions

CNS: Chills, fatigue, fever, headache, malaise

CV: Chest pain, edema, thrombophlebitis

EENT: Epistaxis, glossitis, laryngeal stridor, mucocutaneous candidiasis, stomatitis, throat tightness

GI: Abdominal distention, diarrhea, enterocolitis, flatulence, gastritis, nausea, pseudomembranous colitis, vomiting

GU: Dysuria, urine retention, vaginal candidiasis

HEME: Agranulocytosis, anemia, eosinophilia, leukopenia, thrombocytopenia, thrombocytopenic purpura

SKIN: Erythema multiforme; erythematous, mildly pruritic maculopapular rash or other types of rash; exfoliative dermatitis; pruritus; urticaria

Other: Anaphylaxis, facial edema

Nursing Considerations

* Expect to administer ampicillin for 48 to 72 hours after patient becomes asymptomatic. For streptococcal infection, expect to administer ampicillin for at least 10 days after cultures show streptococcal eradication to reduce the risk of rheumatic fever or glomerulonephritis.
* To dilute ampicillin for intermittent I.V. infusion, add 5 ml of sterile water or bacteriostatic water for injection to each 125-, 250-, or 500-mg vial, or at least 7.4 to 10 ml of diluent to each 1- or 2-g vial. Administer I.V. infusion in suitable diluent in a concentration of less than 30 mg/ml.
* **WARNING** Infuse I.V. solution over 3 to 5 minutes for each 125 or 500 mg, or over 10 to 15 minutes for each 1 or 2 g. More rapid infusion may cause seizures.
* Monitor closely for anaphylaxis, which may be life-threatening. Patients at greatest risk are those with a history of multiple allergies, hypersensitivity to cephalosporins, or a history of asthma, hay fever, or urticaria.
* **WARNING** If ampicillin triggers an anaphylactic reaction, discontinue drug, notify prescriber immediately, and provide appropriate therapy. Anaphylaxis requires immediate treatment with epinephrine as well as airway management and administration of oxygen and I.V. corticosteroids, as needed.
* If long-term or high-dose ampicillin therapy is required, closely monitor results of renal and liver function tests and CBCs.
* Be aware that each gram of ampicillin contains approximately 3.4 mEq of sodium; take this into account when calculating patient's daily sodium intake.
* Know that ampicillin diluted in D_5W to a concentration of 20 mg/ml or less retains its potency for 2 hours at room temperature and for 3 hours when refrigerated.

PATIENT TEACHING

* Instruct patient taking ampicillin to immediately report signs of an allergic reaction, such as shortness of breath, wheezing, rash, chest pain, or facial swelling.

ampicillin sodium and sulbactam sodium

Unasyn

Class and Category

Chemical: Aminopenicillin, beta-lactamase inhibitor
Therapeutic: Broad-spectrum antibiotic
Pregnancy category: B

Indications and Dosages

▶ *To treat skin and soft-tissue infections caused by beta-lactamase–producing strains of* Staphylococcus aureus, Escherichia coli, Klebsiella *species (including* K. pneumoniae*),* Proteus mirabilis, Bacteroides fragilis, Enterobacter *species, and* Acinetobacter calcoaceticus; *intra-abdominal infections caused by beta-lactamase–producing strains of* E. coli, Klebsiella *species (including* K. pneumoniae*),* Bacteroides *species (including* B. fragilis*), and* Enterobacter *species; gynecologic infections caused by beta-lactamase–producing strains of* E. coli *and* Bacteroides *species (including* B. fragilis*)*

I.V. INFUSION

Adults and children age 12 and older who weigh 40 kg (88 lb) or more. 1.5 (1 g of ampicillin and 0.5 g of sulbactam) to 3 g (2 g of ampicillin and 1 g of sulbactam) q 6 hr, up to a maximum of 8 g of ampicillin and 4 g of sulbactam daily.

Children age 1 and older who weigh less than 40 kg. 300 mg/kg (200 mg of ampicillin and 100 mg of sulbactam) daily in divided doses q 6 hr.

DOSAGE ADJUSTMENT Dosing frequency reduced to q 6 to 8 hr for patients with creatinine clearance of 30 ml/min/1.73 m^2 or more, to q 12 hr for patients with creatinine clearance of 15 to 29 ml/min/1.73 m^2, and to q 24 hr for patients with creatinine clearance of 5 to 14 ml/min/1.73 m^2.

Route	Onset	Peak	Duration
I.V.	Immediate	Unknown	Unknown

Mechanism of Action

Inhibits bacterial cell wall synthesis. The rigid, cross-linked cell wall is assembled in several steps. The drug exerts its effects on susceptible bacteria in the final stage of the cross-linking process by binding with and inactivating penicillin-binding proteins (enzymes responsible for linking the cell wall strands). This action causes bacterial cell lysis and death. When ampicillin is administered alone, beta-lactamases may degrade it, making it ineffective. When combined with sulbactam, degradation can't occur. So sulbactam extends ampicillin's bactericidal effects to beta-lactamase–producing bacteria.

Incompatibilities

To prevent mutual inactivation, don't mix ampicillin sodium and sulbactam sodium in the same I.V. bag, bottle, or tubing with an aminoglycoside. If patient must receive both drugs, administer them in separate sites at least 1 hour apart.

Contraindications

Hypersensitivity to ampicillin sodium and sulbactam sodium, its components, or any penicillin

Interactions

DRUGS

allopurinol: Increased risk of rash, particularly in hyperuricemic patient

aminoglycosides: Possibly inactivation of both drugs when given together

heparin, oral anticoagulants: Increased risk of bleeding

oral contraceptives: Possibly reduced contraceptive effectiveness and breakthrough bleeding

probenecid: Possibly increased blood ampicillin level and risk of ampicillin toxicity

tetracyclines: Possibly impaired action of ampicillin sodium and sulbactam sodium

Adverse Reactions

CNS: Chills, fatigue, fever, headache, malaise

CV: Chest pain, edema, thrombophlebitis

EENT: Black "hairy" tongue, epistaxis, glossitis, laryngeal stridor, mucocutaneous candidiasis, stomatitis, throat tightness

GI: Abdominal distention, diarrhea, enterocolitis, flatulence, gastritis, nausea, pseudomembranous colitis, vomiting

GU: Dysuria, urine retention, vaginal candidiasis

HEME: Agranulocytosis, anemia, eosinophilia, leukopenia, thrombocytopenia, thrombocytopenic purpura
SKIN: Erythema multiforme; erythematous, mildly pruritic maculopapular rash or other rash; exfoliative dermatitis; mucosal bleeding; pruritus; urticaria
Other: Anaphylaxis, facial edema

Nursing Considerations

- Avoid administering ampicillin sodium and sulbactam sodium to patients with mononucleosis because of increased risk of a rash.
- Add 3.2 ml of sterile water for injection to each 1.5-g vial or 6.4 ml to each 3-g vial. This provides a total concentration of 375 mg/ml (250 mg/ml of ampicillin and 125 mg/ml of sulbactam). Using a suitable diluent and the concentrations recommended in manufacturer's insert (including sterile water for injection, LR, or $D_5/0.45NS$), further dilute to a final concentration of 3 to 45 mg/ml (2 to 30 mg/ml of ampicillin and 1 to 15 mg/ml of sulbactam).
- Let solution stand to allow foaming to dissipate; inspect for complete solubility before administering.
- Administer I.V. dose by slow injection over 10 to 15 minutes or by infusion over 15 to 30 minutes when diluted further.
- Monitor closely for anaphylaxis, which may be life-threatening. Patients at greatest risk are those with a history of hypersensitivity to penicillin, multiple allergies, hypersensitivity to cephalosporins, or a history of asthma, hay fever, or urticaria.
- **WARNING** If drug triggers an anaphylactic reaction, discontinue drug, notify prescriber immediately, and provide appropriate therapy. Anaphylaxis requires immediate treatment with epinephrine as well as airway management and administration of oxygen and I.V. corticosteroids, as needed.
- Monitor closely for diarrhea, which may signal pseudomembranous colitis. If diarrhea occurs, notify prescriber. If pseudomembranous colitis is diagnosed, expect to discontinue drug and, possibly, administer fluids, electrolytes, protein, and antibiotic effective against *Clostridium difficile*.
- Keep in mind that each 1.5-g dose of ampicillin and sulbactam contains 5 mEq of sodium; take this into account when calculating patient's daily sodium intake.
- Be aware that drug's potency varies, depending on amount and type of diluent used and how solution is stored. For example, dilution with NS for a final concentration of 45 mg/ml (30/15 mg/ml) retains potency for 8 hours when stored at

25° C (77° F) and for 48 hours when stored at 4° C (39° F).
A dilution with NS for a final concentration of 30 mg/ml
(20/10 mg/ml) retains potency for 72 hours when stored at
4° C. See manufacturer's insert for further details.

PATIENT TEACHING

• Instruct patient receiving ampicillin sodium and sulbactam sodium to immediately report sudden or unusual symptoms, such
as shortness of breath, wheezing, rash, chest pain, or facial
swelling. Tell him to notify prescriber immediately if diarrhea
occurs.

anistreplase
(anisoylated plasminogen-streptokinase activator complex)
Eminase

Class and Category
Chemical: p-Anisoylated derivative of the Lys-plasminogen-
streptokinase activator complex
Therapeutic: Thrombolytic enzyme
Pregnancy category: C

Indications and Dosages
▶ *To treat acute MI (to lyse thrombi obstructing coronary arteries,
reduce infarct size, improve ventricular function, and reduce mortality)*
I.V. INFUSION
Adults 30 U injected over 2 to 5 min.

Route	Onset	Peak	Duration
I.V.	Immediate	20 min to 2 hr	4 to 6 hr

Mechanism of Action
Indirectly promotes the conversion of plasminogen to plasmin, an enzyme
that breaks down fibrin clots, fibrinogen, and other plasma proteins, including procoagulant factors V and VIII.

Incompatibilities
Don't add other drugs to anistreplase solution or infuse other
drugs through same I.V. line.

Contraindications

Active internal bleeding, arteriovenous malformation or aneurysm, bleeding diathesis, history of CVA, hypersensitivity to anistreplase or streptokinase, intracranial neoplasm, intracranial or intraspinal surgery or trauma within past 2 months, severe uncontrolled hypertension

Interactions

DRUGS

aspirin, dipyridamole, and other drugs that alter platelet function; heparin; vitamin K antagonists: Possibly increased risk of bleeding if administered before anistreplase

Adverse Reactions

CNS: Dizziness, fever, headache, intracranial hemorrhage
CV: Ankle edema, arrhythmias (especially accelerated idioventricular rhythm, conduction disorders, premature ventricular beats, sinus bradycardia, ventricular fibrillation, ventricular tachycardia), hypotension, vasculitis
EENT: Epistaxis
GI: Abdominal pain or swelling, constipation, GI bleeding, nausea, vomiting
GU: Hematuria, proteinuria, vaginal bleeding
HEME: Bleeding tendency, eosinophilia, mild to severe hemorrhage
MS: Arthralgia, back pain, joint stiffness, myalgia
RESP: Bronchospasm, dyspnea, hemoptysis
SKIN: Flushing, pruritus, rash, urticaria
Other: Anaphylaxis, angioedema

Nursing Considerations

- Obtain appropriate coagulation studies (such as PT, APTT, platelet count, and fibrin-fibrinogen degradation product titer) before initiating anistreplase treatment, if possible.
- To reconstitute anistreplase, slowly direct 5 ml of sterile water for injection or sodium chloride for injection against side of vial. Then gently roll vial to mix dry powder and fluid and minimize foaming. Don't shake vial. The resulting solution should be colorless to pale yellow and transparent.
- Before administering solution, inspect it for particles and discoloration. If present, discard and reconstitute drug from a new vial. Then withdraw entire contents of vial. Don't dilute reconstituted solution further before administration; don't add it to

I.V. fluid. Don't add other drugs to vial or syringe that contains anistreplase. Discard drug if it isn't administered within 30 minutes of reconstitution.

- For maximum effectiveness, expect to administer anistreplase as soon as possible after onset of MI symptoms.
- Closely monitor all puncture sites, such as catheter insertion and needle puncture sites, for bleeding.
- Monitor the following patients for signs and symptoms of bleeding or hemorrhage because they're at increased risk during anistreplase therapy: those with acute pericarditis (risk of hemopericardium, possibly leading to cardiac tamponade); cerebrovascular disease; hemorrhagic ophthalmic conditions; history of major surgery, GI or GU bleeding, or trauma within past 10 days; hypertension; mitral stenosis with atrial fibrillation (risk of embolism); pregnancy; septic thrombophlebitis; severe hepatic or renal disease; or subacute bacterial endocarditis.
- Avoid giving I.M. injections and handling patient unnecessarily during anistreplase therapy. Perform venipuncture only when necessary, using a 23G or smaller needle.
- If an arterial puncture is needed after anistreplase administration, use an arm vessel that allows easy manual compression. Apply manual pressure for 30 minutes. Then apply a pressure dressing and check puncture site frequently for bleeding.
- Use continuous cardiac monitoring because arrhythmias may occur during reperfusion. Keep antiarrhythmics on hand during anistreplase therapy, and manage arrhythmias according to facility policy.
- Keep epinephrine, glucocorticoids, and antihistamines nearby to treat anaphylaxis.
- Know that anistreplase may be less effective if given more than 5 days after previous anistreplase or streptokinase administration. This occurs because patient may have developed antistreptokinase antibodies, which make him more resistant to the drug and make drug therapy less effective. Elevated serum antistreptokinase antibody levels and reduced drug effectiveness can persist for 5 days to 12 months.
- Store drug between 2° and 8° C (36° and 46° F).

PATIENT TEACHING

- Instruct patient receiving anistreplase therapy to report adverse reactions immediately, especially bleeding, dizziness, and chest pain.

antithrombin III, human
(AT-III, heparin co-factor I)
ATnativ, Thrombate III

Class and Category
Chemical: Alpha₂-globulin
Therapeutic: Anticoagulant, antithrombotic
Pregnancy category: C

Indications and Dosages

▶ *To treat patients with hereditary antithrombin III (AT-III) deficiency who are undergoing surgery or obstetric procedures or who have thromboembolism*

I.V. INJECTION

Adults and children. *Initial:* Individualized dosage (based on weight, degree of AT-III deficiency, and desired level of AT-III to be achieved) sufficient to increase AT-III activity to 120% of normal, administered at 50 to 100 IU/min. *Maintenance:* Individualized dosage sufficient to keep AT-III activity at 80% or more of normal, administered q 24 hr for 2 to 8 days, depending on patient's condition and history and prescriber's judgment. A pregnant, immobilized, or postsurgical patient may need more prolonged therapy.

Route	Onset	Peak	Duration
I.V.	Immediate	Unknown	4 days

Mechanism of Action
Inhibits blood coagulation by inactivating thrombin; activated forms of factors IX, X, XI, and XII; and plasmin.

Incompatibilities
Don't mix AT-III with other drugs or solutions.

Interactions
DRUGS
heparin: Enhanced anticoagulant effect

Adverse Reactions
CNS: Chills, dizziness, fever, light-headedness
CV: Chest pain or tightness, hypotension, vasodilation
EENT: Unpleasant taste
GI: Abdominal cramps, bowel fullness, nausea

GU: Diuresis
HEME: Hematoma
RESP: Dyspnea
SKIN: Oozing lesions, urticaria

Nursing Considerations

- Reconstitute AT-III with 10 ml of sterile water for injection (provided by manufacturer) or alternate solution, such as NS or D$_5$W injection. Don't shake vial during reconstitution. Let solution come to room temperature before administration. If desired, dilute reconstituted solution further, using same diluent.
- **WARNING** Don't use diluent that contains benzyl alcohol to reconstitute AT-III for a neonate. This can cause a fatal toxic syndrome characterized by metabolic acidosis, CNS depression, respiratory problems, renal failure, hypotension, seizures, and intracranial hemorrhage.
- Don't refrigerate reconstituted solution. Use it within 3 hours and discard unused solution.
- If after 30 minutes the initial dose doesn't increase AT-III activity to 120% of normal, expect prescriber to increase dosage.
- If patient requires a dosage increase, monitor AT-III activity more frequently and expect to adjust dosage accordingly.
- Expect to reduce heparin dosage to prevent bleeding during AT-III therapy.
- If mild adverse reactions occur, decrease infusion rate, as prescribed. If severe reactions occur, discontinue infusion, as prescribed, until they subside.
- Evaluate serum AT-III level twice a day until dosage is stabilized. After that, evaluate level once daily, immediately before administering a dose.
- Store drug between 2° and 8° C (36° and 46° F).

PATIENT TEACHING
- Inform patient that blood will be drawn periodically during AT-III therapy to guide dosage adjustments.

aprotinin
Trasylol

Class and Category
Chemical: Protease inhibitor
Therapeutic: Antifibrinolytic
Pregnancy category: B

Indications and Dosages

▶ *To reduce blood loss and the need for blood transfusion in patients undergoing repeat coronary artery bypass graft (CABG) surgery and in those undergoing first-time CABG surgery who are at high risk for bleeding or for whom blood transfusion is unavailable or unacceptable*
I.V. INFUSION

Adults. *High-dose regimen:* Test dose of 10,000 KIU (1 ml kalli-krein inactivator units) 10 min before initial dose. If test dose is tolerated, 2,000,000 KIU (200 ml) given over 20 to 30 min, fol-lowed by maintenance dose of 500,000 KIU/hr (50 ml/hr). Pump prime dose of 2,000,000 KIU (200 ml) is added to priming fluid of cardiopulmonary bypass circuit. *Low-dose regimen:* Test dose of 10,000 KIU (1 ml) 10 min before initial dose. If test dose is toler-ated, 1,000,000 KIU (100 ml) given over 20 to 30 min, followed by maintenance dose of 250,000 KIU/hr (25 ml/hr). Pump prime dose of 1,000,000 KIU (100 ml) is added to priming fluid.

Incompatibilities

Don't administer aprotinin with corticosteroids, heparin, tetracy-clines, or nutrient solutions that contain amino acids or fat emul-sions. Don't administer aprotinin through same I.V. line as any other drug; use a different I.V. line or a catheter.

Mechanism of Action

Reduces bleeding, possibly by affecting plasmin and kallikrein, which pre-vents fibrinolysis and may inhibit the early phase of the intrinsic clotting cascade. Aprotinin also increases the resistance of platelets to the damage from elevated plasmin levels and mechanical injury during cardiopulmonary bypass.

Contraindications

Hypersensitivity to aprotinin

Interactions

DRUGS
captopril: Reduced antihypertensive effect
fibrinolytics (such as anistreplase and streptokinase): Inhibited fibrinolysis
heparin: Prolonged activated clotting time

Adverse Reactions

CNS: Confusion, fever

CV: Arrhythmias, cardiac arrest, heart failure, hypertension, hypotension, elevated serum CK level, MI, pericarditis, peripheral edema

ENDO: Hyperglycemia

GI: Diarrhea, elevated liver function test results, nausea, vomiting

GU: Renal failure, UTI

HEME: Leukocytosis, thrombocytopenia

RESP: Apnea, asthma, dyspnea, pleural effusion, pneumonia, pneumothorax

Other: Anaphylaxis, infection, sepsis, shock

Nursing Considerations

- If aprotinin is cloudy or contains precipitate or particles, discard it and obtain a new vial.
- Use aprotinin immediately after opening vial. Discard unused portion.
- To reduce the risk of anaphylaxis, expect to administer an H_1-receptor antagonist, such as diphenhydramine, shortly before giving a loading dose of aprotinin to patient who has received aprotinin previously.
- Administer aprotinin through a central line.
- After patient anesthesia induction and before sternotomy, expect initial aprotinin dose to be given with patient supine. Maintenance dose is given by constant infusion until patient leaves operating room. Before cardiopulmonary bypass begins, the pump prime dose is added to priming fluid of cardiopulmonary bypass circuit by replacing an aliquot of priming fluid with aprotinin.
- **WARNING** Closely monitor all patients, especially those with multiple allergies or a history of previous aprotinin treatments, for signs of anaphylaxis, even during the test dose. If anaphylaxis occurs, discontinue aprotinin immediately and notify prescriber. Then administer oxygen and I.V. epinephrine, antihistamines, and corticosteroids, as prescribed, and maintain a patent airway.
- Be aware that drug may increase the risk of renal failure and even death in patients undergoing deep hypothermic circulatory arrest, especially those over age 65.
- Store drug between 2° and 25° C (36° and 77° F). Don't freeze.

PATIENT TEACHING
- Inform patient that he'll receive aprotinin during surgery, and explain its purpose.

argatroban
Acova

Class and Category
Chemical: N2-substituted derivative of arginine
Therapeutic: Anticoagulant
Pregnancy category: B

Indications and Dosages
▶ *To prevent or treat thrombosis in patients with heparin-induced thrombocytopenia*
I.V. INFUSION
Adults. 2 mcg/kg/min as a continuous infusion. *Maximum:* 10 mcg/kg/min.
DOSAGE ADJUSTMENT Dosage adjusted as prescribed to maintain a therapeutic APTT of 1.5 to 3 times the initial baseline value, not to exceed 100 sec. Initial dosage reduced to 0.5 mcg/kg/min for patients with moderate hepatic impairment.

Route	Onset	Peak	Duration
I.V.	Immediate	3 to 4 hr	Unknown

Mechanism of Action
Forms a tight bond with thrombin, neutralizing this enzyme's actions, even when the enzyme is trapped within clots. Thrombin causes fibrinogen to convert to fibrin, which is essential for clot formation.

Incompatibilities
Don't mix argatroban with other drugs.

Contraindications
Active major bleeding, hypersensitivity to argatroban or its components

Interactions
DRUGS
alteplase, antineoplastic drugs, antiplatelets, antithymocyte globulin, heparin, NSAIDs, reteplase, salicylates, streptokinase, strontium chloride Sr 89, warfarin: Increased risk of bleeding
porfimer: Possibly decreased efficacy of porfimer photodynamic therapy

Adverse Reactions
CNS: Cerebrovascular bleeding, fever, headache
CV: Atrial fibrillation, cardiac arrest, hypotension, unstable angina, ventricular tachycardia
GI: Abdominal pain, anorexia, diarrhea, elevated liver function test results, GI bleeding, nausea, vomiting
GU: Elevated BUN and serum creatinine levels, hematuria (microscopic), UTI
HEME: Hypoprothrombinemia
RESP: Cough, dyspnea, hemoptysis, pneumonia
SKIN: Bleeding at puncture site, rash
Other: Sepsis

Nursing Considerations
- Using NS, D$_5$W, or LR, dilute argatroban to 1 mg/ml before administration.
- Use diluted solution within 24 hours if it has been stored at 15° to 30° C (59° to 86° F), protected from direct sunlight, and kept in ambient indoor light. Use solution within 48 hours if it has been stored between 2° and 8° C (36° and 46° F) and kept in the dark.
- **WARNING** Monitor patients with thrombocytopenia or those receiving daily doses of salicylates greater than 6 g for signs and symptoms of bleeding because they're at increased risk of bleeding from hypoprothrombinemia.
- **WARNING** Expect to perform blood coagulation tests before and 2 hours after start of therapy because of the major risk of bleeding associated with argatroban. Be aware that coagulopathy must be ruled out before therapy is initiated.
- Monitor the following patients for signs and symptoms of bleeding because they're at increased risk during argatroban therapy: actively menstruating females; patients with known vascular or organ abnormalities, such as severe uncontrolled hypertension, advanced renal disease, infective endocarditis, dissecting aortic aneurysm, diverticulitis, hemophilia, hepatic disease (especially if associated with a deficiency of vitamin K–dependent clotting factors), inflammatory bowel disease, or peptic ulcer disease; and those who have recently had a CVA, major surgery (including eye, brain, or spinal cord surgery), large vessel puncture or organ biopsy, lumbar puncture, spinal anesthesia, or major bleeding (including intracranial, GI, intraocular, retroperitoneal, or pulmonary bleeding).

- Whenever possible, avoid I.M. injections in patients receiving argatroban to decrease the risk of bleeding.
- Be aware that thrombin times may not be helpful for monitoring argatroban activity because all thrombin-dependent coagulation tests are affected by the drug.
- Monitor APTT periodically, as ordered, during treatment to verify therapeutic drug levels.
- Expect drug dosage to be tapered before discontinuation to prevent the risk of rebound hypercoagulopathy; drug's effects last for only a short time once drug is discontinued.
- Store unopened vials between 15° and 30° C (59° and 86° F); protect from freezing and light.

PATIENT TEACHING

- Explain to patient receiving argatroban that heparin-induced thrombocytopenia is an antigen-antibody immunologic response that isn't related to dosage of heparin he may have received.
- Inform patient that argatroban is a blood thinner that is administered in the hospital by infusion into a vein. Explain that he'll be switched to another drug before discharge if he requires long-term anticoagulation.
- Advise patient to immediately report unusual or unexplained bleeding, such as blood in urine, easy bruising, nosebleeds, tarry stools, and vaginal bleeding.
- Instruct patient to be careful to avoid injury while receiving argatroban. For example, suggest that he brush his teeth gently, using a soft-bristled toothbrush, and take special care when flossing.
- Inform patient that the risk of bleeding associated with argatroban lasts for only a short time once drug is discontinued.

atenolol

Apo-Atenol (CAN), Novo-Atenol (CAN), Tenormin

Class and Category

Chemical: Beta-adrenergic blocker (beta$_1$ and at high doses beta$_2$)
Therapeutic: Antianginal, antihypertensive
Pregnancy category: D

Indications and Dosages

▶ *To treat acute MI*

I.V. INFUSION, TABLETS

Adults. *Initial:* 5 mg I.V. slowly over 5 min, followed by another 5 mg I.V. 10 min later. After an additional 10 min (if tolerated),

50 mg P.O., followed by another 50 mg P.O. 12 hr later. *Maintenance:* 50 mg P.O. b.i.d. or 100 mg P.O. q.d. for 6 to 9 days or until discharge from hospital.

DOSAGE ADJUSTMENT Dosage reduced to 50 mg/day P.O. for patients with creatinine clearance of of 15 to 35 ml/min/1.73 m^2 and to 25 mg/day for patients with creatinine clearance of less than 15 ml/min/1.73 m^2.

Route	Onset	Peak	Duration
I.V.	Immediate	5 min	12 hr
P.O.	1 hr	2 to 4 hr	24 hr

Mechanism of Action

Inhibits stimulation of beta$_1$-receptor sites, located primarily in the heart, causing a decrease in cardiac excitability, cardiac output, and myocardial oxygen demand. At high doses, atenolol inhibits stimulation of beta$_2$ receptors in the lungs, which may cause bronchoconstriction.

Contraindications

Cardiogenic shock, heart block greater than first degree, hypersensitivity to beta blockers, overt heart failure, sinus bradycardia

Interactions

DRUGS

calcium channel blockers (such as verapamil and diltiazem): Possibly symptomatic bradycardia and conduction abnormalities
catecholamine-depleting drugs (such as reserpine): Additive antihypertensive effect
clonidine: Rebound hypertension

Adverse Reactions

CNS: Depression, disorientation, dizziness, drowsiness, emotional lability, fatigue, fever, lethargy, light-headedness, short-term memory loss, vertigo
CV: Arrhythmias, including bradycardia and heart block; cardiogenic shock; cold arms and legs; heart failure; mesenteric artery thrombosis; mitral insufficiency; myocardial reinfarction; orthostatic hypotension; Raynaud's phenomenon
EENT: Dry eyes, laryngospasm, pharyngitis
GI: Diarrhea, ischemic colitis, nausea
GU: Renal failure
HEME: Agranulocytosis

MS: Leg pain
RESP: Bronchospasm, dyspnea, pulmonary emboli, respiratory distress, wheezing
SKIN: Erythematous rash
Other: Allergic reaction

Nursing Considerations

- Be aware that although its exact mechanism of action is unknown, atenolol improves survival rate in patients with a known or suspected acute MI.
- Dilute atenolol with dextrose, sodium chloride, or dextrose and sodium chloride solution.
- Inspect solution for particles or discoloration before administration.
- During I.V. atenolol therapy, monitor vital signs and cardiac rhythm closely.
- Expect to administer digoxin, a diuretic, or both at first sign of heart failure, and monitor patient closely. If heart failure continues, expect to discontinue atenolol.
- Closely monitor patient with hyperthyroidism because atenolol may mask some signs of thyrotoxicosis. Avoid abrupt withdrawal of atenolol, which may precipitate thyrotoxicosis.
- Assess diabetic patients for signs of hypoglycemia other than tachycardia (such as dizziness and sweating) because atenolol may mask tachycardia caused by hypoglycemia. Unlike other beta-adrenergic blockers, atenolol doesn't mask other signs of hypoglycemia, cause hypoglycemia, or delay the return of blood glucose to a normal level.
- Monitor patients with heart failure controlled by digitalis glycosides or diuretics for exacerbation of heart failure.
- Monitor for adverse effects, such as symptomatic bradycardia or hypotension, in patients with conduction abnormalities or left ventricular dysfunction who are receiving verapamil or diltiazem.
- Monitor for signs of reduced peripheral circulation, such as cold hands and feet, in patients with Raynaud's syndrome or other peripheral vascular disease.
- Because atenolol is excreted by the kidneys, monitor patients with impaired renal function for increased atenolol effects.
- Discard atenolol solution if it isn't used within 48 hours.
- Stop atenolol therapy and notify prescriber if patient develops bradycardia, hypotension, or another serious adverse reaction.

- If patient also receives clonidine, expect to discontinue atenolol several days before gradually withdrawing clonidine. Then expect to restart atenolol therapy several days after clonidine has been discontinued.
- Store drug between 20° and 25° C (68° and 77° F); protect from freezing and light.

PATIENT TEACHING

- Instruct patient not to stop taking atenolol abruptly because angina could worsen and an MI or arrhythmia might occur.
- While patient is being weaned from atenolol, tell him to perform minimal physical activity to prevent chest pain.
- Inform patient that atenolol may alter his blood glucose level and mask symptoms of hypoglycemia.
- Advise patient to report signs of an adverse reaction, such as difficulty breathing, shortness of breath, dizziness, or a rash.

atracurium besylate
Tracrium

Class and Category
Chemical: Biquaternary ammonium ester
Therapeutic: Skeletal muscle relaxant
Pregnancy category: C

Indications and Dosages
▶ *To facilitate endotracheal intubation and induce skeletal muscle relaxation for surgery or mechanical ventilation as adjunct to anesthesia*
I.V. INFUSION OR INJECTION
Adults and children age 2 and older. *Initial:* 0.4 to 0.5 mg/kg by I.V. bolus for nearly complete neuromuscular blockade. *Maintenance:* 0.08 to 0.10 mg/kg 20 to 45 min after initial dose during prolonged surgery. Maintenance doses may be given q 15 to 25 min for patients under balanced anesthesia. For patients undergoing extended surgical procedures, an infusion of 9 to 10 mcg/kg/min may be required after an initial I.V. bolus to counteract the spontaneous return of neuromuscular function, and thereafter 5 to 10 mcg/kg/min is given as a constant infusion.
Children ages 1 month to 2 years who are undergoing halothane anesthesia. *Initial:* 0.3 to 0.4 mg/kg. Frequent maintenance doses may be required.

Route	Onset	Peak	Duration
I.V.	2 to 2.5 min	3 to 5 min	35 to 70 min

Mechanism of Action

Inhibits nerve impulse transmission by competing with acetylcholine for cholinergic receptors on motor end plate.

Incompatibilities

Don't mix atracurium in same syringe or administer it through same I.V. needle as an alkaline solution, such as a barbiturate injection. Don't mix atracurium with lactated Ringer's injection.

Contraindications

Hypersensitivity to atracurium, its components, or benzyl alcohol

Interactions

DRUGS

aminoglycosides, enflurane, furosemide, halothane, isoflurane, lithium, magnesium salts, polymyxin antibiotics, procainamide, quinidine, thiazide diuretics: Possibly enhanced or prolonged atracurium effects
opioid analgesics: Possibly additive histamine release and increased risk and severity of bradycardia and hypotension

Adverse Reactions

CNS: Seizures
CV: Bradycardia, hypertension, hypotension, tachycardia
MS: Inadequate or prolonged neuromuscular blockade
RESP: Apnea, bronchospasm, dyspnea, laryngospasm, wheezing
SKIN: Flushing, rash, urticaria
Other: Anaphylaxis, injection site reaction

Nursing Considerations

- Anticipate using lower doses of atracurium for patients with neuromuscular disease, severe electrolyte disorders, or carcinomatosis because of the risk of enhanced neuromuscular blockade and difficulties with reversal. Lower doses may also be used for patients at risk for adverse reactions associated with histamine release.
- Keep atropine nearby to treat atracurium-induced bradycardia.
- For I.V. infusion, dilute atracurium with NS, D_5W, or D_5NS. To prepare a solution that yields 200 mcg of atracurium/ml, add 2 ml of atracurium to 98 ml of diluent. To prepare a solution that yields 500 mcg/ml, add 5 ml of atracurium to 95 ml of diluent.
- Store prepared solution in refrigerator or at room temperature for up to 24 hours. Discard unused portion after 24 hours.

- Closely monitor blood pressure of patients with hypotension.
- Monitor patient closely for adverse reactions, especially those associated with histamine release. Be aware that atracurium is more likely than other neuromuscular blockers to cause flushing.
- Before use, store undiluted atracurium at 2° to 8° C (36° to 46° F); don't freeze. Use drug within 14 days if stored at room temperature, even if it's refrigerated later.

PATIENT TEACHING
- Explain purpose of atracurium treatment to patient.

atropine sulfate

Class and Category
Chemical: Belladonna alkaloid
Therapeutic: Anticholinergic, antimuscarinic
Pregnancy category: C

Indications and Dosages
▶ *To reduce respiratory tract secretions related to anesthesia*
I.V. INJECTION
Adults. 0.4 to 0.6 mg given preoperatively.
Children. 0.01 mg/kg up to total of 0.4 mg given preoperatively and repeated q 4 to 6 hr, p.r.n.
▶ *To correct bradycardia*
I.V. INJECTION
Adults. 0.4 to 1 mg q 1 to 2 hr, p.r.n. Dosage may be increased up to 2 mg if needed.
Children. 0.01 to 0.03 mg/kg.
▶ *To treat cholinesterase inhibitor (such as neostigmine, pilocarpine, and methacholine) toxicity*
I.V. INJECTION
Adults. 2 to 4 mg, then 2 mg q 5 to 10 min until muscarinic signs (bradycardia, vasodilation, and pupil dilation) disappear or signs of atropine intoxication develop.
Children. 1 mg, then 0.5 to 1 mg q 5 to 10 min until muscarinic signs disappear or signs of atropine intoxication develop.
▶ *To treat mushroom (muscarine) toxicity*
I.V. INJECTION
Adults. 1 to 2 mg q hr until respiratory signs and symptoms (such as bronchoconstriction) subside.

▶ *To treat pesticide (organophosphate) toxicity*
I.V. INJECTION

Adults. 1 to 2 mg, repeated in 20 to 30 min as soon as cyanosis has cleared. Dosage continued until definite improvement is maintained, possibly for 2 or more days.

Route	Onset	Peak	Duration
I.V.	Immediate	2 to 4 min	Brief

Mechanism of Action

Inhibits acetylcholine's muscarinic action at the neuroeffector junctions of smooth muscles, cardiac muscles, exocrine glands, SA and AV nodes, and the urinary bladder. In small doses, atropine inhibits salivary and bronchial secretions and diaphoresis. In moderate doses, it increases impulse conduction through the AV node and causes increased heart rate. In large doses, it decreases GI and urinary tract motility and gastric acid secretion.

Contraindications

Angle-closure glaucoma, asthma, GI obstructive disease (achalasia, pyloric obstruction, pyloroduodenal stenosis), hepatic disease, hypersensitivity to atropine or its components, ileus, intestinal atony, myasthenia gravis, myocardial ischemia, obstructive uropathy, renal disease, severe ulcerative colitis, tachycardia, toxic megacolon, unstable cardiovascular status in acute hemorrhage

Interactions

amantadine, anticholinergics, antidyskinetics, glutethimide, meperidine, muscle relaxants, phenothiazines, tricyclic antidepressants, and other drugs with anticholinergic properties, including antiarrhythmics (disopyramide, quinidine, procainamide), antihistamines, buclizine, and meclizine: Increased atropine effects
antimyasthenics: Reduced intestinal motility
cyclopropane: Risk of ventricular arrhythmias
haloperidol: Decreased antipsychotic effect of haloperidol
ketoconazole: Decreased ketoconazole absorption
metoclopramide: Decreased effect of metoclopramide on GI motility
opioid analgesics: Increased risk of ileus, severe constipation, and urine retention
potassium chloride, especially wax-matrix preparations: Possibly GI ulcers
urinary alkalinizers (calcium or magnesium antacids, carbonic anhydrase inhibitors, citrates, sodium bicarbonate): Delayed excretion and increased risk of adverse effects of atropine

Adverse Reactions

CNS: CNS stimulation (with high doses), confusion, dizziness, drowsiness, headache, insomnia, nervousness, weakness

CV: Bradycardia (with low doses), palpitations, tachycardia (with high doses)

EENT: Altered taste, blurred vision, dry mouth, increased intraocular pressure, mydriasis, nasal congestion, photophobia

GI: Bloating, constipation, dysphagia, heartburn, ileus, nausea, vomiting

GU: Impotence, urinary hesitancy, urine retention

SKIN: Decreased sweating, flushing, urticaria

Other: Anaphylaxis

Nursing Considerations

- Avoid using high-dose atropine therapy in patients with ulcerative colitis because of the risk of toxic megacolon, or in patients with hiatal hernia and reflux esophagitis because of the risk of esophagitis.
- **WARNING** Assess for symptoms of toxic doses of atropine, such as excitement, agitation, drowsiness, and confusion, which are likely to affect elderly patients even with low doses. If these symptoms occur, take safety precautions to prevent patient injury.
- Assess bowel and bladder elimination. Notify prescriber if diarrhea, constipation, urinary hesitancy, or urine retention develops.
- Be aware that atropine may also be administered S.C. and I.M. for some indications.
- Store atropine at 15° to 30° C (59° to 86° F). Don't freeze.

PATIENT TEACHING

- Advise patient receiving atropine therapy to report persistent or severe diarrhea, constipation, or difficulty urinating.

azathioprine sodium

Imuran

azathioprine

Imuran

Class and Category

Chemical: Purine analogue
Therapeutic: Antimetabolite, immunosuppressant
Pregnancy category: D

Indications and Dosages

▶ *To prevent kidney transplant rejection*

I.V. INFUSION, TABLETS

Adults and children. *Initial:* 3 to 5 mg/kg/day I.V. or P.O. as a single dose on or 1 to 3 days before day of transplant, followed by 3 to 5 mg/kg/day I.V. after surgery until P.O. dose is tolerated. *Maintenance:* 1 to 3 mg/kg/day P.O.

DOSAGE ADJUSTMENT Dosage reduced for patients with oliguria (such as from tubular necrosis) after transplantation because their drug or metabolite excretion may be delayed.

Route	Onset	Peak	Duration
I.V., P.O.	4 to 8 wk	Unknown	Several days

Mechanism of Action

May prevent proliferation and differentiation of activated B and T cells by interfering with purine (protein) and nucleic acid (DNA and RNA) synthesis.

Contraindications

Hypersensitivity to azathioprine

Interactions

DRUGS

ACE inhibitors, drugs that affect bone marrow and cell development in bone marrow (such as co-trimoxazole): Possibly severe leukopenia
allopurinol: Possibly increased therapeutic and adverse effects of azathioprine
anticoagulants: Possibly decreased anticoagulant action
cyclosporine: Possibly decreased blood cyclosporine level
methotrexate: Possibly increased blood level of azathioprine metabolite 6-mercaptopurine, which can lead to cell death
neuromuscular blockers: Possibly decreased or reversed action of neuromuscular blocker

Adverse Reactions

CNS: Fever, malaise
GI: Abdominal pain, diarrhea, hepatotoxicity (elevated liver function test results), nausea, pancreatitis, steatorrhea, vomiting
HEME: Leukopenia, macrocytic anemia, pancytopenia, thrombocytopenia
MS: Arthralgia, myalgia

SKIN: Alopecia, rash
Other: Infection, lymphomas and other neoplasms

Nursing Considerations

- Before I.V. administration, add 20 ml of sterile water for injection to azathioprine vial and swirl it until clear solution forms. The resulting drug concentration is 100 mg and can be diluted further, usually in NS or D$_5$W, as prescribed. Calculate infusion rate based on final volume to be infused. Then administer over 30 to 60 minutes or as prescribed (from 5 minutes to 8 hours).
- Obtain results of baseline laboratory tests, including WBC, RBC, and platelet counts. Then expect to monitor results once a week during first month of therapy, twice a month during second and third months of therapy, and once a month or more frequently thereafter.
- Be aware that hematologic reactions typically are dose-related and may occur late in therapy, especially in patients with transplant rejection.
- **WARNING** If WBC count decreases rapidly or remains significantly and consistently low, expect to reduce dosage or discontinue use of azathioprine.
- Periodically monitor liver function test results to detect early signs of hepatotoxicity.
- If patient develops thrombocytopenia, take bleeding precautions, such as avoiding I.M. injections and venipunctures, applying ice to areas of trauma, and checking I.V. infusion sites every 2 hours for bleeding.
- If patient also receives an oral anticoagulant, monitor his PT.
- Know that azathioprine therapy increases the risk of viral, fungal, bacterial, and protozoal infections. Monitor for signs of infection, such as fever, chills, sore throat, and mouth sores. Expect to administer aggressive antibiotic, antiviral, or other drug therapy and to reduce azathioprine dosage.
- Minimize risk of infection. If patient has severe leukopenia, take neutropenic precautions, such as placing him in a private room, limiting visitors, and screening visitors for communicable illnesses.
- If oral azathioprine causes GI upset, administer it in divided doses or with meals.
- Store parenteral form and tablets at 15° to 25° C (59° to 77° F). Keep in a dry place and protect from light.

PATIENT TEACHING
- Advise patient to take oral azathioprine with food or meals to minimize GI upset.
- **WARNING** Teach patient to recognize and report signs of infection, such as sore throat and fever.
- Teach patient how to reduce the risk of bleeding and how to maintain safety so that he doesn't fall.

azithromycin
Zithromax

Class and Category
Chemical: Azalide (subclass of macrolide)
Therapeutic: Antibiotic
Pregnancy category: B

Indications and Dosages
▶ *To treat community-acquired pneumonia*
I.V. INFUSION, CAPSULES, ORAL SUSPENSION, TABLETS
Adults and children age 16 or older. 500 mg I.V. as a single dose daily for at least 2 days, followed by 500 mg P.O. as a single dose daily until patient completes 7 to 10 days of therapy.
▶ *To treat pelvic inflammatory disease*
I.V. INFUSION, CAPSULES, ORAL SUSPENSION, TABLETS
Adults. 500 mg I.V. as a single dose daily for 1 to 2 days, followed by 250 mg P.O. as a single dose daily until patient completes 7 days of therapy.

Mechanism of Action
Inhibits bacterial protein synthesis. Specifically, azithromycin binds to a ribosomal subunit of susceptible bacteria. This blocks peptide translocation, which inhibits RNA-dependent protein synthesis. Azithromycin concentrates in phagocytes, macrophages, and fibroblasts, which release it slowly and may help distribute it to infection sites.

Contraindications
Hypersensitivity to azithromycin, erythromycin, or other macrolide antibiotics

Interactions
DRUGS

aluminum- or magnesium-containing antacids: Possibly decreased peak serum level of azithromycin

carbamazepine, cyclosporine, phenytoin, terfenadine (drugs metabolized by P450 cytochrome system): Possibly increased serum levels of these drugs

digoxin: Possibly increased blood digoxin level

dihydroergotamine, ergotamine: Possibly severe peripheral vasospasm and abnormal sensations (acute ergot toxicity)

HMG-CoA reductase inhibitors: Increased risk of severe myopathy or rhabdomyolysis

pimozide: Possibly sudden death

theophylline: Possibly increased blood theophylline level

triazolam: Possibly decreased excretion and increased therapeutic effects of triazolam

warfarin: Possibly increased anticoagulant effects of warfarin

FOODS

all foods: Dramatically increased absorption rate of azithromycin

Adverse Reactions
CNS: Dizziness, fatigue, headache, somnolence, vertigo

CV: Chest pain, elevated serum CK level, palpitations

EENT: Hearing loss, mucocutaneous candidiasis, tinnitus

ENDO: Hyperglycemia

GI: Abdominal pain, diarrhea, elevated liver function test results, nausea, pseudomembranous colitis, vomiting

GU: Elevated BUN and serum creatinine levels, nephritis, vaginal candidiasis

HEME: Leukopenia, neutropenia, thrombocytopenia

SKIN: Jaundice, photosensitivity, rash, Stevens-Johnson syndrome, toxic epidermal necrolysis, urticaria

Other: Allergic reaction; angioedema; elevated serum phosphorus level; hyperkalemia; infusion site edema, pain, or redness; superinfection

Nursing Considerations
• Obtain culture and sensitivity test results, if possible, before initiating azithromycin therapy.

• Using a 5-ml syringe, add 4.8 ml of sterile water for injection to a 500-mg vial to yield a concentration of 100 mg/ml. Shake vial until all of drug has dissolved.

- Don't use reconstituted drug if you detect particles.
- Dilute further in appropriate diluent, such as NS, D₅W, 0.45NS, D₅/0.45NS, and LR. Recommended amounts of diluent for a 500-mg dose are 500 ml for a 1-mg/ml concentration and 250 ml for a 2-mg/ml concentration.
- Store reconstituted azithromycin at or below 30° C (86° F). Use diluted solution of 1 to 2 mg/ml within 24 hours if stored at or below 30° C or within 7 days if stored at 5° C (41° F). Discard solution if not used within 24 hours.
- **WARNING** Don't give azithromycin as an I.V. bolus or I.M. injection because this may cause a reaction at the infusion site, including erythema, pain, swelling, or tenderness. Instead, infuse it over 60 minutes or longer, as prescribed. (Typical infusion rates are 1 mg/ml over 3 hours and 2 mg/ml over 1 hour.)
- Monitor I.V. site for local reactions, such as redness, pain, and swelling. If site becomes red, discontinue I.V. and restart it at another site. Also, apply warm compresses and elevate affected hand or arm.
- Administer azithromycin capsules or suspension 1 hour before or 2 to 3 hours after food or meals. Give tablets without regard to food.
- Monitor liver function studies in patients with impaired hepatic function because azithromycin is eliminated primarily by the liver.
- Assess for signs of bacterial or fungal superinfection, which may occur with prolonged or repeated therapy. If superinfection occurs, expect to administer another antibiotic or antifungal drug.
- Monitor bowel elimination; if needed, obtain stool culture to rule out pseudomembranous colitis. If this adverse reaction occurs, expect to discontinue azithromycin and administer fluid, electrolytes, and antibiotics that are effective against *Clostridium difficile*.
- Before reconstituting azithromycin, store it at or below 30° C (86° F).

PATIENT TEACHING

- Teach patient to recognize and immediately report signs of an allergic reaction to azithromycin, such as rash, itching, hives, chest tightness, and difficulty breathing.
- Instruct patient to take azithromycin capsules or suspension 1 hour before or 2 to 3 hours after food. Inform him that he can take tablets with or without food.

- **WARNING** Urge patient to contact prescriber before taking any OTC drugs, including antacids, to avoid interactions. If antacids are prescribed, instruct patient to take azithromycin 1 hour before or 2 to 3 hours after antacids.
- Inform patient that abdominal pain and loose, watery stools may occur. If diarrhea persists or becomes severe, urge him to contact prescriber and replace fluids.
- Because azithromycin may destroy normal flora, advise patient to watch for and immediately report signs of superinfection, such as white patches in mouth.

aztreonam

Azactam

Class and Category

Chemical: Monobactam
Therapeutic: Antibiotic
Pregnancy category: B

Indications and Dosages

▶ *To treat infections of the urinary tract, lower respiratory tract, skin, soft tissue, and female reproductive tract; intra-abdominal infections; septicemia; and surgical abscesses caused by susceptible strains of gram-negative bacteria*

I.V. INFUSION OR INJECTION

Adults. 0.5 to 2 g q 8 to 12 hr up to a maximum of 8 g/day. For life-threatening systemic infection, 2 g q 6 to 8 hr up to a maximum of 8 g/day.

Children ages 9 months to 16 years. 30 mg/kg q 6 to 8 hr up to 120 mg/kg/day; 50 mg/kg q 4 to 6 hr (for *Pseudomonas aeruginosa* infection).

DOSAGE ADJUSTMENT For patients with impaired renal function and creatinine clearance between 10 and 30 ml/min/1.73 m^2, initial dose of 1 to 2 g, followed by 50% of the usual dose at the usual interval. For patients with severe renal failure and creatinine clearance less than 10 ml/min/1.73 m^2, initial dose of 500 mg to 2 g, followed by 25% of the usual dose every 6, 8, or 12 hr.

Route	Onset	Peak	Duration
I.V.	Immediate	Immediate	Unknown

Mechanism of Action

Inhibits bacterial cell wall synthesis in susceptible aerobic gram-negative bacteria. These bacteria assemble rigid, cross-linked cell walls in several steps. Aztreonam affects final stage of cross-linking by inactivating penicillin-binding protein 3 (enzyme that links cell wall strands). This action causes bacterial cell lysis and death.

Incompatibilities

Don't mix aztreonam in same I.V. solution as cephradine, metronidazole, or nafcillin sodium.

Contraindications

Hypersensitivity to aztreonam or its components

Interactions

DRUGS

aminoglycosides (prolonged or high-dose therapy): Increased risk of nephrotoxicity and ototoxicity
cefoxitin, imipenem: Possibly antagonized action of aztreonam
furosemide, probenecid: Possibly increased blood aztreonam level

Adverse Reactions

CNS: Confusion, dizziness, fever, headache, insomnia, malaise, paresthesia, seizures, vertigo
CV: Chest pain, hypotension, transient ECG changes
EENT: Altered taste, diplopia, halitosis, mouth ulcers, mucocutaneous candidiasis, nasal congestion, sneezing, tinnitus, tongue numbness
GI: Abdominal cramps, diarrhea, elevated liver function test results, GI bleeding, hepatitis, nausea, pseudomembranous colitis, vomiting
GU: Breast tenderness, elevated serum creatinine level, vaginal candidiasis
HEME: Anemia, eosinophilia, leukocytosis, neutropenia, pancytopenia, positive Coombs' test, prolonged PT and APTT, thrombocytopenia, thrombocytosis
MS: Myalgia
RESP: Bronchospasm, dyspnea, wheezing
SKIN: Diaphoresis, erythema multiforme, exfoliative dermatitis, flushing, jaundice, petechiae, pruritus, purpura, rash, toxic epidermal necrolysis, urticaria
Other: Allergic reaction; injection site pain, phlebitis, swelling, or thrombophlebitis

Nursing Considerations

- Obtain culture and sensitivity test results, if possible, before initiating aztreonam therapy. If patient is acutely ill, expect to begin therapy before results are available.
- Keep in mind that other antimicrobials may be used with aztreonam in seriously ill patients at risk for gram-positive infection.
- Expect to use I.V. route for patients who need single doses over 1 g and those with life-threatening systemic infections, such as septicemia or peritonitis. Be aware that drug may also be administered by I.M. injection.
- To reconstitute aztreonam for I.V. bolus injection, use sterile water for injection.
- Immediately after adding diluent to vial, shake it vigorously to mix it properly. After obtaining correct dose, discard unused solution.
- Be aware that reconstituted solution may turn light pink on standing at room temperature. This doesn't affect drug potency.
- Administer I.V. bolus injection directly into I.V. tubing over 3 to 5 minutes.
- **WARNING** When preparing aztreonam for I.V. infusion, use at least 50 ml of appropriate infusion solution per gram of aztreonam. Then further dilute it in I.V. solution, such as NS, D₅W, D₅NS, LR, or Ringer's solution.
- Be aware that I.V. infusion may be administered over 20 to 60 minutes.
- Flush I.V. tubing with solution, such as NS, before and after administering I.V. infusion to reduce the risk of drug interactions.
- If prescribed, mix aztreonam in same I.V. solution with other antibiotics, such as clindamycin phosphate, gentamicin sulfate, tobramycin sulfate, cefazolin sodium, and ampicillin sodium, or mix it with cloxacillin sodium and vancomycin hydrochloride in peritoneal dialysis solution.
- Be aware that single-dose units of aztreonam are available at 1 g/50 ml and 2 g/50 ml.
- Store single-dose units at −20° C (−4° F). Thaw at room temperature (25° C [77° F]) or in refrigerator at 2° to 8° C (36° to 46° F). Don't refreeze.
- Inspect thawed unit before administering to ensure that all ice crystals have melted. Don't use solution if it's cloudy or contains precipitate, or if plastic bag is leaking.
- Assess for signs of bacterial or fungal superinfection, which may occur with prolonged or repeated therapy. If superinfection occurs, treat it as prescribed.

- Check for loose, watery stools; if needed, obtain stool culture to rule out pseudomembranous colitis. If this adverse reaction occurs, expect to discontinue aztreonam and administer fluid, electrolytes, and antibiotics that are effective against *Clostridium difficile*.
- Be aware that reconstituted solutions with a concentration of 20 mg/ml or less retain potency for 48 hours when stored at 15° to 30° C (59° to 86° F) and for 7 days when refrigerated at 2° to 8° C (36° to 46° F). Solutions with a concentration of more than 20 mg/ml that have been reconstituted with NS or sterile water for injection retain potency for same time frame. Concentratons exceeding 20 mg/ml that have been mixed in other solutions should be used promptly.

PATIENT TEACHING

- Teach patient to recognize and immediately report signs of an allergic reaction to aztreonam, such as rash, itching, hives, chest tightness, and difficulty breathing.
- Inform patient that he may develop abdominal pain and loose, watery stools. If diarrhea persists or becomes severe, urge him to contact prescriber and replace fluids.
- Because aztreonam may destroy normal flora, teach patient to watch for and immediately report signs of superinfection, such as white patches in mouth.

basiliximab

Simulect

Class and Category

Chemical: Chimeric (murine or human) monoclonal antibody
Therapeutic: Immunosuppressant
Pregnancy category: B

Indications and Dosages

▶ *To prevent acute kidney transplant rejection*

I.V. INFUSION OR INJECTION

Adults and adolescents over age 15. 20 mg within 2 hr before
transplant, then 20 mg 4 days after transplant.

Children and adolescents ages 2 to 15. 12 mg/m² within
2 hr before transplant, then 12 mg/m² 4 days after transplant.
Maximum: 20 mg/dose.

Route	Onset	Peak	Duration
I.V.	Unknown	Unknown	22 to 50 days

Mechanism of Action

Initiates immunosuppression by blocking interleukin-2 receptors located on
the surface of activated T cells. Normally, interleukin-2 is released by stimulated T lymphocytes, causing activation and differentiation of other T lymphocytes responsible for cell-mediated immunity.

Incompatibilities

Don't add or infuse any other drugs simultaneously through same
I.V. line as basiliximab.

Contraindications

Hypersensitivity to basiliximab or its components

Interactions

None known.

Adverse Reactions

CNS: Asthenia, dizziness, fever, headache, insomnia, tremor

CV: Hypertension, peripheral edema
EENT: Oral candidiasis, pharyngitis, rhinitis
ENDO: Hyperglycemia
GI: Abdominal pain, constipation, diarrhea, indigestion, nausea, vomiting
GU: Dysuria, increased urinary nitrogen level, UTI
HEME: Anemia
MS: Back pain, leg pain
RESP: Cough, dyspnea, upper respiratory tract infection
SKIN: Acne
Other: Hypercholesterolemia, hyperkalemia, hyperuricemia, hypocalcemia, hypokalemia, hypophosphatemia, impaired wound healing, metabolic acidosis, weight gain

Nursing Considerations

- To reconstitute basiliximab, add 5 ml of sterile water for injection to powder and shake vial gently to dissolve. Further dilute with NS or D₅W for infusion to a volume of 50 ml. Gently invert infusion bag to avoid foaming; don't shake. Drug should appear clear to opalescent and colorless. Don't use if you detect particles.
- Administer reconstituted drug as a bolus dose directly through a central or peripheral I.V. line, or the diluted solution I.V. over 20 to 30 minutes. Be aware that bolus dose may cause nausea, vomiting, and a localized injection site reaction, including pain.
- Monitor blood pressure, heart rate, and respiratory status during drug administration and for a brief period thereafter.
- Expect drug to be given as adjunct to cyclosporine and corticosteroids.
- Don't store reconstituted drug at room temperature for longer than 4 hours; don't refrigerate for longer than 24 hours.
- **WARNING** Be aware that patient may develop hypersensitivity reactions, including anaphylaxis, bronchospasm, dyspnea, hypotension, pruritus, rash, respiratory failure, sneezing, tachycardia, urticaria, and wheezing, on initial exposure or following re-exposure after several months. Notify prescriber immediately if such reactions occur.
- Store unconstituted drug at 2° to 8° C (36° to 46° F).
- PATIENT TEACHING
- Inform patient that second dose of basiliximab will be given 4 days after transplant and that she may also receive cyclosporine and corticosteroid therapy.

• Inform patient that because of drug's immunosuppressant effects, she may experience slower wound healing and be more susceptible to upper respiratory tract infections.

benzquinamide hydrochloride
Emete-Con

Class and Category
Chemical: Benzoquinolizine amide
Therapeutic: Antiemetic
Pregnancy category: Not rated

Indications and Dosages
▶ *To treat nausea and vomiting related to anesthesia or surgery*
I.V. OR I.M. INJECTION
Adults. 25 mg or 0.2 to 0.4 mg/kg by slow infusion (1 ml q 0.5 to 1 min) as a single dose, followed by I.M. doses. Or 50 mg or 0.5 to 1 mg/kg I.M., repeated in 1 hr, then q 3 to 4 hr, p.r.n.

Route	Onset	Peak	Duration
I.V., I.M.	15 min	Unknown	Unknown

Mechanism of Action
Exhibits antiemetic, antihistaminic, mild cholinergic, and sedative effects by unknown mechanism.

Contraindications
Hypersensitivity to benzquinamide or its components

Interactions
DRUGS
vasopressors: Increased hypertensive effects

Adverse Reactions
CNS: Chills, dizziness, drowsiness, excitement, fatigue, fever, headache, insomnia, nervousness, restlessness, tremor, weakness
CV: Atrial fibrillation, hypertension, hypotension, premature atrial or ventricular contractions
EENT: Blurred vision, dry mouth, increased salivation
GI: Anorexia, hiccups, nausea
MS: Muscle twitching
SKIN: Diaphoresis, flushing, rash, urticaria

Nursing Considerations

- **WARNING** Avoid I.V. route when administering benzquinamide to patients with cardiovascular disease because sudden blood pressure increases and transient arrhythmias may occur. Use I.V. route only for patients without cardiovascular disease who aren't receiving a preanesthetic or cardiovascular drug.
- Reconstitute drug with 2.2 ml of sterile water or bacteriostatic water for injection containing benzyl alcohol or methylparaben and propylparaben to yield 2 ml of a 25-mg/ml solution.
- When administering benzquinamide I.M., inject into large, well-developed muscle. Avoid using deltoid muscle unless it's well developed.
- Take safety precautions to reduce the risk of injury from CNS depression.
- Store reconstituted drug at room temperature. Solution retains potency for 14 days.

PATIENT TEACHING

- Advise patient to stay in bed after receiving benzquinamide and to call for assistance to reduce the risk of injury.
- Instruct patient to report whether nausea and vomiting have been relieved.

benztropine mesylate

Apo-Benztropine (CAN), Cogentin, PMS Benztropine (CAN)

Class and Category

Chemical: Tertiary amine
Therapeutic: Antidyskinetic, central-acting anticholinergic
Pregnancy category: C

Indications and Dosages

▶ *As adjunct to treat all forms of Parkinson's disease*
I.V. INJECTION, TABLETS
Adults with Parkinson's disease. 1 to 2 mg/day (usual dose) with a range of 0.5 to 6.0 mg/day.
Adults with idiopathic Parkinson's disease. *Initial:* 0.5 to 1 mg h.s. *Maximum:* 4 to 6 mg/day.
Adults with postencephalitic Parkinson's disease. 2 mg/day in one or more doses; may begin with 0.5 mg h.s. and increase as needed.

▶ *To control extrapyramidal symptoms (except tardive dyskinesia) caused by phenothiazines and other neuroleptic drugs*

I.V. OR I.M. INJECTION
Adults. 1 to 4 mg q.d. or b.i.d.
▶ *To treat acute dystonic reactions*
I.V. OR I.M. INJECTION
Adults. *Initial:* 1 to 2 ml (1 to 2 mg total dose) I.V. or I.M. *Maintenance:* 1 to 2 mg P.O. b.i.d. to prevent recurrence.

Route	Onset	Peak	Duration
I.V., I.M	15 min	Unknown	24 hr
P.O.	1 to 2 hr	Unknown	24 hr

Mechanism of Action

Blocks acetylcholine's action at cholinergic receptor sites. This restores the brain's normal dopamine and acetylcholine balance, which relaxes muscle movement and decreases drooling, rigidity, and tremor. Benztropine also may inhibit dopamine reuptake and storage, which prolongs dopamine's action.

Contraindications

Achalasia, bladder neck obstruction, glaucoma, hypersensitivity to benztropine mesylate or its components, megacolon, myasthenia gravis, prostatic hypertrophy, pyloric or duodenal obstruction, stenosing peptic ulcer

Interactions

DRUGS

amantadine: Possibly increased adverse anticholinergic effects
digoxin: Possibly increased blood digoxin level
haloperidol: Possibly increased schizophrenic symptoms, decreased serum haloperidol level, and development of tardive dyskinesia
levodopa: Possibly decreased levodopa effectiveness
phenothiazines: Possibly reduced phenothiazine effects and increased psychiatric symptoms

Adverse Reactions

CNS: Agitation, confusion, delirium, delusions, depression, disorientation, dizziness, drowsiness, euphoria, excitement, fever, hallucinations, headache, light-headedness, listlessness, memory loss, nervousness, paranoia, psychosis, weakness
CV: Hypotension, mild bradycardia, orthostatic hypotension, palpitations, tachycardia
EENT: Angle-closure glaucoma, blurred vision, diplopia, dry mouth, increased intraocular pressure, mydriasis, suppurative parotitis

GI: Constipation, duodenal ulcer, epigastric distress, ileus, nausea, vomiting
GU: Dysuria, urinary hesitancy, urine retention
MS: Muscle spasms, muscle weakness
SKIN: Decreased sweating, dermatoses, flushing, rash, urticaria

Nursing Considerations

- Expect to administer I.V. or I.M. benztropine when patient needs more rapid response than oral drug can provide. Be aware that I.M. route is commonly used because it provides effects in about same amount of time as I.V. route. Watch for improvement a few minutes after administration. If parkinsonian symptoms reappear, expect to repeat dose.
- Know that therapy generally begins with a low dose followed by gradual increases of 0.5 mg every 5 or 6 days because benztropine has a cumulative action.
- Assess muscle rigidity and tremor as a baseline. Then monitor them frequently for improvement, which indicates the effectiveness of benztropine.
- Administer drug before or after meals based on patient's need and response. If patient has increased salivary secretions, expect to administer benztropine after meals. If patient has dry mouth, plan to give drug before meals unless nausea develops.
- **WARNING** When administering benztropine to patient with drug-induced extrapyramidal reactions, be alert for exacerbation of psychiatric symptoms.
- Know that high-dose benztropine therapy may cause weakness and inability to move specific muscle groups. If this occurs, expect to reduce benztropine dosage.
- Store drug at 15° to 30° C (59° to 86° F). Don't freeze.

PATIENT TEACHING
- Warn patient that benztropine has a cumulative effect, increasing her risk of adverse reactions and overdose.
- Caution patient to avoid driving and similar activities until the effects of benztropineare known because drug may cause blurred vision, dizziness, and drowsiness.
- **WARNING** Because benztropine decreases sweating, urge patient to avoid extremely hot or humid conditions to reduce the risk of heatstroke and severe hyperthermia. This is especially important for elderly patients and those who abuse alcohol or have chronic illnesses or CNS disorders.

• Stress the need for periodic eye examinations and intraocular pressure measurements because benztropine may cause angle-closure glaucoma and increase intraocular pressure.

betamethasone sodium phosphate
Celestone Phosphate, Selestoject

Class and Category
Chemical: Synthetic glucocorticoid
Therapeutic: Anti-inflammatory
Pregnancy category: C

Indications and Dosages
▶ *To treat conditions accompanied by severe inflammation and conditions requiring immunosuppression*
I.V. INJECTION
Adults. *Initial:* Variable (given in emergency situations or when oral therapy isn't possible). *Maximum:* 9 mg/day.
DOSAGE ADJUSTMENT Dosage reduced for elderly patients.

Contraindications
Live virus vaccination, systemic fungal infection

Route	Onset	Peak	Duration
I.V.	Rapid	Unknown	Unknown

Mechanism of Action
Binds to intracellular glucocorticoid receptors and suppresses inflammatory and immune responses by:
• inhibiting neutrophil and monocyte accumulation at inflammation site and suppressing their phagocytic and bactericidal activity
• stabilizing lysosomal membranes
• suppressing antigen response of macrophages and helper T cells
• inhibiting synthesis of inflammatory response mediators, such as cytokines, interleukins, and prostaglandins.

Interactions
DRUGS
anticholinesterase drugs: Possibly antagonized anticholinesterase effects in myasthenia gravis
barbiturates: Possibly decreased effects of betamethasone

cyclosporine: Possibly increased risk of cyclosporine toxicity
digitalis glycosides: Possibly increased risk of digitalis toxicity
estrogens: Possibly decreased excretion of betamethasone
hydantoins, rifampin: Possibly increased excretion and decreased
therapeutic effects of betamethasone
insulin, oral antidiabetic drugs: Possibly increased blood glucose
level
isoniazid: Possibly decreased blood isoniazid level
ketoconazole: Possibly decreased excretion of betamethasone
oral anticoagulants: Possibly increased or decreased action of anticoagulants, requiring adjusted anticoagulant dosage
oral contraceptives: Possibly increased half-life and concentration
and decreased excretion of betamethasone
potassium-wasting diuretics: Increased risk of hypokalemia
salicylates: Possibly decreased blood level and therapeutic effects of
salicylates
somatrem: Possibly inhibition of somatrem's growth-promoting
effects
theophyllines: Possibly changes in effects of both drugs

Adverse Reactions
CNS: Fatigue, headache, increased ICP with papilledema, insomnia, malaise, neuritis, paresthesia, seizures, steroid psychosis, syncope, vertigo
CV: Arrhythmias, ECG changes, fat embolism, heart failure, hypertension, thromboembolism, thrombophlebitis
EENT: Cataracts, exophthalmos, glaucoma, increased intraocular
pressure
ENDO: Cushingoid symptoms (buffalo hump, central obesity, decreased carbohydrate tolerance, fat pad enlargement, moon face),
fluid retention, growth suppression in children, hyperglycemia,
negative nitrogen balance, secondary adrenocortical and pituitary
unresponsiveness (in times of stress)
GI: Abdominal distention, increased appetite, nausea, pancreatitis,
peptic ulcer (possibly with perforation), ulcerative esophagitis,
vomiting
GU: Amenorrhea, glycosuria, menstrual irregularities
HEME: Leukocytosis
MS: Aseptic necrosis of femoral and humeral heads, muscle atrophy or weakness, osteoporosis, spontaneous fractures, tendon
rupture, vertebral compression fractures

SKIN: Acneiform lesions, allergic dermatitis, ecchymosis, facial erythema, hirsutism, increased sweating, petechiae, lupuslike lesions, purpura, subcutaneous fat atrophy, thin and fragile skin, urticaria

Other: Angioedema, hypocalcemia, hypokalemia, impaired wound healing, masking of infection, sodium retention, suppressed skin test reaction, weight gain

Nursing Considerations

- Be aware that betamethasone sodium phosphate is administered I.V. in emergency situations or when oral therapy isn't possible. It's also administered by intra-articular, intrasynovial, intralesional, soft-tissue, or I.M. injection.

- Expect prescriber to order baseline ophthalmic examination before initiating therapy because prolonged betamethasone use may lead to increased intraocular pressure, glaucoma, and subsequent optic nerve damage. Be aware that in patients with ocular herpes simplex, betamethasone may cause corneal perforation.

- Assess for signs of infection before administering betamethasone because drug may mask those signs. Because drug may cause immunosuppression, new infection may develop during therapy. If so, expect to administer appropriate antibiotic.

- Review serum electrolyte levels, as ordered, before initiating therapy. Monitor these levels frequently during therapy to detect imbalances. Sodium and water retention and potassium and calcium depletion may occur with high-dose betamethasone therapy. If so, expect to restrict sodium intake and provide potassium and calcium supplements.

- **WARNING** Monitor ECG tracings for arrhythmias, and evaluate patient for anaphylactic reactions, such as angioedema and seizures, which have been associated with rapid I.V. administration of high-dose corticosteroids.

- Monitor blood glucose levels. Patients who take oral antidiabetic drugs or insulin may require dosage adjustment during betamethasone therapy or when drug is discontinued.

- Monitor blood pressure of elderly patients to detect changes.

- Because betamethasone is linked to peptic ulcer formation, expect to administer it with an antacid or H_2-receptor blocker.

- **WARNING** During long-term betamethasone therapy, assess for signs of adrenal suppression and adrenal insufficiency (fatigue, hypotension, lassitude, nausea, vomiting, and weakness) when patient is exposed to stress. If she exhibits these signs, notify prescriber immediately because adrenal insufficiency can be life-threatening.

• Watch for signs of steroid psychosis, such as delirium, clouded sensorium, euphoria, insomnia, mood swings, personality changes, and severe depression, which may develop 15 to 30 days after therapy begins. Be prepared to discontinue therapy. If this isn't possible, expect to administer psychotropic drugs.

• Monitor for cushingoid symptoms, such as moon face, buffalo hump, central obesity, striae, acne, ecchymosis, and weight gain. If you detect these symptoms, notify prescriber as soon as possible.

• Know that patients on long-term therapy may require increased protein because drug stimulates protein catabolism.

• Store drug at 15° to 30° C (59° to 86° F), and protect from light. Don't freeze.

PATIENT TEACHING
• Reinforce signs of adrenal insufficiency and possible need for increases in betamethasone dosage during stress. Advise patient to notify prescriber immediately if signs of insufficiency occur or if she's exposed to stress.

• Teach patient to recognize and immediately report signs of infection. Urge her to avoid exposure to infections because drug can cause immunosuppression.

biperiden lactate
Akineton Lactate

Class and Category
Chemical: Tertiary amine
Therapeutic: Anticholinergic, antidyskinetic
Pregnancy category: C

Indications and Dosages
▶ *To control extrapyramidal symptoms (except tardive dyskinesia) caused by phenothiazines and other neuroleptic drugs*
I.V. INJECTION
Adults. 2 mg repeated q 30 min until symptoms resolve or maximum of four consecutive doses in 24 hr is reached.

Route	Onset	Peak	Duration
I.V.	15 min	Unknown	1 to 8 hr

Mechanism of Action

Blocks acetylcholine's action at cholinergic receptor sites. This action restores the brain's normal dopamine and acetylcholine balance, which relaxes muscle movement and decreases rigidity and tremors. Biperiden also may inhibit dopamine reuptake and storage, which prolongs dopamine's action.

Contraindications

Achalasia, angle-closure glaucoma, bladder neck obstruction, bowel obstruction, hypersensitivity to biperiden, myasthenia gravis, prostatic hypertrophy, pyloric or duodenal obstruction, stenosing peptic ulcer, toxic megacolon

Interactions

DRUGS

amantadine: Possibly increased adverse anticholinergic effects
digoxin: Possibly increased serum digoxin level
haloperidol: Possibly increased schizophrenic symptoms, decreased serum haloperidol level, and development of tardive dyskinesia
levodopa: Possibly decreased levodopa effectiveness
phenothiazines: Possibly reduced phenothiazine effects and increased psychiatric symptoms

Adverse Reactions

CNS: Agitation, confusion, delirium, delusions, depression, disorientation, dizziness, drowsiness, euphoria, excitement, fever, hallucinations, headache, light-headedness, listlessness, memory loss, nervousness, paranoia, psychosis, weakness
CV: Hypotension, mild bradycardia, orthostatic hypotension, palpitations, tachycardia
EENT: Angle-closure glaucoma, blurred vision, diplopia, dry mouth, increased intraocular pressure, mydriasis, photosensitivity, suppurative parotitis
GI: Constipation, ileus, nausea, vomiting
GU: Dysuria, urinary hesitancy, urine retention
MS: Muscle spasms, muscle weakness
SKIN: Decreased sweating, dermatoses, flushing, rash, urticaria

Nursing Considerations

- Expect to administer I.V. biperiden when patient needs more rapid response than oral drug can provide. Biperiden may also be administered I.M.
- Obtain baseline blood pressure and heart rate. Monitor patient for hypotension and other CV effects, and help patient change position as needed.
- Assess muscle rigidity and tremor as baseline. Then monitor them frequently for improvement, which indicates the effectiveness of biperiden.
- Inspect solution for particles and discoloration before use.
- Administer I.V. biperiden slowly.
- **WARNING** Be alert for exacerbation of psychiatric symptoms during biperiden therapy.
- Store drug at 15° to 30° C (59° to 86° F) and protect from light. Don't freeze.

PATIENT TEACHING
- Teach patient about possible adverse effects of biperiden, including CNS effects. Advise her to report such symptoms as dizziness, depression, confusion, rash, vision changes, and eye pain.
- Instruct patient to avoid sudden position changes.
- Inform patient that she may experience increased eye sensitivity to light during biperiden therapy.

bivalirudin

Angiomax

Class and Category

Chemical: Hirudin analogue
Therapeutic: Anticoagulant
Pregnancy category: B

Indications and Dosages

▶ *As adjunct to provide anticoagulation and to prevent thrombosis in patients with unstable angina who are undergoing percutaneous transluminal coronary angioplasty*

I.V. INFUSION
Adults. *Initial:* 1-mg/kg bolus immediately before angioplasty, then 2.5 mg/kg/hr for 4 hr by continuous infusion, followed by 0.2 mg/kg/hr for up to 20 hr.

DOSAGE ADJUSTMENT Dosage may be reduced by 20% for patients with moderate renal impairment (glomerular filtration rate [GFR] of 30 to 59 ml/min), by 60% for patients with severe renal impairment (GFR of 10 to 29 ml/min), and by 90% for dialysis-dependent patients.

Route	Onset	Peak	Duration
I.V.	Immediate	Unknown	1 hr after end of infusion

Mechanism of Action

Selectively binds to thrombin, including thrombin trapped in established clots. Without thrombin, fibrinogen can't convert to fibrin and clots can't form.

Incompatibilities

Don't mix any other drugs in same I.V. line before or during bivalirudin administration.

Contraindications

Active major bleeding, hypersensitivity to bivalirudin or its components

Interactions

DRUGS

alteplase, antineoplastic drugs, antithymocyte globulin, heparin, NSAIDs, platelet inhibitors, reteplase, streptokinase, strontium chloride Sr 89, warfarin: Additive risk of bleeding

porfimer. Possibly decreased efficacy of porfimer photodynamic therapy

salicylates: Increased risk of hypoprothrombinemia and bleeding

Adverse Reactions

CNS: Headache, intracranial hemorrhage
CV: Hypotension
EENT: Bleeding from mouth, epistaxis
GI: Abdominal cramps, diarrhea, GI or retroperitoneal bleeding, nausea, vomiting
GU: Hematuria, vaginal bleeding
MS: Back pain
RESP: Hemoptysis, hemothorax
SKIN: Ecchymosis
Other: Injection site bleeding, hematoma, or pain

Nursing Considerations

- To reconstitute bivalirudin, add 5 ml of sterile water for injection to each 250-mg vial and swirl gently until dissolved. For initial infusion, further dilute each reconstituted vial in 50 ml of D$_5$W or NS to a final concentration of 5 mg/ml.
- For subsequent low-rate infusion, further dilute reconstituted drug in 500 ml of D$_5$W or NS to a final concentration of 0.5 mg/ml.
- Expect to give patient 300 to 325 mg of aspirin P.O. daily, as prescribed, during bivalirudin therapy.
- Use reconstituted solution within 24 hours if stored between 2° and 8° C (36° and 46° F). Diluted solution is stable for 24 hours when stored at room temperature. Don't freeze reconstituted and diluted solutions.
- Be aware that solution should be colorless to light yellow and appear slightly opalescent. Don't use if you observe particles or discoloration.
- **WARNING** Expect to monitor blood coagulation tests before and regularly during therapy because bleeding is a major risk associated with bivalirudin use.
- **WARNING** Monitor patient frequently for signs and symptoms of bleeding because no specific antidote for bivalirudin is available. If life-threatening bleeding occurs, notify prescriber immediately, discontinue drug therapy, and prepare to monitor APTT and other coagulation tests as ordered. Be aware that blood transfusions may be necessary. Patients with an increased risk of bleeding include actively menstruating females; patients with known vascular or organ abnormalities, such as severe uncontrolled hypertension, advanced renal disease, infective endocarditis, dissecting aortic aneurysm, diverticulitis, hemophilia, hepatic disease (especially if due to a deficiency in vitamin K–dependent clotting factors), inflammatory bowel disease, or peptic ulcer disease; and those who have recently had a CVA, major surgery (including eye, brain, or spinal cord surgery), large vessel or lumbar puncture, organ biopsy, spinal anesthesia, or major bleeding (including intracranial, GI, intraocular, retroperitoneal, or pulmonary bleeding).
- If possible, avoid I.M. injections of any kind in patients receiving bivalirudin to decrease the risk of bleeding.
- Discard any portion of drug that hasn't been used.

PATIENT TEACHING
• Inform patient that bivalirudin is a blood thinner used only in the hospital setting.
• Instruct patient to check her skin for easy bruising or red spots and to immediately report back or stomach pain, difficulty breathing, dizziness or fainting spells, and unusual bleeding, such as black or tarry stools, blood in urine, coughing up blood, heavy menstrual bleeding, or nosebleeds. Drug may need to be discontinued.
• Urge patient to be careful to avoid injury while receiving bivalirudin. For example, suggest that she brush her teeth gently, using a soft-bristled toothbrush, and take special care when flossing.
• Caution patient not to take anti-inflammatory drugs, such as ibuprofen, naproxen, ketoprofen, aspirin, and aspirin-like products, or other blood thinners, such as warfarin, while receiving bivalirudin unless prescriber instructs her to do so.
• Inform patient that the risk of bleeding associated with bivalirudin lasts for only a short time once drug is discontinued.

bleomycin sulfate
Blenoxane

Class and Category
Chemical: Cytotoxic glycopeptide antibiotic mixture
Therapeutic: Antineoplastic antibiotic
Pregnancy category: D

Indications and Dosages
▶ *To treat squamous cell carcinoma of the head and neck (including mouth, tongue, tonsil, sinus, palate, lip, buccal mucosa, gingiva, epiglottis, nasopharynx, oropharynx, and larynx), skin, penis, cervix, and vulva; non-Hodgkin's lymphomas; and testicular carcinoma*
I.V. INJECTION
Adults and adolescents. 0.25 to 0.5 U/kg or 10 to 20 U/m^2 over at least 10 min once or twice a week.
▶ *To treat Hodgkin's disease*
I.V. INJECTION
Adults and adolescents. *Initial:* 0.25 to 0.5 U/kg or 10 to 20 U/m^2 over at least 10 min once or twice a week. *Maintenance:* 1 U/day or 5 U/wk if 50% response occurs. Each dose should be administered over a period of at least 10 minutes.

DOSAGE ADJUSTMENT Patients with Hodgkin's disease or non-Hodgkin's lymphoma are given a test dose of 2 U or less for the first two doses because of the possibility of an anaphylactoid reaction. For patients with renal function impairment (regardless of indication), dosage decreased as follows: to 50% of normal dose if serum creatinine level is 1.5 to 2 mg/dl; to 25% of normal dose if serum creatinine level is 2.5 to 4 mg/dl; to 20% of normal dose if serum creatinine level is 4 to 6 mg/dl; and to 5% to 10% of normal dose if serum creatinine level is 6 to 10 mg/dl.

Mechanism of Action

May inhibit cell's ability to replicate or reproduce by inhibiting DNA synthesis and, to a lesser extent, RNA and protein synthesis. Bleomycin is effective against both cycling and noncycling cells, but it appears to be most effective in the G_2 phase of cell division.

Incompatibilities

Don't mix bleomycin with D_5W or other solutions containing dextrose to avoid a loss in potency.

Contraindications

Hypersensitivity or a history of idiosyncratic reaction to bleomycin

Interactions

DRUGS

antineoplastics: Increased risk of pulmonary and mucosal toxicity and bone marrow depression

cisplatin: Increased risk of bleomycin toxicity due to bleomycin accumulation

digoxin: Decreased blood digoxin level

general anesthetics: Increased risk of pulmonary deterioration and fibrosis

live virus vaccines: Severe and possibly fatal infections

phenytoin: Decreased blood phenytoin level

vincristine: Increased therapeutic effect of bleomycin

Adverse Reactions

CNS: Chills, fever

CV: Pleuropericarditis, Raynaud's phenomenon, vascular toxicity (cerebral arteritis, CVA, MI, thrombotic microangiopathy), vasospasm (when used in combination with vinblastine for testicular cancer)

EENT: Stomatitis
GI: Anorexia, elevated liver function test results, hepatotoxicity, vomiting
GU: Cystitis, elevated BUN and serum creatinine levels, hematuria
HEME: Decreased hemoglobin level, leukopenia, thrombocytopenia
RESP: Pneumonitis progressing to pulmonary fibrosis, pulmonary toxicity (decreased diffusion capacity, lung volume, and vital capacity; dyspnea; crackles)
SKIN: Alopecia, erythema, hyperkeratosis, hyperpigmentation, mucocutaneous toxicity, nail changes, rash, skin tenderness, striae, vesiculation
Other: Idiosyncratic reaction (chills, fever, hypotension, confusion, faintness, wheezing), injection site phlebitis, tumor site pain, weight loss

Nursing Considerations

• Be aware that bleomycin should be administered only under the supervision of a qualified physician where appropriate diagnostic and treatment facilities are available.
• Follow facility protocols for preparation and handling of antineoplastic drugs and appropriate disposal of used equipment.
• Add 5 or 10 ml of sodium chloride for injection to a 15-U or 30-U vial of bleomycin.
• Store reconstituted bleomycin at room temperature and use within 24 hours.
• Be aware that premedication with acetaminophen, steroids, and diphenhydramine may be administered to reduce the risk of anaphylaxis and drug-induced fever.
• Expect pulmonary function tests and chest X-rays to be ordered before initiation of therapy to establish patient's baseline pulmonary status.
• **WARNING** Monitor patient's respiratory status, including auscultation and evaluation of breathing patterns during and after therapy, to assist with early detection of pulmonary toxicity. This complication occurs in about 10% of patients receiving bleomycin, especially elderly patients, those who have received cytotoxic drugs, those who are receiving bleomycin in combination with other antineoplastics, those receiving oxygen therapy during and after surgery, smokers, and patients receiving a total dose greater than 400 U. Expect drug to be discontinued if pulmonary changes are detected. Be aware that pulmonary symptoms can occur up to 1 month after therapy has been discontinued.

- Be aware that patients who have been treated with radiation therapy are at increased risk for pulmonary and mucocutaneous toxicity and bone marrow depression.
- **WARNING** Be aware that patients with lymphoma may develop a severe idiosyncratic reaction (chills, fever, hypotension, confusion, faintness, and wheezing) similar to anaphylaxis, especially after first or second dose. This reaction may occur immediately or several hours after dose is administered. Notify prescriber immediately if such a reaction occurs. Expect to administer antihistamines, corticosteroids, pressor agents, and volume expanders, as prescribed.
- Obtain BUN and serum creatinine levels before initiation of therapy, and monitor for signs and symptoms of renal function deterioration during therapy, especially in patients with significant renal function impairment.
- Monitor for elevated liver function test results, which may indicate drug-induced hepatotoxicity.
- Monitor patient for signs of adverse skin and mucous membrane effects, which occur in 25% to 50% of patients undergoing bleomycin therapy, usually 2 or 3 weeks after administration of 150 to 200 U.
- Be aware that fraction of inspired oxygen (FIO_2) is maintained at 25%—approximately that of room air—during surgery and postoperatively to reduce the risk of pulmonary complications. Expect fluid replacement to be colloid rather than crystalloid during this time.
- Store unreconstituted vials at 2° to 8° C (36° to 46° F).

PATIENT TEACHING

- Teach patient signs and symptoms of adverse reactions associated with bleomycin, and advise her to immediately report any that occur.
- Stress the importance of obtaining periodic chest X-rays, which may be ordered every 1 to 2 weeks, to detect signs of adverse pulmonary reactions.
- Advise patient to inform all health care providers, including dentists, that she is receiving bleomycin.
- Encourage patient to maintain good oral hygiene and adequate nutritional intake. If she develops stomatitis, suggest that she try eating bland, soft foods served cold or at room temperature to decrease irritation.

bretylium tosylate

Bretylate (CAN), Bretylol

Class and Category

Chemical: Bromobenzyl quaternary ammonium compound
Therapeutic: Class III antiarrhythmic
Pregnancy category: C

Indications and Dosages

▶ *To prevent and treat ventricular fibrillation and to treat life-threatening ventricular arrhythmias that don't respond to first-line antiarrhythmics, such as lidocaine*

I.V. INFUSION OR INJECTION

Adults with immediate life-threatening ventricular arrhythmias. *Initial:* 5 mg/kg undiluted by rapid I.V. injection; if ventricular fibrillation persists, 10 mg/kg repeated as often as needed. *Continuous suppression:* 1 to 2 mg/min or 5 to 10 mg/kg of diluted I.V. solution infused over at least 8 min q 6 hr.

Adults with other ventricular arrhythmias. *Initial:* 5 to 10 mg/kg of diluted I.V. solution infused over at least 8 min and repeated q 1 to 2 hr if arrhythmia continues. *Maintenance:* 5 to 10 mg/kg diluted I.V. solution infused over at least 8 min q 6 hr, or 1 to 2 mg/min infused continuously.

DOSAGE ADJUSTMENT Dosing interval increased for patients with impaired renal function because bretylium is excreted primarily by kidneys.

Route	Onset	Peak	Duration
I.V.	5 to 10 min*	6 to 9 hr	6 to 24 hr

Contraindications

Digitalis toxicity, hypersensitivity to bretylium

Interactions

DRUGS

catecholamines (such as dopamine and norepinephrine): Increased vasopressor effects of catecholamines
digoxin: Possibly worsening of digitalis toxicity

---

* For suppression of ventricular fibrillation; 20 to 120 min for suppression of ventricular tachycardia.

Mechanism of Action

Bretylium prolongs the repolarization phase of the action potential and lengthens the effective refractory period, which helps terminate reentry arrhythmias. The drug also acts on adrenergic nerve terminals. Initially, it causes early release of norepinephrine, which increases the heart rate and blood pressure. Then it blocks the release of norepinephrine, as shown above. This reduces the heart rate and blood pressure. Bretylium also increases the ventricular threshold, making the ventricular myocardium less responsive to ectopic impulses and preventing ventricular fibrillation.

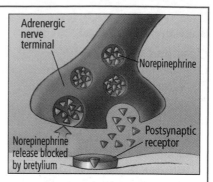

Adverse Reactions

CNS: Anxiety, confusion, dizziness, emotional lability, fever, lethargy, light-headedness, paranoid psychosis, syncope, vertigo
CV: Angina, arrhythmias (including bradycardia and more frequent PVCs), hypotension, orthostatic hypotension, transient hypertension
EENT: Mild conjunctivitis, nasal congestion
GI: Abdominal pain, diarrhea, hiccups, nausea, vomiting
GU: Renal dysfunction
RESP: Dyspnea
SKIN: Diaphoresis, erythematous macular rash, flushing
Other: Injection site pain

Nursing Considerations

- **WARNING** Monitor patients with severe aortic stenosis or pulmonary hypertension for signs of hypotension, a common effect of bretylium therapy.
- Be aware that bretylium is always diluted for I.V. administration *except* when used in life-threatening ventricular fibrillation. In this instance, use *undiluted* bretylium and administer it as quickly as possible.
- Dilute bretylium in a compatible I.V. solution, such as D_5W, D_5NS, D_5LR, NS, 5% sodium bicarbonate, 20% mannitol, 1/6 molar sodium lactate, LR, calcium chloride in D_5W, and potassium chloride in D_5W. Dilute to a concentration of at least 500 mg/50 ml.

- Be aware that bretylium is also available in 5% dextrose; this form should be used for I.V. infusion only.
- For I.V. infusion, dilute bretylium and administer at 1 to 2 mg/ minute, using an infusion pump or other appropriate rate control device.
- **WARNING** Be aware that patient may experience hypotension while supine. Have patient remain supine until tolerance develops. If her supine systolic blood pressure falls below 75 mm Hg, expect to administer dopamine or norepinephrine and monitor her blood pressure closely because vasopressor effects intensify when these drugs are given together.
- Be alert for transient hypertension and increased frequency of arrhythmias because bretylium initially triggers release of norepinephrine. Monitor patient's ECG tracings and blood pressure continuously, and notify prescriber of changes.
- Monitor serum bretylium level. Notify prescriber if level falls outside therapeutic range of 0.5 to 1.5 mcg/ml.
- Store drug at 15° to 30° C (59° to 86° F). Don't freeze.

PATIENT TEACHING
- Advise patient receiving bretylium to immediately report chest pain or pressure, pain at I.V. site, or rash.
- Warn patient that she may feel dizzy or light-headed even when lying down. Instruct her to remain supine and to ask for assistance when attempting to move or sit up. Tell her that this sensation usually subsides in a few days.

bumetanide

Bumex

Class and Category

Chemical: Sulfonamide derivative
Therapeutic: Loop diuretic
Pregnancy category: C

Indications and Dosages

▶ *To treat edema caused by heart failure, hepatic disease, and renal disease, including nephrotic syndrome*

I.V. INFUSION OR INJECTION

Adults. 0.5 to 1 mg over 1 to 2 min q.d.; may repeat q 2 to 3 hr if necessary. *Maximum:* 10 mg/day.

DOSAGE ADJUSTMENT Continuous infusion (12 mg over 12 hr) may be more effective and less toxic than intermittent infusion in patients with severe chronic renal insufficiency.

Route	Onset	Peak	Duration
I.V.	In min	15 to 30 min	3.5 to 4 hr

Mechanism of Action
Inhibits the reabsorption of sodium, chloride, and water in the ascending limb of the loop of Henle, which promotes their excretion and reduces fluid volume.

Contraindications
Anuria, hepatic coma, hypersensitivity to bumetanide or its components, severe electrolyte depletion

Interactions
DRUGS
aminoglycosides: Increased risk of ototoxicity
antihypertensives: Increased antihypertensive effect
indomethacin: Slowed increase in urine and sodium excretion, inhibited plasma renin activity
lithium: Decreased lithium renal clearance, increased risk of lithium toxicity
probenecid: Decreased sodium excretion

Adverse Reactions
CNS: Dizziness, encephalopathy, headache
CV: Chest pain, hypotension
EENT: Ototoxicity
ENDO: Hyperglycemia
GI: Nausea
GU: Azotemia, difficulty maintaining erection, elevated serum creatinine level, premature ejaculation
MS: Muscle spasms
Other: Hyperuricemia, hypocalcemia, hypochloremia, hypokalemia, hyponatremia, hypovolemia

Nursing Considerations
- WARNING Be aware that patients who are hypersensitive to sulfonamides may be hypersensitive to bumetanide. Monitor such patients closely when starting therapy.
- Expect to use parenteral route for patients with impaired GI absorption or those for whom oral route isn't practical. Switch to oral route, as prescribed, as soon as possible.
- Discard unused parenteral solution 24 hours after preparation.

- Assess fluid and electrolyte balance closely because bumetanide is a potent diuretic (40 to 60 times more potent than furosemide). Monitor fluid intake and output once every 8 hours, evaluate serum electrolyte levels when ordered, and assess for imbalances.
- **WARNING** Be aware that high-dose or too-frequent administration can cause profound diuresis and water and electrolyte depletion, especially in elderly patients.
- Monitor serum potassium level regularly to check for hypokalemia, especially if patient takes a digitalis glycoside for heart failure or has hepatic cirrhosis, ascites, aldosteronism, potassium-losing nephropathy, diarrhea, or a history of ventricular arrhythmias.
- Assess for signs of ototoxicity, such as tinnitus, daily. Rarely, bumetanide may cause ototoxicity, especially with I.V. administration, high doses, and increased frequency of administration in a patient with renal impairment.
- Monitor results of renal function tests during bumetanide therapy to detect adverse reactions.
- Store drug at 15° to 30° C (59° to 86° F), and protect from light. Don't freeze.

PATIENT TEACHING
- Inform patient that fluid intake and output will be monitored during bumetanide therapy. Advise her to report signs and symptoms of electrolyte imbalance, such as dizziness, headache, and muscle spasms.
- Teach patient about adverse reactions, and tell her to report any that occur.
- Advise patient to avoid potentially hazardous activities until drug's CNS effects are known.
- Review potassium-rich foods, and encourage patient to include them in her daily diet.
- Inform diabetic patient that her blood glucose level will be monitored regularly; urge her to report signs or symptoms of hyperglycemia.

buprenorphine hydrochloride
Buprenex

Class, Category, and Schedule
Chemical: Opioid, thebaine derivative
Therapeutic: Opioid analgesic

Pregnancy category: C
Controlled substance: Schedule V

Indications and Dosages

▶ *To control moderate to severe pain*
I.V INJECTION
Adults and children age 12 and older. 0.3 mg q 6 or more hr,
p.r.n. A second 0.3-mg dose is given 30 to 60 min after first dose,
if needed.
DOSAGE ADJUSTMENT Dosage reduced by half for elderly
or debilitated patients and for those who have respiratory disease or who also use another CNS depressant.
Children ages 2 to 12. 0.002 to 0.006 mg/kg q 4 to 6 hr, p.r.n.

Route	Onset	Peak	Duration
I.V.	Under 15 min	Under 1 hr	6 to 10 hr*

Mechanism of Action
May bind with and stimulate mu and kappa opiate receptors in the spinal
cord and higher levels in the CNS. In this way, buprenorphine is believed to
alter the perception of and emotional response to pain.

Incompatibilities
Don't administer buprenorphine through same I.V. line as diazepam or lorazepam.

Contraindications
Hypersensitivity to buprenorphine or its components

Interactions
DRUGS
CNS depressants, MAO inhibitors: Additive hypotensive and respiratory and CNS depressant effects of these drugs
other opioid analgesics: Reduced therapeutic effects if buprenorphine is given before another opioid analgesic

Adverse Reactions
CNS: Dizziness, headache, sedation, vertigo
CV: Bradycardia, hypertension, hypotension
EENT: Miosis
GI: Nausea, vomiting
RESP: Hypoventilation

---

* 4 to 5 hr in children ages 2 to 12.

SKIN: Diaphoresis
Other: Injection site edema, pain, or redness

Nursing Considerations

- **WARNING** Administer buprenorphine over at least 2 minutes. Be aware that rapid administration of other opioid analgesics has caused anaphylaxis, severe respiratory depression, hypotension, peripheral circulatory collapse, and cardiac arrest. Keep emergency equipment and drugs nearby.

- Frequently monitor vital signs, respiratory status, and response to drug; take safety precautions, especially after giving first dose.

- Assess respiratory status closely, especially in patients having an acute asthma attack and those with acute respiratory depression, adrenal insufficiency, chronic respiratory disease, hypothyroidism, myxedema, or conditions that increase CSF pressure, because drug causes and may exacerbate respiratory depression. Elderly, extremely ill, or debilitated patients and patients who have recently taken or are currently taking drugs with respiratory depressant effects are also more sensitive to buprenorphine's effects.

- Monitor for signs of drug-induced CNS depression or increased CSF pressure, such as altered LOC, restlessness, and irritability, in patients with a coma, head injury, intracranial lesions, or other conditions that could cause these effects. Patients who are taking or have recently taken drugs that depress the CNS are also more susceptible to these effects. Take appropriate safety precautions.

- Be aware that buprenorphine may induce or exacerbate arrhythmias or seizures in patients with a history of these conditions or may mask symptoms of acute abdominal conditions.

- Monitor patients with renal or hepatic impairment and those receiving a drug that decreases hepatic clearance for signs of increased buprenorphine effects because drug is metabolized in the liver and excreted by the kidneys.

- Monitor patients with prostatic hypertrophy, renal function impairment, recent urinary tract surgery, or urethral stricture for signs of urine retention, such as difficulty voiding or feeling that the bladder isn't empty after voiding, peripheral edema, or weight gain.

- Monitor for prolonged or worsening condition in patients with diarrhea caused by poisoning because drug may slow elimination of toxic material.

- Be aware that buprenorphine should be used cautiously in patients with toxic psychosis or kyphoscoliosis.
- Monitor patients with biliary tract disease for biliary colic (pain in upper midline area that may radiate to the back and right shoulder), which may be caused by increased intracholedochal pressure due to buprenorphine therapy.
- In a physically dependent patient, assess for withdrawal symptoms, which reach peak intensity about 15 days after abrupt withdrawal of drug. Symptoms resemble those of morphine withdrawal (body aches, diaphoresis, diarrhea, nausea, tremor, vomiting), are mild to moderate, and may persist for 1 to 2 weeks. Be aware that patients with a history of drug abuse (including acute alcoholism), emotional instability, or suicidal ideation or attempts are at increased risk for opioid abuse.
- Store drug at 15° to 30° C (59° to 86° F), and protect from prolonged exposure to light. Don't freeze.

PATIENT TEACHING
- Instruct patient to lie down during buprenorphine administration and for a period afterward to lessen drug's hypotensive effects (dizziness, light-headedness) and other adverse effects, such as nausea and vomiting.
- Advise patient to change position slowly and to avoid rising quickly from a sitting or lying position.
- Advise patient to avoid potentially hazardous activities until drug's CNS effects are known.

butorphanol tartrate
Stadol

Class, Category, and Schedule
Chemical: Opioid
Therapeutic: Anesthesia adjunct, opioid analgesic
Pregnancy category: C
Controlled substance: Schedule II

Indications and Dosages
▶ *To manage pain*
I.V. INJECTION
Adults. 0.5 to 2 mg (usually 1 mg) q 3 to 4 hr, p.r.n.
▶ *As adjunct to provide preoperative anesthesia*
I.V. INJECTION
Adults. Individualized; average of 2 mg 60 to 90 min before surgery.

▶ *As adjunct to provide anesthesia*
I.V. INJECTION
Adults. Individualized; average of 1 to 4 mg initially and then supplemental doses of 0.5 to 1 mg, p.r.n. Total usually required during surgery is 60 to 180 mcg/kg (0.06 to 0.18 mg/kg).
DOSAGE ADJUSTMENT Dosage reduced by half for elderly patients and those with impaired hepatic or renal function.

Route	Onset	Peak	Duration
I.V.	2 to 3 min	30 min	2 to 4 hr

Mechanism of Action

May bind with and stimulate mu and kappa opiate receptors in the spinal cord and higher levels in the CNS. In this way, butorphanol is believed to alter the perception of and emotional response to pain.

Contraindications

Acute respiratory depression, diarrhea due to poisoning, hypersensitivity to butorphanol or its components (including the preservative benzethonium chloride)

Interactions

DRUGS
CNS depressants: Additive CNS depression
ACTIVITIES
alcohol use: Additive CNS depression

Adverse Reactions

CNS: Anxiety, confusion, difficulty performing purposeful movements, difficulty speaking, dizziness, euphoria, floating feeling, headache, lethargy, nervousness, paresthesia, somnolence, syncope, tremor, vertigo
CV: Chest pain, hypotension, palpitations, tachycardia, vasodilation
EENT: Blurred vision, dry mouth, tinnitus
GI: Anorexia, constipation, epigastric pain, nausea, vomiting
RESP: Apnea, respiratory depression, shallow breathing
SKIN: Clammy skin, pruritus, sensation of warmth

Nursing Considerations

• Administer butorphanol slowly, over several minutes. Be aware that rapid administration may cause anaphylaxis, severe respiratory depression, hypotension, peripheral circulatory collapse, and cardiac arrest. Keep emergency equipment and drugs nearby.

- Assess respiratory status closely, especially in patients having an acute asthma attack and those with chronic respiratory disease, hypothyroidism, or conditions that increase CSF pressure, because drug causes respiratory depression. Pediatric, elderly, extremely ill, or debilitated patients and those who have recently taken or are currently taking drugs with respiratory depressant effects are also more sensitive to butorphanol's effects.
- Frequently monitor blood pressure after giving butorphanol. If severe hypertension develops (rare), stop drug at once and notify prescriber. If patient isn't opioid-dependent, expect to administer naloxone to reverse drug's effects.
- Monitor for signs of drug-induced CNS depression or increased CSF pressure, such as altered LOC, restlessness, and irritability, in patients with a head injury, intracranial lesions, or other conditions that could cause these effects. Patients who are taking or have recently taken drugs that depress the CNS are also more susceptible to these effects. Take appropriate safety precautions.
- Because butorphanol can increase cardiac workload, use it with extreme caution in patients with acute MI, ventricular dysfunction, or coronary insufficiency.
- Be aware that butorphanol may induce or exacerbate arrhythmias or seizures in patients with a history of these conditions and may mask symptoms of acute abdominal conditions.
- Monitor patients with renal or hepatic impairment and those receiving a drug that decreases hepatic clearance for signs of increased butorphanol effects because drug is metabolized in the liver and excreted by the kidneys.
- Be aware that patients with a history of drug abuse (including acute alcoholism), emotional instability, or suicidal ideation or attempts are at increased risk for opioid abuse; however, the risk of drug dependence from butorphanol is lower than with some other opioid analgesics.
- Monitor patients with prostatic hypertrophy, renal function impairment, recent urinary tract surgery, or urethral stricture for signs of urine retention, such as difficulty voiding or feeling that the bladder isn't empty after voiding, peripheral edema, or weight gain.
- Store drug at 15° to 30° C (59° to 86° F), and protect from light. Don't freeze.

PATIENT TEACHING
• Instruct patient to lie down during butorphanol administration and for a period afterward to lessen drug's hypotensive effects (dizziness, light-headedness) and other adverse effects, such as nausea and vomiting.
• Advise patient to change position slowly and to avoid rising quickly from a sitting or lying position.
• Advise patient to avoid potentially hazardous activities until drug's CNS effects are known.
• Tell patient to avoid alcohol and other CNS depressants, including OTC drugs, during butorphanol therapy because of possible additive CNS depression.

calcitriol
(1,25-dihydroxycholecalciferol)
Calcijex

Class and Category
Chemical: Sterol derivative, vitamin D analogue
Therapeutic: Antihypocalcemic, antihypoparathyroid
Pregnancy category: C

Indications and Dosages
▶ *To treat hypocalcemia in patients undergoing long-term renal dialysis, to reduce parathyroid hormone levels*
I.V. INJECTION
Adults. *Initial:* 1 to 2 mcg 3 times/wk q.o.d. (Initial dose may range from 0.5 to 4 mcg 3 times/wk q.o.d.) Each dose increased by 0.5 to 1 mcg at 2- to 4-wk intervals, if needed.

Mechanism of Action
Binds to specific receptors of the intestinal mucosa to increase calcium absorption from the intestines. Calcitriol also may regulate calcium ion transfer from bone to blood and stimulate calcium reabsorption in the distal renal tubules, making more calcium available in the body.

Contraindications
Hypercalcemia, vitamin D toxicity

Interactions
DRUGS
cholestyramine: Decreased calcitriol absorption
digitalis glycosides: Possibly arrhythmias
ketoconazole: Decreased blood calcitriol level
magnesium-containing antacids: Hypermagnesemia
mineral oil: Decreased blood calcitriol level (with prolonged use of mineral oil)
phenobarbital, phenytoin: Decreased synthesis and blood level of calcitriol
thiazide diuretics: Hypercalcemia

Adverse Reactions

None with the usual dosages.

Nursing Considerations

- Inspect calcitriol for particles and discoloration before use.
- Monitor serum calcium and phosphorus levels at least twice a week during the initial phase of therapy. Also monitor serum magnesium, alkaline phosphate, and 24-hour urinary calcium and phosphorus levels periodically.
- For patients treated for hypoparathyroidism, expect dosage to be titrated in response to parathyroid hormone level changes.
- Know that drug should be discontinued if hypercalcemia occurs or if serum calcium–times–phosphate product (calcium × phosphate) is greater than 70.
- Make sure patient has adequate calcium intake during therapy.
- Be alert for vitamin D toxicity in patients who receive high-dose or long-term calcitriol therapy. Early signs and symptoms include bone pain, constipation, dry mouth, headache, metallic taste, myalgia, nausea, somnolence, vomiting, and weakness. Late signs and symptoms include albuminuria, anorexia, arrhythmias, azotemia, conjunctivitis (calcific), decreased libido, elevated AST and ALT levels, elevated BUN level, generalized vascular calcification, hypercholesterolemia, hypertension, hyperthermia, irritability, mild acidosis, nephrocalcinosis, nocturia, pancreatitis, photophobia, polydipsia, polyuria, pruritus, rhinorrhea, and weight loss.
- Store drug at 15° to 30° C (59° to 86° F), and protect from heat and direct light.

PATIENT TEACHING

- Warn patient not to take other forms of vitamin D while receiving calcitriol.
- Advise patient to notify prescriber immediately if signs of toxicity, such as headache, irritability, nausea, photophobia, vomiting, weakness, and weight loss, develop.

calcium chloride
Calciject (CAN)

calcium gluceptate
Calcium Stanley (CAN)

calcium gluconate

Class and Category
Chemical: Elemental cation

Therapeutic: Antihypermagnesemic agent, antihypocalcemic agent, calcium replacement, cardiotonic agent
Pregnancy category: C

Indications and Dosages

▶ *To replace calcium in hypocalcemia*
I.V. INFUSION (CALCIUM CHLORIDE)
Adults. 0.5 to 1 g q 1 to 3 days, infused at less than 1 ml/min.
Children. 25 mg/kg given over several minutes.
I.V. INJECTION (CALCIUM GLUCEPTATE)
Adults and children. 1.1 to 4.4 g I.V. at a rate not to exceed 2 ml (36 mg)/min.
I.V. INJECTION (CALCIUM GLUCONATE)
Adults. 970 mg given slowly and repeated if needed until tetany is controlled.
Children. 200 to 500 mg as a single dose given slowly and repeated if needed until tetany is controlled.
▶ *As adjunct to treat magnesium intoxication*
I.V. INJECTION (CALCIUM CHLORIDE)
Adults. 500 mg promptly and repeated p.r.n., based on response.
▶ *As adjunct in cardiac resuscitation*
I.V. INJECTION (CALCIUM CHLORIDE)
Adults. 0.5 to 1 g.
Children. 0.2 ml/kg.
▶ *As adjunct in exchange transfusion*
I.V. INJECTION (CALCIUM GLUCONATE)
Adults. 1.35 mEq after each 100 ml of citrated blood is exchanged.
Neonates. 0.45 mEq after each 100 ml of citrated blood is exchanged.
I.V. INJECTION (CALCIUM GLUCEPTATE)
Neonates. 110 mg after each 100 ml of citrated blood is exchanged.

Mechanism of Action

Increases levels of intracellular and extracellular calcium, which is needed to maintain homeostasis, especially in the nervous and musculoskeletal systems. Also plays a role in normal cardiac and renal function, respiration, coagulation, and cell membrane and capillary permeability. Helps regulate the release and storage of neurotransmitters and hormones.

Incompatibilities

To avoid precipitation, don't administer I.V. calcium chloride, gluceptate, or gluconate through the same I.V. line as bicarbonates, carbonates, phosphates, sulfates, or tartrates. Don't mix with tetracyclines to avoid rendering tetracyclines inactive.

Contraindications

Hypercalcemia, hypersensitivity to calcium salts or their components, hypophosphatemia, renal calculi, ventricular fibrillation

Interactions

DRUGS

atenolol: Decreased blood atenolol level and beta blockade

calcitonin: Possibly antagonized effects of calcitonin in hypercalcemia treatment

calcium supplements, magnesium-containing preparations: Increased serum calcium or magnesium level, especially in patients with impaired renal function

cellulose sodium phosphate: Decreased effectiveness of cellulose sodium phosphate in preventing hypercalciuria

digitalis glycosides: Increased risk of arrhythmias

estrogens, oral contraceptives (estrogen-containing): Increased calcium absorption

etidronate: Decreased etidronate absorption

fluoroquinolones: Reduced fluoroquinolone absorption by calcium carbonate

gallium nitrate: Antagonized effects of gallium nitrate

iron salts: Decreased gastric absorption of iron

magnesium sulfate (parenteral): Neutralized effects of magnesium by parenteral calcium salts

neuromuscular blockers (except succinylcholine): Possibly reversal of neuromuscular blockade by parenteral calcium salts; enhanced or prolonged neuromuscular blockade induced by tubocurarine

norfloxacin: Decreased norfloxacin bioavailability

phenytoin: Decreased bioavailability of phenytoin and calcium

potassium phosphates, potassium and sodium phosphates: Increased risk of calcium deposition in soft tissue

sodium bicarbonate: Possibly milk-alkali syndrome

sodium fluoride: Reduced fluoride and calcium absorption

sodium polystyrene sulfonate: Possibly metabolic alkalosis if patient has renal impairment

tetracyclines: Decreased tetracycline absorption and blood level, leading to decreased anti-infective response

thiazide diuretics: Possibly hypercalcemia
verapamil: Reversed verapamil effects
vitamin A (more than 25,000 U/day): Possibly stimulation of bone loss, decreased effects of calcium supplementation, and hypercalcemia
vitamin D (high doses): Excessively increased calcium absorption
FOODS
caffeine: Possibly decreased calcium absorption
ACTIVITIES
alcohol use (excessive), smoking: Possibly decreased calcium absorption

Adverse Reactions

CNS: Paresthesia
CV: Hypotension, irregular heartbeat
GI: Nausea, vomiting
SKIN: Diaphoresis, flushing, or sensation of warmth
Other: Hypercalcemia; injection site burning, pain, rash, or redness

Nursing Considerations

• **WARNING** Be aware that calcium chloride injection contains three times as much calcium per milliliter as calcium gluconate injection.
• Warm solution to room temperature before administration.
• Don't use calcium gluceptate if you detect crystals.
• If you observe crystals in calcium gluconate, you can dissolve them by warming solution to 30° to 40° C (86° to 104° F).
• Administer I.V. calcium through an infusing I.V. solution, using a small-bore needle inserted into a large vein to minimize irritation. Give calcium slowly to prevent excess calcium from reaching the heart and causing adverse cardiovascular reactions. Adverse reactions often result from too-rapid administration. If ECG tracings are abnormal or patient reports injection site discomfort, expect to temporarily discontinue administration.
• Maintain patient in a recumbent position for 30 minutes after administration to prevent dizziness from hypotension.
• Assess regularly for extravasation because calcium causes necrosis. If infiltration occurs, discontinue I.V. calcium and notify prescriber immediately.
• Regularly monitor serum calcium level and evaluate therapeutic response by assessing for Chvostek's and Trousseau's signs, which shouldn't appear. Be aware that patients with dehydration, electrolyte imbalance, renal function impairment, or sar-

coidosis are at increased risk for hypercalcemia. Patients with diarrhea or GI malabsorption may have increased fecal calcium excretion.

• Monitor vital signs and ECG tracings as appropriate. Calcium administration may cause a temporary increase in blood pressure, especially in elderly or hypertensive patients.

• Assess for arrhythmias in patients with cardiac disease, those receiving digitalis glycosides, and those with a history of ventricular fibrillation during cardiac resuscitation.

• Monitor for signs of calculi formation, such as pain radiating from the lumbar region, in patients with a history of renal calculi.

• Store calcium at 15° to 30° C (59° to 86° F), and protect from heat, moisture, and direct light. Don't freeze.

PATIENT TEACHING

• Instruct patient to immediately report pain at calcium injection site.

• Tell patient to avoid excessive use of tobacco and excessive consumption of alcoholic beverages and caffeine-containing products because these substances may decrease calcium absorption.

• Teach patient with hypocalcemia about the need for sufficient calcium and vitamin D intake as well as weight-bearing exercise.

capreomycin sulfate
Capastat

Class and Category
Chemical: Polypeptide antibiotic isolated from *Streptomyces capreolus*
Therapeutic: Antitubercular agent
Pregnancy category: C

Indications and Dosages
▶ *As adjunct to treat pulmonary tuberculosis caused by* Mycobacterium tuberculosis *when primary drugs have been ineffective or can't be used because of toxicity*
I.V. INFUSION, I.M. INJECTION
Adults. 1 g q.d. for 60 to 120 days, followed by 1 g 2 or 3 times/ wk for 12 to 24 mo. *Maximum:* 20 mg/kg/day.

Mechanism of Action
May interfere with lipid and nucleic acid biosynthesis in actively growing tubercle bacilli.

Contraindications
Hypersensitivity to capreomycin or its components

Interactions
DRUGS
aminoglycosides (parenteral): Increased risk of ototoxicity, nephrotoxicity, and neuromuscular blockade
nephrotoxic drugs (such as amphotericin B): Increased risk of nephrotoxicity
neuromuscular blockers: Enhanced neuromuscular blockade
ototoxic drugs (such as quinidine): Increased risk of ototoxicity
polymyxins (parenteral): Increased risk of nephrotoxicity and neuromuscular blockade

Adverse Reactions
CNS: Dizziness, vertigo
EENT: Ototoxicity
GI: Elevated liver function test results
GU: Nephrotoxicity
HEME: Leukocytosis, leukopenia
SKIN: Maculopapular rash, sterile abscess (with I.M. injection), urticaria
Other: Injection site pain, induration, or bleeding

Nursing Considerations
- Expect capreomycin dosage to be decreased for patients with reduced renal clearance.
- Reconstitute sterile capreomycin powder with 0.9% sodium chloride injection or sterile water for injection. Add 2, 2.15, 2.63, 3.3, or 4.3 ml of diluent to a 1-g vial of capreomycin to yield a concentration of 370, 350, 300, 250, or 200 mg/ml, respectively. Let stand for 2 to 3 minutes to allow for complete dissolution.
- Dilute reconstituted drug for I.V. injection with 100 ml of NS. Administer over 60 minutes.
- To reconstitute drug for I.M. injection, add 2 ml of sodium chloride for injection or sterile water for injection to each 1-g vial. Allow 2 to 3 minutes for complete dissolution.

- Inject I.M. form deep into a large muscle mass, such as the gluteus maximus.
- Observe injection site for excessive bleeding or sterile abscess.
- Store reconstituted capreomycin at 2° to 8° C (36° to 46° F) for up to 24 hours. Be aware that a color change to pale straw color with subsequent darkening doesn't indicate loss of potency or development of toxicity.
- Monitor results of renal function tests and assess urine for sediment to detect signs of renal injury or nephrotoxicity.
- Assess patient for changes in hearing. Ensure that he receives audiometric testing and vestibular function assessments regularly.
- Monitor closely for signs of a hypersensitivity reaction, such as urticaria and maculopapular rash, especially in patients with a history of hypersensitivity reactions to other drugs.

PATIENT TEACHING
- Advise patient receiving capreomycin to report excessive bleeding at injection site.
- Instruct patient to notify prescriber immediately if he develops hearing loss or ringing in ears.
- Explain the need for frequent laboratory tests to monitor renal function.
- Tell patient that tuberculosis therapy lasts for 12 to 24 months and that another drug will also be prescribed.
- Explain that noncompliance may decrease effectiveness and increase duration of treatment.

caspofungin acetate
Cancidas

Class and Category
Chemical: Echinocandins
Therapeutic: Antifungal
Pregnancy category: C

Indications and Dosages
▶ *To treat invasive aspergillosis in patients who are refractory to or intolerant of other therapies*
I.V. INFUSION
Adults. *Initial:* 70 mg on day 1, followed by 50 mg q.d. *Maximum:* 70 mg/day.

DOSAGE ADJUSTMENT Dosage reduced to 35 mg q.d. after initial 70-mg loading dose for patients with moderate hepatic insufficiency.

Mechanism of Action
Caspofungin acetate interferes with fungal cell membrane synthesis by inhibiting the synthesis of β (1,3)-D-glucan. A polypeptide, β (1,3)-D-glucan is the essential component of the fungal cell membrane that makes it rigid and protective. Without it, fungal cells rupture and die. This mechanism of action is most effective against susceptible filamentous fungi, such as *Aspergillus*.

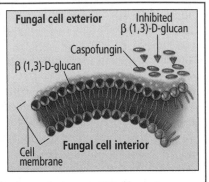

Incompatibilities
Don't mix or infuse caspofungin with other drugs. Don't admix with diluents containing dextrose.

Contraindications
Hypersensitivity to caspofungin acetate or its components

Interactions
DRUGS
carbamazepine, dexamethasone, efavirenz, nelfinavir, nevirapine, phenytoin, rifampin: Possibly decreased blood caspofungin level
cyclosporine: Transient increases in ALT and AST levels
tacrolimus: Possibly decreased blood tacrolimus level

Adverse Reactions
CNS: Fever
CV: Edema
GI: Nausea, vomiting
RESP: Dyspnea, stridor
SKIN: Flushing, pruritus, rash, sensation of warmth
Other: Facial edema, infusion site pain or redness

Nursing Considerations

- Be aware that caspofungin acetate should not be given to a patient also receiving the antirejection drug cyclosporine unless prescriber determines that the potential benefit outweighs the potential risk of liver damage to patient.
- To prepare the 70-mg loading dose, allow vial of drug to reach room temperature. To reconstitute, add 10.5 ml of NS to vial. Further dilute for administration by transferring 10 ml of reconstituted drug to 250 ml of NS.
- To prepare the 70-mg loading dose from two 50-mg vials, add 10.5 ml of NS to each vial; then transfer 14 ml of prepared solution to 250 ml of NS.
- To prepare the daily 50-mg infusion, allow vial of drug to reach room temperature. To reconstitute, add 10.5 ml of NS to vial. Further dilute for administration by transferring only 10 ml of reconstituted drug to 250 ml of NS.
- To prepare the daily 50-mg infusion at reduced volume, add 10 ml of reconstituted drug to 100 ml of NS.
- To prepare a 35-mg daily dose for patients with moderate hepatic insufficiency, reconstitute 50-mg vial with 10.5 ml of NS. Further dilute for administration by transferring only 7 ml of reconstituted drug to 250 ml of NS or, if medically necessary, to 100 ml of NS.
- When preparing powder for reconstitution, mix gently until you obtain a clear solution. Reconstituted solution may be stored below 25° C (77° F) for 1 hour before further dilution. Final diluted solution may be stored below 25° C for 24 hours.
- Don't use solution if it's cloudy or contains precipitates.
- Infuse drug slowly over approximately 1 hour.
- Expect to increase daily dose to 70 mg, as prescribed, for patients who are receiving carbamazepine, dexamethasone, efavirenz, nelfinavir, nevirapine, phenytoin, or rifampin and who are not responding clinically.
- Monitor skin for flushing, and frequently assess patient for unexplained temperature elevation.
- Assess for airway patency if patient develops excessive facial edema or respiratory stridor. Be prepared to intervene with emergency airway management if complete obstruction occurs.
- Before reconstituting drug, store it at 2° to 8° C (36° to 46° F).

PATIENT TEACHING
• Inform patient that he may experience sensations of warmth during caspofungin infusion. Advise him to notify prescriber if sensation becomes intolerable.
• Urge patient to immediately report difficulty talking, swallowing, or breathing during drug administration.

cefamandole nafate
Mandol

Class and Category
Chemical: Second-generation cephalosporin, 7-aminocephalosporanic acid
Therapeutic: Antibiotic
Pregnancy category: B

Indications and Dosages
▶ *To treat lower respiratory tract infections, including pneumonia, caused by beta-hemolytic streptococci,* Haemophilus influenzae, Klebsiella *species,* Proteus mirabilis, Staphylococcus aureus, *and* Streptococcus pneumoniae; *peritonitis caused by* Enterobacter *species and* Escherichia coli; *septicemia caused by* E. coli, H. influenzae, Klebsiella *species,* S. aureus, S. pneumoniae, *and* Streptococcus pyogenes; *and bone and joint infections caused by* S. aureus
I.V. INFUSION OR INJECTION
Adults. 0.5 to 1 g q 4 to 8 hr; for uncomplicated pneumonia, 0.5 g q 6 hr; for severe infections, 1 g q 4 to 6 hr; for life-threatening infections or infections caused by less susceptible organisms, 2 g q 4 hr. *Maximum:* 12 g/day.
Children. 50 to 100 mg/kg/day in equally divided doses q 4 to 8 hr. For severe infections, 150 mg/kg/day. *Maximum:* Maximum adult dosage.
▶ *To treat soft-tissue infections caused by* E. coli, Enterobacter *species,* H. influenzae, P. mirabilis, S. aureus, *and* S. pyogenes
I.V. INFUSION OR INJECTION
Adults. 500 mg q 6 hr.
Children. 50 to 100 mg/kg/day in equally divided doses q 4 to 8 hr. For severe infections, 150 mg/kg/day. *Maximum:* Maximum adult dosage.
▶ *To treat UTIs caused by* E. coli, Enterobacter *species, group D streptococci,* Klebsiella *species,* Proteus *species, and* Staphylococcus epidermidis

I.V. INFUSION OR INJECTION

Adults. 500 to 1,000 mg q 8 hr.

Children. 50 to 100 mg/kg/day in equally divided doses q 4 to 8 hr. For severe infections, 150 mg/kg/day. *Maximum:* Maximum adult dosage.

▶ *To provide surgical prophylaxis*

I.V. INFUSION OR INJECTION

Adults. 1 to 2 g 30 to 60 min before surgery followed by 1 to 2 g q 6 hr for 24 to 48 hr (or for 72 hr for prosthetic arthroplasty).

Children age 3 months or older. 50 to 100 mg/kg/day in divided doses with first dose given 30 to 60 min before surgery and then q 6 hr for 24 to 48 hr.

DOSAGE ADJUSTMENT After initial dose of 1 to 2 g, dosage reduced for patients with creatinine clearance of 50 to 80 ml/min/1.73 m^2 to 1.5 g q 4 hr or 2 g q 6 hr for life-threatening infections, and to 0.75 to 1.5 g q 6 hr for less severe infections; for those with creatinine clearance of 25 to 50 ml/min/1.73 m^2, dosage reduced to 1.5 g q 6 hr or 2 g q 8 hr for life-threatening infections, and to 0.75 to 1.5 g q 8 hr for less severe infections; for those with creatinine clearance of 10 to 25 ml/min/1.73 m^2, dosage reduced to 1 g q 6 hr or 1.25 g q 8 hr for life-threatening infections, and to 0.5 to 1 g q 8 hr for less severe infections; for those with creatinine clearance of 2 to 10 ml/min/1.73 m^2, dosage reduced to 0.67 g q 8 hr or 1 g q 12 hr for life-threatening infections, and to 0.5 to 0.75 g q 12 hr for less severe infections; and for those with creatinine clearance of less than 2 ml/min/1.73 m^2, dosage reduced to 0.5 g q 8 hr or 0.75 g q 12 hr for life-threatening infections, and to 0.25 to 0.5 g q 12 hr for less severe infections.

Mechanism of Action

Interferes with bacterial cell wall synthesis by inhibiting the final step in the cross-linking of peptidoglycan strands. Peptidoglycan makes cell membranes rigid and protective. Without it, bacterial cells rupture and die.

Incompatibilities

To prevent mutual inactivation, don't mix cefamandole with aminoglycosides. Also don't mix drug with Ringer's solution or lactated Ringer's solution.

Contraindications

Hypersensitivity to cephalosporins or their components

Interactions

DRUGS

aminoglycosides, loop diuretics: Increased risk of nephrotoxicity
oral anticoagulants, other drugs that affect blood clotting: Increased anticoagulant effect

ACTIVITIES

alcohol use: Disulfiram-like reaction from acetaldehyde accumulation

Adverse Reactions

CNS: Chills, fever, headache, seizures
CV: Edema
EENT: Hearing loss, oral candidiasis
GI: Abdominal cramps, diarrhea, elevated liver function test results, hepatic failure, hepatomegaly, nausea, pseudomembranous colitis, vomiting
GU: Elevated BUN level, nephrotoxicity, renal failure, vaginal candidiasis
HEME: Eosinophilia, hemolytic anemia, hypoprothrombinemia, neutropenia, thrombocytopenia, unusual bleeding
MS: Arthralgia
RESP: Dyspnea
SKIN: Ecchymosis, erythema, erythema multiforme, pruritus, rash, Stevens-Johnson syndrome
Other: Anaphylaxis, infusion site thrombophlebitis, superinfection

Nursing Considerations

- If possible, obtain culture and sensitivity test results, as ordered, before giving cefamandole.
- For direct intermittent I.V. injection, dilute each gram of drug with 10 ml of sterile water for injection, 5% dextrose injection, or sodium chloride for injection. Slowly inject solution over 3 to 5 minutes through tubing of a flowing compatible I.V. solution.
- For continuous I.V. infusion, dilute each gram of drug with 10 ml of sterile water for injection and add to compatible I.V. solution, such as NS or D_5W. (See manufacturer's guidelines for complete listing.)
- After drug reconstitution, don't fill syringe until immediately before use because carbon dioxide develops and may cause leakage or may dislodge rubber closure of syringe.

- Don't use solution if it contains particles or is discolored (other than a pale yellow to amber color).
- Be aware that a solution of 1 g cefamandole in 2 ml sterile water for injection is isotonic.
- Store reconstituted cefamandole for up to 24 hours at room temperature (25° C [77° F]), or refrigerate it for up to 96 hours.
- Be aware that cefamandole that has been reconstituted with sterile water for injection, 0.9% sodium chloride for injection, or 5% dextrose injection may be stored at −20° C (−4° F) in original container for up to 6 months. The solution may be warmed to a maximum 37° C (98.6° F), but be careful not to heat once thawing is complete. Don't refreeze.
- Monitor BUN and serum creatinine levels for early signs of nephrotoxicity. Also monitor fluid intake and output; decreasing urine output may indicate nephrotoxicity.
- Monitor for signs of an allergic reaction, such as difficulty breathing or a rash, especially in patients who are hypersensitive to penicillin, because cross-sensitivity has occurred in about 10% of such patients. Be aware that an allergic reaction may occur a few days after therapy starts.
- Assess bowel pattern daily; severe diarrhea may indicate pseudomembranous colitis.
- Assess for signs of superinfection, such as perineal itching, fever, malaise, redness, pain, swelling, drainage, rash, diarrhea, and cough or sputum changes.
- Assess for pharyngitis, ecchymosis, bleeding, and arthralgia, which may indicate a blood dyscrasia. Patients with a history of bleeding disorders are at increased risk. Monitor PT and bleeding time as appropriate. Be prepared to administer vitamin K, if ordered, to treat hypoprothrombinemia.

PATIENT TEACHING

- Advise patient receiving cefamandole to immediately report severe diarrhea or signs of blood dyscrasia or superinfection. Inform him that yogurt or buttermilk can help decrease diarrhea.
- Review with patient other possibly serious adverse reactions, including difficulty breathing, rash, and chest tightness, and tell him to report any that occur.

cefazolin sodium

Ancef, Kefzol

Class and Category

Chemical: First-generation cephalosporin, 7-aminocephalosporanic acid
Therapeutic: Antibiotic
Pregnancy category: B

Indications and Dosages

▶ *To treat respiratory tract infections caused by group A beta-hemolytic streptococci,* Haemophilus influenzae, Klebsiella *species,* Staphylococcus aureus, *and* Streptococcus pneumoniae; *skin and soft-tissue infections caused by* S. aureus, *group A beta-hemolytic and other strains of streptococci; biliary tract infections caused by* Escherichia coli, Klebsiella *species,* Proteus mirabilis, S. aureus, *and various strains of streptococci; bone and joint infections caused by* S. aureus; *genital infections, such as epididymitis and prostatitis, caused by* E. coli, Klebsiella *species,* P. mirabilis, *and some strains of enterococci; septicemia caused by* E. coli, Klebsiella *species,* P. mirabilis, S. aureus, *and* S. pneumoniae; *and endocarditis caused by group A beta-hemolytic streptococci and* S. aureus

I.V. INFUSION OR INJECTION

Adults. For mild infections, 250 to 500 mg q 8 hr; for moderate to severe infections, 500 to 1,000 mg q 6 to 8 hr; and for life-threatening infections, 1,000 to 1,500 mg q 6 hr. *Maximum:* 6 g/day.

Children. For mild to moderate infections, 25 to 50 mg/kg/day divided equally and given t.i.d. or q.i.d.; for severe infections, 100 mg/kg/day divided equally and given t.i.d. or q.i.d.

▶ *To treat pneumococcal pneumonia*

I.V. INFUSION OR INJECTION

Adults. 500 mg q 12 hr.

▶ *To treat acute uncomplicated UTIs caused by* E. coli, Klebsiella *species,* P. mirabilis, *and some strains of* Enterobacter *and* Enterococcus

I.V. INFUSION OR INJECTION

Adults. 1 g q 12 hr.

▶ *To provide surgical prophylaxis*

I.V. INFUSION OR INJECTION

Adults. 1 g 30 to 60 min before surgery, 0.5 to 1 g during surgery if procedure lasts 2 hr or longer, then 0.5 to 1 g q 6 to 8 hr for 24 hr after surgery.

DOSAGE ADJUSTMENT After initial loading dose appropriate to severity of infection, dosage interval restricted to at least 8 hr for adults with creatinine clearance of 35 to 54 ml/min/1.73 m^2; dosage reduced by 50% and given q 12 hr for adults with creatinine clearance of 11 to 34 ml/min/1.73 m^2; and dosage reduced by 50% and given q 18 to 24 hr for adults with creatinine clearance of 10 ml/min/1.73 m^2 or less. Dosage reduced to 60% and given q 12 hr for children with creatinine clearance of 40 to 70 ml/min/1.73 m^2; dosage reduced to 25% and given q 12 hr for children with creatinine clearance of 20 to 40 ml/min/1.73 m^2; and dosage reduced to 10% and given q 24 hr for children with creatinine clearance of 5 to 20 ml/min/1.73 m^2.

Mechanism of Action

Interferes with bacterial cell wall synthesis by inhibiting the final step in the cross-linking of peptidoglycan strands. Peptidoglycan makes cell membranes rigid and protective. Without it, bacterial cells rupture and die.

Incompatibilities

To prevent mutual inactivation, don't mix cefazolin with aminoglycosides. Also avoid mixing cefazolin with other drugs, including pentamidine isethionate.

Contraindications

Hypersensitivity to cephalosporins or their components

Interactions

DRUGS

aminoglycosides, loop diuretics: Additive nephrotoxicity
probenecid: Increased and prolonged blood cefazolin level

Adverse Reactions

CNS: Chills, fever, headache, seizures
CV: Edema
EENT: Hearing loss, oral candidiasis
GI: Abdominal cramps, diarrhea, elevated liver function test results, hepatic failure, hepatomegaly, nausea, pseudomembranous colitis, vomiting
GU: Elevated BUN level, nephrotoxicity, renal failure, vaginal candidiasis
HEME: Eosinophilia, hemolytic anemia, hypoprothrombinemia, neutropenia, thrombocytopenia, unusual bleeding

MS: Arthralgia
RESP: Dyspnea
SKIN: Ecchymosis, erythema, erythema multiforme, pruritus, rash, Stevens-Johnson syndrome
Other: Anaphylaxis, infusion site thrombophlebitis, superinfection

Nursing Considerations

• If possible, obtain culture and sensitivity test results, as ordered, before giving cefazolin.
• Reconstitute 500-mg vial of cefazolin for injection with 2 ml of sterile water for injection (or 1-g vial with 2.5 ml). Shake well until dissolved.
• For direct I.V. injection, further dilute reconstituted solution with at least 5 ml of sterile water for injection. Inject slowly over 3 to 5 minutes through tubing of a flowing compatible I.V. solution.
• For intermittent I.V. infusion, dilute 500 to 1,000 mg of reconstituted cefazolin in 50 to 100 ml of NS, D_5W, $D_{10}W$, D_5LR, $D_5/0.2NS$, $D_5/0.45NS$, D_5NS, LR, 5% or 10% invert sugar in sterile water for injection, 5% sodium bicarbonate (Ancef), or Ringer's solution.
• Store reconstituted cefazolin for up to 24 hours at room temperature or for up to 10 days under refrigeration.
• Be aware that cefazolin also comes in a plastic container with a concentration of 500 mg or 1 g in 50 ml. Store container at $-25°$ to $-10°$ C ($-13°$ to $14°$ F). Thaw at room temperature or under refrigeration. Don't use water bath or microwave to thaw. Don't refreeze. Drug inside plastic container retains potency for 48 hours when stored at room temperature and for 30 days when refrigerated.
• Monitor I.V. site for irritation, phlebitis, and extravasation.
• Monitor BUN and serum creatinine levels for early signs of nephrotoxicity, especially in patients with impaired renal function. Also monitor fluid intake and output; decreasing urine output may indicate nephrotoxicity.
• Monitor for signs of an allergic reaction, such as difficulty breathing or a rash, especially in patients who are hypersensitive to penicillin, because cross-sensitivity has occurred in about 10% of such patients. Be aware that an allergic reaction may occur a few days after therapy starts.
• Assess bowel pattern daily; severe diarrhea may indicate pseudomembranous colitis. Patients with a history of GI disease, particularly colitis, are at increased risk.

- Assess for signs of superinfection, such as perineal itching, fever, malaise, redness, pain, swelling, drainage, rash, diarrhea, and cough or sputum changes.
- Assess for pharyngitis, ecchymosis, bleeding, and arthralgia, which may indicate a blood dyscrasia. Monitor PT and bleeding time as ordered.
- Before reconstituting drug, store it at 15° to 30° C (59° to 86° F).

PATIENT TEACHING
- Advise patient receiving cefazolin to immediately report severe diarrhea or signs of blood dyscrasia or superinfection. Inform him that yogurt or buttermilk can help decrease diarrhea.
- Review with patient other possibly serious adverse reactions, including difficulty breathing, rash, and chest tightness, and tell him to report any that occur.

cefepime hydrochloride
Maxipime

Class and Category
Chemical: Fourth-generation cephalosporin, 7-aminocephalosporanic acid
Therapeutic: Antibiotic
Pregnancy category: B

Indications and Dosages
▶ *To treat mild to moderate UTIs caused by* Escherichia coli, Klebsiella pneumoniae, *and* Proteus mirabilis
I.V. INFUSION
Adults and children age 12 and older. 500 to 1,000 mg q 12 hr for 7 to 10 days.
▶ *To treat severe UTIs caused by* E. coli *or* K. pneumoniae *and moderate to severe skin and soft-tissue infections caused by* Staphylococcus aureus *or* Streptococcus pyogenes
I.V. INFUSION
Adults and children age 12 and older. 2 g q 12 hr for 10 days.
▶ *To treat moderate to severe pneumonia caused by* Enterobacter species, K. pneumoniae, Pseudomonas aeruginosa, *or* Streptococcus pneumoniae
I.V. INFUSION
Adults and children age 12 and older. 1 to 2 g q 12 hr for 10 days.

▶ *To treat febrile neutropenia*
I.V. INFUSION
Adults and children age 12 and older. 2 g q 8 hr for 7 days or until neutropenia resolves.

▶ *To treat complicated intra-abdominal infections (together with metronidazole) caused by alpha-hemolytic streptococci,* Bacteroides fragilis, E. coli, Enterobacter *species,* K. pneumoniae, *or* P. aeruginosa
I.V. INFUSION
Adults and children age 12 and older. 2 g q 12 hr for 7 to 10 days.

DOSAGE ADJUSTMENT Dosing interval increased from 12 to 24 hr or from 8 to 12 hr for patients with creatinine clearance of 30 to 60 ml/min/1.73 m^2; dosing interval increased from q 8 or 12 hr to q 24 hr and dosage decreased from 2 g q 12 hr to 1 g q 24 hr (all other doses remain unchanged) for patients with creatinine clearance of 11 to 29 ml/min/1.73 m^2; dosage decreased from 500 mg q 12 hr to 250 mg q 24 hr, from 1,000 mg q 12 hr to 250 mg q 24 hr, from 2,000 mg q 12 hr to 500 mg q 24 hr, and from 2 g q 8 hr to 1 g q 24 hr if creatinine clearance is less than 11 ml/min/1.73 m^2.

Mechanism of Action
Interferes with bacterial cell wall synthesis by inhibiting the final step in the cross-linking of peptidoglycan strands. Peptidoglycan makes cell membranes rigid and protective. Without it, bacterial cells rupture and die.

Incompatibilities
Don't add cefepime to solutions that contain ampicillin in a concentration of more than 40 mg/ml. Don't add drug to solutions that contain aminophylline, gentamicin, metronidazole, netilmicin sulfate, tobramycin, or vancomycin.

Contraindications
Hypersensitivity to cephalosporins or their components

Interactions
DRUGS
aminoglycosides, loop diuretics: Increased risk of renal failure in patients with renal disease
probenecid: Increased and prolonged blood cefepime level

Adverse Reactions
CNS: Chills, fever, headache, seizures
CV: Edema

EENT: Hearing loss, oral candidiasis
GI: Abdominal cramps, diarrhea, elevated liver function test results, hepatic failure, hepatomegaly, nausea, pseudomembranous colitis, vomiting
GU: Elevated BUN level, nephrotoxicity, renal failure, vaginal candidiasis
HEME: Eosinophilia, hemolytic anemia, hypoprothrombinemia, neutropenia, thrombocytopenia, unusual bleeding
MS: Arthralgia
RESP: Dyspnea
SKIN: Ecchymosis, erythema, erythema multiforme, pruritus, rash, Stevens-Johnson syndrome
Other: Anaphylaxis, infusion site thrombophlebitis, superinfection

Nursing Considerations

- If possible, obtain culture and sensitivity test results, as ordered, before giving cefepime.
- Reconstitute according to manufacturer's guidelines. Administer over 30 minutes.
- Be aware that after drug reconstitution, concentrations of 1 to 40 mg/ml retain potency for up to 24 hours if stored at 20° to 25° C (68° to 77° F) and for 7 days if refrigerated at 2° to 8° C (36° to 46° F).
- Monitor BUN and serum creatinine levels for early signs of nephrotoxicity, especially in patients with impaired renal function. Also monitor fluid intake and output; decreasing urine output may indicate nephrotoxicity.
- Monitor for signs of an allergic reaction, such as difficulty breathing or a rash, especially in patients who are hypersensitive to penicillin, because cross-sensitivity has occurred in about 10% of such patients. Be aware that an allergic reaction may occur a few days after therapy starts.
- Assess bowel pattern daily; severe diarrhea may indicate pseudomembranous colitis. Patients with a history of GI disease, particularly colitis, are at increased risk.
- Assess for signs of superinfection, such as perineal itching, fever, malaise, redness, pain, swelling, drainage, rash, diarrhea, and cough or sputum changes.
- Assess for pharyngitis, ecchymosis, bleeding, and arthralgia, which may indicate a blood dyscrasia. Monitor PT and bleeding time as ordered.
- Before reconstituting drug, store it between 2° and 25° C (36° and 77° F), and protect from light.

PATIENT TEACHING
- Advise patient receiving cefepime to immediately report severe diarrhea or signs of blood dyscrasia or superinfection. Inform him that yogurt or buttermilk can help decrease diarrhea.
- Review with patient other possibly serious adverse reactions, including difficulty breathing, rash, and chest tightness, and tell him to report any that occur.

cefmetazole sodium
Zefazone

Class and Category
Chemical: Second-generation cephalosporin, 7-aminocephalosporanic acid
Therapeutic: Antibiotic
Pregnancy category: B

Indications and Dosages
▶ *To treat UTIs caused by* Escherichia coli; *lower respiratory tract infections, such as bronchitis and pneumonia, caused by* E. coli, Haemophilus influenzae, Staphylococcus aureus, *and* Streptococcus pneumoniae; *skin and soft-tissue infections caused by* Bacteroides fragilis, B. melaninogenicus, E. coli, Klebsiella oxytoca, Klebsiella pneumoniae, Morganella morganii, Proteus mirabilis, Proteus vulgaris, S. aureus, Staphylococcus epidermidis, Streptococcus agalactiae, *and* Streptococcus pyogenes; *and intra-abdominal infections caused by* B. fragilis, Clostridium perfringens, E. coli, K. oxytoca, *and* K. pneumoniae

I.V. INFUSION
Adults. 2 g q 6 to 12 hr for 5 to 14 days.

DOSAGE ADJUSTMENT Dosage reduced to 1 to 2 g q 12 hr for patients with creatinine clearance of 50 to 90 ml/min/1.73 m^2; 1 to 2 g q 16 hr for patients with creatinine clearance of 30 to 49 ml/min/1.73 m^2; 1 to 2 g q 24 hr for patients with creatinine clearance of 10 to 29 ml/min/1.73 m^2; and 1 to 2 g q 48 hr for patients with creatinine clearance of less than 10 ml/min/1.73 m^2.

▶ *To provide surgical prophylaxis for vaginal hysterectomy*
I.V. INFUSION
Adults. 2 g as a single dose 30 to 90 min before surgery, or 1 g 30 to 90 min before surgery and repeated 8 and 16 hr later.

▶ *To provide surgical prophylaxis for abdominal hysterectomy and for high-risk cholecystectomy*
I.V. INFUSION
Adults. 1 g 30 to 90 min before surgery and repeated 8 and 16 hr later.

▶ *To provide surgical prophylaxis for cesarean section*
I.V. INFUSION
Adults. 2 g as a single dose after cord is clamped or 1 g after cord is clamped and then repeated 8 and 16 hr later.

▶ *To provide surgical prophylaxis for colorectal surgery*
I.V. INFUSION
Adults. 2 g as a single dose 30 to 90 min before surgery, or 2 g 30 to 90 min before surgery and repeated 8 and 16 hr later.

Mechanism of Action
Interferes with bacterial cell wall synthesis by inhibiting the final step in the cross-linking of peptidoglycan strands. Peptidoglycan makes cell membranes rigid and protective. Without it, bacterial cells rupture and die.

Contraindications
Hypersensitivity to cephalosporins or their components

Interactions
DRUGS
aminoglycosides, loop diuretics: Increased risk of nephrotoxicity
anticoagulants: Possibly increased anticoagulant effect
probenecid: Increased and prolonged blood cefmetazole level
ACTIVITIES
alcohol use: Possibly disulfiram-like reaction

Adverse Reactions
CNS: Chills, fever, headache, seizures
CV: Edema
EENT: Hearing loss, oral candidiasis
GI: Abdominal cramps, diarrhea, elevated liver function test results, hepatic failure, hepatomegaly, nausea, pseudomembranous colitis, vomiting
GU: Elevated BUN level, nephrotoxicity, renal failure, vaginal candidiasis

HEME: Eosinophilia, hemolytic anemia, hypoprothrombinemia, neutropenia, thrombocytopenia, unusual bleeding
MS: Arthralgia
RESP: Dyspnea
SKIN: Ecchymosis, erythema, erythema multiforme, pruritus, rash, Stevens-Johnson syndrome
Other: Anaphylaxis, infusion site thrombophlebitis, superinfection

Nursing Considerations

- If possible, obtain culture and sensitivity test results, as ordered, before giving cefmetazole.
- Reconstitute drug with sterile water for injection, bacteriostatic water for injection, or 0.9% sodium chloride for injection.
- Store reconstituted solution for up to 24 hours at room temperature or for up to 7 days when refrigerated. Solution may also be frozen at −20° C (−4° F) or less for up to 6 weeks.
- Dilute primary solution as needed to 1 to 20 mg/ml in D_5W, NS, LR, or 1% lidocaine solution without epinephrine. Diluted solution remains potent for 24 hours if stored at room temperature, for 7 days if refrigerated, and for 6 weeks if frozen.
- Monitor for signs of an allergic reaction, such as difficulty breathing or a rash, especially in patients who are hypersensitive to penicillin, because cross-sensitivity has occurred in about 10% of such patients.
- Monitor BUN and serum creatinine levels to detect early signs of nephrotoxicity, especially in patients with impaired renal function. Also monitor fluid intake and output; decreasing urine output may indicate nephrotoxicity.
- Assess bowel pattern daily; severe diarrhea may indicate pseudomembranous colitis. Patients with a history of GI disease, particularly colitis, are at increased risk.
- Assess for signs of superinfection, such as perineal itching, fever, malaise, redness, pain, swelling, drainage, rash, diarrhea, and cough or sputum changes.
- Assess for pharyngitis, ecchymosis, bleeding, and arthralgia, which may indicate a blood dyscrasia. Monitor PT and bleeding time as ordered.
- Don't refreeze thawed solutions.

PATIENT TEACHING
- Advise patient receiving cefmetazole to immediately report severe diarrheaor signs of blood dyscrasia or superinfection. Inform him that yogurt or buttermilk can help decrease diarrhea.

- Instruct patient to avoid alcohol during therapy and for at least 3 days after taking last dose.
- Review with patient other possibly serious adverse reactions, including difficulty breathing, rash, and chest tightness, and tell him to report any that occur.

cefonicid sodium

Monocid

Class and Category

Chemical: Second-generation cephalosporin, 7-aminocephalosporanic acid
Therapeutic: Antibiotic
Pregnancy category: B

Indications and Dosages

▶ *To treat lower respiratory tract infections caused by* Escherichia coli, Haemophilus influenzae, Klebsiella pneumoniae, *and* Streptococcus pneumoniae; *UTIs caused by* E. coli, K. pneumoniae, Morganella morganii, Proteus mirabilis, Proteus vulgaris, *and* Providencia rettgeri; *skin and soft-tissue infections caused by* Staphylococcus aureus, Staphylococcus epidermidis, Streptococcus agalactiae, *and* Streptococcus pyogenes; *septicemia caused by* E. coli *and* S. pneumoniae; *and bone and joint infections caused by* S. aureus

I.V. INFUSION OR INJECTION

Adults. For mild to moderate infections, 1 g q 24 hr; for severe or life-threatening infections, 2 g q 24 hr.

▶ *To treat uncomplicated UTIs*

I.V. INFUSION OR INJECTION

Adults. 500 mg q 24 hr.

DOSAGE ADJUSTMENT Initial dose reduced to 75 mg/kg in patients with impaired renal function. Then dosage reduced to 10 to 25 mg/kg q 24 hr if creatinine clearance ranges from 60 to 79 ml/min/1.73 m^2; 8 to 20 mg/kg q 24 hr if creatinine clearance ranges from 40 to 59 ml/min/1.73 m^2; 4 to 15 mg/kg q 24 hr if creatinine clearance ranges from 20 to 39 ml/min/1.73 m^2; 4 to 15 mg/kg q 48 hr if creatinine clearance ranges from 10 to 19 ml/min/1.73 m^2; 4 to 15 mg/kg q 3 to 5 days if creatinine clearance ranges from 5 to 9 ml/minute/1.73 m^2; and 3 to 4 mg/kg q 3 to 5 days if creatinine clearance is less than 5 ml/min/1.73 m^2.

▶ *To provide surgical prophylaxis*
I.V. INFUSION OR INJECTION
Adults. 1 g 60 min before surgery. Dose repeated once daily, if needed, for 2 days after prosthetic arthroplasty or open-heart surgery.

Mechanism of Action
Interferes with bacterial cell wall synthesis by inhibiting the final step in the cross-linking of peptidoglycan strands. Peptidoglycan makes cell membranes rigid and protective. Without it, bacterial cells rupture and die.

Incompatibilities
To prevent mutual inactivation, don't mix cefonicid with aminoglycosides.

Contraindications
Hypersensitivity to cephalosporins or their components

Interactions
DRUGS
aminoglycosides, loop diuretics: Increased risk of nephrotoxicity
probenecid: Increased and prolonged blood cefonicid level

Adverse Reactions
CNS: Chills, fever, headache, seizures
CV: Edema
EENT: Hearing loss, oral candidiasis
GI: Abdominal cramps, diarrhea, elevated liver function test results, hepatic failure, hepatomegaly, nausea, pseudomembranous colitis, vomiting
GU: Elevated BUN level, nephrotoxicity, renal failure, vaginal candidiasis
HEME: Eosinophilia, hemolytic anemia, hypoprothrombinemia, neutropenia, thrombocytopenia, unusual bleeding
MS: Arthralgia
RESP: Dyspnea
SKIN: Ecchymosis, erythema, erythema multiforme, pruritus, rash, Stevens-Johnson syndrome
Other: Anaphylaxis, infusion site thrombophlebitis, superinfection

Nursing Considerations
• If possible, obtain culture and sensitivity test results, as ordered, before giving cefonicid.

- Reconstitute each 500-mg vial of drug with 2 ml of sterile water for injection (or each 1-g vial with 2.5 ml).
- For I.V. infusion, dilute further in 50 to 100 ml of compatible solution, such as D_5W, $D_{10}W$, $D_5/0.2NS$, $D_5/0.45NS$, or D_5NS.
- Be aware that 1 g of cefonicid/18 ml of sterile water for injection is an isotonic solution.
- Store reconstituted solution at room temperature for up to 24 hours or under refrigeration for up to 72 hours.
- Administer I.V. injection slowly over 3 to 5 minutes through tubing of a flowing compatible I.V. solution.
- Monitor for signs of an allergic reaction, such as difficulty breathing or a rash, especially in patients who are hypersensitive to penicillin, because cross-sensitivity has occurred in about 10% of such patients.
- Monitor BUN and serum creatinine levels to detect early signs of nephrotoxicity, especially in patients with impaired renal function. Also monitor fluid intake and output; decreasing urine output may indicate nephrotoxicity.
- Assess bowel pattern daily; severe diarrhea may indicate pseudomembranous colitis. Patients with a history of GI disease, particularly colitis, are at increased risk.
- Assess for signs of superinfection, such as perineal itching, fever, malaise, redness, pain, swelling, drainage, rash, diarrhea, and cough or sputum changes.
- Assess for pharyngitis, ecchymosis, bleeding, and arthralgia, which may indicate a blood dyscrasia. Monitor PT and bleeding time as ordered.
- Before reconstituting drug, store it at 2° to 8° C (36° to 46° F). Protect from light.

PATIENT TEACHING
- Advise patient receiving cefonicid to immediately report severe diarrhea or signs of blood dyscrasia or superinfection. Inform him that yogurt or buttermilk can help decrease diarrhea.
- Review with patient other possibly serious adverse reactions, including difficulty breathing, rash, and chest tightness, and tell him to report any that occur.

cefoperazone sodium
Cefobid

Class and Category
Chemical: Third-generation cephalosporin, 7-aminocephalosporanic acid

Therapeutic: Antibiotic
Pregnancy category: B

Indications and Dosages

▶ *To treat respiratory tract infections caused by* Enterobacter *species,* Escherichia coli, Haemophilus influenzae, Klebsiella pneumoniae, Proteus mirabilis, Pseudomonas aeruginosa, Staphylococcus aureus, Streptococcus pneumoniae, Streptococcus pyogenes, *and other streptococci (excluding enterococci); UTIs caused by* E. coli *and* P. aeruginosa; *uncomplicated gonorrhea caused by* Neisseria gonorrhoeae; *gynecologic infections caused by anaerobic gram-positive cocci,* Bacteroides *species,* Clostridium *species,* E. coli, Staphylococcus epidermidis, *and* Streptococcus agalactiae; *bacterial septicemia caused by* E. coli, Klebsiella *species,* S. aureus, Serratia marcescens, *and streptococci; skin and soft-tissue infections caused by* P. aeruginosa, S. aureus, *and* S. pyogenes; *and intra-abdominal infections caused by anaerobic gram-negative bacilli,* E. coli, *and* P. aeruginosa

I.V. INFUSION

Adults. 1 to 2 g q 12 hr. For severe infections or those caused by less sensitive organisms, 6 to 12 g/day divided into equal doses and given b.i.d., t.i.d., or q.i.d. *Maximum:* 12 g/day.

Mechanism of Action

Interferes with bacterial cell wall synthesis by inhibiting the final step in the cross-linking of peptidoglycan strands. Peptidoglycan makes cell membranes rigid and protective. Without it, bacterial cells rupture and die.

Incompatibilities

To prevent mutual inactivation, don't mix cefoperazone with aminoglycosides. Also avoid mixing cefoperazone with other drugs, including pentamidine isethionate.

Contraindications

Hypersensitivity to cephalosporins or their components

Interactions

DRUGS

aminoglycosides, loop diuretics: Increased risk of nephrotoxicity
oral anticoagulants, other drugs that affect blood clotting: Increased anticoagulant effect

ACTIVITIES

alcohol use: Disulfiram-like reaction from acetaldehyde accumulation

Adverse Reactions

CNS: Chills, fever, headache, seizures

CV: Edema

EENT: Hearing loss, oral candidiasis

GI: Abdominal cramps, diarrhea, elevated liver function test results, hepatic failure, hepatomegaly, nausea, pseudomembranous colitis, vomiting

GU: Elevated BUN level, nephrotoxicity, renal failure, vaginal candidiasis

HEME: Eosinophilia, hemolytic anemia, hypoprothrombinemia, neutropenia, thrombocytopenia, unusual bleeding

MS: Arthralgia

RESP: Dyspnea

SKIN: Ecchymosis, erythema, erythema multiforme, pruritus, rash, Stevens-Johnson syndrome

Other: Anaphylaxis, infusion site thrombophlebitis, superinfection

Nursing Considerations

- Expect cefoperazone dosage to be reduced for patients with combined renal and hepatic function impairment. Monitor serum drug levels in patients with impaired hepatic function or biliary obstruction who are receiving more than 4 g/day; dosage may need to be reduced.
- If possible, obtain culture and sensitivity test results, as ordered, before giving drug.
- Reconstitute cefoperazone for injection with required amount of diluent; then dilute further in compatible solution, such as D_5W, $D_{10}W$, D_5LR, $D_5/0.2NS$, D_5NS, LR, NS, Normosol M and D_5W, or Normosol R. (See manufacturer's guidelines for details.)
- After drug reconstitution, let foam dissipate and inspect solution to ensure complete dissolution.
- Store reconstituted solution of cefoperazone for injection at room temperature for 24 hours.
- Be aware that cefoperazone also comes in a minibag (cefoperazone injection) with a concentration of 1 or 2 g/50 ml. Before use, store minibag at −25° to −10° C (−13° to 14 ° F). Thaw at room temperature of 25° C (77° F) or under refrigeration at

5° C (41° F). Don't thaw with warm bath or microwave. Make sure that all ice crystals have melted before use.

- After thawing minibag, use it within 48 hours if stored at room temperature or within 14 days if refrigerated. Don't refreeze. Discard solution if it's cloudy or contains precipitate.
- To prevent air embolism, don't administer minibags (cefoperazone injection) using I.V. lines with series connections.
- Administer I.V. drug as intermittent infusion over 15 to 30 minutes or as continuous infusion. Direct bolus injection isn't recommended.
- Monitor BUN and serum creatinine levels to detect early signs of nephrotoxicity. Also monitor fluid intake and output; decreasing urine output may indicate nephrotoxicity.
- Monitor for signs of an allergic reaction, such as difficulty breathing or a rash, especially in patients who are hypersensitive to penicillin, because cross-sensitivity has occurred in about 10% of such patients.
- Assess bowel pattern daily; severe diarrhea may indicate pseudomembranous colitis. Patients with a history of GI disease, particularly colitis, are at increased risk.
- Assess for pharyngitis, ecchymosis, bleeding, and arthralgia, which may indicate a blood dyscrasia. Monitor PT and bleeding time as ordered. Be prepared to administer vitamin K, if ordered, to treat hypoprothrombinemia.
- Assess for signs of superinfection, such as perineal itching, fever, malaise, redness, pain, swelling, drainage, rash, diarrhea, and cough or sputum changes.
- Before reconstituting cefoperazone for injection, store at 15° to 30° C (59° to 86° F). Protect from light.

PATIENT TEACHING
- Ask patient to avoid alcohol during cefoperazone therapy and for at least 3 days after taking the last dose.
- Instruct patient to immediately report severe diarrhea or signs of blood dyscrasia or superinfection. Inform him that yogurt or buttermilk can help decrease diarrhea.
- Review with patient other possibly serious adverse reactions, including difficulty breathing, rash, and chest tightness, and tell him to report any that occur.

cefotaxime sodium
Claforan

Class and Category
Chemical: Third-generation cephalosporin, 7-aminocephalosporanic acid
Therapeutic: Antibiotic
Pregnancy category: B

Indications and Dosages
▶ *To provide perioperative prophylaxis*
I.V. INFUSION OR INJECTION
Adults and children who weigh 50 kg (110 lb) or more. 1 g 30 to 90 min before surgery.
▶ *To provide perioperative prophylaxis related to cesarean section*
I.V. INFUSION OR INJECTION
Adults. 1 g as soon as cord is clamped. Then 1 g q 6 hr up to two doses.
▶ *To treat disseminated gonorrhea*
I.V. INFUSION OR INJECTION
Adults and children who weigh 50 kg or more. 1 g q 8 hr.
▶ *To treat uncomplicated infections caused by susceptible organisms*
I.V. INFUSION OR INJECTION
Adults and children who weigh 50 kg or more. 1 g q 12 hr.
Children ages 1 month to 12 years who weigh less than 50 kg. 50 to 180 mg/kg/day in four to six divided doses.
Infants ages 1 to 4 weeks. 50 mg/kg q 8 hr.
Infants up to 1 week old. 50 mg/kg q 12 hr.
▶ *To treat moderate to severe infections caused by susceptible organisms*
I.V. INFUSION OR INJECTION
Adults and children who weigh 50 kg or more. 1 to 2 g q 8 hr.
Children ages 1 month to 12 years who weigh less than 50 kg. 50 to 180 mg/kg/day in four to six divided doses. For more serious infections, including meningitis, higher dosages are used.
Infants ages 1 to 4 weeks. 50 mg/kg q 8 hr.
Infants up to 1 week old. 50 mg/kg q 12 hr.

▶ *To treat septicemia and other infections that commonly require antibiotics in higher doses than those used to treat moderate to severe infections*

I.V. INFUSION OR INJECTION

Adults and children who weigh 50 kg or more. 2 g q 6 to 8 hr.

▶ *To treat life-threatening infections caused by susceptible organisms*

I.V. INFUSION OR INJECTION

Adults and children who weigh 50 kg or more. 2 g q 4 hr. *Maximum:* 12 g/day.

Children ages 1 month to 12 years who weigh less than 50 kg. 50 to 180 mg/kg/day in four to six divided doses.

Infants ages 1 to 4 weeks. 50 mg/kg q 8 hr.

Infants up to 1 week old. 50 mg/kg q 12 hr.

DOSAGE ADJUSTMENT Dosage reduced by 50% for patients with estimated creatinine clearance below 20 ml/min/1.73 m^2.

Mechanism of Action

Interferes with bacterial cell wall synthesis by inhibiting the final step in the cross-linking of peptidoglycan strands. Peptidoglycan makes cell membranes rigid and protective. Without it, bacterial cells rupture and die.

Incompatibilities

To prevent mutual inactivation, don't mix cefotaxime with aminoglycosides. Also avoid mixing cefotaxime with other drugs, including pentamidine isethionate.

Contraindications

Hypersensitivity to cephalosporins or their components

Interactions

DRUGS

aminoglycosides, loop diuretics: Increased risk of nephrotoxicity
probenecid: Increased and prolonged blood cefotaxime level

Adverse Reactions

CNS: Chills, fever, headache, seizures
CV: Edema
EENT: Hearing loss
GI: Abdominal cramps, diarrhea, elevated liver function test results, hepatic failure, hepatomegaly, nausea, oral candidiasis, pseudomembranous colitis, vomiting

GU: Elevated BUN level, nephrotoxicity, renal failure, vaginal candidiasis
HEME: Eosinophilia, hemolytic anemia, hypoprothrombinemia, neutropenia, thrombocytopenia, unusual bleeding
MS: Arthralgia
RESP: Dyspnea
SKIN: Ecchymosis, erythema, erythema multiforme, pruritus, rash, Stevens-Johnson syndrome
Other: Anaphylaxis, insertion site thrombophlebitis, superinfection

Nursing Considerations

• If possible, obtain culture and sensitivity test results, as ordered, before giving cefotaxime.
• **WARNING** When preparing drug for administration to a neonate, don't use diluents that contain benzyl alcohol because these have been linked to a fatal toxic syndrome.
• Reconstitute each 0.5-, 1-, or 2-g vial of cefotaxime for injection with 10 ml of sterile water for injection. Shake to dissolve.
• For intermittent I.V. infusion, further dilute in 50 to 100 ml of D_5W or NS.
• Be aware that cefotaxime also comes in a minibag (cefotaxime injection) with a concentration of 1 or 2 g/50 ml. Before use, store minibag at −25° to −10° C (−13° to 14° F). Thaw at room temperature or in refrigerator. Don't use warm bath or microwave to thaw.
• Discard minibag after 24 hours if stored at room temperature or after 10 days if refrigerated. Don't refreeze. Don't use solution if it's cloudy or contains precipitate.
• To prevent air embolism, don't administer minibags (cefotaxime injection) using I.V. lines with series connections.
• Administer cefotaxime by I.V. injection slowly over 3 to 5 minutes through tubing of a flowing compatible I.V. solution. Temporarily stop other solutions being given through same I.V. site.
• Discard unused portion of cefotaxime for injection after 12 hours (for a 2-g vial) or 24 hours (for a 500-mg or 1-g vial) if stored at room temperature. Discard after 5 days if refrigerated in plastic syringes or after 7 days if refrigerated in original container.
• Protect cefotaxime powder and solution from light and heat. Darkening of solution doesn't affect potency.
• Monitor I.V. sites for signs of phlebitis or extravasation. Rotate I.V. sites every 72 hours.

- Monitor BUN and serum creatinine levels for early signs of nephrotoxicity, especially in patients with impaired renal function. Also monitor fluid intake and output; decreasing urine output may indicate nephrotoxicity.
- Monitor for signs of an allergic reaction, such as difficulty breathing or a rash, especially in patients who are hypersensitive to penicillin, because cross-sensitivity has occurred in about 10% of such patients. Be aware that an allergic reaction may occur a few days after therapy starts.
- Assess bowel pattern daily; severe diarrhea may indicate pseudomembranous colitis. Patients with a history of GI disease, particularly colitis, are at increased risk.
- Assess for pharyngitis, ecchymosis, bleeding, and arthralgia, which may indicate a blood dyscrasia. Monitor PT and bleeding time as ordered.
- Be aware that 1 g of cefotaxime/14 ml of sterile water for injection is an isotonic solution.

PATIENT TEACHING
- Advise patient receiving cefotaxime to immediately report severe diarrhea or signs of blood dyscrasia or superinfection. Inform him that yogurt or buttermilk can help decrease diarrhea.
- Review with patient other possibly serious adverse reactions, including difficulty breathing, rash, and chest tightness, and tell him to report any that occur.

cefotetan disodium
Cefotan

Class and Category
Chemical: Second-generation cephalosporin, 7-aminocephalosporanic acid
Therapeutic: Antibiotic
Pregnancy category: B

Indications and Dosages
▶ *To provide surgical prophylaxis*
I.V. INJECTION
Adults. 1 to 2 g 30 to 60 min before surgery or, if cesarean section, as soon as cord is clamped.
▶ *To treat lower respiratory tract infections caused by* Escherichia coli, Haemophilus influenzae, Klebsiella species, Proteus mirabilis, Serratia marcescens, Staphylococcus aureus, *and* Streptococcus pneumoniae; *gynecologic infections caused by*

Bacteroides *species (excluding* B. distasonis, B. ovatus, *and* B. thetaiotaomicron*),* E. coli, Fusobacterium *species, gram-positive anaerobic cocci,* Neisseria gonorrhoeae, P. mirabilis, S. aureus, Staphylococcus epidermidis, *and* Streptococcus *species (excluding enterococci); intra-abdominal infections caused by* Bacteroides *species (excluding* B. distasonis, B. ovatus, *and* B. thetaiotaomicron*),* Clostridium *species,* E. coli, Klebsiella *species, and* Streptococcus *species (excluding enterococci); and bone and joint infections caused by* S. aureus

I.V. INFUSION OR INJECTION

Adults. For mild to moderate infections, 1 or 2 g q 12 hr; for severe infections, 2 g q 12 hr; for life-threatening infections, 3 g q 12 hr.

▶ *To treat UTIs caused by* E. coli, Klebsiella *species, and* Proteus *species*

I.V. INFUSION OR INJECTION

Adults. 0.5 to 2 g q 12 hr or 1 or 2 g q 24 hr.

▶ *To treat skin and soft-tissue infections caused by* E. coli, Klebsiella pneumoniae, Peptostreptococcus *species,* S. aureus, S. epidermidis, Streptococcus pyogenes, *and other* Streptococcus *species (excluding enterococci)*

I.V. INFUSION OR INJECTION

Adults. For mild to moderate infections due to *K. pneumoniae,* 1 or 2 g q 12 hr; for mild to moderate infections caused by other organisms, 1 g q 12 hr or 2 g q 24 hr; for severe infections, 2 g q 12 hr. **DOSAGE ADJUSTMENT** Dosing interval reduced to 24 hr for patients with creatinine clearance of 10 to 30 ml/min/ 1.73 m² and to 48 hr for patients with creatinine clearance below 10 ml/min/1.73 m².

Mechanism of Action

Like all cephalosporins, cefotetan interferes with bacterial cell wall synthesis by inhibiting the final step in the cross-linking of peptidoglycan strands. Peptidoglycan makes the cell membrane rigid and protective. Without it, bacterial cells rupture and die. This mechanism of action is most effective against bacteria that divide rapidly, including many gram-positive and gram-negative bacteria.

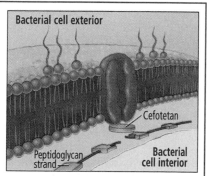

Bacterial cell exterior

Cefotetan

Peptidoglycan strand

Bacterial cell interior

Incompatibilities
Don't mix cefotetan with aminoglycosides to prevent mutual inactivation.

Contraindications
Hypersensitivity to cephalosporins or their components

Interactions
DRUGS
aminoglycosides, loop diuretics: Increased risk of nephrotoxicity
oral anticoagulants, other drugs that affect blood clotting: Enhanced anticoagulant effect
probenecid: Increased and prolonged blood cefotetan level
ACTIVITIES
alcohol use: Disulfiram-like reaction

Adverse Reactions
CNS: Chills, fever, headache, seizures
CV: Edema
EENT: Hearing loss
GI: Abdominal cramps, diarrhea, elevated liver function test results, hepatic failure, hepatomegaly, nausea, oral candidiasis, pseudomembranous colitis, vomiting
GU: Elevated BUN level, nephrotoxicity, renal failure, vaginal candidiasis
HEME: Eosinophilia, hemolytic anemia, hypoprothrombinemia, neutropenia, thrombocytopenia, unusual bleeding
MS: Arthralgia
RESP: Dyspnea
SKIN: Ecchymosis, erythema, erythema multiforme, pruritus, rash, Stevens-Johnson syndrome
Other: Anaphylaxis; infusion site pain, redness, and swelling; superinfection

Nursing Considerations
• If possible, obtain culture and sensitivity test results, as ordered, before giving cefotetan.
• Reconstitute each 1-g vial of cefotetan for injection with 10 ml of sterile water for injection. For each 2-g vial, use 10 to 20 ml of diluent. For I.V. infusion, further dilute solution in 50 to 100 ml of D_5W or NS.
• Protect reconstituted solution from light; store for up to 24 hours at room temperature or for up to 96 hours if refrigerated.

• For direct I.V. injection, administer drug slowly, over 3 to 5 minutes, through tubing of a flowing compatible I.V. solution.
• Be aware that cefotetan also comes in a minibag (cefotetan injection) with a concentration of 1 or 2 g/50 ml. Before using minibag, store it at –20° C (–4° F). Thaw at room temperature or in refrigerator. Don't use warm bath or microwave to thaw.
• Discard minibag after 48 hours if stored at room temperature or after 21 days if refrigerated. Don't refreeze. Don't use solution if it contains precipitate or is cloudy.
• To prevent air embolism, don't administer minibag using I.V. lines with series connections.
• Monitor I.V. site for signs of phlebitis and extravasation; rotate sites every 72 hours.
• Monitor for signs of an allergic reaction, such as difficulty breathing or a rash, especially in patients who are hypersensitive to penicillin, because cross-sensitivity has occurred in about 10% of such patients. Be aware that an allergic reaction may occur a few days after therapy starts.
• Monitor BUN and serum creatinine levels for early signs of nephrotoxicity, especially in patients with impaired renal function. Also monitor fluid intake and output; decreasing urine output may indicate nephrotoxicity.
• If patient receives long-term therapy, monitor CBC and serum AST, ALT, bilirubin, LD, and alkaline phosphatase levels.
• Assess bowel elimination pattern daily; severe diarrhea may indicate pseudomembranous colitis. Patients with a history of GI disease, particularly colitis, are at increased risk.
• Assess for pharyngitis, ecchymosis, bleeding, and arthralgia, which may indicate a blood dyscrasia. Monitor PT and bleeding time as ordered. Be prepared to administer vitamin K, if ordered, to treat hypoprothrombinemia.
• Assess for signs of superinfection, including perineal itching, fever, malaise, redness, swelling, rash, and change in cough or sputum.
• Before reconstituting cefotetan for injection, store it below 22° C (72° F).

PATIENT TEACHING
• Instruct patient receiving cefotetan to immediately report severe diarrhea or signs of blood dyscrasias or superinfection. Inform him that yogurt or buttermilk can help maintain intestinal flora and decrease diarrhea.

- Review with patient other possibly serious adverse reactions, such as difficulty breathing, rash, and chest tightness, and tell him to report any that occur.
- Urge patient to avoid alcohol during cefotetan therapy and for at least 3 days after taking last dose.

cefoxitin sodium

Mefoxin

Class and Category

Chemical: Second-generation cephalosporin, 7-aminocephalosporanic acid
Therapeutic: Antibiotic
Pregnancy category: B

Indications and Dosages

▶ *To provide surgical prophylaxis*
I.V. INFUSION OR INJECTION
Adults. 2 g 30 to 60 min before surgery and then 2 g q 6 hr after first dose for up to 24 hr.
Children age 3 months and older. 30 to 40 mg/kg 30 to 60 min before surgery and then q 6 hr after first dose for up to 24 hr.
▶ *To provide surgical prophylaxis for cesarean section*
I.V. INFUSION OR INJECTION
Adults. 2 g as a single dose as soon as cord is clamped, or 2 g as soon as cord is clamped followed by 2 g 4 and 8 hr after initial dose.
▶ *To provide surgical prophylaxis for transurethral prostatectomy*
I.V. INFUSION OR INJECTION
Adults. 1 g 30 to 60 min before surgery and then 1 g q 8 hr for up to 5 days.
▶ *To treat infections, such as septicemia, gynecologic infections, intra-abdominal infections, UTIs, and infections of the lower respiratory tract, skin, soft tissue, bones, and joints caused by anaerobes (including* Bacteroides *species,* Clostridium *species,* Fusobacterium *species,* Peptococcus niger, *and* Peptostreptococcus *species), gram-negative organisms (including* Escherichia coli, Haemophilus influenzae *[also ampicillin-resistant strains],* Klebsiella, *and* Proteus *species), and gram-positive organisms (including* Staphylococcus aureus *[penicillinase- and non-penicillinase-producing strains],* Staphylococcus epidermidis, Streptococcus agalactiae, Streptococcus pneumoniae, *and* Streptococcus pyogenes)

I.V. INFUSION OR INJECTION

Adults. For uncomplicated infections, 1 g q 6 to 8 hr; for moderate to severe infections, 1 g q 4 hr or 2 g q 6 to 8 hr; for infections that commonly require high-dose antibiotics (such as gas gangrene), 2 g q 4 hr or 3 g q 6 hr.

Children age 3 months and older. 80 to 160 mg/kg/day given in equal doses q 4 to 6 hr (with higher dosages used for more severe infections). *Maximum:* 12 g/day.

DOSAGE ADJUSTMENT Dosage reduced to 1 to 2 g q 8 to 12 hr for patients with creatinine clearance of 30 to 50 ml/min/1.73 m^2; to 1 to 2 g q 12 to 24 hr for patients with creatinine clearance of 10 to 29 ml/min/1.73 m^2; to 0.5 to 1 g q 12 to 24 hr for patients with creatinine clearance of 5 to 9 ml/min/1.73 m^2; and to 0.5 to 1 g q 24 to 48 hr for patients with creatinine clearance of less than 5 ml/min/1.73 m^2.

Mechanism of Action

Interferes with bacterial cell wall synthesis by inhibiting the final step in the cross-linking of peptidoglycan strands. Peptidoglycan makes cell membranes rigid and protective. Without it, bacterial cells rupture and die.

Incompatibilities

Don't mix cefoxitin with aminoglycosides to prevent mutual inactivation. Also avoid mixing cefoxitin with other drugs, including pentamidine isethionate.

Contraindications

Hypersensitivity to cephalosporins or their components

Interactions

DRUGS

aminoglycosides, loop diuretics: Increased risk of nephrotoxicity
probenecid: Increased and prolonged blood cefoxitin level

Adverse Reactions

CNS: Chills, fever, headache, seizures
CV: Edema
EENT: Hearing loss
GI: Abdominal cramps, diarrhea, elevated liver function test results, hepatic failure, hepatomegaly, nausea, oral candidiasis, pseudomembranous colitis, vomiting
GU: Elevated BUN level, nephrotoxicity, renal failure, vaginal candidiasis

HEME: Eosinophilia, hemolytic anemia, hypoprothrombinemia, neutropenia, thrombocytopenia, unusual bleeding
MS: Arthralgia
RESP: Dyspnea
SKIN: Ecchymosis, erythema, erythema multiforme, pruritus, rash, Stevens-Johnson syndrome
Other: Anaphylaxis; infusion site pain, redness, and swelling; superinfection

Nursing Considerations

- If possible, obtain culture and sensitivity test results, as ordered, before giving cefoxitin.
- **WARNING** When preparing drug for administration to neonates or premature infants, don't use diluents that contain benzyl alcohol because they have been linked to a fatal toxic syndrome characterized by CNS, respiratory, circulatory, and renal impairment and metabolic acidosis.
- Reconstitute 1 g of cefoxitin for injection with 10 ml of sterile water for injection or 2 g of cefoxitin for injection with 10 to 20 ml of diluent.
- Administer I.V. injection slowly, over 3 to 5 minutes, through tubing of a flowing compatible I.V. solution.
- When administering drug by intermittent infusion, further dilute it with 50 to 100 ml of D_5W or NS.
- When administering drug by continuous high-dose infusion, add cefoxitin to I.V. solution of D_5W, NS, or D_5NS.
- Discard unused drug after 24 hours if stored at room temperature or after 1 week if refrigerated.
- Be aware that cefoxitin also comes in a minibag (cefoxitin injection) with a concentration of 1 or 2 g/50 ml. Before using minibag, store it between –25° and –10° C (–13° and 14° F). Thaw it at room temperature or in refrigerator. Don't use warm bath or microwave to thaw.
- Discard minibag after 24 hours if stored at room temperature or after 21 days if refrigerated. Don't refreeze. Don't use solution if it contains precipitate or is cloudy.
- To prevent air embolism, don't administer minibag using I.V. lines with series connections.
- Be aware that powder or solution may darken during storage, a change that doesn't reflect altered potency.
- Monitor for signs of an allergic reaction, such as difficulty breathing or a rash, especially in patients who are hypersensitive to penicillin, because cross-sensitivity has occurred in about

10% of such patients. Be aware that an allergic reaction may occur a few days after therapy starts.

• Monitor BUN and serum creatinine levels for early signs of nephrotoxicity, especially in patients with impaired renal function. Also monitor fluid intake and output; decreasing urine output may indicate nephrotoxicity.

• Assess bowel elimination pattern daily; severe diarrhea may indicate pseudomembranous colitis. Patients with a history of GI disease, particularly colitis, are at increased risk.

• Assess for pharyngitis, ecchymosis, bleeding, and arthralgia, which may indicate a blood dyscrasia. Monitor PT and bleeding time as ordered.

• Assess for signs of superinfection, such as perineal itching, fever, malaise, redness, swelling, rash, and change in cough or sputum.

• Before using cefoxitin for injection, store it at 15° to 30° C (59° to 86° F).

PATIENT TEACHING

• Instruct patient receiving cefoxitin to immediately report severe diarrhea or signs of blood dyscrasias or superinfection. Inform him that yogurt and buttermilk can help maintain intestinal flora and decrease diarrhea.

• Review with patient other possibly serious adverse reactions, such as difficulty breathing, rash, and chest tightness, and tell him to report any that occur.

ceftazidime

Ceptaz, Fortaz, Tazicef, Tazidime

Class and Category

Chemical: Third-generation cephalosporin, 7-aminocephalosporanic acid

Therapeutic: Antibiotic

Pregnancy category: B

Indications and Dosages

▶ *To treat infections caused by gram-negative organisms, including* Acinetobacter, Citrobacter, Enterobacter, Escherichia coli, Haemophilus influenzae, Klebsiella, Neisseria, Proteus mirabilis, Proteus vulgaris, Pseudomonas aeruginosa, Salmonella, Serratia, *and* Shigella; *gram-positive organisms, including* Streptococcus agalactiae, Streptococcus pneumoniae, *and* Streptococcus pyogenes *(group B streptococci); as well as*

Staphylococcus aureus *(penicillinase- and non-penicillinase-producing strains)*
I.V. INFUSION
Adults and children over age 12. 1 g q 8 to 12 hr.
Children ages 1 month to 12 years. 30 to 50 mg/kg q 8 hr. *Maximum:* 6 g/day.
Neonates up to age 1 month. 30 mg/kg q 12 hr.
▶ *To treat uncomplicated UTIs*
I.V. INFUSION
Adults and children over age 12. 250 mg q 12 hr.
▶ *To treat complicated UTIs*
I.V. INFUSION
Adults and children over age 12. 500 mg q 8 to 12 hr.
▶ *To treat uncomplicated pneumonia and mild skin and soft-tissue infections*
I.V. INFUSION
Adults and children over age 12. 0.5 to 1 g q 8 hr.
▶ *To treat bone and joint infections*
I.V. INFUSION
Adults and children over age 12. 2 g q 12 hr.
▶ *To treat serious gynecologic and intra-abdominal infections, meningitis, and life-threatening infections, especially in immunocompromised patients*
I.V. INFUSION
Adults and children over age 12. 2 g q 8 hr.
▶ *To treat pseudomonal lung infection in patients with cystic fibrosis and normal renal function*
I.V. INFUSION
Adults and children age 1 month and older. 30 to 50 mg/kg q 8 hr. *Maximum:* 6 g/day.
Neonates up to age 1 month. 30 mg/kg q 12 hr.
DOSAGE ADJUSTMENT Dosage reduced to 1 g q 12 hr if creatinine clearance is 31 to 50 ml/min/1.73 m^2; to 1 g q 24 hr if creatinine clearance is 16 to 30 ml/min/1.73 m^2; to 0.5 g q 24 hr if creatinine clearance is 6 to 15 ml/min/1.73 m^2; and to 0.5 g q 48 hr if creatinine clearance is less than 6 ml/min/1.73 m^2.

Mechanism of Action
Interferes with bacterial cell wall synthesis by inhibiting the final step in the cross-linking of peptidoglycan strands. Peptidoglycan makes the cell membrane rigid and protective. Without it, bacterial cells rupture and die.

Incompatibilities

Don't mix ceftazidime with aminoglycosides to prevent mutual inactivation. Don't mix ceftazidime with vancomycin because they're physically incompatible and a precipitate may form; if these two drugs must be given through the same I.V. line, flush tubing between infusions. Also avoid mixing ceftazidime with other drugs, including pentamidine isethionate.

Contraindications

Hypersensitivity to cephalosporins or their components

Interactions

DRUGS

aminoglycosides, loop diuretics: Increased risk of nephrotoxicity

Adverse Reactions

CNS: Chills, fever, headache, seizures
CV: Edema
EENT: Hearing loss
GI: Abdominal cramps, diarrhea, elevated liver function test results, hepatic failure, hepatomegaly, nausea, oral candidiasis, pseudomembranous colitis, vomiting
GU: Elevated BUN level, nephrotoxicity, renal failure, vaginal candidiasis
HEME: Eosinophilia, hemolytic anemia, hypoprothrombinemia, neutropenia, thrombocytopenia, unusual bleeding
MS: Arthralgia
RESP: Dyspnea
SKIN: Ecchymosis, erythema, erythema multiforme, pruritus, rash, Stevens-Johnson syndrome
Other: Anaphylaxis; infusion site pain, redness, and swelling; superinfection

Nursing Considerations

• If possible, obtain culture and sensitivity test results, as ordered, before giving ceftazidime.
• Be aware that use of ceftazidime L-arginine formulation (Ceptaz) is not recommended for children under age 12.
• Protect ceftazidime powder and reconstituted drug from heat and light; both tend to darken during storage.
• **WARNING** When preparing drug for administration to neonates or premature infants, don't use diluents that contain benzyl alcohol because they have been linked to a fatal toxic syndrome characterized by CNS, respiratory, circulatory, and renal impairment and metabolic acidosis.

- When preparing I.V. bolus, reconstitute 1 to 2 g of drug with 10 ml of sterile water for injection, D_5W, or sodium chloride for injection. Shake to dissolve. Administer I.V. injection slowly, over 3 to 5 minutes, through tubing of a flowing compatible I.V. fluid.
- When preparing intermittent infusion, further dilute drug in 50 to 100 ml of D_5W or NS. During ceftazidime administration, temporarily stop other solutions being given at same I.V. site.
- Avoid using sodium bicarbonate injection as a diluent because drug is least stable in it.
- If frozen solution (minibag of ceftazidime injection in concentration of 1 or 2 g/50 ml) is delivered from pharmacy, thaw it only at room temperature. Don't use water bath or microwave to thaw. Store thawed solution for up to 24 hours at room temperature or 7 days in a refrigerator; don't refreeze.
- To prevent air embolism, don't administer minibag using I.V. lines with series connections. Don't use solution if it contains precipitate or is cloudy.
- Rotate I.V. sites every 72 hours. Assess for phlebitis and extravasation.
- Monitor for signs of an allergic reaction, such as difficulty breathing or a rash, especially in patients who are hypersensitive to penicillin, because cross-sensitivity has occurred in about 10% of such patients. Be aware that an allergic reaction may occur a few days after therapy starts.
- Monitor BUN and serum creatinine levels to detect early signs of nephrotoxicity, especially in patients with impaired renal function. Also monitor fluid intake and output; decreasing urine output may indicate nephrotoxicity.
- Assess bowel elimination pattern daily; severe diarrhea may indicate pseudomembranous colitis. Patients with a history of GI disease, particularly colitis, are at increased risk.
- Monitor CBC, hematocrit, and serum AST, ALT, bilirubin, LD, and alkaline phosphatase levels during long-term therapy.
- Assess for signs of superinfection, such as perineal itching, fever, malaise, redness, swelling, rash, and change in cough or sputum.
- Assess for pharyngitis, ecchymosis, bleeding, and arthralgia, which may indicate a blood dyscrasia. Monitor PT and bleeding time as ordered.
- Before reconstituting ceftazidime for injection, store it at room temperature (specific range varies with manufacturer).

PATIENT TEACHING

• Instruct patient receiving ceftazidime to immediately report severe diarrhea or signs of blood dyscrasias or superinfection. Inform him that yogurt and buttermilk can help maintain intestinal flora and decrease diarrhea.
• Review with patient other possibly serious adverse reactions, such as difficulty breathing, rash, and chest tightness, and tell him to report any that occur.

ceftizoxime sodium

Cefizox

Class and Category

Chemical: Third-generation cephalosporin, 7-aminocephalosporanic acid
Therapeutic: Antibiotic
Pregnancy category: B

Indications and Dosages

▶ *To treat mild to moderate infections of the lower respiratory tract, skin, soft tissue, bones, and joints; septicemia; meningitis; and intra-abdominal infections caused by anaerobes (such as* Bacteroides *species,* Peptococcus, *and* Peptostreptococcus*), gram-negative organisms (including* Escherichia coli, Haemophilus influenzae, Klebsiella, *and* Proteus mirabilis*), and gram-positive organisms (including* Enterobacter *species,* Serratia *species,* Staphylococcus aureus, Staphylococcus epidermidis, Streptococcus agalactiae, Streptococcus pneumoniae, *and* Streptococcus pyogenes*)*

I.V. INFUSION OR INJECTION

Adults and children age 12 and older. 1 to 2 g q 8 to 12 hr.

▶ *To treat severe or refractory infections of the type listed above*

I.V. INFUSION OR INJECTION

Adults and children age 12 and older. 1 g q 8 hr or 2 g q 8 to 12 hr.

▶ *To treat life-threatening infections of the type listed above*

I.V. INFUSION OR INJECTION

Adults and children age 12 and older. 3 to 4 g q 8 hr or, if required, up to 2 g q 4 hr.

▶ *To treat bacterial infections in children*

I.V. INFUSION OR INJECTION

Children age 6 months and older. 50 mg/kg q 6 to 8 hr.

▶ *To treat uncomplicated UTIs*
I.V. INFUSION OR INJECTION
Adults. 500 mg q 12 hr.
▶ *To treat pelvic inflammatory disease*
I.V. INFUSION OR INJECTION
Adults. 2 g q 8 hr.
DOSAGE ADJUSTMENT Dosage reduced to 0.5 g q 8 hr for less severe infections and 0.75 to 1.5 g q 8 hr for life-threatening infections if creatinine clearance is 50 to 79 ml/min/1.73 m^2; to 0.25 to 0.5 g q 12 hr for less severe infections and 0.5 to 1 g q 12 hr for life-threatening infections if creatinine clearance is 5 to 49 ml/min/1.73 m^2; and to 0.5 g q 48 hr or 0.25 g q 24 hr for less severe infections and 0.5 to 1 g q 48 hr or 0.5 g q 24 hr for life-threatening infections if creatinine clearance is 4 ml/min/1.73 m^2 or less.

Mechanism of Action
Interferes with bacterial cell wall synthesis by inhibiting the final step in the cross-linking of peptidoglycan strands. Peptidoglycan makes the cell membrane rigid and protective. Without it, bacterial cells rupture and die.

Incompatibilities
Don't mix ceftizoxime with aminoglycosides to prevent mutual inactivation.

Contraindications
Hypersensitivity to cephalosporins or their components

Interactions
DRUGS
aminoglycosides, loop diuretics: Increased risk of nephrotoxicity
probenecid: Increased and prolonged blood ceftizoxime level

Adverse Reactions
CNS: Chills, fever, headache, seizures
CV: Edema
EENT: Hearing loss
GI: Abdominal cramps, diarrhea, elevated liver function test results, hepatic failure, hepatomegaly, nausea, oral candidiasis, pseudomembranous colitis, vomiting
GU: Elevated BUN level, nephrotoxicity, renal failure, vaginal candidiasis

HEME: Eosinophilia, hemolytic anemia, hypoprothrombinemia, neutropenia, thrombocytopenia, unusual bleeding
MS: Arthralgia
RESP: Dyspnea
SKIN: Ecchymosis, erythema, erythema multiforme, pruritus, rash, Stevens-Johnson syndrome
Other: Anaphylaxis; infusion site pain, redness, and swelling; superinfection

Nursing Considerations

- If possible, obtain culture and sensitivity test results, as ordered, before giving ceftizoxime.
- Reconstitute ceftizoxime for injection with sterile water for injection as follows: for 500-mg vial, add 5 ml; for 1-g vial, add 10 ml; and for 2-g vial, add 20 ml. Shake well. Dilute reconstituted solution further with 50 to 100 ml of a compatible solution, such as NS or D_5W, before I.V. infusion.
- Be aware that reconstituted drug may be stored for 24 hours at room temperature or 96 hours if refrigerated.
- Administer I.V. injection slowly over 3 to 5 minutes through tubing of a flowing compatible I.V. fluid.
- Be aware that ceftizoxime also comes in a minibag (ceftizoxime injection) with a concentration of 1 or 2 g/50 ml. Before using minibag, store it at −25° to −10° C (−13° to 14° F). Thaw it at room temperature or in refrigerator.
- Discard minibag after 48 hours if stored at room temperature or after 28 days if refrigerated. Don't refreeze. Don't use solution if it contains precipitate or is cloudy.
- To prevent air embolism, don't administer minibag using I.V. lines with series connections.
- Assess I.V. site for extravasation and phlebitis.
- Monitor BUN and serum creatinine levels to detect early signs of nephrotoxicity, especially in patients with impaired renal function. Also monitor fluid intake and output; decreasing urine output may indicate nephrotoxicity.
- Assess bowel elimination pattern daily; severe diarrhea may indicate pseudomembranous colitis. Patients with a history of GI disease, particularly colitis, are at increased risk.
- Monitor for signs of an allergic reaction, such as difficulty breathing or a rash, especially in patients who are hypersensitive to penicillin, because cross-sensitivity has occurred in about 10% of such patients. Be aware that an allergic reaction may occur a few days after therapy starts.

- Assess CBC, hematocrit, and serum AST, ALT, bilirubin, LD, and alkaline phosphatase levels during long-term therapy.
- Assess for pharyngitis, ecchymosis, bleeding, and arthralgia, which may indicate a blood dyscrasia. Monitor PT and bleeding time as ordered.
- Assess for signs of superinfection, such as perineal itching, fever, redness, swelling, rash, and change in cough or sputum.
- Before reconstituting drug, store it at 15° to 30° C (59° to 86° F).

PATIENT TEACHING
- Advise patient receiving ceftizoxime to immediately report severe diarrhea or signs of blood dyscrasias or superinfection. Inform him that yogurt and buttermilk can help maintain intestinal flora and decrease diarrhea.
- Review with patient other possibly serious adverse reactions, such as difficulty breathing, rash, and chest tightness, and tell him to report any that occur.

ceftriaxone sodium
Rocephin

Class and Category
Chemical: Third-generation cephalosporin, 7-aminocephalosporanic acid
Therapeutic: Antibiotic
Pregnancy category: B

Indications and Dosages
▶ *To treat infections of the lower respiratory tract, skin, soft tissue, urinary tract, bones, and joints; sinusitis; intra-abdominal infections; and septicemia caused by anaerobes (including* Bacteroides bivius, B. fragilis, B. melaninogenicus, *and* Peptostreptococcus *species), gram-negative organisms (including* Citrobacter *species,* Enterobacter aerogenes, Escherichia coli, Haemophilus influenzae, Klebsiella *species,* Neisseria *species,* Proteus mirabilis, Proteus vulgaris, Providencia *species,* Salmonella *species,* Serratia marcescens, Shigella, *and some strains of* Pseudomonas aeruginosa), *and gram-positive organisms (including* Staphylococcus aureus, Streptococcus pneumoniae, *and* Streptococcus pyogenes)*

I.V. INFUSION
Adults. 1 to 2 g q.d. or in equally divided doses b.i.d. *Maximum:* 4 g/day.
Children. 50 to 75 mg/kg/day in divided doses q 12 hr. *Maximum:* 2 g/day.

▶ *To treat meningitis*
I.V. INFUSION
Children. Initial: 100 mg/kg on first day, then 100 mg/kg q.d. or in divided doses q 12 hr for 7 to 14 days. *Maximum:* 4 g/day.
▶ *To treat disseminated gonococcal infection and pelvic inflammatory disease*
I.V. INFUSION
Adults. 1 g q 24 hr.
▶ *To treat gonococcal meningitis and endocarditis*
I.V. INFUSION
Adults. 1 to 2 g q 12 hr for 10 to 14 days (meningitis) or for 4 wk or longer (endocarditis).
▶ *To provide surgical prophylaxis*
I.V. INFUSION
Adults. 1 g 30 min to 2 hr before surgery.

Mechanism of Action
Interferes with bacterial cell wall synthesis by inhibiting the final step in the cross-linking of peptidoglycan strands. Peptidoglycan makes the cell membrane rigid and protective. Without it, bacterial cells rupture and die.

Incompatibilities
Don't mix ceftriaxone with other antibiotics, such as aminoglycosides or penicillins, to prevent mutual inactivation. Also avoid mixing ceftriaxone with other drugs, including pentamidine isethionate and labetalol hydrochloride.

Contraindications
Hypersensitivity to cephalosporins or their components

Interactions
DRUGS
aminoglycosides, loop diuretics: Increased risk of nephrotoxicity

Adverse Reactions
CNS: Chills, fever, headache, seizures
CV: Edema
EENT: Hearing loss
GI: Abdominal cramps, diarrhea, elevated liver function test results, hepatic failure, hepatomegaly, nausea, oral candidiasis, pseudolithiasis, pseudomembranous colitis, vomiting
GU: Elevated BUN level, nephrotoxicity, renal failure, vaginal candidiasis

HEME: Eosinophilia, hemolytic anemia, hypoprothrombinemia, neutropenia, thrombocytopenia, unusual bleeding
MS: Arthralgia
RESP: Dyspnea
SKIN: Ecchymosis, erythema, erythema multiforme, pruritus, rash, Stevens-Johnson syndrome
Other: Anaphylaxis; infusion site pain, redness, and swelling; superinfection

Nursing Considerations

- If possible, obtain culture and sensitivity results, as ordered, before giving ceftriaxone.
- Protect powder from light before reconstitution.
- Reconstitute with an appropriate diluent, such as sterile water for injection or sodium chloride for injection, as follows: 250-mg vial, add 2.4 ml; 500-mg vial, add 4.8 ml; 1-g vial, add 9.6 ml; and 2-g vial, add 19.2 ml to yield a concentration of 100 mg/ml. For piggyback bottles, reconstitute with 10 ml of diluent indicated above for 1-g bottle and 20 ml for 2-g bottle. After reconstituting drug, further dilute it to 50 to 100 ml with diluent indicated above and administer as an infusion over 30 minutes.
- Be aware that ceftriaxone also comes in a minibag (ceftriaxone injection) with a concentration of 1 or 2 g/50 ml. Before using minibag, store at −25° to −10° C (−13° to 14° F). Thaw at room temperature and ensure that ice crystals are melted before use.
- To prevent air embolism, don't administer minibag using I.V. lines with series connections. Don't use solution if it contains precipitate or is cloudy.
- Monitor BUN and serum creatinine levels to detect early signs of nephrotoxicity, especially in patients with impaired renal function. Also monitor fluid intake and output; decreasing urine output may indicate nephrotoxicity.
- Monitor for signs of an allergic reaction, such as difficulty breathing or a rash, especially in patients who are hypersensitive to penicillin, because cross-sensitivity has occurred in about 10% of such patients. Be aware that an allergic reaction may occur a few days after therapy starts.
- Assess CBC, hematocrit, and serum AST, ALT, bilirubin, LD, and alkaline phosphatase levels during long-term therapy.
- Assess bowel elimination pattern daily; severe diarrhea may indicate pseudomembranous colitis. Patients with a history of GI disease, particularly colitis, are at increased risk.

- Assess for signs of superinfection, such as perineal itching, fever, malaise, redness, swelling, rash, and change in cough or sputum.
- Assess for pharyngitis, ecchymosis, bleeding, and arthralgia, which may indicate a blood dyscrasia. Monitor PT and bleeding time as ordered.
- Before reconstituting ceftriaxone for injection, store it at 15° to 30° C (59° to 86° F).

PATIENT TEACHING
- Instruct patient receiving ceftriaxone to immediately report severe diarrhea or signs of blood dyscrasias or superinfection. Inform him that yogurt and buttermilk can help maintain intestinal flora and decrease diarrhea.
- Review with patient other possibly serious adverse reactions, such as difficulty breathing, rash, and chest tightness, and tell him to report any that occur.

cefuroxime sodium
Kelurox, Zinacef

Class and Category
Chemical: Second-generation cephalosporin, 7-aminocephalosporanic acid
Therapeutic: Antibiotic
Pregnancy category: B

Indications and Dosages
▶ *To treat uncomplicated skin and soft-tissue infections, uncomplicated UTIs, uncomplicated pneumonia, and disseminated gonococcal infections*
I.V. INFUSION OR INJECTION
Adults. 750 mg q 8 hr.
▶ *To treat bone and joint infections*
I.V. INFUSION OR INJECTION
Adults. 1.5 g q 8 hr.
Children over age 3 months. 50 to 150 mg/kg/day in divided doses q 8 hr. *Maximum:* Adult dose.
▶ *To treat bacterial meningitis*
I.V. INFUSION
Adults. 1.5 to 3 g q 8 hr.
Children over age 1 month. 50 to 80 mg/kg q 6 to 8 hr.
Neonates up to age 1 month. 33.3 to 50 mg/kg q 8 to 12 hr.

▶ *To treat moderate infections other than those listed above*

I.V. INFUSION OR INJECTION

Adults. 750 mg q 8 hr for 5 to 10 days.

Children over age 3 months. 50 mg/kg/day in equally divided doses q 6 to 8 hr.

▶ *To treat severe or complicated infections other than those listed above*

I.V. INFUSION OR INJECTION

Adults. 1.5 g q 8 hr.

Children over age 3 months. 100 mg/kg/day in equally divided doses q 6 to 8 hr.

▶ *To treat life-threatening infections other than those listed above*

I.V. INFUSION OR INJECTION

Adults. 1.5 g q 6 hr.

▶ *To provide perioperative prophylaxis*

I.V. INFUSION OR INJECTION

Adults. For open-heart surgery, 1.5 g at induction of anesthesia and then 1.5 g q 12 hr for total of 6 g; for other types of surgery, 1.5 g 30 to 60 min before surgery and then 0.75 g q 8 hr thereafter.

DOSAGE ADJUSTMENT Dosage reduced to 0.75 g q 12 hr for patients with creatinine clearance of 10 to 20 ml/min/1.73 m^2 and to 0.75 g q 24 hr for patients with creatinine clearance of less than 10 ml/min/1.73 m^2.

Mechanism of Action

Interferes with bacterial cell wall synthesis by inhibiting the final step in the cross-linking of peptidoglycan strands. Peptidoglycan makes the cell membrane rigid and protective. Without it, bacterial cells rupture and die.

Incompatibilities

Don't mix cefuroxime with other antibiotics, such as aminoglycosides, to prevent mutual inactivation. If they must be administered concurrently, don't mix them in the same I.V. bag or bottle.

Contraindications

Hypersensitivity to cephalosporins or their components

Interactions

DRUGS

aminoglycosides, loop diuretics: Increased risk of nephrotoxicity

probenecid: Increased and prolonged blood cefuroxime level

Adverse Reactions

CNS: Chills, fever, headache, seizures
CV: Edema
EENT: Hearing loss
GI: Abdominal cramps, diarrhea, elevated liver function test results, hepatic failure, hepatomegaly, nausea, oral candidiasis, pseudomembranous colitis, vomiting
GU: Elevated BUN level, nephrotoxicity, renal failure, vaginal candidiasis
HEME: Eosinophilia, hemolytic anemia, hypoprothrombinemia, neutropenia, thrombocytopenia, unusual bleeding
MS: Arthralgia
RESP: Dyspnea
SKIN: Ecchymosis, erythema, erythema multiforme, pruritus, rash, Stevens-Johnson syndrome
Other: Anaphylaxis; injection site pain, redness, and swelling; superinfection

Nursing Considerations

- If possible, obtain culture and sensitivity results, as ordered, before giving cefuroxime.
- Following manufacturer's instructions, reconstitute cefuroxime for injection according to type of preparation available. Solution ranges in color from light yellow to amber.
- Store reconstituted drug for up to 24 hours at room temperature or 96 hours in refrigerator.
- Administer I.V. injection over 3 to 5 minutes through tubing of a flowing compatible I.V. fluid.
- If using a container of frozen parenteral solution (cefuroxime injection in a concentration of 750 mg or 1.5 g/50 ml), thaw at room temperature or under refrigeration before administration; make sure all ice crystals have melted. Don't thaw in water bath or microwave. Thawed solutions may be stable for 24 hours at room temperature or 28 days if refrigerated.
- To prevent air embolism, don't administer minibag using I.V. lines with series connections. Don't use solution if it contains precipitate or is cloudy.
- Monitor I.V. site for extravasation and phlebitis.
- Monitor for signs of an allergic reaction, such as difficulty breathing or a rash, especially in patients who are hypersensitive to penicillin, because cross-sensitivity has occurred in about 10% of such patients. Be aware that an allergic reaction may occur a few days after therapy starts.

- Monitor BUN and serum creatinine levels to detect early signs of nephrotoxicity, especially in patients with impaired renal function. Also monitor fluid intake and output; decreasing urine output may indicate nephrotoxicity.
- Assess bowel elimination pattern daily; severe diarrhea may indicate pseudomembranous colitis. Patients with a history of GI disease, particularly colitis, are at increased risk.
- Assess for pharyngitis, ecchymosis, bleeding, and arthralgia, which may indicate a blood dyscrasia. Monitor PT and bleeding time as ordered.
- Assess CBC, hematocrit, and serum AST, ALT, bilirubin, LD, and alkaline phosphatase levels during long-term therapy.
- Before reconstituting cefuroxime for injection, store it at 15° to 30° C (59° to 86° F) and protect from light.

PATIENT TEACHING
- Instruct patient receiving cefuroxime to immediately report severe diarrhea or signs of blood dyscrasias or superinfection. Inform him that yogurt and buttermilk can help maintain intestinal flora and decrease diarrhea.
- Review with patient other possibly serious adverse reactions, such as difficulty breathing, rash, and chest tightness, and tell him to report any that occur.

cephapirin sodium
Cefadyl

Class and Category
Chemical: First-generation cephalosporin, 7-aminocephalosporanic acid
Therapeutic: Antibiotic
Pregnancy category: B

Indications and Dosages
▶ *To treat respiratory tract infections, skin and soft-tissue infections, UTIs, septicemia, endocarditis, and osteomyelitis caused by gram-negative organisms (including* Escherichia coli, Haemophilus influenzae, Klebsiella *species, and* Proteus mirabilis*) and gram-positive organisms (including group A beta-hemolytic streptococci,* Streptococcus pneumoniae, *and staphylococci, including coagulase-positive, coagulase-negative, and penicillinase-producing—but not methicillin-resistant—strains of* Staphylococcus aureus*)*

I.V. INFUSION OR INJECTION

Adults. 0.5 to 1 g q 4 to 6 hr. *Maximum:* 12 g/day.

Children older than age 3 months. 40 to 80 mg/kg/day divided into four equal doses and given q 6 hr. *Maximum:* 12 g/day.

▶ *To provide surgical prophylaxis*

I.V. INFUSION OR INJECTION

Adults. 1 to 2 g 30 to 60 min before surgery, 1 to 2 g during long procedure, and 1 to 2 g q 6 hr after surgery for 24 hr.

DOSAGE ADJUSTMENT For open-heart surgery or prosthetic arthroplasty, prophylaxis continued for 3 to 5 days after procedure, if needed.

Mechanism of Action

Interferes with bacterial cell wall synthesis by inhibiting the final step in the cross-linking of peptidoglycan strands. Peptidoglycan makes the cell membrane rigid and protective. Without it, bacterial cells rupture and die.

Contraindications

Hypersensitivity to cephalosporins or their components

Interactions

DRUGS

aminoglycosides, loop diuretics: Increased risk of nephrotoxicity

probenecid: Increased and prolonged blood cephapirin level

Adverse Reactions

CNS: Chills, fever, headache, seizures

CV: Edema

EENT: Hearing loss

GI: Abdominal cramps, diarrhea, elevated liver function test results, hepatic failure, hepatomegaly, nausea, oral candidiasis, pseudomembranous colitis, vomiting

GU: Elevated BUN level, nephrotoxicity, renal failure, vaginal candidiasis

HEME: Eosinophilia, hemolytic anemia, hypoprothrombinemia, neutropenia, thrombocytopenia, unusual bleeding

MS: Arthralgia

RESP: Dyspnea

SKIN: Ecchymosis, erythema, erythema multiforme, pruritus, rash, Stevens-Johnson syndrome

Other: Anaphylaxis; infusion site pain, redness, and swelling; superinfection

Nursing Considerations

- If possible, obtain culture and sensitivity test results, as ordered, before giving cephapirin.
- For I.V. injection, reconstitute 1 g with 10 ml or more of appropriate diluent, such as sterile water for injection. Administer I.V. injection slowly over 3 to 5 minutes through tubing of a flowing compatible I.V. fluid.
- For I.V. infusion, dilute further in 50 ml of D$_5$W or NS and infuse over 15 to 30 minutes. Stop primary I.V. solution during cephapirin administration.
- Store reconstituted drug for 12 to 48 hours (depending on diluent used) at room temperature or for 10 days in refrigerator.
- Don't administer a cloudy solution.
- Assess I.V. site for extravasation and phlebitis.
- Monitor BUN and serum creatinine levels to detect early signs of nephrotoxicity, especially in patients with impaired renal function. Also monitor fluid intake and output; decreasing urine output may indicate nephrotoxicity.
- Monitor for signs of an allergic reaction, such as difficulty breathing or a rash, especially in patients who are hypersensitive to penicillin, because cross-sensitivity has occurred in about 10% of such patients. Be aware that an allergic reaction may occur a few days after therapy starts.
- Assess CBC, hematocrit, and serum AST, ALT, bilirubin, LD, and alkaline phosphatase levels during long-term therapy.
- Assess bowel elimination pattern daily; severe diarrhea may indicate pseudomembranous colitis. Patients with a history of GI disease, particularly colitis, are at increased risk.
- Assess for pharyngitis, ecchymosis, bleeding, and arthralgia, which may indicate a blood dyscrasia. Monitor PT and bleeding time, as ordered.
- Assess for furry tongue, perineal itching, and loose, foul-smelling stools, any of which may indicate superinfection.
- Before reconstituting cephapirin for injection, store it at 15° to 30° C (59° to 86° F).

PATIENT TEACHING

- Instruct patient receiving cephapirin to immediately report severe diarrhea or signs of blood dyscrasias or superinfection. Inform him that yogurt and buttermilk can help maintain intestinal flora and decrease diarrhea during therapy.
- Review with patient other possibly serious adverse reactions, such as difficulty breathing, rash, and chest tightness, and tell him to report any that occur.

chloramphenicol sodium succinate
Chloromycetin

Class and Category
Chemical: Dichloroacetic acid derivative
Therapeutic: Antibiotic
Pregnancy category: Not rated

Indications and Dosages
▶ *To treat serious infections for which less potentially dangerous drugs are ineffective or contraindicated*
I.V. INFUSION
Adults. 12.5 mg/kg q 6 hr. *Maximum:* 4 g/day.
Children. 12.5 mg/kg q 6 hr.
Full-term infants age 2 weeks and older. 12.5 mg/kg q 6 hr or 25 mg/kg q 12 hr.
Preterm and full-term infants up to age 2 weeks. 6.25 mg/kg q 6 hr.
▶ *To treat bacteremia or meningitis*
I.V. INFUSION
Children. 50 to 100 mg/kg/day in divided doses q 6 hr.
DOSAGE ADJUSTMENT Dosage limited to 25 mg/kg/day for infants and children with immature metabolic processes.

Mechanism of Action
Produces a bacteriostatic effect on susceptible organisms by inhibiting protein synthesis, thereby preventing amino acids from being transferred to growing polypeptide chains.

Contraindications
Hypersensitivity to chloramphenicol or its components

Interactions
DRUGS
alfentanil: Prolonged alfentanil effect
barbiturates: Increased blood barbiturate level; decreased blood chloramphenicol level
blood-dyscrasia–causing drugs (such as captropil and cephalosporins), bone marrow depressants (including colchicine and methotrexate): Increased bone marrow depression
chlorpropamide, tolbutamide: Increased hypoglycemic effects of these drugs

clindamycin, erythromycin, lincomycin: Decreased antibacterial effects of these drugs

cyclophosphamide: Decreased or delayed activation of cyclophosphamide, increased bone marrow depression

hepatic enzyme inducers (including rifampin): Decreased blood chloramphenicol level

hydantoins: Increased blood hydantoin level, possibly resulting in toxicity, including increased bone marrow depression; decreased blood chloramphenicol level

iron salts: Increased serum iron level

oral anticoagulants: Enhanced anticoagulant effect

oral contraceptives containing estrogen: Decreased contraceptive effect with prolonged chloramphenicol use

penicillins: Decreased penicillin activity, synergistic effects with treatment of certain microorganisms

vitamin B_{12}: Antagonized hematopoietic response to vitamin B_{12}

Adverse Reactions

CNS: Confusion, delirium, depression, fever, headache, peripheral neuropathy

CV: Gray syndrome in neonates

EENT: Glossitis, optic neuritis, stomatitis

GI: Diarrhea, nausea, vomiting

HEME: Aplastic anemia, bone marrow depression, granulocytopenia, hypoplastic anemia, leukopenia, reticulocytopenia, thrombocytopenia

SKIN: Macular or vesicular rash, urticaria

Other: Anaphylaxis, angioedema

Nursing Considerations

- **WARNING** Keep in mind that chloramphenicol should never be used to treat minor infections or for prophylaxis because of the many serious toxicities associated with its use.
- Be aware that patients with impaired or immature renal function (especially neonates and infants) may require reduced dosage. Monitor chloramphenicol concentrations, as ordered.
- Prepare a 10% solution by adding 10 ml of sterile water for injection or D_5W to each 1-g vial of chloramphenicol. Administer over at least 1 minute.
- Know that diluted I.V. solution is stable for 24 to 48 hours when stored at room temperature or refrigerated (depending on manufacturer's recommendation). Don't use if it's cloudy.

- Monitor CBC as ordered for signs of blood dyscrasias, including leukopenia and thrombocytopenia.
- Assess for fever, sore throat, tiredness, unusual bleeding, or ecchymosis, which may indicate a blood dyscrasia.
- Perform neurologic assessments regularly, looking for signs and symptoms of peripheral neuropathy.
- **WARNING** If early signs of gray syndrome (failure to feed, pallor, cyanosis, abdominal distention, irregular respirations, and vasomotor collapse) appear, notify prescriber and be prepared to stop drug immediately.
- Be aware that chloramphenicol may increase bone marrow depression in patients receiving radiation therapy.
- Be aware that administering chloramphenicol at term or during labor puts neonate at risk for gray syndrome and administering drug to breast-feeding woman may have toxic effects on infant.
- Before reconstituting chloramphenicol, store it at 15° to 25° C (59° to 77° F).

PATIENT TEACHING
- Instruct patient receiving chloramphenicol to immediately report signs of blood dyscrasias.
- **WARNING** Advise patient to be alert for signs of potentially fatal, irreversible bone marrow depression, which leads to aplastic anemia and is characterized by fever, pallor, pharyngitis, severe fatigue and weakness, and unusual bleeding or bruising. Bone marrow depression may occur weeks to months after therapy and seems unrelated to administration route. Stress the importance of follow-up care.
- Encourage patient to use a soft-bristled toothbrush and to avoid using toothpicks or dental floss because of increased risk of infection and gingival bleeding due to drug's effects on blood counts.

chlordiazepoxide hydrochloride
Librium

Class, Category, and Schedule
Chemical: Benzodiazepine
Therapeutic: Antianxiety agent
Pregnancy category: Not rated
Controlled substance: Schedule IV

Indications and Dosages

▶ *To provide short-term management of severe anxiety*
I.V. INJECTION
Adults. *Initial:* 50 to 100 mg. Then 25 to 50 mg t.i.d. or q.i.d., p.r.n. *Maximum:* 300 mg/day.

▶ *To provide short-term treatment of acute alcohol withdrawal*
I.V. INJECTION
Adults. *Initial:* 50 to 100 mg. Repeated in 2 to 4 hr, followed by individualized oral dosage if needed to control symptoms. *Maximum:* 300 mg/day.

DOSAGE ADJUSTMENT Dosage reduced to 25 to 50 mg for elderly or debilitated patients and for children age 12 and older.

Mechanism of Action

May potentiate the effects of gamma-aminobutyric acid (GABA) and other inhibitory neurotransmitters by binding to specific benzodiazepine receptors in the limbic and cortical areas of the CNS. By binding to these receptors, chlordiazepoxide increases GABA's inhibitory effects and blocks cortical and limbic arousal, which helps control emotional behavior. It also helps relieve symptoms of alcohol withdrawal by causing CNS depression.

Contraindications

Hypersensitivity to chlordiazepoxide or its components

Interactions

DRUGS
cimetidine, disulfiram, fluoxetine, isoniazid, ketoconazole, metoprolol, oral contraceptives, propoxyphene, propranolol, valproic acid: Increased blood chlordiazepoxide level
CNS depressants: Increased CNS effects
digoxin: Increased blood digoxin level and risk of digitalis toxicity
levodopa: Decreased efficacy of levodopa's antiparkinsonian effects
neuromuscular blockers: Potentiated, counteracted, or diminished effects of neuromuscular blockers
phenytoin: Possibly increased phenytoin toxicity
probenecid: Shortened onset of action or prolonged effect of chlordiazepoxide
rifampin: Decreased chlordiazepoxide effects
theophyllines: Antagonized sedative effects of chlordiazepoxide
ACTIVITIES
alcohol use: Increased CNS effects

Adverse Reactions

CNS: Ataxia, confusion, depression, drowsiness
CV: ECG changes, hypotension, tachycardia
GI: Hepatic dysfunction
HEME: Agranulocytosis
SKIN: Jaundice
Other: Infusion site pain, redness, and swelling

Nursing Considerations

- **WARNING** Be aware that prolonged use of therapeutic doses of chlordiazepoxide can lead to dependence.
- Reconstitute ampule contents with 5 ml of sterile water for injection or sodium chloride for injection. Agitate gently until completely dissolved. Administer slowly over 1 minute immediately after reconstitution. Discard unused portions.
- **WARNING** Don't use supplied diluent (provided for I.M. use) to prepare drug for I.V. use because air bubbles form on the surface.
- Be aware that rapid I.V. administration may cause apnea, hypotension, bradycardia, and cardiac arrest. Keep emergency equipment and drugs nearby. Observe patient for 5 hours or longer, as needed.
- Monitor patients with porphyria for signs of an exacerbation, such as fever, photosensitivity, abdominal pain, and neuropathy.
- Monitor patient for adverse reactions, especially if he has hypoalbuminemia, which increases drug's sedative effects.
- Observe for signs of phlebitis or thrombophlebitis after I.V. administration.
- Monitor patients with impaired hepatic or renal function for signs of increased CNS effects due to slowed chlordiazepoxide metabolism or excretion because drug is metabolized by liver and excreted by kidneys.
- Monitor a hyperactive, aggressive child or any patient who has a history of psychiatric disorders for paradoxical reactions, such as excitement, stimulation, and acute rage, during first 2 weeks of therapy.
- Before reconstituting chlordiazepoxide, store it at 15° to 30° C (59° to 86° F).

PATIENT TEACHING

- Caution patient about possible drowsiness, and advise him to avoid activities requiring alertness until chlordiazepoxide's full CNS effects are known.

chlorothiazide sodium

Diuril

Class and Category

Chemical: Sulfonamide derivative
Therapeutic: Antihypertensive, diuretic
Pregnancy category: B

Indications and Dosages

▶ *To manage hypertension*

I.V. INFUSION OR INJECTION

Adults. 500 mg to 1 g as a single dose or in two divided doses.

▶ *To produce diuresis*

I.V. INFUSION OR INJECTION

Adults. 250 mg q 6 to 12 hr.

Route	Onset	Peak	Duration
I.V.	15 min	4 hr	6 to 12 hr

Contraindications

Anuria; hepatic coma; hypersensitivity to chlorothiazide or its components, sulfonamides, or related thiazide diuretics; renal failure

Interactions

DRUGS

allopurinol: Increased risk of allopurinol hypersensitivity

amiodarone: Increased risk of arrhythmias from hypokalemia

amphotericin B, corticosteroids: Intensified electrolyte depletion

anesthetics: Potentiated effects of anesthetics

anticholinergics: Increased chlorothiazide absorption

anticoagulants, methenamines, sulfonylureas: Decreased effects of these drugs

antihypertensives: Increased antihypertensive effects

antineoplastics: Prolonged antineoplastic-induced leukopenia

calcium: Possibly increased blood calcium level

cholestyramine, colestipol: Decreased chlorothiazide absorption

diazoxide: Hyperglycemia, hypotension

digitalis glycosides: Increased risk of digitalis-induced arrhythmias

dopamine: Increased diuretic effect of both drugs

lithium: Increased risk of lithium toxicity

loop diuretics: Synergistic effects, resulting in profound diuresis and serious electrolyte imbalances

methyldopa: Potential development of hemolytic anemia

neuromuscular blockers: Increased neuromuscular blockade
NSAIDs: Possibly reduced diuretic effect of chlorothiazide
sympathomimetics: Possibly inhibited antihypertensive effect of
chlorothiazide
vitamin D: Enhanced vitamin D action

Mechanism of Action

A thiazide diuretic, chlorothiazide inhibits sodium (Na^+) reabsorption and promotes the movement of Na^+, chloride (Cl^-), and water (H_2O) from blood in the peritubular capillaries into the nephron's distal convoluted tubule, as shown below. Initially, chlorothiazide may decrease extracellular fluid volume, plasma volume, and cardiac output, which helps explain blood pressure reduction. It also may reduce blood pressure by causing direct dilation of arteries. After several weeks, extracellular fluid volume, plasma volume, and cardiac output return to normal, and peripheral vascular resistance remains decreased.

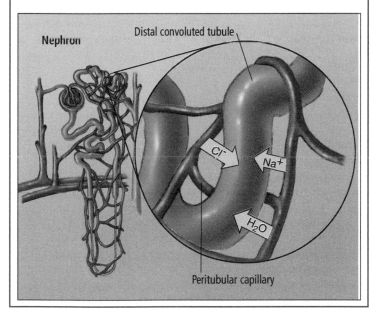

Adverse Reactions

CNS: Dizziness, headache, paresthesia, restlessness, vertigo, weakness
CV: Orthostatic hypotension
ENDO: Hyperglycemia

GI: Abdominal cramps, anorexia, constipation, diarrhea, gastric irritation, nausea, pancreatitis, vomiting
GU: Glycosuria, hematuria, impotence, interstitial nephritis, renal dysfunction or failure
HEME: Agranulocytosis, aplastic anemia, hemolytic anemia, leukopenia, thrombocytopenia
MS: Muscle spasms
SKIN: Jaundice, photosensitivity, purpura, rash, urticaria
Other: Anaphylaxis, hypercalcemia, hyperuricemia, hypochloremic alkalosis, hypokalemia, hypomagnesemia, hyponatremia, hypovolemia

Nursing Considerations

- Don't give parenteral form of chlorothiazide by I.M. or S.C. route.
- Reconstitute with at least 18 ml of sterile water for injection. Discard unused solution after 24 hours. Reconstituted solution is compatible with dextrose solution or NS for infusion.
- Monitor I.V. site closely to detect signs of extravasation. If extravasation occurs, stop drug administration and notify prescriber immediately.
- Weigh patient daily to assess fluid loss and drug effectiveness. Monitor fluid intake and output. Also, check blood pressure frequently if drug is used to treat hypertension; antihypertensive effects may not appear for days.
- Monitor elderly patients for increased sensitivity to drug's effects.
- Monitor for electrolyte imbalances, especially hypokalemia.
- Assess for signs of hypokalemia, such as muscle spasms or weakness.
- Monitor BUN and serum creatinine levels regularly.
- Frequently monitor blood glucose level of patients with diabetes, and expect to increase antidiabetic drug dosage as needed.
- Before reconstituting chlorothiazide, store it at 15° to 30° C (59° to 86° F).

PATIENT TEACHING

- Encourage patient to eat a high-potassium diet during chlorothiazide therapy.
- Instruct patient to rise slowly to minimize effects of orthostatic hypotension.
- Advise patient to immediately notify prescriber if any of these signs and symptoms occur: weakness, cramps, nausea, vomiting, restlessness, excessive thirst, drowsiness, tiredness, increased heart rate, diarrhea, sudden joint pain, or dizziness.

- Inform patient with diabetes mellitus that his blood glucose level will be monitored and that his oral antidiabetic drug dosage may need to be increased.

chlorpromazine hydrochloride

Largactil (CAN), Thorazine

Class and Category

Chemical: Propylamine derivative of phenothiazine
Therapeutic: Antiemetic, antipsychotic, tranquilizer
Pregnancy category: Not rated

Indications and Dosages

▶ *To provide intraoperative control of nausea and vomiting*

I.V. INJECTION

Adults. 25 mg diluted to 1 mg/ml with sodium chloride for injection and given at a rate not to exceed 2 mg q 2 min. *Maximum:* 25 mg.

Children age 6 months and older. 0.275 mg/kg diluted to at least 1 mg/ml with sodium chloride for injection and given at a rate not to exceed 1 mg q 2 min. *Maximum:* 75 mg/day for children ages 5 to 12 years or weighing 50 to 100 lb; 40 mg/day for children up to age 5 years or weighing up to 50 lb.

▶ *To treat intractable hiccups*

I.V. INFUSION

Adults. 25 to 50 mg diluted in 500 to 1,000 ml of NS and administered at a rate of 1 mg/min with patient in supine position.

▶ *To treat tetanus (usually as adjunct to barbiturates)*

I.V. INFUSION

Adults. 25 to 50 mg diluted to at least 1 mg/ml and given at a rate not to exceed 1 mg/min.

Children age 6 months and older. 0.55 mg/kg q 6 to 8 hr, diluted to at least 1 mg/ml and given at a rate not to exceed 1 mg/2 min. *Maximum:* 75 mg/day for children ages 5 to 12 or weighing 50 to 100 lb; 40 mg/day for children up to age 5 or weighing up to 50 lb.

DOSAGE ADJUSTMENT Dosage possibly reduced for patients with hepatic dysfunction. Dosage reduced to one-third to one-half the normal adult dosage for elderly or debilitated patients.

Mechanism of Action

Depresses areas of the brain that control activity and aggression, including the cerebral cortex, hypothalamus, and limbic system, by an unknown mechanism. Chlorpromazine prevents nausea and vomiting by inhibiting or blocking dopamine receptors in the medullary chemoreceptor trigger zone and peripherally by blocking the vagus nerve in the GI tract. It may relieve anxiety by causing indirect reduction in arousal and increased filtering of internal stimuli to the reticular activating system in the brain stem.

Incompatibilities

Don't mix chlorpromazine with thiopental, atropine, or solutions that don't have a pH of 4 to 5 because a precipitate will form. Don't mix chlorpromazine injection in same syringe with other drugs.

Contraindications

Comatose states; hypersensitivity to chlorpromazine, phenothiazines, or their components; use of large amounts of CNS depressants

Interactions

DRUGS

amphetamines: Decreased amphetamine effectiveness, decreased antipsychotic effectiveness of chlorpromazine
barbiturates: Decreased plasma level and, possibly, effectiveness of chlorpromazine
CNS depressants: Prolonged and intensified CNS depression
metrizamide: Possibly lowered seizure threshold
oral anticoagulants: Decreased anticoagulant effect
phenytoin: Interference with phenytoin metabolism, increased risk of phenytoin toxicity
propranolol: Increased plasma levels of both drugs
thiazide diuretics: Possibly increased orthostatic hypotension
ACTIVITIES
alcohol use: Prolonged and intensified CNS depression

Adverse Reactions

CNS: Drowsiness, extrapyramidal reactions (dystonia, fever, motor restlessness, pseudoparkinsonism, and tardive dyskinesia), neuroleptic malignant syndrome, seizures
CV: ECG changes, such as nonspecific, usually reversible Q- and T-wave changes; orthostatic hypotension; tachycardia
EENT: Blurred vision, dry mouth, nasal congestion, ocular changes (fine particle deposits in lens and cornea) with long-term therapy

ENDO: Gynecomastia, hyperglycemia, hypoglycemia, lactation, moderate breast engorgement
GI: Constipation, ileus, nausea
GU: Amenorrhea, ejaculation disorders, impotence, priapism, urine retention
HEME: Agranulocytosis, aplastic anemia, eosinophilia, hemolytic anemia, leukopenia, pancytopenia, thrombocytopenic purpura
SKIN: Exfoliative dermatitis, jaundice, photosensitivity, tissue necrosis, urticaria

Nursing Considerations

- Protect chlorpromazine solution from light. Solution should be clear and colorless to pale yellow. Discard markedly discolored solution.
- Don't inject drug by S.C. route because it can cause severe tissue necrosis.
- Wear gloves when working with liquid or injectable form because parenteral solution may cause contact dermatitis.
- For I.V. injection, dilute chlorpromazine with sodium chloride for injection to a concentration that yields 1 mg/ml before administration.
- **WARNING** Be aware that chlorpromazine contains benzyl alcohol, which can cause a fatal toxic syndrome in neonates or immature infants, characterized by CNS, respiratory, circulatory, and renal impairment and metabolic acidosis. Dosage has not been established for infants younger than age 6 months.
- **WARNING** Be alert for possible suppressed cough reflex, which increases patient's risk of aspirating vomitus.
- **WARNING** If neuroleptic malignant syndrome (hyperpyrexia, muscle rigidity, altered mental status, autonomic instability) develops, notify prescriber immediately and expect to discontinue drug and begin intensive medical treatment. Monitor carefully for recurrence if patient resumes antipsychotic therapy.
- Monitor patients (especially children) with chronic respiratory disorders (such as severe asthma or emphysema) or acute respiratory tract infections for exacerbations of these conditions caused by chlorpromazine's CNS depressant effects. Be aware that patients with cardiovascular, hepatic, or renal disease are at increased risk for developing hypotension, heart failure, and arrhythmias.

- Monitor patients with a history of hepatic encephalopathy from cirrhosis for increased sensitivity to drug's CNS effects.
- Because of chlorpromazine's anticholinergic effects, monitor patients with a history of or predisposition to glaucoma for signs and symptoms of this disorder, such as eye pain, vision changes, or nausea and vomiting from increased intraocular pressure.
- Be aware that drug should be used cautiously in those who are exposed to organophosphorus insecticides.
- Monitor patients who have been exposed to extreme heat for heatstroke due to drug-induced suppression of temperature regulation. Symptoms include tachycardia, fever, and confusion.
- Be aware that pediatric and elderly patients are at increased risk for developing hypotension amd extrapyramidal reactions, especially if they're acutely ill or debilitated.
- Before reconstituting chlorpromazine, store it at 15° to 30° C (59° to 86° F).

PATIENT TEACHING
- Because chlorpromazine may cause drowsiness, dizziness, and blurred vision (especially during the first few days of therapy), advise patient to avoid potentially hazardous activities until drug's CNS effects are known.
- Advise patient, especially if elderly, to rise slowly from a supine or seated position to avoid dizziness, light-headedness, and fainting.
- Urge patient to avoid alcohol because of possible additive effects and hypotension.
- Inform patient that drug may reduce body's response to heat and cold; advise him to avoid temperature extremes, as in very cold or hot showers.
- If patient reports dry mouth, suggest sugarless chewing gum, hard candy, and fluids.
- Urge patient to report sudden sore throat or other signs of infection.

cidofovir
Vistide

Class and Category
Chemical: Synthetic purine nucleotide analogue
Therapeutic: Antiviral
Pregnancy category: C

Indications and Dosages
I.V. INFUSION

▶ *To treat cytomegalovirus (CMV) retinitis in patients with AIDS*
Adults. Induction dose of 5 mg/kg infused over 1 hr once q wk for
2 wk. *Maintenance:* 5 mg/kg infused over 1 hr once q 2 wk. Probenecid should be administered before and after each cidofovir dose.
DOSAGE ADJUSTMENT Maintenance dosage reduced to
3 mg/kg if serum creatinine level increases by 0.3 or 0.4 mg/dl
above baseline.

Mechanism of Action
Is ultimately converted by pyrimidine nucleoside monophosphate kinase and
other cellular enzymes to cidofovir diphosphate. Cidofovir diphosphate suppresses cytomegalovirus (CMV) replication by incorporation into and termination of the growing DNA chain, and by selective inhibition and inactivation of viral DNA polymerase, an enzyme used in the viral DNA replication
process.

Incompatibilities
Don't add other drugs or supplements to cidofovir solutions.

Contraindications
Concurrent administration within 7 days of other nephrotoxic
drugs; direct intraocular injection; hypersensitivity to cidofovir or
severe hypersensitivity to probenecid or other sulfa-containing
drugs; serum creatinine level greater than 1.5 mg/dl, calculated
creatinine clearance less than or equal to 55 ml/min/1.73 m^2, or
urine protein level greater than or equal to 100 mg/dl (proteinuria greater than or equal to +2)

Interactions
DRUGS

*nephrotoxic drugs (such as aminoglycosides, amphotericin B, foscarnet,
NSAIDs, and pentamidine):* Increased risk of nephrotoxicity

Adverse Reactions
CNS: Asthenia, fever, headache
EENT: Iritis, ocular hypotony, uveitis, vision changes
GI: Anorexia, diarrhea, nausea, vomiting
GU: Elevated serum creatinine level, nephrotoxicity, proteinuria
HEME: Neutropenia
Other: Decreased serum sodium bicarbonate levels, metabolic
acidosis

Nursing Considerations

- **WARNING** Be aware that cidofovir is for I.V. infusion only and is not for direct intraocular injection.
- Monitor serum creatinine and urine protein levels within 48 hours of an upcoming cidofovir dose, as ordered. Expect maintenance dosage to be decreased if serum creatinine level increases by 0.3 or 0.4 mg/dl above baseline. Expect therapy to be discontinued if serum creatinine level increases by at least 0.5 mg/dl above baseline or if patient develops proteinuria of 3+ or more.
- Monitor WBC count with differential before a scheduled cidofovir dose to detect drug-induced neutropenia. Also, assess patient for signs of neutropenia, including fever, chills, and sore throat.
- Expect to administer 2 g of probenecid 3 hours before each dose of cidofovir and 1 g 2 hours and 8 hours after each dose—for a total of 4 g—to minimize the risk of nephrotoxicity.
- Administer at least 1 L of NS over a 1- to 2-hour period immediately before cidofovir administration. An additional infusion of 1 L of NS over 1 to 3 hours may be prescribed for patients who can tolerate the extra fluid, to be initiated at beginning of cidofovir infusion or immediately afterward.
- Be aware that adverse reactions can vary when cidofovir is administered in combination therapy. Review information for all drugs administered as part of a specific regimen, including drug interactions and adverse effects.
- Be aware that an antiemetic may be prescribed to help reduce nausea from probenecid. Also, be prepared to administer prophylactic or therapeutic antihistamines or acetaminophen if patient develops an allergic or hypersensitivity reaction.
- Be aware that cidofovir has mutagenic properties. Follow facility protocol for preparation and handling of such drugs and for appropriate disposal of used equipment. Thoroughly wash any skin exposed to cidofovir with soap and water.
- Inspect each vial of cidofovir before administration; discard it if you detect particles or discoloration. Dilute each dose of cidofovir with 100 ml of NS. Administer within 24 hours. Diluted solutions not used immediately may be stored at 2° to 8° C (36° to 46° F) but must be used within the original 24-hour period. Allow refrigerated solution to return to room temperature before administration.

- Administer cidofovir at a constant rate over a 1-hour period, using an infusion pump.
- Assess patient for changes in vision, such as decreased vision, which may indicate decreased intraocular pressure. Ensure that patient's intraocular pressure is measured periodically.

PATIENT TEACHING

- Instruct patient to eat some food before each dose of probenecid to help reduce drug-related nausea and vomiting.
- Stress the importance of taking the full course of probenecid with each dose of cidofovir to decrease the risk of adverse reactions.
- Advise patient to comply with follow-up ophthalmic exams to assess drug effectiveness and monitor for adverse reactions. Inform patient that CMV retinitis may continue to progress during and following treatment.
- Inform patient who is also receiving zidovudine that a dosage adjustment or temporary discontinuation of zidovudine may be needed on the day of cidofovir therapy.
- If patient develops neutropenia, urge him to avoid sports and other activities that increase the risk of accidental injury. Also advise him to take measures to avoid infection, such as maintaining good oral hygiene (for example, by using a soft-bristled toothbrush) and washing hands before touching eyes or nose.

cimetidine hydrochloride

Novo-Cimetine (CAN), Tagamet

Class and Category

Chemical: Imidazole derivative
Therapeutic: Antiulcer agent, gastric acid secretion inhibitor, H_2-receptor antagonist
Pregnancy category: B

Indications and Dosages

▶ *To treat and prevent recurrence of duodenal ulcer*

I.V. INJECTION

Adults. *Initial:* 300 mg q 6 to 8 hr. Dosage increased, if needed, by increasing frequency. *Maximum:* 2,400 mg/day.

▶ *To treat active, benign gastric ulcer*

I.V. INJECTION

Adults and adolescents. *Initial:* 300 mg q 6 to 8 hr. Dosage increased, if needed, by increasing frequency. *Maximum:* 2,400 mg/day.

▶ *To treat pathologic hypersecretory conditions, such as Zollinger-Ellison syndrome*
I.V. INJECTION
Adults and adolescents. *Initial:* 300 mg q 6 to 8 hr. Dosage increased, if needed, by increasing frequency. *Maximum:* 2,400 mg/day.
▶ *To prevent stress-related upper GI bleeding during hospitalization*
I.V. INFUSION
Adults. 50 mg/hr by continuous infusion for 7 days.

Route	Onset	Peak	Duration
I.V.	Unknown	Unknown	4 to 5 hr

Mechanism of Action
Blocks histamine's action at H_2-receptor sites on the stomach's parietal cells. This action reduces gastric fluid volume and acidity. Cimetidine also decreases the amount of gastric acid that's secreted in response to food, caffeine, insulin, betazole, or pentagastrin.

Incompatibilities
Don't mix cimetidine in same I.V. solution with aminophylline or barbiturates. Don't mix drug in same syringe with pentobarbital sodium.

Contraindications
Hypersensitivity to cimetidine or its components

Interactions
DRUGS
antacids, anticholinergics, metoclopramide: Decreased cimetidine absorption
benzodiazepines, calcium channel blockers, carbamazepine, chloroquine, labetalol, lidocaine, metoprolol, metronidazole, moricizine, pentoxifylline, phenytoin, propafenone, propranolol, quinidine, quinine, sulfonylureas, tacrine, theophyllines, triamterene, tricyclic antidepressants, valproic acid, warfarin: Reduced metabolism and increased blood levels and effects of these drugs, possibly toxicity from these drugs
carmustine: Increased carmustine myelotoxicity
digoxin, fluconazole: Possibly decreased blood levels of these drugs
ferrous salts, indomethacin, ketoconazole, tetracyclines: Decreased effects of these drugs
flecainide: Increased flecainide effects

fluorouracil: Increased blood fluorouracil level after long-term cimetidine use

ketoconazole: Decreased blood ketoconazole level

opioid analgesics: Increased toxic effects of opioid analgesics

oral anticoagulants: Increased anticoagulant effect

procainamide: Increased blood procainamide level

succinylcholine: Increased neuromuscular blockade

tocainide: Decreased tocainide effects

FOODS

caffeine: Reduced metabolism and increased blood level and effects of caffeine

ACTIVITIES

alcohol use: Possibly increased blood alcohol level

Adverse Reactions

CNS: Confusion, dizziness, hallucinations, headache, peripheral neuropathy, somnolence

ENDO: Mild gynecomastia if used longer than 1 month

GI: Mild and transient diarrhea

GU: Impotence, transiently elevated serum creatinine level

SKIN: Rash

Nursing Considerations

- Don't use cimetidine if solution is discolored or contains precipitate.
- For I.V. injection, dilute cimetidine in NS to a total volume of 20 ml. Inject drug over 5 minutes or more.
- Use diluted solution within 48 hours when stored at room temperature.
- **WARNING** Be aware that rapid administration of cimetidine can increase patient's risk of developing arrhythmias and hypotension.
- For intermittent I.V. infusion, dilute drug in at least 50 ml of D_5W or other compatible I.V. solution. Infuse over 15 to 20 minutes.
- Be especially alert for confusion in elderly or debilitated patients who receive cimetidine.
- Before using cimetidine, store it at 15° to 30° C (59° to 86° F).

PATIENT TEACHING

- Advise patient to avoid alcohol during cimetidine therapy to prevent interactions.
- Caution patient that cigarette smoking increases gastric acid secretion and can worsen gastric disease.

ciprofloxacin
Cipro I.V.

Class and Category
Chemical: Fluoroquinolone derivative
Therapeutic: Antibiotic
Pregnancy category: C

Indications and Dosages
▶ *To prevent inhalation anthrax after exposure or to treat inhalation anthrax*
I.V. INFUSION
Adults and adolescents. 400 mg q 12 hr for 60 days.
Children. 10 mg/kg q 12 hr for 60 days. *Maximum:* 400 mg/dose or 800 mg/day.
▶ *To treat acute sinusitis caused by gram-negative organisms (including* Campylobacter jejuni, Citrobacter diversus, Citrobacter freundii, Enterobacter cloacae, Escherichia coli, Haemophilus influenzae, Haemophilus parainfluenzae, Klebsiella pneumoniae, Morganella morganii, Neisseria gonorrhoeae, Proteus mirabilis, Proteus vulgaris, Providencia rettgeri, Providencia stuartii, Pseudomonas aeruginosa, Serratia marcescens, Shigella flexneri, *and* Shigella sonnei) *and gram-positive organisms (including* Enterococcus faecalis, Staphylococcus aureus, Staphylococcus epidermidis, *and* Streptococcus pneumoniae)
I.V. INFUSION
Adults. For mild to moderate infections, 400 mg q 12 hr.
▶ *To treat bone and joint infections caused by susceptible organisms listed above*
I.V. INFUSION
Adults. For mild to moderate infections, 400 mg q 12 hr for 4 to 6 wk; for severe or complicated infections, 400 mg q 8 hr.
▶ *To treat skin and soft-tissue infections caused by susceptible organisms listed above*
I.V. INFUSION
Adults. For mild to moderate infections, 400 mg q 12 hr; for severe or complicated infections, 400 mg q 8 hr.
▶ *To treat chronic bacterial prostatitis caused by susceptible organisms listed above*
I.V. INFUSION
Adults. 400 mg q 12 hr.

▶ *To treat UTIs caused by susceptible organisms listed above*
I.V. INFUSION
Adults. For mild to moderate infections, 200 mg q 12 hr; for severe or complicated infections, 400 mg q 12 hr.
▶ *To treat lower respiratory tract infections caused by susceptible organisms listed above*
I.V. INFUSION
Adults. For mild to moderate infections, 400 mg q 12 hr; for severe or complicated infections, 400 mg q 8 hr.
▶ *To treat intra-abdominal infections caused by susceptible organisms listed above*
I.V. INFUSION
Adults. 400 mg q 8 hr along with parenteral metronidazole.
▶ *To treat mild to severe nosocomial pneumonia caused by susceptible organisms listed above*
I.V. INFUSION
Adults. 400 mg q 8 hr.
DOSAGE ADJUSTMENT Dosage reduced to 250 to 500 mg q 12 hr for patients with creatinine clearance of 30 to 50 ml/min/ 1.73 m^2 and to 200 to 400 mg I.V. q 18 hr for patients with creatinine clearance of 5 to 29 ml/min/1.73 m^2.

Mechanism of Action
Inhibits the enzyme DNA gyrase, which is responsible for the unwinding and supercoiling of bacterial DNA before it replicates. By inhibiting this enzyme, ciprofloxacin causes bacterial cells to die.

Incompatibilities
Don't mix ciprofloxacin with aminophylline, amoxicillin, cefepime, clindamycin, dexamethasone, floxacillin, furosemide, heparin, or phenytoin. If ciprofloxacin must be given concurrently with other drugs, administer them separately.

Contraindications
Hypersensitivity to ciprofloxacin, quinolones, or their components

Interactions
DRUGS
cyclosporine: Elevated serum creatinine and cyclosporine levels
glyburide: Severe hypoglycemia
oral anticoagulants: Enhanced anticoagulant effects
phenytoin: Increased or decreased blood phenytoin level

probenecid: Increased blood ciprofloxacin level, possibly toxicity
theophylline: Increased blood level, half-life, and risk of adverse effects of theophylline
FOODS
caffeine: Increased caffeine effects

Adverse Reactions
CNS: Confusion, headache, restlessness, seizures
CV: Orthostatic hypotension
EENT: Oral candidiasis
GI: Abdominal pain, constipation, diarrhea, elevated liver function test results, flatulence, indigestion, nausea, pseudomembranous colitis, vomiting
GU: Crystalluria, hematuria, increased serum creatinine level, nephrotoxicity, renal calculi, vaginal candidiasis
SKIN: Exfoliative dermatitis, photosensitivity, rash, Stevens-Johnson syndrome, toxic epidermal necrolysis

Nursing Considerations
- Obtain culture and sensitivity test results, as ordered, before giving ciprofloxacin.
- Dilute ciprofloxacin concentrate to 1 to 2 mg/ml, using D_5W or sodium chloride for injection. Before I.V. infusion, don't dilute solutions that come from the manufacturer in D_5W. Infuse slowly over 1 hour.
- Monitor for signs of CNS stimulation or toxicity, such as agitation, confusion, and headache, especially in patients with CNS disorders, such as seizure disorders. Patients with a history of seizures or alcohol abuse and those who are receiving theophylline concurrently with ciprofloxacin may be at risk for seizures.
- Store reconstituted solution for up to 14 days at room temperature or under refrigeration.
- Keep patient well hydrated to help prevent nephrotoxicity.
- Before using ciprofloxacin, store it at room temperature (20° to 25° C [68° to 77° F]) or in a cool place (8° to 15° C [46° to 59° F]).

PATIENT TEACHING
- Encourage patient to drink plenty of fluids during therapy.
- Explain enhanced effects of caffeine caused by ciprofloxacin.
- Instruct patient to notify prescriber immediately at first sign of an allergic reaction, such as rash.
- Advise patient to avoid potentially hazardous activities until drug's CNS effects are known.

cisplatin

Platinol (CAN), Platinol-AQ

Class and Category

Chemical: Inorganic metal complex
Therapeutic: Alkylating-like antineoplastic
Pregnancy category: D

Indications and Dosages

▶ *To treat metastatic testicular tumors*

I.V. INFUSION

Adults. 20 mg/m² q.d. for 5 days q 21-day cycle. *Maximum:* 120 mg/m² for each course.

▶ *To treat metastatic ovarian tumors*

I.V. INFUSION

Adults also receiving cyclophosphamide sequentially. 75 to 100 mg/m² per cycle q 4 wk. *Maximum:* 120 mg/m² for each course.

Adults not receiving cyclophosphamide. 100 mg/m² per cycle q 4 wk. *Maximum:* 120 mg/m² for each course.

Adults also receiving paclitaxel. 75 mg/m² q 3 wk for 6 courses. *Maximum:* 120 mg/m² for each course.

▶ *To treat advanced bladder cancer*

I.V. INFUSION

Adults: 50 to 70 mg/m² per cycle q 3 or 4 wk. *Maximum:* 120 mg/m² for each course.

Mechanism of Action

May bind to DNA within the cell, thus interfering with DNA function and synthesis. May also have a smaller effect on RNA synthesis. Cisplatin's actions are cell-cycle-phase–nonspecific.

Incompatibilities

Don't use needles or I.V. sets containing aluminum to administer cisplatin because a precipitate could form and potency could be decreased.

Contraindications

Hearing impairment, hypersensitivity to cisplatin or other platinum-containing drugs, myelosuppression

Interactions

DRUGS

antihistamines, buclizine, cyclizine, loxapine, meclizine, phenothiazines, thioxanthenes, trimethobenzamide: Possible masking of ototoxicity symptoms

bleomycin: Increased risk of bleomycin toxicity

blood-dyscrasia–causing drugs (including ACE inhibitors, cephalosporins, and NSAIDs): Increased leukopenic and thrombocytopenic effects of cisplatin

bone marrow depressants (such as amphotericin B, colchicine, and paclitaxel): Increased effects of these drugs

nephrotoxic drugs (such as acyclovir, aminoglycosides, and penicillamine): Potentiated risk of nephrotoxicity

ototoxic drugs (such as capreomycin, furosemide, and NSAIDs): Increased risk of ototoxicity

vaccines, killed virus: Possibly decreased antibody response to vaccine

vaccines, live virus: Possibly increased adverse effects of vaccine virus, life-threatening infection, and decreased antibody response to vaccine

Adverse Reactions

CNS: Neurotoxicity

EENT: Optic neuritis, ototoxicity, papilledema, stomatitis, vision changes

ENDO: Syndrome of inappropriate ADH secretion

GI: Anorexia, nausea, vomiting

GU: Nephrotoxicity, uric acid nephropathy

HEME: Anemia, hemolytic anemia, leukopenia, thrombocytopenia

SKIN: Extravasation

Other: Anaphylaxis, hyperuricemia, hypocalcemia, hypomagnesemia

Nursing Considerations

- Be aware that cisplatin should be administered only under the supervision of a qualified physician or nurse in settings where appropriate diagnostic and treatment facilities are available.
- **WARNING** Make sure that emergency equipment and drugs, such as antihistamines, epinephrine, and I.V. corticosteroids, are available in case of anaphylaxis.
- Follow facility protocols for preparation and handling of antineoplastic drugs and appropriate disposal of used equipment.
- **WARNING** To decrease the risk of inadvertent overdose, contact prescriber if cumulative cisplatin dose for each cycle exceeds 100 mg/m^2.

- Monitor creatinine clearance, serum uric acid, and BUN levels, as ordered, before initiating cisplatin therapy and before each subsequent course to detect early signs of nephrotoxicity. Expect dosage to be reduced for patients with impaired renal function.
- Monitor CBC, including hematocrit, platelet count, and WBC count with differential, before and periodically during therapy.
- Monitor serum electrolyte levels, including magnesium, sodium, potassium, and calcium levels, before initiating therapy and before each subsequent course. Be aware that tetany associated with hypocalcemia and hypomagnesemia has been reported.
- Hydrate patient, as ordered, with 1 to 2 L of fluid 8 to 12 hours before cisplatin administration.
- **WARNING** Wear gloves when handling cisplatin. If cisplatin comes in contact with skin or mucosa, immediately and thoroughly wash skin with soap and water and flush mucosa with water.
- Dilute prescribed dose of cisplatin with 2 L of D_5/0.45NS or D_5/0.3NS that contains 37.5 g of mannitol.
- **WARNING** Don't expose cisplatin to needles or administration sets containing aluminum because a precipitate will form and drug potency will be decreased.
- Anticipate dosage reduction if patient is also receiving radiation therapy or a drug that depresses bone marrow.
- Reconstitute cisplatin for injection (available in Canada only) by adding 10 or 50 ml of sterile water for injection to 10- or 50-mg vial, respectively. Further dilute using D_5/0.45NS or D_5/0.3NS. Diluted solution is stable for 20 hours at 27° C (80° F). Protect from light if not used within 6 hours of removal from vial.
- Administer an antiemetic, as prescribed, before initiation of cisplatin therapy. Infuse cisplatin as prescribed. Protect from light if diluted cisplatin is not administered within 6 hours.
- Be prepared to hydrate patient for 24 hours after cisplatin administration, and assess for adequate urine output.
- Observe patient for signs of leukopenia or infection, including fever, chills, pharyngitis, tiredness or weakness, and unusual bleeding or ecchymosis.
- Perform neurologic assessment to check for signs of neurotoxicity, such as paresthesia of the hands and feet, loss of taste or motor function, seizures, muscle spasms, and areflexia. Expect to discontinue cisplatin therapy if neurotoxicity occurs.

- Monitor serum uric acid level, especially in patients with a history of gout or urate calculi. Be aware that allopurinol may be prescribed to help prevent uric acid nephropathy. Expect antigout drug dosage to be adjusted if blood uric acid level is elevated from cisplatin therapy.
- Assess for signs of extravasation at I.V. infusion site, such as redness, swelling, or pain. Be aware that concentrations greater than 0.5 mg/ml put the patient at increased risk for tissue cellulitis, fibrosis, and necrosis.
- Be aware that effects of radiation therapy or bone marrow depressants may be increased when these treatments are administered concurrently with cisplatin. Patients with a history of bone marrow depression, chickenpox (including recent exposure), or herpes zoster are at increased risk for severe generalized disease.
- Monitor patient for signs and symptoms of syndrome of inappropriate ADH secretion, including dizziness, confusion, agitation, and tiredness or weakness.
- Expect subsequent courses of cisplatin therapy to be initiated after an appropriate time interval when serum creatinine level is below 1.5 mg/dl or BUN level is below 25 mg/dl (or both); platelet count is above or equal to $100,000/mm^3$; WBC count is greater than or equal to $4,000/mm^3$; and audiometric testing indicates hearing is within normal limits.
- Store cisplatin injection at 15° to 25° C (59° to 77° F); don't refrigerate.
- Store cisplatin for injection (available in Canada only) at 15° to 30° C (39° to 86° F), and protect from light.

PATIENT TEACHING
- Instruct patient receiving cisplatin to immediately report unusual bruising or bleeding; black, tarry stools; blood in urine or stools; pinpoint red spots on skin; numbness or tingling in fingers or toes; and ringing in ears or hearing loss.
- Urge patient not to receive live or killed virus vaccines during cisplatin therapy and for 3 months to 1 year after completion of therapy, unless approved by prescriber. Instruct him to avoid people who have received such vaccines or to wear a protective mask when he's around them.
- Caution patient to avoid sports and other activities that increase the risk of accidental injury. Also advise him to take measures to avoid infection, such as maintaining good oral hygiene (for

example, by using soft-bristled toothbrush) and washing hands before touching eyes or nose.
* Stress the importance of keeping scheduled follow-up appointments and undergoing prescribed diagnostic tests, such as neurologic function studies and audiometric testing, before each course of cisplatin to monitor for adverse drug effects.
* Suggest that patient with stomatitis eat soft, bland foods served cold or at room temperature to decrease irritation.

clindamycin phosphate
Cleocin, Dalacin C Phosphate (CAN)

Class and Category
Chemical: Lincosamide
Therapeutic: Antibacterial and antiprotozoal antibiotic
Pregnancy category: B

Indications and Dosages
▶ *To treat serious respiratory tract infections caused by anaerobes such as occur with anaerobic pneumonitis, empyema, and lung abscess and those caused by pneumococci, staphylococci, and streptococci; serious skin and soft-tissue infections caused by anaerobes, staphylococci, and streptococci; septicemia caused by anaerobes; intra-abdominal infections caused by anaerobes such as occur with intra-abdominal abscess and peritonitis; infections of the female pelvis and genital tract caused by anaerobes such as occur with endometritis, nongonococcal tubo-ovarian abscess, pelvic cellulitis, and postsurgical vaginal cuff infection; bone and joint infections caused by* Staphylococcus aureus; *as adjunct therapy in chronic bone and joint infections*
I.V. INFUSION
Adults and adolescents age 16 and older. For serious infections, 600 to 1,200 mg/day in equally divided doses b.i.d. to q.i.d.; for severe infections, 1,200 to 2,700 mg/day in equally divided doses b.i.d. to q.i.d.; for life-threatening infections, 4,800 mg/day in equally divided doses b.i.d. to q.i.d.
Children ages 1 month to 16 years. 20 to 40 mg/kg/day in equally divided doses t.i.d. or q.i.d., depending on severity of infection.
Neonates less than age 1 month. 15 to 20 mg/kg/day in equally divided doses t.i.d. or q.i.d., depending on severity of infection.

Mechanism of Action
Inhibits protein synthesis in susceptible bacteria by binding to the 50S subunits of bacterial ribosomes and preventing peptide bond formation, which causes bacterial cells to die.

Incompatibilities
Don't administer clindamycin with aminophylline, ampicillin, barbiturates, calcium gluconate, magnesium sulfate, or phenytoin because these drugs are physically incompatible.

Contraindications
Hypersensitivity to clindamycin or lincomycin

Interactions
DRUGS
chloramphenicol, erythromycin: Possibly antagonized effects of clindamycin
neuromuscular blockers: Increased neuromuscular blockade

Adverse Reactions
CNS: Fatigue, headache
CV: Hypotension
EENT: Glossitis, metallic or unpleasant taste, stomatitis
GI: Abdominal pain, diarrhea, esophagitis, nausea, pseudomembranous colitis, vomiting
HEME: Agranulocytosis, eosinophilia, leukopenia, neutropenia, thrombocytopenic purpura
SKIN: Pruritus, rash, urticaria
Other: Anaphylaxis, infusion site thrombophlebitis, superinfection

Nursing Considerations
- Expect to obtain a specimen for culture and sensitivity testing before giving first dose of clindamycin.
- Administer I.V. dose by infusion only; don't give bolus dose. Dilute 300 mg of clindamycin in 50 ml of diluent and administer over 10 minutes. Dilute 600 mg of clindamycin in 100 ml of diluent and administer over 20 minutes. Dilute 900 mg of clindamycin in 100 ml of diluent and administer over 30 minutes.
- Store diluted parenteral solution for up to 24 hours at room temperature.

- **WARNING** When preparing clindamycin for administration to neonates or premature infants, don't use drug that contains benzyl alcohol because it may cause a fatal toxic syndrome characterized by CNS, respiratory, circulatory, and renal impairment and metabolic acidosis.
- Be aware that drug should be used cautiously in patients with atopy, significant allergies, or a history of asthma.
- Check I.V. site frequently for phlebitis and irritation.
- Monitor results of liver function tests, CBC, and platelet counts during prolonged therapy.
- Monitor serum drug levels, as ordered, in patients with impaired hepatic or renal function who are receiving high doses. A dosage adjustment may be necessary.
- Observe patient for signs of superinfection, such as vaginal itching and sore mouth, and for signs of pseudomembranous colitis, which may occur 2 to 9 days after therapy begins. Patients with a history of GI disease, particularly colitis or regional enteritis, are at increased risk for colitis. Be aware that antibiotic-related diarrhea and colitis are more common and may be more severe and less well tolerated in elderly patients.
- Before diluting drug, store it at 15° to 30° C (59° to 86° F).

PATIENT TEACHING

- Advise patient receiving clindamycin to immediately report signs or symptoms of colitis (severe diarrhea and abdominal cramps) or superinfection (an inflamed mouth or vagina), as well as rash or lesions.

codeine phosphate

Class, Category, and Schedule
Chemical: Phenanthrene derivative
Therapeutic: Opioid analgesic
Pregnancy category: C
Controlled substance: Schedule II

Indications and Dosages
▶ *To treat mild to moderate pain*
I.V. INJECTION
Adults. 15 to 60 mg q 4 hr. *Usual:* 30 mg/dose.

Mechanism of Action

May produce analgesia through partial metabolism to morphine. Codeine binds with mu, delta, and kappa receptors in the spinal cord and with mu_1 and $kappa_3$ receptors at higher levels in the CNS, altering the perception of—and emotional response to—pain. By binding with these receptors, the drug decreases levels of intracellular cAMP, which inhibits adenylate cyclase activity. This action prevents the release of pain neurotransmitters, such as substance P and dopamine.

Contraindications

Hypersensitivity to codeine, other opioids, or their components; significant respiratory depression

Interactions

DRUGS

anticholinergics, paregoric: Increased risk of severe constipation
antihypertensives, diuretics: Potentiated hypotensive effects
buprenorphine: Decreased effectiveness of codeine
CNS depressants: Additive CNS effects
hydroxyzine: Increased codeine analgesic effect, increased CNS depressant and hypotensive effects
MAO inhibitors: Increased risk of unpredictable, severe, and sometimes fatal reactions
metoclopramide: Antagonized effect of metoclopramide on GI motility
naloxone: Antagonized codeine analgesic effect
naltrexone: Precipitated withdrawal symptoms in codeine-dependent patients
neuromuscular blockers: Additive respiratory depressant effects
other opioid analgesics: Additive CNS and respiratory depressant effects and hypotensive effects

ACTIVITIES

alcohol use: Additive CNS effects

Adverse Reactions

CNS: Coma, delirium, depression, disorientation, dizziness, drowsiness, euphoria, hallucinations, headache, lack of coordination, lethargy, light-headedness, mental and physical impairment, mood changes, restlessness, sedation, seizures, tremor
CV: Bradycardia, heart block, orthostatic hypotension, palpitations, tachycardia

EENT: Altered taste, blurred vision, diplopia, dry mouth, laryngeal edema, laryngospasm, miosis
GI: Abdominal cramps and pain, anorexia, constipation, flatulence, ileus, nausea, vomiting
GU: Decreased libido, difficult ejaculation, dysuria, impotence, oliguria, ureteral spasm, urinary incontinence, urine retention
MS: Muscle rigidity
RESP: Apnea, bronchoconstriction, bronchospasm, depressed cough reflex, respiratory depression
SKIN: Diaphoresis, flushing, pallor, pruritus, rash, urticaria
Other: Anaphylaxis, facial edema, physical and psychological dependence

Nursing Considerations

- Instruct patient to lie down during codeine administration and for a period afterward to lessen dizziness, light-headedness, nausea, and vomiting.
- **WARNING** Administer diluted codeine solution slowly over several minutes. Rapid administration may cause serious adverse reactions, including anaphylaxis, severe respiratory depression, hypotension, peripheral circulatory collapse, and cardiac arrest. Make sure emergency equipment and drugs are available.
- Evaluate for therapeutic response, including decreased pain and facial grimacing.
- Monitor respiratory depth, effort, and rate. Notify prescriber immediately if respiratory rate drops below 10 breaths/minute; patients having an acute asthma attack and those with chronic respiratory disease are at increased risk. Pediatric, elderly, debilitated, or extremely ill patients are at increased risk for drug's respiratory depressant effects.
- Monitor for signs of drug-induced CNS depression or increased CSF pressure, such as altered LOC, restlessness, and irritability, in patients with a head injury, intracranial lesions, or other conditions that could cause these effects. Patients who are taking or have recently taken drugs that cause CNS depression are also more susceptible to these effects. Take appropriate safety precautions.
- Be aware that codeine may induce or exacerbate arrhythmias or seizures in patients with a history of these conditions and may mask symptoms of acute abdominal conditions.
- **WARNING** Assess patient for signs of physical and psychological dependence.

- Be aware that patients with a history of drug abuse (including acute alcoholism), emotional instability, or suicidal ideation or attempts are at increased risk for opioid abuse; however, the risk of drug dependence is lower with codeine than with some other opioid analgesics.
- Assess urine output; decreasing output may signal urine retention.
- Store drug at 15° to 30° C (59° to 86° F). Protect from freezing and light.

PATIENT TEACHING
- Advise patient to avoid alcohol and other CNS depressants, including OTC preparations, during codeine therapy because of possible additive CNS effects.
- Advise patient to avoid potentially hazardous activities until drug's CNS effects are known.
- Caution patient to get up slowly from a sitting or lying position.
- To prevent constipation, encourage patient to consume plenty of fluids and high-fiber foods, if not contraindicated by another condition.
- Advise patient to notify prescriber if he becomes short of breath or has difficulty breathing.

colchicine

Class and Category
Chemical: Colchicum alkaloid derivative
Therapeutic: Antigout agent, anti-inflammatory
Pregnancy category: D

Indications and Dosages
▶ *To prevent gouty arthritis attacks*
I.V. INFUSION OR INJECTION
Adults. 0.5 to 1 mg q.d. or b.i.d. *Maximum:* 4 mg/day.
▶ *To treat acute gouty arthritis*
I.V. INFUSION OR INJECTION
Adults. 2 mg over 2 to 5 min; then 0.5 mg q 6 hr or 1 mg q 6 to 12 hr until pain decreases. *Maximum:* 4 mg/day.
DOSAGE ADJUSTMENT For elderly patients, maximum dosage reduced to 2 mg/24 hr. After initial course of therapy, patient should receive no further colchicine in any form for 21 days.

Route	Onset	Peak	Duration
I.V.	In 6 to 12 hr	Unknown	Unknown

Mechanism of Action

In gouty arthritis, leukocytes re-lease chemotactic factors, deg-radation enzymes, and other in-flammatory substances through phagocytosis of urate crystals in affected joints. Colchicine helps stop this process, probably by disrupting microtubules within leukocytes.

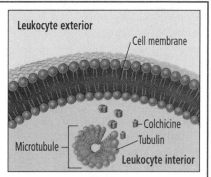

Normally, microtubules con-tribute to cell structure and movement. When colchicine binds to tubulin (the protein from which microtubules are made), the microtubule falls apart, as shown. This process disrupts cell function and prevents leukocytes from in-vading joints and producing inflammation.

Contraindications

Blood dyscrasias; hypersensitivity to colchicine or its components; serious cardiac, GI, hepatic, or renal disorders

Incompatibilities

Don't combine colchicine with bacteriostatic agents, any solution or injection that contains D_5W, or any other solution that may change colchicine's pH because precipitation may occur.

Interactions

DRUGS

anticoagulants (such as heparin), platelet aggregation inhibitors (such as aspirin), thrombolytics (such as alteplase): Possibly significantly in-creased risk of GI ulceration or hemorrhage

antineoplastics: Possibly increased serum uric acid level and de-creased therapeutic effectiveness of colchicine

cyclosporine: Increased blood cyclosporine level

NSAIDs (such as phenylbutazone): Possibly increased risk of bone mar-row depression, GI bleeding, leukopenia, or thrombocytopenia

vitamin B_{12}: Possibly impaired absorption of and increased dosage requirements for vitamin B_{12}

ACTIVITIES

alcohol use: Increased risk of adverse GI effects

Adverse Reactions

CNS: Peripheral neuropathy
CV: Arrhythmias
GI: Abdominal pain, diarrhea, nausea, vomiting
HEME: Agranulocytosis, aplastic anemia, thrombocytopenia
MS: Myopathy
SKIN: Alopecia, rash
Other: Injection site pain and tenderness, median nerve neuritis in affected arm, and skin and soft-tissue necrosis if extravasation occurs

Nursing Considerations

- **WARNING** To prevent extravasation, ensure that the I.V. catheter is patent and correctly positioned before administering colchicine. Throughout therapy, check I.V. injection site frequently for pain, tenderness, and skin peeling. Consult prescriber about switching to oral form as soon as possible. Avoid S.C. or I.M. administration of colchicine because these routes may cause tissue necrosis and sloughing.
- **WARNING** Don't give colchicine by any route within 7 days after a full I.V. course (4 mg) because of the risk of toxicity. Be aware that elderly or debilitated patients and those with a history of cardiac disease or impaired renal or hepatic function are at increased risk for cumulative toxicity.
- Expect to monitor CBC and platelet and reticulocyte counts at baseline and every 3 months after therapy starts.
- Dilute drug with 10 to 20 ml of NS. Don't use a diluent that contains a bacteriostatic agent. Alternatively, administer colchicine through a free-flowing I.V. line with NS into a large vein. Don't use colchicine if solution is cloudy or contains sediment.
- Administer I.V. form over 2 to 5 minutes.
- Notify prescriber immediately and expect to stop therapy if patient develops signs or symptoms of colchicine toxicity, such as abdominal pain, diarrhea, nausea, or vomiting.
- Store drug at 15° to 30° C (59° to 86° F); protect from freezing and light.

PATIENT TEACHING

- Instruct patient to return for blood tests every 3 months, as ordered, during colchicine therapy.
- Explain that gouty arthritis pain and swelling typically subside in 24 to 48 hours after therapy begins.

- Advise patient to immediately report abdominal pain, diarrhea, nausea, or vomiting.

co-trimoxazole
(sulfamethoxazole and trimethoprim)
Bactrim, Septra

Class and Category
Chemical: Sulfonamide derivative (sulfamethoxazole), dihydrofolic acid analogue (trimethoprim)
Therapeutic: Antibiotic
Pregnancy category: C

Indications and Dosages
▶ *To treat acute otitis media, shigellosis, UTIs, and other infections caused by gram-negative organisms (including* Enterobacter *species,* Escherichia coli, Haemophilus ducreyi, Haemophilus influenzae, *indole-positive* Proteus *species,* Klebsiella pneumoniae, Neisseria gonorrhoeae, Proteus mirabilis, Providencia *species,* Salmonella *species,* Serratia *species, and* Shigella *species) and gram-positive organisms (including group A beta-hemolytic streptococci,* Nocardia *species,* Staphylococcus aureus, *and* Streptococcus pneumoniae)

I.V. INFUSION
Adults and children over age 2 months. 40 to 50 mg/kg of sulfamethoxazole (SMZ) and 8 to 10 mg/kg of trimethoprim (TMP) daily in divided doses q 6, 8, or 12 hr for up to 5 days for shigellosis and 14 days for UTIs.

▶ *To treat* Pneumocystis carinii *pneumonia*
I.V. INFUSION
Adults and children over age 2 months. 75 to 100 mg/kg of SMZ and 15 to 20 mg/kg of TMP daily in three or four divided doses q 6 to 8 hr for up to 14 days.

Mechanism of Action
Blocks two consecutive steps in the formation of essential nucleic acids and proteins in susceptible organisms. Sulfamethoxazole inhibits synthesis of dihydrofolic acid (a nucleic acid) by competing with para-aminobenzoic acid. Trimethoprim inhibits the action of the enzyme dihydrofolate reductase, thus blocking production of tetrahydrofolic acid.

Incompatibilities
Don't mix co-trimoxazole with other drugs or solutions.

Contraindications
Age less than 2 months; hypersensitivity to sulfamethoxazole, sulfonamides, trimethoprim, or their components; megaloblastic anemia caused by folate deficiency

Interactions
DRUGS

cyclosporine: Decreased blood level and therapeutic effectiveness of cyclosporine, increased risk of nephrotoxicity

dapsone: Possibly increased blood levels of co-trimoxazole and dapsone

diuretics: Increased risk of thrombocytopenic purpura in elderly patients

methotrexate: Increased blood methotrexate level and risk of methotrexate toxicity

oral anticoagulants: Increased anticoagulant effects

phenytoin: Possibly decreased hepatic clearance and prolonged half-life of phenytoin

sulfonylureas: Possibly increased hypoglycemic effects of sulfonylureas

zidovudine: Possibly increased blood zidovudine level

Adverse Reactions
CNS: Anxiety, aseptic meningitis, ataxia, chills, depression, fatigue, hallucinations, headache, insomnia, seizures, vertigo
EENT: Glossitis, stomatitis
GI: Abdominal pain, anorexia, diarrhea, hepatitis, nausea, pancreatitis, pseudomembranous colitis, vomiting
GU: Crystalluria, renal failure, toxic nephrosis
HEME: Agranulocytosis, eosinophilia, hemolytic anemia, leukopenia, methemoglobinemia, neutropenia, thrombocytopenia
RESP: Cough, dyspnea
SKIN: Dermatitis, erythema, photosensitivity, rash, Stevens-Johnson syndrome, toxic epidermal necrolysis, urticaria
Other: Anaphylaxis, infusion site inflammation and pain

Nursing Considerations
- Expect to obtain culture and sensitivity test results before beginning co-trimoxazole therapy, as ordered.
- Dilute each 5 ml of co-trimoxazole with 125 ml of D_5W (75 ml if fluid restriction is needed) before administration. Don't use other solutions.

- Don't refrigerate diluted solutions. Use within 6 hours if diluted in 125 ml of D₅W and within 2 hours if diluted in 75 ml of D₅W.
- Discard solution if it becomes cloudy or contains crystals.
- **WARNING** When preparing drug for administration to neonates or premature infants, don't use diluents that contain benzyl alcohol because they have been linked to a fatal toxic syndrome characterized by CNS, respiratory, circulatory, and renal impairment and metabolic acidosis.
- Infuse drug slowly, over 60 to 90 minutes.
- Monitor bowel elimination pattern daily; severe diarrhea may indicate pseudomembranous enterocolitis.
- Assess for evidence of blood dyscrasia, including bleeding, ecchymosis, joint pain, and pharyngitis.

PATIENT TEACHING
- Instruct patient receiving co-trimoxazole to notify prescriber immediately if rash, severe diarrhea, or other serious adverse reactions occur. Be aware that elderly patients, especially those taking diuretics, are at increased risk for severe skin and hematologic reactions.
- Inform patient that yogurt and buttermilk can help minimize diarrhea during therapy.
- To minimize photosensitivity, advise patient to avoid direct sunlight and to use sunscreen and wear protective clothing when outdoors.

cyclophosphamide

Cytoxan, Neosar, Procytox (CAN)

Class and Category

Chemical: Nitrogen mustard derivative
Therapeutic: Alkylating antineoplastic
Pregnancy category: D

Indications and Dosages

▶ *To treat acute lymphocytic or nonlymphocytic leukemia, chronic myelocytic or lymphocytic leukemia, neuroblastoma, retinoblastoma, and Hodgkin's disease or non-Hodgkin's lymphoma*

I.V. INFUSION OR INJECTION

Adults. *Initial:* 40 to 50 mg/kg in divided doses over 2 to 5 days, or 10 to 15 mg/kg q 7 to 10 days, or 3 to 5 mg/kg 2 times a week. *Maintenance:* Varies with diagnosis and patient's clinical and hematologic response to, and tolerance of, therapy.

Children. *Initial:* 2 to 8 mg/kg or 60 to 250 mg/m² q wk or in divided doses for 6 or more days. *Maintenance:* 10 to 15 mg/kg q 7 to 10 days, or 30 mg/kg q 3 to 4 wk or when bone marrow recovery occurs.

▶ *To treat breast, epithelial, or ovarian cancer; multiple myeloma; and mycosis fungoides*

I.V. INFUSION OR INJECTION

Adults. *Initial:* 40 to 50 mg/kg in divided doses over 2 to 5 days, or 10 to 15 mg/kg q 7 to 10 days, or 3 to 5 mg/kg 2 times a week. *Maintenance:* Varies with diagnosis and patient's clinical and hematologic response and tolerance to therapy.

DOSAGE ADJUSTMENT Dosage varies, depending on regimen used. Dosage may be reduced when cyclophosphamide is used in combination with other cytotoxic drugs.

Mechanism of Action

After biotransformation in the liver, crosslinks with strands of DNA and RNA to interfere with the growth of susceptible, rapidly proliferating malignant cells. Cyclophosphamide inhibits protein synthesis within the cell and also has immunosuppressive qualities. Its actions are cell-cycle-phase–nonspecific.

Contraindications

Hypersensitivity to cyclophosphamide, severely depressed bone marrow

Interactions

DRUGS

allopurinol: Increased toxic effects of cyclophosphamide on bone marrow

blood-dyscrasia–causing drugs (such as cephalosporins and cisplatin): Increased leukopenic and thrombocytopenic effects of cyclophosphamide

bone marrow depressants (such as colchicine and methotrexate): Increased bone marrow depression

busulfan: Decreased cyclophosphamide clearance, possibly leading to cyclophosphamide toxicity

chloramphenicol: Decreased cyclophosphamide effectiveness

cocaine: Increased risk of prolonged cocaine effects and cocaine toxicity

cytarabine: Cardiomyopathy and risk of death

daunorubicin, doxorubicin: Risk of increased cardiotoxicity

hepatic enzyme inducers (such as allopurinol and erythromycin): Decreased half-life and increased activity of cyclophosphamide
immunosuppressants (such as azathioprine, chlorambucil, corticosteroids, and cyclosporine): Increased risk of infection and development of neoplasms
lovastatin: Increased risk of rhabdomyolysis and acute renal failure in heart transplant patients
oral anticoagulants: Decreased or increased anticoagulant activity
pentostatin, trastuzumab: Increased risk of cardiotoxicity
phenobarbital: Increased metabolism and leukopenic activity of cyclophosphamide
succinylcholine: Enhanced neuromuscular blockade effects of succinylcholine
tamoxifen: Increased risk of thromboembolism
thiazide diuretics: Increased risk of granulocytopenia
vaccines, killed virus: Possibly decreased antibody response to vaccine
vaccines, live virus: Possibly increased adverse effects of vaccine, severe infection, and decreased antibody response to vaccine

Adverse Reactions

CNS: Dizziness, headache
CV: Cardiotoxicity (including acute myopericarditis and cardiomyopathy)
EENT: Stomatitis
ENDO: Condition resembling syndrome of inappropriate ADH secretion (SIADH), hyperglycemia
GI: Anorexia, diarrhea, epigastric pain, hemorrhagic colitis, hepatitis, nausea, vomiting
GU: Amenorrhea, azoospermia, hemorrhagic and nonhemorrhagic cystitis, infertility, nephrotoxicity, oligospermia, uric acid nephropathy
HEME: Anemia, leukopenia, thrombocytopenia
RESP: Interstitial pulmonary fibrosis, pneumonitis
SKIN: Alopecia, darkened nails, diaphoresis, flushing or erythema of face, hyperpigmentation, pruritus, rash, urticaria
Other: Anaphylaxis, hyperkalemia, hyperuricemia, hyponatremia, impaired wound healing, infection, injection site edema, pain, or redness

Nursing Considerations

• Follow facility protocol for preparation and handling of antineoplastic drugs and for appropriate disposal of used equipment.

- Anticipate dosage reduction if patient is also receiving radiation therapy or a drug that depresses bone marrow.
- Monitor liver and renal function test results before and periodically during therapy because drug is metabolized in the liver and excreted by the kidneys.
- Monitor CBC, including hematocrit, platelet count, and WBC count with differential, before and periodically during therapy.
- Be prepared to hydrate patient before and after therapy to minimize the risk of hemorrhagic cystitis and to help eliminate drug-induced uric acid accumulation.
- Prepare a solution with a concentration of 20 mg/ml by adding appropriate amount of sterile water for injection or bacteriostatic water for injection (paraben-preserved only) if specified by manufacturer. Shake until dissolved. Be aware that nonlyophilized form of cyclophosphamide for injection may take up to 6 minutes to dissolve; lyophilized form takes about 45 seconds.
- **WARNING** When preparing drug for administration to neonates or premature infants, don't use diluents that contain benzyl alcohol because they have been linked to a fatal toxic syndrome characterized by CNS, respiratory, circulatory, and renal impairment and metabolic acidosis.
- Solution may be diluted further for I.V. infusion with D_5W, D_5NS, D_5LR, LR, 0.45NS, or sodium lactate injection. Use within 24 hours if stored at room temperature or within 6 days if refrigerated.
- Be aware that adverse reactions can vary when cyclophosphamide is administered in combination therapy. Review information for all drugs administered as part of a specific regimen, including drug interactions and adverse effects.
- Assess patient for signs of hemorrhagic cystitis, including hematuria and dysuria, and expect to discontinue cyclophosphamide therapy if you detect them.
- Monitor serum uric acid level, especially in patients with a history of gout or urate calculi. Expect a dosage adjustment of antigout drugs if blood uric acid level is elevated from cyclophosphamide therapy. Be aware that uricosuric antigout drugs may increase the risk of uric acid nephropathy.
- Observe patient for signs of leukopenia or infection, including fever, chills, pharyngitis, tiredness or weakness, and unusual bleeding or ecchymosis.
- Monitor patients who have undergone an adrenalectomy for increased toxic effects of cyclophosphamide. Expect dosages of replacement steroids and cyclophosphamide to be adjusted.

- Be aware that effects of radiation therapy or bone marrow depressants may be increased when these therapies are administered concurrently with cyclophosphamide. Patients with a history of bone marrow depression, chickenpox (including recent exposure), or herpes zoster are at increased risk for severe generalized disease.
- Assess urine output and urinary specific gravity to assess for a syndrome resembling SIADH. Obtain urine specimen, as ordered, for microscopic examination for hematuria periodically during therapy and for several hours after a large dose.
- Monitor patient for signs of dizziness, confusion, and agitation, which could indicate a syndrome similar to SIADH. Tiredness and weakness are also symptoms.
- Be aware that some patients receiving cyclophosphamide have developed a second malignancy, such as leukemia or bladder or renal cancer; however, a causal relationship hasn't been established.
- Store unopened cyclophosphamide below 25° C (77° F).

PATIENT TEACHING

- Tell patient receiving cyclophosphamide to immediately report unusual bruising or bleeding; black, tarry stools; blood in urine or stools; or pinpoint red spots on the skin.
- Review with patient the need for adequate fluid intake and frequent urination (including at least once at night) to help prevent hemorrhagic cystitis and to aid in elimination of excess uric acid, which may result from cyclophosphamide treatment.
- Instruct patient to consult prescriber if he requires dental surgery or emergency treatment with general anesthesia within 10 days of cyclophosphamide treatment.
- Advise patient not to receive live or killed virus vaccines during therapy and for 3 months to 1 year after completion of cyclophosphamide therapy, unless approved by prescriber. Urge patient to avoid people who have received such vaccines or to wear a protective mask when he's around them.
- Caution patient to avoid sports and other activities that increase the risk of accidental injury. Also advise him to take measures to avoid infection, such as maintaining good oral hygiene (for example, by using soft-bristled toothbrush) and washing hands before touching eyes or nose.
- Advise patient with thrombocytopenia to avoid alcohol and aspirin to reduce the risk of GI bleeding.
- Suggest that patient with stomatitis eat soft, bland foods served cold or at room temperature to decrease irritation.

- Inform patient that his hair should grow back following treatment but that color and texture may be different.
- Inform patient that although cyclophosphamide may reduce sperm count and function and ovarian function, he should use a barrier method of birth control during therapy.

cyclosporine
(cyclosporin A)
Neoral, Sandimmune, SangCya

Class and Category
Chemical: Tolypocladium inflatum Gams–derived or *Cylindrocarpon lucidum* Booth–derived polypeptide
Therapeutic: Immunosuppressant
Pregnancy category: C

Indications and Dosages
▶ *To prevent or treat organ rejection in allogenic kidney, liver, or heart transplantation*
I.V. INFUSION
Adults. 2 to 6 mg/kg/day, beginning 4 to 12 hr before surgery and continuing postoperatively until patient can tolerate oral form.
CAPSULES, MODIFIED CAPSULES, MODIFIED ORAL SOLUTION, ORAL SOLUTION
Adults and children. *Initial:* 12 to 15 mg/kg/day in divided doses q 12 hr, beginning 4 to 12 hr before surgery and continuing for 1 to 2 wk postoperatively. Then, dosage reduced by 5%/wk to maintenance dose. *Maintenance:* 5 to 10 mg/kg/day in divided doses q 12 hr.

Mechanism of Action
Causes immunosuppression by inhibiting the proliferation of T lymphocytes, the production and release of lymphokines, and the release of interleukin-2.

Contraindications
Abnormal renal function, neoplastic diseases, and uncontrolled hypertension in patients with psoriasis or rheumatoid arthritis (modified capsules and oral solution); hypersensitivity to cyclosporine, its components, or polyoxyethylated castor oil (with I.V. infusion)

Interactions

DRUGS

aminoglycosides, amphotericin B, NSAIDs: Increased risk of nephrotoxicity

amiodarone, calcium channel blockers, chloroquine, clarithromycin, erythromycin, itraconazole, ketoconazole, miconazole, oral contraceptives, verapamil: Increased blood cyclosporine level and risk of nephrotoxicity

anabolic steroids, androgens: Increased blood cyclosporine level and risk of toxicity

carbamazepine, phenytoin, rifabutin, rifampin: Decreased blood cyclosporine level and therapeutic response

colchicine: Increased risk of adverse GI, hepatic, neuromuscular, and renal effects

corticosteroids: Increased risk of cyclosporine toxicity

co-trimoxazole, sulfonamides: Decreased blood cyclosporine level, increased risk of nephrotoxicity

digoxin: Increased blood digoxin level and risk of digitalis toxicity

etoposide: Decreased renal clearance of etoposide, increased risk of etoposide toxicity

foscarnet: Increased risk of renal failure

HMG-CoA reductase inhibitors: Risk of irreversible myopathy and rhabdomyolysis

imipenem and cilastatin: Increased risk of CNS toxicity

metoclopramide: Increased cyclosporine bioavailability and risk of toxicity

probucol: Possibly decreased blood level and effects of cyclosporine

terbinafine: Increased metabolism and decreased blood level of cyclosporine

vaccines, killed virus: Possibly decreased antibody response to vaccine

vaccines, live virus: Possibly increased adverse effects of vaccine, severe infection, and decreased antibody response to vaccine

FOODS

grapefruit juice: Increased risk of nephrotoxicity (with oral drug)

Adverse Reactions

CNS: Confusion, headache, paresthesia, seizures, tremor

CV: Chest pain, hypertension

EENT: Gingival hyperplasia, oral candidiasis

ENDO: Gynecomastia

GI: Diarrhea, nausea, pancreatitis, vomiting

GU: Albuminuria, hematuria, proteinuria, renal failure

HEME: Anemia, leukopenia, thrombocytopenia

SKIN: Acne, flushing, hirsutism, rash
Other: Anaphylaxis, hyperkalemia, hypomagnesemia, lymphoma

Nursing Considerations

- Prepare I.V. infusion by diluting each milliliter of cyclosporine concentrate in 20 to 100 ml of NS or D₅W. Use glass containers because of possible leaching of diethylhexyphthalate from polyvinyl chloride (PVC) bags into cyclosporine solution.
- Use solutions reconstituted with D₅W within 24 hours. Use solutions reconstituted with NS within 6 hours if in PVC container or within 12 hours if in a glass container.
- Administer I.V. infusion over 2 to 6 hours or, if needed, over 24 hours.
- **WARNING** Closely monitor for anaphylaxis during at least first 30 minutes of I.V. administration. Make sure emergency equipment and drugs are immediately available.
- **WARNING** Be aware that rapid I.V. infusion may cause acute nephrotoxicity.
- Don't draw blood to measure cyclosporine level through same I.V. tubing used to administer drug, even if line was flushed after administration. Blood level may be falsely elevated.
- Monitor blood pressure, especially in patients with a history of hypertension, because drug can exacerbate this condition.
- Monitor results of hepatic and renal function tests, as ordered, to detect signs of decreased function.
- Be aware that cyclosporine use may result in increased serum cholesterol levels.
- Be aware that cyclosporine capsules and oral solution aren't interchangeable with modified capsules and modified oral solution. Modified forms have greater bioavailability than nonmodified forms.
- Be aware that oral solution contains alcohol and shouldn't be administered to patient who drinks heavily or has a history of alcohol dependence.
- Don't add water to oral solution because it will alter drug's effectiveness.
- Avoid giving oral forms of cyclosporine with grapefruit juice, which may raise trough level, increasing risk of nephrotoxicity.
- Store capsules at 25° C (77° F) and in prepackaged foil wrap to protect them from light.
- Before diluting cyclosporine concentrate for injection, store it below 30° C (86° F); don't freeze.

PATIENT TEACHING

• Instruct patient receiving cyclosporine to immediately report any serious adverse reactions, such as difficulty breathing, a rash, or chest tightness.

• Caution patient to avoid contact with people who have infections during therapy because cyclosporine causes immunosuppression.

• Urge patient to maintain good dental hygiene because of risk of gingival hyperplasia.

• Advise patient not to stop taking drug without consulting prescriber.

• Instruct patient not to receive live or killed virus vaccines during therapy. Urge him to avoid people who have received such vaccines or to wear a protective mask when he's around them.

• Instruct patient to take oral drug at same time each day and in same relation to type and timing of food intake to help increase compliance and maintain steady blood level.

• Advise patient to mix oral solution in a glass—not plastic—container with milk, chocolate milk, orange juice, or apple juice to improve flavor. Also advise him to avoid grapefruit juice because it alters drug metabolism.

• Instruct patient to use syringe supplied by manufacturer to ensure accurate measurement of oral solution dose and to wipe syringe—not rinse it—after use to prevent cloudiness.

• Advise patient to discard oral solution after it has been opened for 2 months.

daclizumab
(dacliximab)
Zenapax

Class and Category
Chemical: Monoclonal antibody
Therapeutic: Immunosuppressant
Pregnancy category: C

Indications and Dosages
▶ *To prevent acute organ rejection after kidney transplantation*
I.V. INFUSION
Adults and children. 1 mg/kg given in five doses: dose 1 given no more than 24 hr before transplantation; doses 2 through 5, at 14-day intervals.

Mechanism of Action
Inhibits interleukin-2–mediated activation of lymphocytes, which prevents WBCs from attacking the transplanted kidney. Daclizumab also reduces the body's infection-fighting ability.

Contraindications
Hypersensitivity to daclizumab or its components

Interactions
None known.

Adverse Reactions
CNS: Anxiety, chills, depression, dizziness, fatigue, fever, headache, insomnia, paresthesia, tremor, weakness
CV: Chest pain, edema, hypertension, hypotension, tachycardia, thrombosis
EENT: Blurred vision, pharyngitis, rhinitis
ENDO: Hyperglycemia
GI: Abdominal distention and pain, constipation, diarrhea, flatulence, gastritis, heartburn, hemorrhoids, indigestion, nausea, vomiting

GU: Dysuria, hematuria, hydronephrosis, oliguria, renal insufficiency, renal tubular necrosis, urine retention
HEME: Bleeding
MS: Arthralgia, back pain, leg cramps, myalgia
RESP: Atelectasis, cough, crackles, dyspnea, hypoxia, lung congestion, pleural effusion, pulmonary edema
SKIN: Acne, diaphoresis, hirsutism, impaired wound healing, night sweats, pruritus, rash
Other: Dehydration, fluid overload, injection site pain and redness, lymphocele

Nursing Considerations
• Avoid shaking vial of daclizumab before use. Dilute calculated dose of daclizumab in 50 ml of NS. Gently invert bag to mix; don't shake it to prevent foaming.
• Don't use solution if it contains particles or is discolored.
• Use room temperature solution within 4 hours or refrigerated solution within 24 hours; discard unused solution.
• Because daclizumab's compatibility with other drugs isn't known, don't add or simultaneously infuse other drugs through same I.V. line.
• Administer drug through a peripheral or central vein over 15 minutes.
• Monitor blood glucose level for increases during therapy.
• **WARNING** Although daclizumab seldom causes severe hypersensitivity reactions, keep drugs that treat such reactions readily available.
• Before using drug, store it at 2° to 8° C (36° to 46° F). Don't freeze or shake; protect from direct light.
PATIENT TEACHING
• Urge patient to complete full course of daclizumab therapy and to return for scheduled follow-up visits.

dantrolene sodium
Dantrium, Dantrium Intravenous

Class and Category
Chemical: Hydantoin derivative, imidazolidinedione sodium salt
Therapeutic: Malignant hyperthermia therapy adjunct
Pregnancy category: C (parenteral), not rated (oral)

Indications and Dosages

▶ *To prevent malignant hyperthermia before surgery*
I.V. INFUSION
Adults and children. *Initial:* 2.5 mg/kg infused over 1 hr 60 to 75 min before anesthesia. Additional individualized doses given as needed during surgery.
CAPSULES
Adults and children. 4 to 8 mg/kg/day in divided doses t.i.d. or q.i.d. 1 or 2 days before surgery, with last dose given 3 to 4 hr before surgery.
▶ *To treat malignant hyperthermia*
I.V. INJECTION
Adults and adolescents. *Initial:* 1 mg/kg by rapid bolus, repeated as needed until symptoms subside or cumulative dose of 10 mg/kg has been reached. Dose repeated if symptoms reappear.
▶ *To treat postmalignant hyperthermic crisis*
I.V. INJECTION
Adults and children. *Initial:* Individualized dosage beginning with 1 mg/kg or more as needed if oral therapy can't be used. *Maximum:* 10 mg/kg total dose.
CAPSULES
Adults and children. 4 to 8 mg/kg/day in divided doses q.i.d. for 1 to 3 days.

Mechanism of Action
Prevents calcium release from the sarcoplasmic reticulum of skeletal muscle cells. Blocked calcium release inhibits the activation of acute catabolism associated with malignant hyperthermia.

Incompatibilities
Don't administer dantrolene with acidic solutions, including D_5W and NS.

Contraindications
For oral drug only: Active hepatic disease (such as cirrhosis and hepatitis), conditions in which spasticity helps maintain upright posture and improve balance or function, skeletal muscle spasms caused by rheumatic disorders

Interactions
DRUGS
calcium channel blockers (especially verapamil): Possibly hyperkalemia, life-threatening arrhythmias, and shock

sedatives: Possibly profound sedation
ACTIVITIES
alcohol use: Possibly increased CNS depression

Adverse Reactions

CNS: Dizziness, drowsiness, fatigue, light-headedness, malaise, slurred speech or other speech problems, weakness
CV: Heart failure (I.V. form), pericarditis
GI: Abdominal cramps, diarrhea, dysphagia, hepatitis, hepatotoxicity, nausea, vomiting
GU: Enuresis
MS: Decreased grip strength, myalgia
RESP: Dyspnea, feeling of suffocation, pleural effusion
SKIN: Erythema (I.V. form), extravasation with tissue damage, urticaria
Other: Thrombophlebitis

Nursing Considerations

- Reconstitute each vial of dantrolene with 60 ml of sterile water for injection (without a bacteriostatic agent). Shake vial until clear. Store reconstituted solution at room temperature, protected from direct sunlight. Discard after 6 hours.
- To prevent precipitation of reconstituted drug, transfer it to a plastic I.V. bag, rather than a glass bottle, for infusion. Don't use solution if it contains precipitate or is cloudy.
- Because drug has a high pH, infuse into a central vein, if possible, to avoid tissue damage from extravasation.
- Monitor blood pressure and heart rate frequently during drug administration to detect tachycardia and blood pressure changes.
- Monitor results of liver function tests—especially ALT, AST, alkaline phosphatase, and total bilirubin levels—to detect hepatotoxicity.
- Be aware that oral form of dantrolene is also used to treat chronic spastic conditions. Consult manufacturer's insert for additional dosage guidelines, nursing considerations, and adverse reactions associated with long-term oral use.
- Before reconstituting dantrolene, store it at 15° to 30° C (59° to 86° F), and avoid prolonged exposure to light.

PATIENT TEACHING
- Inform patient that dantrolene may weaken her grip strength as well as muscles used for walking and climbing stairs. Advise her to be careful when eating to avoid problems due to difficulty swallowing.

- Caution patient about drug's sedating effects. Instruct her to avoid sedatives, unless prescribed, and other sedating substances, such as alcohol.
- Advise patient to report yellow skin or sclerae, itching, or fatigue.

darbepoetin alfa
Aranesp

Class and Category
Chemical: 165–amino acid glycoprotein similar to human erythropoietin
Therapeutic: Antianemic agent
Pregnancy category: C

Indications and Dosages
▶ *To treat anemia from chronic renal failure*
I.V. INJECTION
Adults. *Initial:* 0.45 mcg/kg as a single dose q wk. *Maintenance:* Dosage individualized and titrated once a month to maintain a hemoglobin level of no more than 12 g/dl.
DOSAGE ADJUSTMENT Dosage reduced by approximately 25% if hemoglobin level increases and approaches 12 g/dl. If hemoglobin level continues to increase, doses temporarily withheld until hemoglobin level begins to decrease, at which point therapy is restarted at a dose approximately 25% below previous dose. Dosage reduced by approximately 25% if hemoglobin level increases by more than 1 g/dl in a 2-wk period. Dosage increased by approximately 25% of previous dose if hemoglobin increase is less than 1 g/dl over 4 wk, but only if serum ferritin level is 100 mcg/L or greater and serum transferrin saturation is 20% or greater. Further increases made q 4 wk until specified hemoglobin level is obtained.
DOSAGE ADJUSTMENT For patients being converted from epoetin alfa to darbepoetin alfa, dose administered q wk for those who previously received epoetin alfa 2 to 3 times/wk and darbepoetin alfa dosage adjusted as follows: 6.25 mcg/wk for patients who received less than 2,500 U/wk of epoetin alfa; 12.5 mcg/wk for patients who received 2,500 to 4,999 U/wk of epoetin alfa; 25 mcg/wk for patients who received 5,000 to 10,999 U/wk of epoetin alfa; 40 mcg/wk for patients who received 11,000 to 17,999 U/wk of epoetin alfa; 60 mcg/wk for patients who received 18,000 to 33,999 U/wk of epoetin alfa; 100 mcg/wk for patients who received 34,000 to 89,999 U/wk

of epoetin alfa; and 200 mcg/wk for patients who received 90,000 U/wk or more of epoetin alfa. Preceding adjusted dosages of darbepoetin administered once q 2 wk for patients who previously received epoetin alfa once q wk.

Route	Onset	Peak	Duration
I.V.	In 2 to 6 wk	Unknown	Unknown

Mechanism of Action
Stimulates the release of reticulocytes from the bone marrow into the bloodstream, where they develop into mature RBCs.

Incompatibilities
Don't mix darbepoetin alfa with any other drug.

Contraindications
Hypersensitivity to human albumin or products made from mammal cells, uncontrolled hypertension

Interactions
None known.

Adverse Reactions
CNS: Asthenia, dizziness, fatigue, fever, headache, seizures
CV: Arrhythmias, chest pain, heart failure, hypertension, hypotension, peripheral edema, vascular access hemorrhage or thrombosis
GI: Abdominal pain, constipation, diarrhea, nausea, vomiting
MS: Arthralgia, back or limb pain, myalgia
RESP: Bronchitis, cough, dyspnea, upper respiratory tract infection
SKIN: Rash, urticaria
Other: Death, fluid overload, flulike symptoms, infection, injection site pain, sepsis

Nursing Considerations
• Before beginning darbepoetin alfa therapy, expect to correct folic acid or vitamin B_{12} deficiencies because these conditions may interfere with the drug's effectiveness.
• To ensure effective drug response, expect to obtain serum ferritin level and serum transferrin saturation before beginning and during therapy, as ordered. If serum ferritin level is less than 100 mcg/L or serum transferrin saturation is less than 20%, expect to begin supplemental iron therapy.

- Don't shake vial during preparation to avoid denaturing drug and rendering it biologically inactive.
- Discard drug if you observe particles or discoloration.
- Don't dilute drug before administration.
- Discard unused portion of drug because it contains no preservatives.
- Monitor blood pressure frequently during therapy for signs of hypertension. Expect to reduce dosage or withhold drug if blood pressure is poorly controlled with antihypertensive and dietary measures.
- Monitor hemoglobin level weekly, as ordered, until hemoglobin stabilizes and maintenance dosage has been achieved. Thereafter, monitor hemoglobin regularly, as ordered. After each dosage adjustment, expect to monitor hemoglobin level weekly for 4 weeks until hemoglobin stabilizes in response to dosage change.
- **WARNING** Be aware that the risk of cardiac arrest, seizures, stroke, exacerbation of hypertension, heart failure, vascular thrombosis, vascular ischemia, vascular infarction, acute MI, and fluid overload with peripheral edema increases if hemoglobin level increases by more than approximately 1 g/dl during any 2-week period. Expect to decrease darbepoetin dosage.
- Institute seizure precautions according to facility policy.
- Expect to administer lower dosage to patients with chronic renal failure who *aren't* receiving dialysis than to patients who *are* receiving dialysis. Also, monitor renal function test results and fluid and electrolyte balance in these patients to detect signs of deteriorating renal function.
- Store drug at 2° to 8° C (36° to 46° F); protect from freezing and light.

PATIENT TEACHING
- Inform patient that the risk of seizures is highest during first few months of darbepoetin alfa therapy. Advise her not to engage in potentially hazardous activities during this time.
- Stress the importance of complying with the dosage regimen and keeping follow-up doctor's appointments and appointments for laboratory tests.
- Advise patient to undergo periodic blood pressure monitoring with prescriber.

- Encourage patient to eat iron-rich foods.
- If patient will self-administer darbepoetin, teach her and her caregiver the proper administration technique.
- Instruct patient and caregiver not to reuse needles or syringes and to discard any unused portion of drug after each dose. Thoroughly instruct them in proper needle and syringe disposal using a puncture-resistant container.
- Review possible adverse reactions, and urge patient to notify prescriber if she experiences chest pain, headache, rash, seizures, shortness of breath, or swelling.

desmopressin acetate
DDAVP Injection, Octostim (CAN)

Class and Category
Chemical: Synthetic ADH analogue
Therapeutic: Antidiuretic, antihemorrhagic
Pregnancy category: B

Indications and Dosages
▶ *To control symptoms of central diabetes insipidus*
I.V. INFUSION
Adults. 2 to 4 mcg/day in divided doses b.i.d. Dosage adjusted as needed.
▶ *To prevent or manage bleeding episodes in hemophilia A or mild to moderate type I von Willebrand's disease*
I.V. INFUSION
Adults and children who weigh more than 10 kg (22 lb). 0.3 mcg/kg diluted in 50 ml of NS and infused over 15 to 30 min. If used preopcratively, dose is given 30 min before procedure.
Children who weigh 10 kg or less. 0.3 mcg/kg diluted in 10 ml of NS and infused over 15 to 30 min. If used preoperatively, dose is given 30 min before procedure.

Route	Onset	Peak	Duration
I.V.	15 to 30 min*	30 to 60 min*	3 hr†

* For antihemorrhagic effect.
† For von Willebrand's disease; 4 to 20 hr for mild hemophilia A.

Mechanism of Action

Exerts an antidiuretic effect similar to that of vasopressin by increasing the cellular permeability of renal collecting ducts and distal tubules, thereby enhancing water reabsorption. This action results in reduced urine flow and increased osmolality. As an antihemorrhagic, desmopressin increases the blood concentration of clotting factor VIII (antihemophilic factor) and the activity of von Willebrand's factor. It also may increase platelet aggregation and adhesion at injury sites by exerting a direct effect on blood vessel walls.

Contraindications

Hypersensitivity to desmopressin or its components

Interactions

DRUGS

carbamazepine, chlorpropamide, clofibrate: Possibly potentiated antidiuretic effect of desmopressin

demeclocycline, lithium: Possibly decreased antidiuretic effect of desmopressin

vasopressors: Possibly potentiated vasopressor effect of desmopressin

Adverse Reactions

CNS: Asthenia, chills, dizziness, headache
CV: Hypertension (with high doses), tachycardia, transient hypotension
GI: Nausea
GU: Vulvar pain
SKIN: Flushing
Other: Allergic reaction, anaphylaxis, hyponatremia, injection site pain and redness, water intoxication

Nursing Considerations

• Monitor serum sodium and chloride levels, as ordered, during desmopressin therapy. Also monitor fluid intake and output and urine osmolality, and weigh patient daily. Assess for signs and symptoms of hyponatremia, including anxiety, hypotension, muscle twitching, oliguria, and tachycardia. Be aware that patients with conditions associated with fluid and electrolyte imbalances, such as cystic fibrosis, are at increased risk for hyponatremia.
• Monitor blood pressure and pulse rate frequently during therapy.
• Be aware that comparable antidiuretic parenteral dose is about one-tenth the intranasal dose.

- Assess laboratory values, as ordered, including APTT, bleeding time, coagulation factor assay, von Willebrand's factor antigen, and von Willebrand's factor assay.

PATIENT TEACHING

- To prevent hyponatremia and water intoxication in a child or an elderly patient during desmopressin therapy, instruct family to restrict fluids as prescribed.
- Urge patient to report adverse reactions, including difficulty breathing and wheezing.

dexamethasone sodium phosphate

Cortastat, Dalalone, Decadrol, Decadron Phosphate, Decaject, Dexacorten, Dexasone, Dexone, Hexadrol Phosphate, Primethasone, Solurex

Class and Category

Chemical: Synthetic adrenocortical steroid
Therapeutic: Anti-inflammatory, diagnostic aid, immunosuppressant
Pregnancy category: C

Indications and Dosages

▶ *To treat endocrine disorders, such as congenital adrenal hyperplasia, hypercalcemia associated with cancer, and nonsuppurative thyroiditis; acute episodes or exacerbations of rheumatic disorders; collagen diseases, such as systemic lupus erythematosus and acute rheumatic carditis; severe dermatologic diseases; severe allergic conditions, such as seasonal or perennial allergic rhinitis, bronchial asthma, laryngeal edema, serum sickness, and drug hypersensitivity reactions; respiratory diseases, such as symptomatic sarcoidosis, Löffler's syndrome, berylliosis, fulminating or disseminated pulmonary tuberculosis, and aspiration pneumonitis; hematologic disorders, such as idiopathic thrombocytopenic purpura and secondary thrombocytopenia in adults, autoimmune hemolytic anemia, aplastic crisis, and congenital hypoplastic anemia; tuberculous meningitis and trichinosis with neurologic or myocardial involvement*
▶ *To manage leukemia and lymphoma in adults and acute leukemia in children; to induce diuresis or remission of proteinuria in idiopathic nephrotic syndrome without uremia or nephrotic syndrome caused by systemic lupus erythematosus*
▶ *To provide palliative therapy during acute exacerbations of GI diseases, such as ulcerative colitis and regional enteritis*

I.V. INJECTION

Adults. Highly individualized dosage based on severity of disorder. *Usual:* 0.75 to 9 mg/day as a single dose or in divided doses.

▶ *To manage adrenocortical insufficiency*
I.V. INJECTION
Adults. 0.5 to 9 mg/day as a single dose or in divided doses.
▶ *To distinguish Cushing's syndrome related to pituitary corticotropin excess from Cushing's syndrome related to other causes*
I.V. OR I.M. INJECTION
Adults. 10 mg I.V., followed by 4 mg I.M. q 6 hr. Decreased after 2 to 4 days, if needed, gradually tapering off over 5 to 7 days unless inoperable or recurring brain tumor is present. If such a tumor is present, dosage gradually decreased after 2 to 4 days to maintenance dosage of 2 mg I.M. q 8 to 12 hr and switched to P.O. regimen as soon as possible.
▶ *To treat unresponsive shock*
I.V. INFUSION AND INJECTION
Adults. 20 mg as a single dose, followed by 3 mg/kg over 24 hr as a continuous infusion; 40 mg as a single dose, followed by 40 mg q 2 to 6 hr, as needed; or 1 mg/kg as a single dose. All regimens used for no more than 3 days.

Mechanism of Action
Binds to intracellular glucocorticoid receptors and suppresses inflammatory and immune responses by:
- inhibiting neutrophil and monocyte accumulation at inflammation site and suppressing their phagocytic and bactericidal activity
- stabilizing lysosomal membranes
- suppressing antigen response of macrophages and helper T cells
- inhibiting synthesis of inflammatory response mediators, such as cytokines, interleukins, and prostaglandins.

Contraindications
Administration of live virus vaccine to patient or family member, hypersensitivity to dexamethasone or its components (including sulfites), idiopathic thrombocytopenic purpura (I.M. use), systemic fungal infections

Interactions
DRUGS
aminoglutethimide, barbiturates, hydantoins, mitotane, rifampin: Decreased dexamethasone effectiveness
amphotericin B (parenteral), carbonic anhydrase inhibitors: Risk of hypokalemia

anticholinesterases: Decreased anticholinesterase effectiveness in myasthenia gravis
digoxin: Increased risk of digitalis toxicity related to hypokalemia
ephedrine: Decreased half-life and increased clearance of dexamethasone
estrogens, ketoconazole: Decreased dexamethasone clearance
isoniazid: Decreased blood isoniazid level
neuromuscular blockers: Possibly potentiated or counteracted neuromuscular blockade
oral anticoagulants: Altered coagulation times, requiring reduction of anticoagulant dosage
oral contraceptives: Increased half-life and concentration of dexamethasone
potassium-wasting diuretics: Increased potassium loss and risk of hypokalemia
salicylates: Decreased blood level and effectiveness of salicylates
somatrem: Possibly inhibition of somatrem's growth-promoting effect
theophyllines: Altered effects of either drug
toxoids, vaccines: Decreased antibody response
ACTIVITIES
alcohol use: Increased risk of GI bleeding

Adverse Reactions

CNS: Depression, euphoria, fever, headache, increased ICP, insomnia, light-headedness, malaise, paresthesia, psychosis, seizures, syncope, tiredness, vertigo, weakness
CV: Arrhythmias, edema, fat embolism, heart failure, hypercholesterolemia, hyperlipidemia, hypertension, myocardial rupture, thromboembolism, thrombophlebitis
EENT: Cataracts, glaucoma, papilledema, vision changes
ENDO: Cushingoid symptoms, decreased iodine uptake, growth suppression in children, hyperglycemia, menstrual irregularities
GI: Abdominal distention, bloody stools, heartburn, increased appetite, indigestion, melena, nausea, pancreatitis, peptic ulcer with possible perforation, ulcerative esophagitis, vomiting
GU: Glycosuria, increased or decreased number and motility of spermatozoa, perineal irritation, urinary frequency
HEME: Leukocytosis, leukopenia
MS: Muscle atrophy or weakness, myalgia, osteoporosis, pathologic fracture of long bones, tendon rupture, vertebral compression fractures
RESP: Bronchospasm, dyspnea

SKIN: Acne, allergic dermatitis, diaphoresis, ecchymosis, erythema, flushing, hirsutism, necrotizing vasculitis, petechiae, subcutaneous fat atrophy, striae, thin and fragile skin, urticaria

Other: Aggravated or masked signs of infection, anaphylaxis, angioedema, hypernatremia, hypocalcemia, hypokalemia, hypokalemic alkalosis, impaired wound healing, metabolic acidosis, sodium and fluid retention, suppressed skin test reaction, weight gain

Nursing Considerations

- Give once-daily dose of dexamethasone in the morning to coincide with the body's natural cortisol secretion.
- Inject undiluted I.V. dose directly into I.V. tubing of infusing compatible solution over 30 seconds or less, as prescribed. Use solutions diluted with D_5W or NS within 24 hours.
- Be aware that dosage forms with a concentration of 24 mg/ml are for I.V. use only.
- Shake I.M. solution before injecting deep into large muscle mass.
- **WARNING** Avoid S.C. injection; it may cause atrophy and sterile abscess.
- Expect to taper drug rather than stopping it abruptly; prolonged use can cause adrenal suppression.
- Assess for hypersensitivity reactions after administration because dexamethasone sodium phosphate may contain bisulfites or parabens, inactive ingredients to which some people are allergic. Be aware that some preparations also contain benzyl alcohol, which may cause a fatal toxic syndrome in neonates and immature infants.
- Monitor fluid intake and output and daily weight, and assess for crackles, dyspnea, peripheral edema, and steady weight gain.
- Test stool for occult blood.
- Monitor results of hematology studies as well as blood glucose and serum electrolyte, cholesterol, and lipid levels. Dexamethasone may cause hyperglycemia, hypernatremia, hypocalcemia, hypokalemia, or leukopenia; may increase serum cholesterol and lipid levels; and may decrease iodine uptake by the thyroid.
- Assess for evidence of osteoporosis, Cushing's syndrome, and other systemic effects during long-term use.
- Monitor neonate for signs of hypoadrenocorticism if mother received dexamethasone during pregnancy.
- Store dexamethasone at 15° to 30° C (59° to 86° F); protect from freezing and light.

PATIENT TEACHING

- Inform patient that symptoms won't subside for several days after starting dexamethasone therapy.
- Caution patient to avoid alcoholic beverages during therapy because they increase the risk of GI bleeding.
- Advise patient to follow a low-sodium, high-potassium, high-protein diet, if prescribed, to help minimize weight gain (common with this drug). Instruct her to inform prescriber if she's on a special diet.
- Instruct patient not to stop using drug abruptly.
- Encourage patient to keep regularly scheduled follow-up appointments, even after therapy stops.
- Advise patient to notify prescriber if condition recurs or worsens after dosage is reduced or therapy stops.
- Urge patient to have regular eye examinations during long-term use.
- Advise patient receiving long-term therapy to carry medical identification and to notify all health care providers that she takes dexamethasone.
- Instruct patient to avoid close contact with anyone who has chickenpox or measles and to notify prescriber immediately if exposure occurs.
- Advise patient and family members to avoid live virus vaccinations during therapy unless prescriber approves.
- Inform diabetic patient that drug may affect her blood glucose level.
- Advise patient to report anorexia, depression, light-headedness, malaise, muscle pain, nausea, vomiting, and signs of early hyperadrenocorticism (abdominal distention, amenorrhea, easy bruising, extreme weakness, facial hair, increased appetite, moon face, weight gain). Inform patient and family about possible changes in appearance.
- Instruct patient to report illness, surgery, or changes in stress level.

dexrazoxane
Zinecard

Class and Category

Chemical: Piperazinedione
Therapeutic: Cardioprotective agent, chelating agent
Pregnancy category: C

Indications and Dosages

▶ *To prevent or reduce severity of cardiomyopathy associated with doxorubicin therapy in women with metastatic breast cancer*

I.V. INJECTION

Adults. 500 mg/m^2 for every 50 mg/m^2 of doxorubicin q 3 wk.

Mechanism of Action

Rapidly enters cardiac cells and acts as an intracellular heavy metal chelator. In cardiac tissues, anthracyclines such as doxorubicin form complexes with iron or copper, resulting in damage to cardiac cell membranes and mitochondria. Dexrazoxane combines with intracellular iron and protects against anthracycline-induced free radical damage to the myocardium. It also prevents the conversion of ferrous ions back to ferric ions for use by free radicals.

Incompatibilities

Don't mix dexrazoxane in same I.V. line with other drugs.

Contraindications

Hypersensitivity to dexrazoxane or its components; use with chemotherapy regimens that don't contain an anthracycline (such as daunorubicin, doxorubicin, epirubicin, idarubicin, or mitoxantrone)

Interactions

DRUGS

bone marrow depressants: Possibly enhanced bone marrow depression

Adverse Reactions

HEME: Myelosuppression, including granulocytopenia, leukopenia, or thrombocytopenia

Other: Injection site pain

Nursing Considerations

• **WARNING** Use gloves when preparing reconstituted solution. If dexrazoxane powder or solution comes in contact with your skin or mucosa, immediately and thoroughly wash with soap and water.

• Reconstitute drug by mixing with 25 or 50 ml of 0.167 molar sodium lactate, supplied by the manufacturer, to produce a final concentration of 10 mg/ml. Administer reconstituted solution by slow I.V. push, or further dilute with either NS or D$_5$W to a concentration of 1.3 to 5 mg/ml, as prescribed, for rapid I.V. infusion.

- After reconstituting or further diluting drug, store it for up to 6 hours at room temperature of 15° to 30° C (59° to 86° F) or refrigerated at 2° to 8° C (36° to 46° F).
- Be aware that dexrazoxane may interfere with tumor response to doxorubicin, especially in patients receiving drug at beginning of fluorouracil-doxorubicin-cyclophosphamide (FAC) therapy.
- Monitor patient with preexisting immunosuppression or decreased bone marrow reserves resulting from prior chemotherapy or radiation therapy to prevent worsening of her condition. Notify prescriber if condition deteriorates.
- Before reconstituting dexrazoxane, store it at 15° to 30° C (59° to 86° F).

PATIENT TEACHING

- Inform patient that dexrazoxane is used to protect the heart from damage caused by myeolosuppression and that she'll be given the drug by a health care professional in the hospital or clinic before receiving chemotherapy.
- Inform patient that dexrazoxane and chemotherapy may make her feel generally unwell, but urge her to continue treatment unless prescriber tells her to stop.
- Instruct patient to report such symptoms as fever, chills, sore throat, mouth sores, unusual bleeding or bruising, unusual tiredness or weakness, pain at injection site, and vomiting because these symptoms may require a change in dosage or discontinuation of drug.
- Inform patient that drug may exacerbate symptoms of bone marrow suppression caused by anthracycline chemotherapy, including increased risk of infection.
- Emphasize to patient the importance of avoiding injury and infection during dexrazoxane therapy. For example, advise her to use a soft-bristled toothbrush to prevent damage to teeth and gums; to avoid people with colds, the flu, or bronchitis; and to avoid anyone who has recently had a live virus vaccine because of the increased risk of infection from the live virus.

dextrose
glucose
2.5% Dextrose Injection, 5% Dextrose Injection, 10% Dextrose Injection, 20% Dextrose Injection, 25% Dextrose Injection, 30% Dextrose Injection, 40% Dextrose Injection, 50% Dextrose Injection, 60% Dextrose Injection, 70% Dextrose Injection

Class and Category
Chemical: Monosaccharide
Therapeutic: Antihypoglycemic, nutritional supplement
Pregnancy category: C

Indications and Dosages
▶ *To treat insulin-induced hypoglycemia*
I.V. INFUSION OR INJECTION
Adults and children. *Initial:* 20 to 50 ml of 50% solution given at 3 ml/min. *Maintenance:* 10% to 15% solution by continuous infusion until blood glucose level reaches therapeutic range.
Infants and neonates. 2 ml/kg of 10% to 25% solution until blood glucose level reaches therapeutic range.
▶ *To replace calories*
I.V. INFUSION
Adults and children. Individualized dosage of 2.5%, 5%, or 10% solution, based on need for fluids or calories and given through peripheral I.V. line. Or a 10% to 70% solution given through a large central vein, if needed, and typically mixed with amino acids or other solutions.

Route	Onset	Peak	Duration
I.V.	2 to 3 min	Unknown	Unknown

Mechanism of Action
Prevents protein and nitrogen loss, promotes glycogen deposition, prevents or decreases ketosis, and, in large amounts, acts as an osmotic diuretic. Dextrose is readily metabolized and undergoes oxidation to carbon dioxide and water.

Incompatibilities
Don't give dextrose through same infusion set as blood or blood products because pseudoagglutination of RBCs may occur.

Contraindications
For all solutions: Diabetic coma with excessively elevated blood glucose level
For concentrated solutions: Anuria, alcohol withdrawal syndrome in dehydrated patient, glucose-galactose malabsorption syndrome, hepatic coma, intracranial or intraspinal hemorrhage, overhydration

Interactions
DRUGS
corticosteroids, corticotropin: Increased risk of fluid and electrolyte imbalance if dextrose solution contains sodium ions

Adverse Reactions
CNS: Confusion, fever
GU: Glycosuria
Other: Dehydration; hyperosmolar coma; hypervolemia; hypovolemia; injection site extravasation with tissue necrosis, infection, phlebitis, and venous thrombosis

Nursing Considerations
• Give highly concentrated dextrose solution by central venous catheter, not by S.C. or I.M. route.
• Assess infusion site regularly for signs of infiltration, such as pain, redness, and swelling.
• Monitor blood glucose and electrolyte levels, as appropriate.
• Assess for glucosuria by using a urine reagent strip or collecting a urine sample and reviewing urinalysis results.
• When discontinuing a concentrated solution, expect to give a 5% to 10% dextrose infusion to avoid rebound hypoglycemia.
• Monitor for signs of hypervolemia, such as jugular vein distention and crackles.
PATIENT TEACHING
• Inform patient that her blood glucose level will be monitored as directed during dextrose therapy.
• Stress the importance of reporting discomfort, pain, or signs of infection at I.V. site.

dezocine
Dalgan

Class and Category
Chemical: Aminotetralin, synthetic opioid
Therapeutic: Opioid analgesic
Pregnancy category: C

Indications and Dosages
▶ *To relieve pain*
I.V. INJECTION
Adult. *Initial:* 5 mg, followed by 2.5 to 10 mg q 2 to 4 hr, p.r.n. *Maximum:* 120 mg/day.

Route	Onset	Peak	Duration
I.V.	In 15 min	30 min	2 to 4 hr

Mechanism of Action
Binds with opioid receptors at many CNS sites, which alters the perception of, and emotional response to, pain.

Contraindications
Hypersensitivity to dezocine or its components

Interactions
DRUGS
CNS depressants, general anesthetics, hypnotics, sedatives, tranquilizers: Increased CNS depression
other opioid analgesics: Possibly decreased therapeutic effects of other opioid and withdrawal symptoms in patient receiving long-term opioid therapy
ACTIVITIES
alcohol use: Increased CNS depression

Adverse Reactions
CNS: CNS toxicity (delirium, delusions, mental depression), dizziness, sedation, vertigo
CV: Chest pain, hypertension, hypotension, irregular heartbeat
GI: Nausea, vomiting
GU: Decreased urine output, dysuria, urinary frequency
RESP: Atelectasis, cough, dyspnea, respiratory depression
Other: Injection site redness and swelling

Nursing Considerations
• Have patient lie down during dezocine administration and for a period afterward to lessen drug's hypotensive effects (dizziness, light-headedness) and other adverse effects, such as nausea and vomiting.
• **WARNING** Administer dezocine slowly. Rapid administration of other opioid analgesics has caused anaphylaxis, severe respiratory depression, hypotension, peripheral circulatory collapse, and cardiac arrest. Keep emergency equipment and drugs nearby.
• Be aware that dosage reduction may be required for patients with respiratory disease (to avoid decreased respiratory drive and increased airway resistance); impaired hepatic function, including cirrhosis (because elimination half-life may be pro-

longed); or impaired renal function as well as for elderly, debilitated, or severely ill patients (who may be more sensitive to drug's effects).

- Discard solution if it contains precipitate.
- Frequently monitor blood pressure and pulse and respiratory rates after giving first dose.
- **WARNING** Avoid administering dezocine to a patient who is opioid-dependent. Doing so may precipitate withdrawal symptoms because drug can antagonize opioid effects. Patients with a history of drug abuse (including acute alcoholism), emotional instability, or suicidal ideation or attempts are at increased risk for abuse.
- Assess for pain relief and document findings frequently.
- Assess respiratory status in patients with acute respiratory depression because dezocine can exacerbate this condition. Patients having an acute asthma attack and those with chronic disease are at increased risk for respiratory depression.
- Monitor patients with a history of common bile duct disorders for signs of increased biliary pressure, such as pain in upper midline area that may radiate to back and right shoulder.
- Monitor for worsening condition in patients with diarrhea caused by poisoning or pseudomembranous colitis.
- Assess urine output; decreasing output may signal urine retention.
- Monitor for signs of drug-induced CNS depression or increased CSF pressure, such as altered LOC, restlessness, and irritability, in patients with a head injury, intracranial lesions, or other conditions that could cause these effects. Patients who are taking or have recently taken drugs that cause CNS depression are also more susceptible to these effects. Take appropriate safety precautions.
- Be aware that patients with hypothyroidism are at increased risk for respiratory depression and prolonged CNS depression.
- Be aware that dezocine may affect GI motility or mask symptoms of acute abdominal conditions.

PATIENT TEACHING
- Instruct patient to report if dezocine doesn't relieve pain within 1 hour.
- Advise patient to avoid potentially hazardous activities until drug's CNS effects are known.
- Advise patient to change position slowly to minimize dizziness and light-headedness.
- Urge patient to avoid alcohol and other drugs that cause CNS depression during dezocine therapy.

diazepam

Diazemuls, Dizac, Valium

Class, Category, and Schedule

Chemical: Benzodiazepine
Therapeutic: Anticonvulsant, anxiolytic, sedative-hypnotic, skeletal muscle relaxant
Pregnancy category: D
Controlled substance: Schedule IV

Indications and Dosages

▶ *To relieve anxiety*

I.V. INJECTION

Adults. 2 to 5 mg q 3 to 4 hr, p.r.n., for moderate anxiety; 5 to 10 mg q 3 to 4 hr, p.r.n., for severe anxiety.

Children. Individualized dosage. *Maximum:* 0.25 mg/kg given over 3 min and repeated after 15 to 30 min if needed and after another 15 to 30 min if needed.

▶ *To treat symptoms of acute alcohol withdrawal*

I.V. INJECTION

Adults. 10 mg and then 5 to 10 mg in 3 to 4 hr, if needed.

▶ *To provide muscle relaxation, sedation*

I.V. INJECTION

Adults. 5 to 10 mg and then 5 to 10 mg in 3 to 4 hr, if needed.

DOSAGE ADJUSTMENT Dosage reduced to 2 to 5 mg/dose and increased as needed and tolerated for debilitated patients.

▶ *To treat status epilepticus and severe recurrent seizures*

I.V. INJECTION

Adults. 5 to 10 mg repeated q 10 to 15 min, as needed, up to a cumulative dose of 30 mg. Regimen repeated, if needed, in 2 to 4 hr. (Use I.M. route if I.V. access is impossible.)

Children age 5 and older. 1 mg repeated q 2 to 5 min, as needed, up to a cumulative dose of 10 mg. Regimen repeated, if needed, in 2 to 4 hr.

Children ages 1 month to 5 years. 0.2 to 0.5 mg repeated q 2 to 5 min, as needed, up to a cumulative dose of 5 mg. Regimen repeated, if needed, in 2 to 4 hr.

▶ *To provide preoperative sedation*

I.V. INJECTION

Adults. 5 to 10 mg 30 min before surgery.

▶ *To reduce anxiety before cardioversion*

I.V. INJECTION

Adults. 5 to 15 mg 5 to 10 min before procedure.

▶ *To reduce anxiety before endoscopic procedures*
I.V. INJECTION
Adults. Up to 20 mg titrated to desired sedation and administered immediately before procedure.
▶ *To treat tetanus*
I.V. INJECTION
Adults and children age 5 and older. *Initial:* 5 to 10 mg repeated q 3 to 4 hr, if needed. Sometimes larger doses are needed for adults.
DOSAGE ADJUSTMENT For debilitated patients, initial dose reduced to 2 to 5 mg and increased gradually as needed and tolerated.
Children ages 1 month to 5 years. 1 to 2 mg repeated q 3 to 4 hr, as needed.

Mechanism of Action

May potentiate the effects of gamma-aminobutyric acid (GABA) and other inhibitory neurotransmitters by binding to specific benzodiazepine receptors in the limbic and cortical areas of the CNS. GABA inhibits excitatory stimulation, which helps control emotional behavior. The limbic system contains a highly dense area of benzodiazepine receptors, which may explain the drug's anti-anxiety effects. Diazepam also suppresses the spread of seizure activity caused by seizure-producing foci in the cortex, thalamus, and limbic structures.

Incompatibilities

Don't mix diazepam injection with aqueous solutions. Don't mix diazepam emulsion with morphine or glycopyrrolate or administer it through an infusion set that contains polyvinyl chloride.

Contraindications

Acute angle-closure glaucoma, hypersensitivity to diazepam or its components, untreated open-angle glaucoma

Interactions

DRUGS
cimetidine, disulfiram, fluoxetine, isoniazid, itraconazole, ketoconazole, metoprolol, oral contraceptives, propoxyphene, propranolol, valproic acid: Decreased diazepam metabolism, increased blood level and risk of adverse effects of diazepam
CNS depressants: Increased CNS depression
digoxin: Increased serum digoxin level and risk of digitalis toxicity
levodopa: Decreased antidyskinetic effect of levodopa

probenecid: Faster onset or more prolonged effects of diazepam
ranitidine: Delayed elimination and increased blood level of diazepam
rifampin: Decreased blood diazepam level
theophyllines: Antagonized sedative effect of diazepam
ACTIVITIES
alcohol use: Increased CNS depression

Adverse Reactions

CNS: Anterograde amnesia, anxiety, ataxia, confusion, depression, dizziness, drowsiness, fatigue, headache, insomnia, lethargy, light-headedness, sedation, sleepiness, slurred speech, tremor, vertigo
CV: Hypotension, palpitations, phlebitis, tachycardia, thrombophlebitis
EENT: Blurred vision, diplopia, increased salivation
GI: Anorexia, constipation, diarrhea, nausea, vomiting
GU: Libido changes, urinary incontinence, urine retention
RESP: Respiratory depression
SKIN: Dermatitis
Other: Physical and psychological dependence

Nursing Considerations

• Protect diazepam injection from light. Don't use solution if it is more than slightly yellow or contains precipitate.
• Don't mix emulsion form with anything other than its emulsion base. Otherwise, it may become unstable and increase the risk of serious adverse reactions.
• Before administering emulsion form, ask if patient is allergic to soybeans because this form contains soybean oil.
• Administer diazepam directly into an I.V. line inserted in a large vein or through I.V. tubing as close to insertion site as possible at a rate of at least 5 mg/minute. For an infant or a child, administer I.V. injection slowly over 3 minutes.
• Administer emulsion form within 6 hours of opening ampule because this form contains no preservatives and allows rapid microbial growth. Use polyethylene-lined or glass infusion sets and polyethylene or polypropylene plastic syringes for administration. Don't use a filter with a pore size of less than 5 microns because it may break down the emulsion.
• **WARNING** Be aware that patients with a history of seizure disorders may experience seizures when diazepam therapy is initiated or suddenly withdrawn. Monitor patients with Lennox-Gastaut syndrome or absence seizures for tonic status epilepticus.

- Monitor for increased sedation, especially in patients with hypoalbuminemia.
- Monitor hepatic and renal function blood test results in patients with impaired renal or hepatic function because diazepam is metabolized in the liver and excreted by the kidneys.
- **WARNING** Observe for signs of physical and psychological dependence: a strong desire or need to continue taking diazepam, a need to increase dosage to maintain drug effects, and posttherapy withdrawal symptoms, such as abdominal cramps, insomnia, irritability, nervousness, and tremor.
- Observe for signs of phlebitis or thrombophlebitis after administration.
- Store diazepam injection at 15° to 30° C (59° to 86° F). Store diazepam emulsion below 25° C (77° F). Protect from freezing and light.

PATIENT TEACHING
- Inform patient that diazepam may cause drowsiness, and advise her to avoid activities requiring alertness until drug's CNS effects are known.
- Urge patient to avoid CNS depressants and alcohol during therapy.
- Instruct patient not to take drug more often, in greater quantities, or for a longer time than prescribed. Inform her that physical and psychological dependence can occur, and teach her to recognize signs of dependence.
- Instruct patient not to abruptly stop taking drug without prescriber supervision. Caution patient with a history of seizures that abrupt drug withdrawal may trigger them.

diazoxide
Hyperstat

Class and Category
Chemical: Benzothiadiazine derivative
Therapeutic: Antihypertensive, antihypoglycemic
Pregnancy category: C

Indications and Dosages
▶ *To treat severe hypertension in hospitalized patients*
I.V. INJECTION
Adults and children. *Initial:* 1 to 3 mg/kg by rapid bolus, repeated q 5 to 15 min until diastolic pressure falls below 100 mm Hg. Re-

peated in 4 hr and again in 24 hr, if needed, until oral antihypertensive therapy begins. *Maximum:* 150 mg/dose, 1.2 g/day.

Route	Onset	Peak	Duration
I.V.	1 min	2 to 5 min	2 to 12 hr

Mechanism of Action
Directly affects smooth muscle cells of peripheral arteries and arterioles, causing them to dilate. This action decreases peripheral resistance, which helps reduce blood pressure. Diazoxide also inhibits insulin release from the pancreas, stimulates catecholamine release, and increases hepatic glucose release.

Contraindications
Acute aortic dissection; hypersensitivity to diazoxide, thiazides, other sulfonamide derivatives, or their components; treatment of compensatory hypertension (as occurs with aortic coarctation)

Interactions
DRUGS
allopurinol, colchicine, probenecid, sulfinpyrazone: Increased serum uric acid level
antihypertensives: Additive hypotensive effects
beta blockers: Increased hypotensive effects of diazoxide
diuretics (especially thiazides): Potentiated hyperglycemic, hyperuricemic, and antihypertensive effects of diazoxide
estrogens, NSAIDs, sympathomimetics: Antagonized hypotensive effects of diazoxide
insulin, oral antidiabetic drugs: Possibly decreased effectiveness of these drugs
oral anticoagulants: Increased anticoagulant effects
peripheral vasodilators, ritodrine (I.V.): Additive, possibly severe, hypotensive effects

Adverse Reactions
CNS: Anxiety, apprehension, cerebral ischemia, confusion, dizziness, euphoria, headache, insomnia, light-headedness, malaise, somnolence, weakness
CV: Bradycardia, chest pain, hypotension, orthostatic hypotension, palpitations, peripheral edema, tachycardia, transient hypertension
EENT: Blurred vision, dry mouth, increased salivation, taste perversion, tinnitus, transient hearing loss

ENDO: Transient hyperglycemia
GI: Abdominal pain, anorexia, constipation, diarrhea, ileus, nausea, vomiting
HEME: Thrombocytopenia
MS: Gout
SKIN: Diaphoresis, flushing, pruritus, rash, sensation of warmth
Other: Allergic reaction, extravasation with injection site cellulitis and pain; fluid and sodium retention

Nursing Considerations

- Administer diazoxide undiluted over 10 to 30 seconds. Don't give drug by I.M. or S.C. route.
- Keep patient supine during I.V. injection and for 1 hour afterward.
- Monitor blood pressure throughout treatment to check for hypertension. Before ending surveillance, measure patient's standing blood pressure if she's ambulatory.
- Monitor patients with uncompensated heart failure for signs of fluid retention and worsening heart failure due to diazoxide's effects.
- Monitor patients with impaired cardiac or cerebral circulation for exacerbations caused by drug-related abrupt blood pressure reduction, mild tachycardia, and decreased blood perfusion.
- Frequently assess I.V. site for extravasation because the alkaline drug can irritate tissue.
- If diabetic patient receives diazoxide to treat hypertension, monitor for signs and symptoms of hyperglycemia because parenteral form commonly causes transient hyperglycemia.
- Be aware that patients with impaired renal function may require reduced dosage because drug effects may be prolonged.
- Monitor patients with a history of gout for signs of exacerbation, such as joint redness or swelling and hyperuricemia.
- Monitor blood glucose level of all patients who receive diazoxide to determine if drug has raised blood glucose level to normal.
- Store drug at 15° to 30° C (59° to 86° F); protect from freezing and light.

PATIENT TEACHING
- Inform patient that she'll be on bed rest until oral diazoxide therapy starts.
- Caution patient not to take antidiabetic drugs unless prescribed.
- Advise patient to report signs of hyperglycemia, such as increased urinary frequency, increased thirst, and fruity breath.

digoxin

Lanoxin Injection, Lanoxin Injection Pediatric

Class and Category

Chemical: Digitalis glycoside
Therapeutic: Antiarrhythmic, cardiotonic
Pregnancy category: C

Indications and Dosages

▶ *To treat heart failure, atrial flutter, atrial fibrillation, and paroxysmal atrial tachycardia with rapid digitalization*

I.V. INJECTION

Adults. *Loading:* 10 to 15 mcg/kg in 3 divided doses q 6 to 8 hr, with first dose equal to 50% of total dose. *Maintenance:* 125 to 350 mcg/day q.d. or b.i.d.

Children over age 10. *Loading:* 8 to 12 mcg/kg in 3 or more divided doses, with first dose equal to 50% of total dose. Subsequent doses given q 6 to 8 hr. *Maintenance:* 2 to 3 mcg/kg/day q.d.

Children ages 6 to 10. *Loading:* 15 to 30 mcg/kg in 3 or more divided doses, with first dose equal to 50% of total dose. Subsequent doses given q 6 to 8 hr. *Maintenance:* 4 to 8 mcg/kg/day in 2 divided doses.

Children ages 2 to 5. *Loading:* 25 to 35 mcg/kg in 3 or more divided doses, with first dose equal to 50% of total dose. Subsequent doses given q 6 to 8 hr. *Maintenance:* 6 to 9 mcg/kg/day in 2 divided doses.

Infants ages 1 to 24 months. *Loading:* 30 to 50 mcg/kg in 3 or more divided doses, with first dose equal to 50% of total dose. Subsequent doses given q 6 to 8 hr. *Maintenance:* 7.5 to 12 mcg/kg/day in 2 divided doses.

Full-term neonates. *Loading:* 20 to 30 mcg/kg in 3 or more divided doses, with first dose equal to 50% of total dose. Subsequent doses given q 6 to 8 hr. *Maintenance:* 5 to 8 mcg/kg/day in 2 divided doses.

Premature neonates. *Loading:* 15 to 25 mcg/kg in 3 or more divided doses, with first dose equal to 50% of total dose. Subsequent doses given q 6 to 8 hr. *Maintenance:* 4 to 6 mcg/kg/day in 2 divided doses.

DOSAGE ADJUSTMENT Dosage carefully adjusted for elderly or debilitated patients and those who have implanted pacemakers because they may develop toxicity at doses tolerated by most patients.

Route	Onset	Peak	Duration
I.V.	5 to 30 min	1 to 5 hr	3 to 4 days

Mechanism of Action

Increases the force and velocity of myocardial contraction, resulting in positive inotropic effects. Digoxin produces antiarrhythmic effects by decreasing the conduction rate and increasing the effective refractory period of the AV node.

Incompatibilities

Don't mix digoxin in the same container or I.V. line as other other drugs.

Contraindications

Hypersensitive carotid sinus syndrome, hypersensitivity to digoxin, presence or history of digitalis toxicity or idiosyncratic reaction to digoxin, ventricular fibrillation, ventricular tachycardia unless heart failure unrelated to digoxin therapy occurs

Interactions

DRUGS

amiodarone, propafenone: Elevated blood digoxin level, possibly to toxic level

antacids: Inhibited digoxin absorption

antiarrhythmics, pancuronium, parenteral calcium salts, rauwolfia alkaloids, sympathomimetics: Possibly increased risk of arrhythmias

diltiazem, verapamil: Increased blood digoxin level, possibly excessive bradycardia

edrophonium: Excessive slowing of heart rate

erythromycin, neomycin, tetracycline: Possibly increased blood digoxin level

hypokalemia-causing drugs, potassium-wasting diuretics: Increased risk of digitalis toxicity from hypokalemia

indomethacin: Decreased renal clearance and increased blood level of digoxin

magnesium sulfate (parenteral): Possibly cardiac conduction changes and heart block

quinidine, quinine: Increased blood digoxin level

spironolactone: Increased half-life and risk of adverse effects of digoxin

succinylcholine: Increased risk of digoxin-induced arrhythmias

sucralfate: Decreased digoxin absorption

Adverse Reactions
CNS: Anxiety, confusion, depression, drowsiness, extreme weakness, hallucinations, headache, syncope
CV: Arrhythmias, heart block
EENT: Blurred vision, colored halos around objects
GI: Abdominal discomfort or pain, anorexia, diarrhea, nausea, vomiting
SKIN: Rash
Other: Electrolyte imbalances

Nursing Considerations
- Before giving each dose of digoxin, take patient's apical pulse and notify prescriber if pulse is below 60 beats/minute (or other specified level).
- Administer drug undiluted, or dilute with a fourfold or greater volume of sterile water for injection, NS, or D_5W for I.V. administration. Once diluted, administer immediately over at least 5 minutes. Discard if solution is markedly discolored or contains precipitate.
- Monitor closely for signs of digitalis toxicity: altered mental status, arrhythmias, heart block, nausea, vision disturbances, and vomiting. If they appear, notify prescriber, check serum digoxin level as ordered, and expect to withhold drug until level is known. Monitor ECG tracing continuously.
- If patient has acute or unstable chronic atrial fibrillation, assess for drug effectiveness. Ventricular rate may not normalize even when serum drug level falls within therapeutic range; raising the dosage probably won't produce a therapeutic effect and may lead to toxicity.
- Frequently obtain ECG tracings as ordered in elderly patients because of their smaller body mass and reduced renal clearance. Elderly patients, especially those with coronary insufficiency, are more susceptible to arrhythmias—particularly ventricular fibrillation—if digitalis toxicity occurs.
- Monitor serum electrolyte—especially potassium—levels regularly because hypokalemia predisposes patient to digitalis toxicity and serious arrhythmias. Also monitor potassium levels frequently if patient is receiving potassium salts in addition to digoxin because hyperkalemia in such a patient can be fatal.
- Store drug at 15° to 25° C (59° to 77° F); protect from freezing and light.

PATIENT TEACHING
• Urge patient to report adverse reactions, such as GI distress, palpitations, or pulse changes.

digoxin immune Fab (ovine)
Digibind

Class and Category
Chemical: Digoxin-specific antigen-binding fragments
Therapeutic: Digitalis glycoside antidote
Pregnancy category: C

Indications and Dosages
▶ *To treat acute toxicity from a known amount of digoxin elixir or tablets*
I.V. INJECTION
Adults and children. Individualized dosage based on amount ingested. Dose (mg) = dose ingested (mg) multiplied by 0.8 and then divided by 0.5, multiplied by 38, and rounded up to next whole vial.
▶ *To treat acute toxicity from a known quantity of digoxin capsules, digitoxin tablets, or I.V. injection of digoxin or digitoxin*
I.V. INJECTION
Adults and children. Individualized dosage based on amount ingested. Dose (mg) = dose ingested (mg) divided by 0.5, then multiplied by 38 and rounded up to next whole vial.
▶ *To treat acute toxicity from an unknown amount of digoxin or digitoxin during long-term therapy*
I.V. INJECTION
Adults and children. Individualized dosage for digoxin toxicity: Dose (mg) = serum digoxin level (ng/ml) multiplied by body weight (kg), then divided by 100, and then multiplied by 38. Individualized dosage for digitoxin toxicity: Dose (mg) = serum digitoxin level (ng/ml) multiplied by body weight (kg) and then divided by 1,000, multiplied by 38, and rounded up to next whole vial.
DOSAGE ADJUSTMENT Higher dose administered, as prescribed, if the dose based on ingested amount differs substantially from the dose based on serum digoxin or digitoxin level. Dose repeated after several hours, if needed.

Route	Onset	Peak	Duration
I.V.	15 to 30 min	Unknown	8 to 12 hr

> ## Mechanism of Action
> Binds with digoxin or digitoxin molecules. The resulting complex is excreted through the kidneys. As the free serum digoxin level declines, tissue-bound digoxin enters the serum and also is bound and excreted.

Contraindications
Hypersensitivity to digoxin immune Fab

Interactions
None known.

Adverse Reactions
CV: Increased ventricular rate (in atrial fibrillation), worsening of heart failure or low cardiac output
Other: Allergic reaction (difficulty breathing, urticaria), febrile reaction, hypokalemia

Nursing Considerations
- Expect each 38-mg vial of purified digoxin immune Fab to bind with about 0.5 mg of digoxin or digitoxin.
- Reconstitute by dissolving 38 mg of drug in 4 ml of sterile water for injection to yield 9.5 mg/ml. Mix gently. Further dilute with NS to a convenient volume for I.V. infusion. For very small doses, reconstituted 38-mg vial may be diluted with 34 ml of NS to yield 1 mg/ml. Use reconstituted solution promptly or, if necessary, store it for up to 4 hours at 2° to 8° C (36° to 46° F).
- **WARNING** Before administering digoxin immune Fab to high-risk patient, test for allergic reaction as prescribed by diluting 0.1 ml of reconstituted drug in 9.9 ml of sodium chloride for injection and then injecting 0.1 ml (9.5 mcg/0.1 ml) intradermally. After 20 minutes, observe for an urticarial wheal surrounded by erythema. Alternatively, perform a scratch test by placing one drop of 9.5 mcg/0.1 ml dilution on patient's skin and making a ¼" scratch through drop with a sterile needle. Inspect site in 20 minutes. Test is considered positive if it produces a wheal surrounded by erythema. If test causes a systemic reaction, apply tourniquet above test site, notify prescriber, and prepare to respond to anaphylaxis. Be aware that if a skin or systemic reaction occurs, additional drug shouldn't be given unless essential; if more of the drug must be given, expect prescriber to pretreat patient with corticosteroids and diphenhydramine. Prescriber should be on standby to treat anaphylaxis.

- When preparing digoxin immune Fab for an infant, reconstitute drug as ordered and administer with a tuberculin syringe.
- When administering drug to a child, monitor for fluid volume overload.
- When giving a large dose, expect a faster onset but watch closely for febrile reaction. Monitor body temperature and ECG tracing during treatment. Make sure emergency equipment and drugs are readily available.
- Administer I.V. infusion through a 0.22-micron membrane filter over 30 minutes. Keep in mind that drug may be given by rapid I.V. injection if cardiac arrest is imminent.
- Monitor serum potassium level frequently, especially during first few hours of therapy, because potassium level may drop rapidly.
- Be aware that patient may not be redigitalized for several days or even longer, until fragments of digoxin immune Fab have been eliminated from body. This process may be delayed in patients with impaired renal function because drug is eliminated by kidneys.

PATIENT TEACHING
- Teach patient the purpose of digoxin immune Fab and how it will be administered.
- Advise patient to notify you immediately if she experiences adverse reactions, especially difficulty breathing and urticaria.

dihydroergotamine mesylate
D.H.E. 45, Dihydroergotamine-Sandoz (CAN)

Class and Category
Chemical: Semisynthetic ergot alkaloid
Therapeutic: Antimigraine agent
Pregnancy category: X

Indications and Dosages
▶ *To treat acute migraine with or without an aura*
I.V. INJECTION
Adults. 1 mg, repeated in 1 hr, if needed. *Maximum:* 6 mg/wk.

Route	Onset	Peak	Duration
I.V.	In 5 min	15 min to 2 hr	About 8 hr

Mechanism of Action

Produces intracranial and peripheral vasoconstriction by binding to all known 5-hydroxytryptamine$_1$ (5-HT$_1$) receptors, alpha$_1$- and alpha$_2$-adrenergic receptors, and dopaminergic receptors. Activation of 5-HT$_1$ receptors on intracranial blood vessels probably constricts large intracranial arteries and closes arteriovenous anastomoses to relieve migraine headache. Activation of 5-HT$_1$ receptors on sensory nerves in the trigeminal system also may inhibit the release of pro-inflammatory neuropeptides.

Peripherally, dihydroergotamine causes vasoconstriction by stimulating alpha-adrenergic receptors. At therapeutic doses, it inhibits norepinephrine reuptake, increasing vasoconstriction. The drug constricts veins more than arteries, increasing venous return while decreasing venous stasis and pooling.

Contraindications

Coronary artery disease, hemiplegic or basilar migraine, hepatic or renal impairment, hypersensitivity to dihydroergotamine or other ergot alkaloids, malnutrition, peripheral vascular disease or vascular surgery, sepsis, severe pruritus, uncontrolled hypertension, use within 24 hours of sumatriptan or other ergot drugs

Interactions

DRUGS

beta blockers: Possibly peripheral vasoconstriction and peripheral ischemia, increased risk of gangrene

macrolides: Possibly increased risk of vasospasm, acute ergotism with peripheral ischemia

nitrates: Decreased antianginal effects of nitrates

other ergot drugs (including ergoloid mesylates, ergonovine, methylergonovine, and methysergide): Increased risk of serious adverse effects

sumatriptan: Increased risk of coronary artery vasospasm, possibly increased effects of dihydroergotamine

systemic vasoconstrictors: Risk of severe hypertension

ACTIVITIES

smoking: Increased risk of vasoconstriction

Adverse Reactions

CNS: Anxiety, confusion, dizziness, fatigue, headache, paresthesia, somnolence, weakness

CV: Bradycardia, chest pain, peripheral vasospasm (calf or heel pain with exertion, cool and cyanotic hands and feet, leg weakness, weak or absent pulses), tachycardia

EENT: Abnormal vision, dry mouth, miosis, pharyngitis, sinusitis, taste perversion
GI: Diarrhea, nausea, vomiting
MS: Muscle stiffness
SKIN: Localized edema of face, feet, fingers, and lower legs; pruritus; sensation of heat or warmth; sudden diaphoresis

Nursing Considerations

- Inspect dihydroergotamine before use; discard if solution isn't clear and colorless. Also discard drug if not used within 1 hour of opening ampule.
- Monitor blood pressure before and after repeat administration of drug; a rise in blood pressure may require treatment.
- Maintain ECG monitoring during first few doses for a patient over age 60 who is receiving multiple doses.
- **WARNING** Monitor for signs of dihydroergotamine overdose, such as abdominal pain, confusion, delirium, dizziness, dyspnea, headache, nausea, pain in legs or arms, paresthesia, seizures, and vomiting.
- Assess peripheral pulses, skin sensation, warmth, and capillary refill. Monitor for signs of blood vessel constriction and adverse reactions caused by decreased circulation to many body areas, such as ischemic bowel disease from decreased arterial blood flow. Also monitor for signs and symptoms of angina, such as chest pain, which can result from coronary artery spasm.
- Store drug below 25° C (77° F), but don't refrigerate or freeze. Store in light-resistant container and protect from light.

PATIENT TEACHING

- Encourage patient to lie down in a quiet, dark room after receiving dihydroergotamine.
- Instruct patient to notify you if her headache returns or worsens or if she experiences a headache that's different from her usual migraines.
- Advise patient to avoid alcohol, which can exacerbate or cause headaches.
- Warn patient about possible dizziness during or after a migraine for which she received dihydroergotamine.
- Advise patient to report adverse reactions, such as chest pain, itching, numbness or tingling in arms or legs, and swelling of face, fingers, feet, or legs.

diltiazem hydrochloride

Cardizem

Class and Category

Chemical: Benzothiazepine derivative
Therapeutic: Antiarrhythmic
Pregnancy category: C

Indications and Dosages

▶ *To treat atrial fibrillation, atrial flutter, and paroxysmal supraventricular tachycardia*

I.V. INFUSION OR INJECTION

Adults and adolescents. 0.25 mg/kg given by bolus over 2 min. If response is inadequate after 15 min, 0.35 mg/kg given by bolus over 2 min. Then 10 mg/hr for continued reduction of heart rate after bolus dose, increased by 5 mg/hr, as needed. *Maximum:* 15 mg/hr for up to 24 hr.

Route	Onset	Peak	Duration
I.V.	In 3 min	2 to 7 min	30 min to 10 hr*

Mechanism of Action

Diltiazem inhibits calcium movement into coronary and vascular smooth-muscle cells by blocking slow calcium channels in cell membranes, as shown. This action decreases intracellular calcium, which:

- inhibits smooth-muscle cell contractions

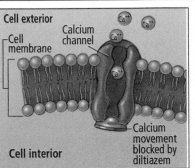

- decreases myocardial oxygen demand by relaxing coronary and vascular smooth muscle, reducing peripheral vascular resistance and systolic and diastolic blood pressures
- slows AV conduction time and prolongs AV nodal refractoriness
- interrupts the reentry circuit in AV nodal reentrant tachycardias.

* For infusion; 1 to 3 hr for injection.

Incompatibilities

Don't give diltiazem through same I.V. line as acetazolamide, acyclovir, aminophylline, ampicillin sodium and sulbactam sodium, cefamandole, cefoperazone, diazepam, furosemide, heparin, hydrocortisone sodium succinate, methylprednisolone sodium succinate, mezlocillin, nafcillin, phenytoin, rifampin, or sodium bicarbonate. Don't mix diltiazem in same container as other drugs.

Contraindications

Acute MI; cardiogenic shock; Lown-Ganong-Levine or Wolff-Parkinson-White syndrome, second- or third-degree AV block, and sick sinus syndrome, unless artificial pacemaker is in place; pulmonary edema; systolic blood pressure below 90 mm Hg; ventricular tachycardia (wide complex)

Interactions

DRUGS

anesthetics (hydrocarbon inhalation): Additive hypotension
beta blockers: Possibly increased risk of adverse cardiovascular effects
carbamazepine, cyclosporine, quinidine, theophyllines: Decreased hepatic clearance and increased blood levels of these drugs, leading to toxicity
cimetidine: Decreased diltiazem metabolism, increased blood diltiazem level
digoxin: Increased blood digoxin level
lithium: Possibly neurotoxicity
NSAIDs: Possibly antagonized antihypertensive effect of diltiazem
prazocin: Possibly increased risk of hypotension
procainamide: Possibly increased risk of prolonged QT interval

Adverse Reactions

CNS: Abnormal gait, amnesia, depression, dizziness, dream disturbances, extrapyramidal reactions, hallucinations, headache, insomnia, nervousness, paresthesia, personality change, somnolence, syncope, tremor, weakness
CV: Angina, atrial flutter, AV block (first-, second-, and third-degree), bradycardia, bundle-branch block, ECG changes, heart failure, hypotension, palpitations, peripheral edema, PVCs, sinus arrest, sinus tachycardia, ventricular fibrillation, ventricular tachycardia
EENT: Amblyopia, dry mouth, epistaxis, eye irritation, gingival bleeding and hyperplasia, gingivitis, nasal congestion, retinopathy, taste perversion, tinnitus

ENDO: Hyperglycemia

GI: Anorexia, constipation, diarrhea, elevated liver function test results, indigestion, nausea, thirst

GU: Acute renal failure, impotence, nocturia, polyuria, sexual dysfunction

HEME: Hemolytic anemia, leukopenia, prolonged bleeding time, thrombocytopenia

MS: Arthralgia, muscle spasms, myalgia

RESP: Dyspnea

SKIN: Alopecia, diaphoresis, erythema multiforme, exfoliative dermatitis, flushing, leukocytoclastic vasculitis, petechiae, photosensitivity, pruritus, purpura, Stevens-Johnson syndrome, toxic epidermal necrolysis, urticaria

Other: Angioedema, hyperuricemia, weight gain

Nursing Considerations

- For I.V. infusion, dilute diltiazem in a compatible solution, such as NS, D_5W, or $D_5/0.45NS$. Before using diluted solution, store it at 15° to 30° C (59° to 86° F) or refrigerate it at 2° to 8° C (36° to 46° F) for up to 24 hours.
- Monitor hepatic and renal function test results, as appropriate, especially in patients with impaired hepatic or renal function, because drug is metabolized mainly in liver and excreted by kidneys.
- **WARNING** Monitor blood pressure, pulse rate, and heart rate and rhythm by continuous ECG, as appropriate, during diltiazem therapy. Keep emergency equipment and drugs readily available.
- Assess for signs of heart failure, such as sudden and unexplained weight gain, dyspnea, and peripheral edema.
- If patient also receives digoxin, monitor for signs of digitalis toxicity, such as nausea, vomiting, halo vision, and elevated serum digoxin level.
- Expect to discontinue drug if adverse skin reactions, which are usually transient, persist.
- Store drug at 2° to 8° C or for up to 1 month at room temperature; then discard.

PATIENT TEACHING
- Urge patient to notify prescriber if she experiences chest pain, difficulty breathing, dizziness, fainting, irregular heartbeat, rash, or swollen ankles during diltiazem therapy.
- Inform patient that blood pressure and pulse rate will be monitored regularly.

dimenhydrinate

Dinate, Dramanate, Gravol (CAN), Hydrate

Class and Category

Chemical: Ethanolamine derivative
Therapeutic: Antiemetic, antihistamine, antivertigo agent
Pregnancy category: B

Indications and Dosages

▶ *To treat nausea, vomiting, dizziness, or vertigo associated with motion sickness*

I.V. INFUSION OR INJECTION

Adults and adolescents. 50 mg in 10 ml of NS administered slowly, over at least 2 min, q 4 hr p.r.n.
Children. 1.25 mg/kg or 37.5 mg/m^2 in 10 ml of NS administered slowly, over at least 2 min, q 6 hr p.r.n. *Maximum:* 300 mg/day.

Route	Onset	Peak	Duration
I.V.	Immediate	Unknown	3 to 6 hr

Mechanism of Action

May inhibit vestibular stimulation and labyrinthine stimulation and function by acting on the otolith system and, with larger doses, on the semicircular canals.

Contraindications

Hypersensitivity to dimenhydrinate or its components, premature and full-term neonates

Interactions

DRUGS

aminoglycosides and other ototoxic drugs: Masked symptoms of ototoxicity
anticholinergics and drugs with anticholinergic activity: Potentiated anticholinergic effects of dimenhydrinate
apomorphine: Possibly decreased emetic response to apomorphine in treatment of poisoning
barbiturates and other CNS depressants: Possibly increased CNS depression
MAO inhibitors: Increased anticholinergic and CNS depressant effects of dimenhydrinate

ACTIVITIES

alcohol use: Possibly increased CNS depression

Adverse Reactions

CNS: Confusion, drowsiness, hallucinations, nervousness, paradoxical stimulation
CV: Hypotension, palpitations, tachycardia
EENT: Blurred vision, diplopia, dry eyes, dry mouth, nasal congestion
GI: Anorexia, constipation, diarrhea, epigastric discomfort, nausea, vomiting
GU: Dysuria
HEME: Hemolytic anemia
RESP: Thickening of bronchial secretions, wheezing
SKIN: Photosensitivity, rash, urticaria
Other: Anaphylaxis

Nursing Considerations

- **WARNING** Don't administer dimenhydrinate to premature or full-term neonates. Some I.V. preparations may contain benzyl alcohol, which can cause a fatal toxic syndrome characterized by CNS, respiratory, circulatory, and renal impairment and metabolic acidosis.
- **WARNING** Be aware that 50-mg/ml concentration of dimenhydrinate is intended for I.M. use. For I.V. administration, the solution *must* be diluted further with at least 10 ml of diluent, such as D₅W or NS, for each milliliter of dimenhydrinate.
- Monitor patients with prostatic hypertrophy, stenosing peptic ulcer, pyloroduodenal obstruction, bladder neck obstruction, narrow angle glaucoma, bronchial asthma, or cardiac arrhythmias for signs and symptoms of exacerbation of these conditions resulting from drug's anticholinergic effects.
- Monitor elderly patients for signs of increased sensitivity to dimenhydrinate, such as excessive drowsiness, confusion, and restlessness.
- Assess for signs of paradoxical stimulation, such as nightmares, unusual excitement, nervousness, restlessness, or irritability, especially in children and elderly patients.
- Store drug at 15° to 30° C (59° to 86° F); don't freeze.

PATIENT TEACHING

- Because dimenhydrinate may cause drowsiness, instruct patient to avoid potentially hazardous activities until drug's CNS effects are known.

- Advise patient to inform health care providers of dimenhydrinate therapy, especially if she's being evaluated for medical conditions that are affected by this drug, such as appendicitis.
- Instruct patient to avoid alcohol, sedatives, and tranquilizers while receiving this drug.
- Encourage patient to use sunscreen to prevent photosensitivity reactions.

diphenhydramine hydrochloride
Benadryl, Hyrexin

Class and Category
Chemical: Ethanolamine derivative
Therapeutic: Antianaphylactic adjunct, antidyskinetic, antiemetic, antihistamine, antivertigo agent
Pregnancy category: B

Indications and Dosages
▶ *To treat hypersensitivity reactions, such as perennial and seasonal allergic rhinitis, vasomotor rhinitis, allergic conjunctivitis, uncomplicated allergic skin eruptions, and transfusion reactions*
I.V. INJECTION
Adults and adolescents. 10 to 50 mg q 4 to 6 hr up to 100 mg/dose, if needed. *Maximum:* 400 mg/day.
Children. 1.25 mg/kg q 4 to 6 hr. *Maximum:* 300 mg/day.
▶ *To prevent motion sickness or treat vertigo*
I.V. INJECTION
Adults and adolescents. *Initial:* 10 mg; increased to 20 to 50 mg q 2 to 3 hr, if needed. *Maximum:* 100 mg/dose, 400 mg/day.
Children. 1 to 1.5 mg/kg I.M. q 4 to 6 hr, p.r.n. *Maximum:* 300 mg/day.
▶ *To treat symptoms of Parkinson's disease and drug-induced extrapyramidal reactions in elderly patients who can't tolerate more potent antidyskinetic drugs*
I.V. INJECTION
Adults and adolescents. 10 to 50 mg q.i.d., as needed. *Maximum:* 100 mg/dose, 400 mg/day.

Route	Onset	Peak	Duration
I.V.	Immediate	1 to 3 hr	6 to 8 hr

Mechanism of Action

Binds to central and peripheral H_1 receptors, competing with histamine for these sites and preventing it from reaching its site of action. By blocking histamine, diphenhydramine produces antihistamine effects: inhibiting respiratory, vascular, and GI smooth-muscle contraction; decreasing capillary permeability, which reduces wheals, flares, and itching; and decreasing salivary and lacrimal gland secretions.

Diphenhydramine also produces antidyskinetic effects, possibly by inhibiting acetylcholine in the CNS. The drug's antiemetic and antivertigo effects may be related to its ability to bind to CNS muscarinic receptors and depress vestibular stimulation and labyrinthine function.

Contraindications

Bladder neck obstruction, hypersensitivity to diphenhydramine or its components, lower respiratory tract symptoms (including asthma), narrow-angle glaucoma, pyloroduodenal obstruction, stenosing peptic ulcer, symptomatic benign prostatic hyperplasia, use within 14 days of MAO inhibitor therapy

Interactions

DRUGS

anticholinergics and drugs with anticholinergic activity: Potentiated anticholinergic effects of diphenhydramine

apomorphine: Possibly decreased emetic response to apomorphine in treatment of poisoning

barbiturates, other CNS depressants: Possibly increased CNS depression

MAO inhibitors: Increased anticholinergic and CNS depressant effects of diphenhydramine

ACTIVITIES

alcohol use: Possibly increased CNS depression

Adverse Reactions

CNS: Confusion, dizziness, drowsiness
CV: Arrhythmias, palpitations, tachycardia
EENT: Blurred vision, diplopia
GI: Epigastric distress, nausea
HEME: Agranulocytosis, hemolytic anemia, thrombocytopenia
RESP: Thickened bronchial secretions
SKIN: Photosensitivity

Nursing Considerations

• Expect to give parenteral form of diphenhydramine only when oral ingestion isn't possible.

- Don't exceed a rate of 25 mg/minute when administering diphenhydramine.
- Expect to discontinue drug at least 72 hours before skin tests for allergies because drug may inhibit cutaneous histamine response, thus producing false-negative results.
- Store drug at 15° to 30° C (59° to 86° F); protect from freezing and light.

PATIENT TEACHING
- Because diphenhydramine may cause drowsiness, advise patient to avoid potentially hazardous activities until its CNS effects are known.
- Urge patient to avoid alcohol and other CNS depressants, such as sedatives and tranquilizers, while receiving diphenhydramine.
- Instruct her to use sunscreen to prevent photosensitivity reactions.

dipyridamole
Persantine

Class and Category
Chemical: Pyrimidine
Therapeutic: Diagnostic aid
Pregnancy category: B

Indications and Dosages
▶ *To aid diagnosis during thallium perfusion imaging of myocardium*
I.V. INFUSION
Adults. 0.57 mg/kg in 50 ml of D$_5$W infused over 4 min. *Maximum:* 60 mg.

Route	Onset	Peak	Duration
I.V.	Unknown	3.8 to 8.7 min*	Unknown

Mechanism of Action
May increase the intraplatelet level of adenosine, which causes coronary vasodilation and inhibits platelet aggregation. Vasodilation and increased blood flow occur preferentially in nondiseased coronary vessels, which results in redistribution of blood away from significantly diseased vessels. Changes in the perfusion of myocardial areas served by diseased and nondiseased vessels are observed during thallium imaging studies.

* After start of infusion, for increased velocity of coronary artery blood flow.

Contraindications

Asthma, hypersensitivity to dipyridamole or its components, hypotension, unstable angina pectoris

Interactions

DRUGS

adenosine: Potentiated effects of adenosine

cefamandole, cefoperazone, cefotetan, plicamycin, valproic acid: Possibly hypoprothrombinemia and increased risk of bleeding

heparin, NSAIDs, thrombolytics: Possibly increased risk of bleeding

theophylline: Reversal of coronary vasodilation caused by dipyridamole, possibly false-negative thallium imaging result

Adverse Reactions

CNS: Dizziness, headache

CV: Angina, arrhythmias, ECG changes (specifically ST-segment and T-wave changes)

GI: Abdominal pain, diarrhea, nausea, vomiting

RESP: Bronchospasm, dyspnea

SKIN: Flushing, pruritus, rash

Other: Allergic reaction

Nursing Considerations

- Protect dipyridamole I.V. solution from direct light and freezing.
- Don't administer drug undiluted. Use an antecubital vein to avoid irritating smaller veins.
- Monitor blood pressure, pulse rate and rhythm, and breath sounds every 10 to 15 minutes during I.V. infusion.
- Keep parenteral aminophylline available to relieve adverse reactions to dipyridamole infusion.
- When drug is given at therapeutic doses, expect adverse reactions to be minimal and transient. They typically resolve with long-term use.
- Store drug at 15° to 25° C (59° to 77° F); protect from freezing and light.

PATIENT TEACHING

- Instruct patient to seek immediate emergency treatment if she develops chest pain or other adverse reactions during dipyridamole therapy.

dobutamine hydrochloride

Dobutrex

Class and Category

Chemical: Synthetic catecholamine

Therapeutic: Cardiac stimulant
Pregnancy category: Not rated

Indications and Dosages

▶ *To treat low cardiac output and heart failure*

I.V. INFUSION

Adults. 2.5 to 10 mcg/kg/min as continuous infusion, adjusted according to hemodynamic response.

Children. 5 to 20 mcg/kg/min as continuous infusion, adjusted according to hemodynamic response.

Route	Onset	Peak	Duration
I.V.	1 to 2 min	Unknown	Under 5 min

Mechanism of Action

Primarily stimulates beta$_1$-adrenergic receptors and mildly stimulates beta$_2$- and alpha$_1$-adrenergic receptors. Beta$_1$-receptor stimulation produces a positive inotropic effect on the myocardium. This increases cardiac output by boosting myocardial contractility and stroke volume. Increased myocardial contractility raises coronary blood flow and myocardial oxygen consumption. Systolic blood pressure typically rises as a result of increased stroke volume. Other hemodynamic effects include decreased systemic vascular resistance, which reduces afterload, and decreased ventricular filling pressure, which reduces preload.

Incompatibilities

Don't combine dobutamine with cefamandole, cefazolin, cephalothin, ethacrynate sodium, heparin sodium, hydrocortisone sodium succinate, or penicillin because these drugs are incompatible. Don't mix dobutamine with alkaline solutions, such as sodium bicarbonate, because of possible incompatibility. Don't use diluents that contain sodium bisulfite or ethanol. Don't mix dobutamine in same solution with other drugs.

Contraindications

Hypersensitivity to dobutamine or its components, idiopathic hypertrophic subaortic stenosis

Interactions

DRUGS

beta blockers: Possibly increased alpha-adrenergic activity and peripheral resistance

bretylium: Potentiated vasopressor activity, possibly arrhythmias

cyclopropane, halothane: Possibly serious arrhythmias
guanethidine: Decreased hypotensive effect of guanethidine, possibly resulting in severe hypertension
thyroid hormones: Increased cardiovascular effects of thyroid hormones or dobutamine
tricyclic antidepressants: Possibly potentiated cardiovascular and vasopressor effects of dobutamine, resulting in arrhythmias, hyperpyrexia, or severe hypertension

Adverse Reactions

CNS: Fever, headache, nervousness, restlessness
CV: Angina, bradycardia, hypertension, hypotension, palpitations, PVCs, tachycardia
GI: Nausea, vomiting
RESP: Dyspnea
SKIN: Extravasation with tissue necrosis and sloughing, rash
Other: Allergic reaction, hypokalemia

Nursing Considerations

• Avoid giving dobutamine to patients with uncorrected hypovolemia. Expect prescriber to order whole blood or plasma volume expanders to correct hypovolemia. Also avoid giving dobutamine to patients with acute MI because it can intensify or extend myocardial ischemia.
• Dilute concentrate with at least 50 ml of compatible I.V. solution. A common dilution is 500 mg (40 ml from 250-ml bag) in 210 ml of D₅W or NS to yield 2,000 mcg/ml. Or dilute 1,000 mg (80 ml from 250-ml bag) in 170 ml of D₅W or NS to yield 4,000 mcg/ml. Adjust maximum concentration according to patient's fluid requirements, as prescribed. Don't exceed a concentration of 5,000 mcg/ml. Discard solution after 24 hours.
• Inspect parenteral solution for particles and discoloration before administering it.
• Administer drug using an infusion pump.
• Monitor patients who are allergic to sulfites because commercially available dobutamine injections contain sodium bisulfite and may cause anaphylaxis-like signs and symptoms.
• Keep in mind that patients with atrial fibrillation should be adequately digitalized before administration. Monitor such patients for signs of increased AV conduction, such as increased heart rate.
• Monitor blood pressure frequently during therapy, preferably by continuous intra-arterial monitoring; a systolic pressure increase

of 10 to 20 mm Hg may indicate a dobutamine-induced increase in cardiac output.

- If hypotension develops, expect to reduce dosage or discontinue drug.
- Monitor heart rate and rhythm continuously for PVCs, which may result from drug's stimulatory effect on the heart's conduction system, and sinus tachycardia, which results from positive chronotropic effect of beta stimulation and may increase the heart rate by 5 to 15 beats/minute.
- Monitor hemodynamic parameters, such as central venous pressure, pulmonary artery wedge pressure, and cardiac output, as indicated, to assess drug's effectiveness.
- **WARNING** Monitor serum potassium level to check for hypokalemia, a rare result of beta$_2$ stimulation that causes electrolyte imbalances.
- Monitor urine output hourly, as appropriate, to assess for improved renal blood flow.
- Be aware that dobutamine isn't indicated for long-term treatment of heart failure because it may not be effective and may increase the risk of hospitalization and death.
- Before diluting drug, store it at 15° to 30° C (59° to 86° F).

PATIENT TEACHING
- Explain the need for frequent hemodynamic monitoring during dobutamine therapy.

dolasetron mesylate
Anzemet

Class and Category
Chemical: Carboxylate monomethanesulfonate
Therapeutic: Antiemetic
Pregnancy category: B

Indications and Dosages
▶ *To prevent nausea and vomiting due to chemotherapy*
I.V. INJECTION
Adults and children over age 16. 1.8 mg/kg or 100 mg as a single dose within 30 min before chemotherapy.
Children ages 2 to 16. 1.8 mg/kg as a single dose within 30 min before chemotherapy. *Maximum:* 100 mg.

ORAL SOLUTION

Adults and children over age 16. 100 mg within 1 hr before chemotherapy.

Children ages 2 to 16. 1.8 mg/kg within 1 hr before chemotherapy. *Maximum:* 100 mg.

▶ *To prevent postoperative nausea and vomiting*

I.V. INJECTION

Adults and children over age 16. 12.5 mg 15 min before end of anesthesia.

Children ages 2 to 16. 0.35 mg/kg 15 min before end of anesthesia. *Maximum:* 12.5 mg/dose.

ORAL SOLUTION

Adults and children over age 16. 100 mg within 2 hr before surgery.

Children ages 2 to 16. 1.2 mg/kg within 2 hr before surgery. *Maximum:* 100 mg.

▶ *To treat postoperative nausea and vomiting*

I.V. INJECTION

Adults and children over age 16. 12.5 mg as a single dose as soon as symptoms develop.

Children ages 2 to 16. 0.35 mg/kg as a single dose as soon as symptoms develop. *Maximum:* 12.5 mg/dose.

Mechanism of Action

With its active metabolite hydrodolasetron, prevents activation of the serotonin 5-HT$_3$ receptors located peripherally on the vagal nerve terminals and centrally in the chemoreceptor trigger zone, thereby decreasing the vomiting reflex.

Contraindications

Hypersensitivity to dolasetron or its components

Interactions

DRUGS

atenolol: Possibly decreased clearance of dolasetron

cimetidine: Possibly increased blood dolasetron level

rifampin: Possibly decreased blood dolasetron level

Adverse Reactions

CNS: Headache

CV: Bradycardia, ECG changes, hypertension, hypotension, tachycardia

GI: Diarrhea
SKIN: Rash
Other: Anaphylaxis, injection site pain

Nursing Considerations

- Administer up to 100 mg of dolasetron I.V. in 30 seconds or dilute drug in NS, D₅W, D₅/0.45NS, or lactated Ringer's solution and infuse for up to 15 minutes, as prescribed.
- Flush I.V. line with compatible solution before and after drug administration.
- Expect to prepare an oral solution of dolasetron for patients unable to swallow tablets by diluting injection solution with apple or apple-grape juice.
- **WARNING** Monitor patients receiving dolasetron for ECG changes, including prolonged PR, QTc, and JT intervals and widened QRS complex.
- Store drug at 20° to 25° C (68° to 77° F) and protect from light.

PATIENT TEACHING

- Advise parents of pediatric patients and patients who have difficulty swallowing that oral solution can be prepared by diluting injection form of dolasetron with apple or apple-grape juice.
- Inform patient that oral solution may be refrigerated for up to 48 hours but should be discarded after 2 hours at room temperature.

dopamine hydrochloride

Intropin, Revimine (CAN)

Class and Category

Chemical: Catecholamine
Therapeutic: Cardiac stimulant, vasopressor
Pregnancy category: C

Indications and Dosages

▶ *To correct hypotension that is unresponsive to adequate fluid volume replacement or occurs as part of shock syndrome caused by bacteremia, chronic cardiac decompensation, drug overdose, MI, open-heart surgery, renal failure, trauma, or other major systemic illnesses; to improve low cardiac output*

I.V. INFUSION

Adults. 0.5 to 3 mcg/kg/min for vasodilation of renal arteries; 2 to 10 mcg/kg/min for positive inotropic effects and increased cardiac output; 10 mcg/kg/min, increased gradually according to patient's response, for increased systolic and diastolic blood pressures.

Children. 0.5 to 3 mcg/kg/min for vasodilation of renal arteries; 5 to 20 mcg/kg/min for increased cardiac output and systolic and diastolic blood pressures.

DOSAGE ADJUSTMENT Initial dosage reduced to 10% of usual amount if patient has received an MAO inhibitor in previous 2 to 3 wk.

Route	Onset	Peak	Duration
I.V.	In 5 min	Unknown	Up to 10 min

Mechanism of Action

Stimulates dopamine$_1$ (D$_1$) and dopamine$_2$ (D$_2$) postsynaptic receptors. D$_1$ receptors mediate vasodilation in renal, mesenteric, coronary, and cerebral blood vessels. D$_2$ receptors, when stimulated, inhibit norepinephrine release. In higher doses, dopamine also stimulates alpha$_1$ and alpha$_2$ receptors, causing vascular smooth-muscle contraction.

At doses of 0.5 to 3 mcg/kg/min, this naturally occurring catecholamine mainly affects dopaminergic receptors in renal, mesenteric, coronary, and cerebral vessels, resulting in vasodilation, increased renal blood flow, improved GFR, and increased urine output. At doses of 2 to 10 mcg/kg/min, dopamine stimulates beta$_1$-adrenergic receptors, increasing cardiac output while maintaining dopaminergic-induced vasodilation. At doses of 10 mcg/kg/min or more, alpha-adrenergic agonism takes over, causing increased peripheral vascular resistance and renal vasoconstriction.

Incompatibilities

Don't add dopamine to 5% sodium bicarbonate, alkaline I.V. solutions, oxidizing agents, or iron salts.

Contraindications

Pheochromocytoma, uncorrected ventricular fibrillation, ventricular tachycardia and other tachyarrhythmias

Interactions

DRUGS

alpha blockers, haloperidol, loxapine, phenothiazines, thioxanthenes: Antagonized peripheral vasoconstriction with high doses of dopamine

anesthetics (such as chloroform, enflurane, halothane, isoflurane, and methoxyflurane): Increased risk of severe atrial and ventricular arrhythmias

antihypertensives, diuretics used as antihypertensives: Possibly decreased antihypertensive effects of these drugs
beta blockers: Antagonized beta receptor–mediated inotropic effects of dopamine
digitalis glycosides: Possibly increased risk of arrhythmias and additive inotropic effects
diuretics: Possibly increased diuretic effects of dopamine or diuretic
doxapram: Possibly increased vasopressor effects of dopamine or doxapram
ergot alkaloids: Enhanced peripheral vasoconstriction
guanadrel, guanethidine: Possibly decreased antihypertensive effects of these drugs and potentiated vasopressor response to dopamine, resulting in hypertension and arrhythmias
levodopa: Possibly increased risk of arrhythmias
MAO inhibitors: Prolonged and intensified cardiac stimulation and vasopressor effect of dopamine
maprotiline, tricyclic antidepressants: Possibly potentiated cardiovascular and vasopressor effects of dopamine, resulting in arrhythmias, hyperpyrexia, or severe hypertension
mecamylamine, methyldopa: Possibly decreased hypotensive effects of these drugs and enhanced vasopressor effect of dopamine
methylphenidate: Possibly potentiated vasopressor effect of dopamine
nitrates: Possibly decreased antianginal effect of nitrates; possibly decreased vasopressor effect of dopamine, resulting in hypotension
oxytoxic drugs: Possibly severe hypertension
phenoxybenzamine: Possibly antagonized peripheral vasoconstriction of dopamine, causing hypotension and tachycardia
phenytoin: Possibly sudden bradycardia and hypotension
rauwolfia alkaloids: Possibly decreased hypotensive effects of these drugs
sympathomimetics: Possibly increased adverse cardiovascular and other effects
thyroid hormones: Increased risk of coronary insufficiency

Adverse Reactions
CNS: Headache
CV: Angina, bradycardia, hypertension, hypotension, palpitations, peripheral vasoconstriction, sinus tachycardia, ventricular arrhythmias
GI: Nausea, vomiting
RESP: Dyspnea
SKIN: Extravasation with tissue necrosis
Other: Allergic reaction

Nursing Considerations

- If possible, avoid giving dopamine to patients with occlusive vascular disease, such as atherosclerosis, Buerger's disease, diabetic endarteritis, or Raynaud's disease, because of the risk of decreased peripheral circulation.
- Inspect parenteral solution for particles and discoloration before administration.
- Dilute dopamine concentrate with a compatible I.V. solution before administering. Typical dilution is 400 mg in 250 ml to yield 1.6 mg/ml. Don't exceed 3.2 mg/ml.
- Be aware that drug also comes premixed with D_5W in concentrations of 800 mcg, 1.6 mg, and 3.2 mg. Monitor for elevated glucose levels, as ordered, in patients with subclinical or overt diabetes mellitus because this finding may signal an exacerbation.
- If patient has hypovolemia, ensure adequate fluid resuscitation before giving drug.
- Give drug by I.V. infusion using an infusion pump.
- **WARNING** When the infusion rate exceeds 20 mcg/kg/minute, monitor for excessive vasoconstriction and loss of renal vasodilating effects. Don't exceed an infusion rate of 50 mcg/kg/minute.
- If you must infuse more than 20 mcg/kg/minute of dopamine to maintain blood pressure, expect to infuse norepinephrine as prescribed.
- Administer infusion through a central catheter to avoid extravasation and tissue necrosis. If you must administer drug through a peripheral line, inspect site frequently for signs of extravasation and necrosis. If you detect such signs, start a new I.V. line for dopamine infusion, discontinue previous I.V. line, and notify prescriber immediately.
- If drug extravasates, expect prescriber to give 5 to 10 mg of phentolamine diluted in 10 to 15 ml of NS, as prescribed. Phentolamine infiltrates directly into area to antagonize vasoconstriction and minimize sloughing and tissue necrosis.
- Titrate dopamine gradually to minimize hypotension, especially after a high infusion rate.
- Monitor blood pressure continuously with an intra-arterial line, as indicated.
- Place patient on continuous ECG monitoring, and assess heart rate and rhythm for arrhythmias.

- Assess patients with cardiac disease, particularly coronary artery disease, for signs of exacerbation or adverse cardiac reactions because dopamine increases myocardial oxygen demand.
- Monitor hemodynamic parameters, such as central venous pressure, pulmonary artery wedge pressure, and cardiac output, as indicated, to assess drug's effectiveness.
- Monitor urine output hourly as appropriate to assess for improved renal blood flow.
- Monitor patients who are allergic to sulfites for signs of an allergic reaction because some forms of dopamine contain sulfites.
- Store dopamine at 15° to 30° C (59° to 86° F); don't freeze.

PATIENT TEACHING
- Explain the need for frequent hemodynamic monitoring during dopamine therapy.

doxapram hydrochloride
Dopram

Class and Category
Chemical: Pyrrolidinone derivative
Therapeutic: Respiratory stimulant
Pregnancy category: B

Indications and Dosages
▶ *To stimulate respiration in COPD-related acute respiratory insufficiency*
I.V. INFUSION
Adults and adolescents. 1 to 2 mg/min, titrated according to respiratory response. *Maximum:* 3 mg/min for up to 2 hr.
▶ *To treat respiratory depression after anesthesia*
I.V. INFUSION
Adults and adolescents. 5 mg/min until desired response occurs and then reduced to 1 to 3 mg/min. *Maximum:* Cumulative dose of 4 mg/kg or 300 mg.
I.V. INJECTION
Adults and adolescents. 0.5 to 1 mg/kg, repeated q 5 min, if needed. *Maximum:* 1.5 mg/kg as a single dose or 2 mg/kg q 5 min.

Route	Onset	Peak	Duration
I.V.	20 to 40 sec	1 to 2 min	5 to 12 min

Mechanism of Action

Activates peripheral carotid, aortic, and other chemoreceptors to stimulate respiration, resulting in increased tidal volume and respiratory rate. Doxapram also may increase respiratory rate and tidal volume by directly stimulating the respiratory center in the medulla oblongata.

Incompatibilities

To avoid precipitation and gas formation, don't mix doxapram with alkaline solutions, such as aminophylline, sodium bicarbonate, or 2.5% thiopental.

Contraindications

CVA; head injury; hypersensitivity to doxapram or its components; mechanical disorders of ventilation, including acute asthma, flail chest, muscle paresis, pneumothorax, and pulmonary fibrosis; seizure disorder; severe cardiovascular disorder; severe hypertension; use in neonates

Interactions

DRUGS

anesthetics (such as chloroform, cyclopropane, enflurane, halothane, isoflurane, methoxyflurane, and trichloroethylene): Possibly adverse myocardial effects if doxapram given within 10 minutes of these drugs

CNS stimulants: Possibly excessive CNS stimulation, resulting in arrhythmias, insomnia, irritability, nervousness, or seizures

MAO inhibitors, sympathomimetics: Additive vasopressor effects

skeletal muscle relaxants: Masked residual effects of muscle relaxants

Adverse Reactions

CNS: Disorientation, dizziness, headache

CV: Arrhythmias, including sinus tachycardia; hypertension

GI: Diarrhea, hiccups, nausea, vomiting

GU: Urine retention

RESP: Bronchospasm, cough, dyspnea

SKIN: Diaphoresis

Other: Injection site pain, redness, swelling, and thrombophlebitis

Nursing Considerations

• Avoid giving doxapram to patients receiving mechanical ventilation.

• Maintain a patent airway, and assess for optimal oxygenation before administering drug. Monitor ABG levels before and every 30 minutes during infusion, as ordered.

- **WARNING** Don't administer doxapram faster than recommended rate to avoid hemolysis.
- Monitor I.V. insertion site for extravasation and signs of thrombophlebitis or local skin irritation.
- If hypertension or dyspnea develops suddenly, stop infusion as directed.
- When drug is administered to treat respiratory depression after anesthesia, monitor patient for signs of recurrent narcosis (such as stupor) for 30 to 60 minutes after she becomes alert.
- Assess for early signs of overdose, including enhanced deep tendon reflexes, skeletal muscle hyperactivity, and tachycardia.
- Store drug at 15° to 30° C (59° to 86° F); don't freeze.

PATIENT TEACHING
- Explain the need for frequent pulse and blood pressure monitoring during doxapram therapy.

doxorubicin hydrochloride
Adriamycin PFS, Adriamycin RDF, Rubex

Class and Category
Chemical: Anthracycline glycoside
Therapeutic: Antibiotic antineoplastic
Pregnancy category: D

Indications and Dosages
▶ *To treat disseminated neoplastic conditions, such as acute lymphoblastic or acute myeloblastic leukemia; Wilms' tumor; neuroblastoma; soft-tissue and bone sarcomas; breast, bronchogenic, gastric, ovarian, transitional cell bladder, or thyroid cancer; Hodgkin's disease; or malignant lymphoma*

I.V. INFUSION OR INJECTION
Adults. 60 to 75 mg/m^2 administered over at least 3 to 5 min q 21 days when given as a single agent, or 40 to 60 mg/m^2 administered over at least 3 to 5 min q 21 to 28 days when given in combination therapy.
Children. 30 mg/m^2 for 3 days q 4 wk.
DOSAGE ADJUSTMENT Dosage varies, depending on regimen used. Dosage may be reduced when doxorubicin is used in combination with other cytotoxic drugs. Dosage reduced by 50% when plasma bilirubin level is 1.2 to 3 mg/ml and by 75% when plasma bilirubin level is 3.1 to 5 mg/ml.

Mechanism of Action
Binds directly to DNA by inserting (intercalating) itself between two DNA bases, which inhibits the synthesis of DNA and RNA and produces single-strand breaks in DNA. In addition, doxorubicin undergoes an enzymatic reduction, resulting in the multi-step production of a hydroxyl radical, which may lead to cell death by reacting with DNA, RNA, cell membranes, and proteins. Doxorubicin is active in all phases of the cell cycle, though cell cycle phase S is most sensitive.

Incompatibilities
Don't mix doxorubicin with heparin or fluorouracil because a precipitate will form. Don't mix doxorubicin with other drugs or with bacteriostatic agents.

Contraindications
Patients who've received maximum acceptable doses of doxorubicin, daunorubicin, idarubicin, or other anthracyclines and anthracenes; marked myelosuppression from prior antitumor therapy or radiation therapy

Interactions
DRUGS

actinomycin D: Acute "recall" pneumonitis after local radiation therapy in children

blood-dyscrasia–causing drugs (such as cephalosporins and cisplatin): Increased leukopenic and thrombocytopenic effects of doxorubicin

bone marrow depressants (such as colchicine and methotrexate): Increased bone marrow depression

carbamazepine: Decreased blood carbamazepine level

cisplatin: Risk of leukemia

cyclophosphamide: Potentiated cyclophosphamide-induced hemorrhagic cystitis, increased risk of doxorubicin-induced cardiotoxicity

cyclosporine: Possibly decreased doxorubicin metabolism; increased risk of severe and prolonged hematologic toxicity, coma, and seizures

cytarabine: Possibly necrotizing colitis

dactinomycin, mitomycin, nifedipine, and other calcium channel blockers: Increased risk of doxorubicin-induced cardiotoxicity

digoxin: Decreased absorption of digoxin

fosphenytoin, phenytoin: Possibly decreased blood phenytoin level

methotrexate and other hepatotoxic drugs: Possibly impaired hepatic function, increased risk of doxorubicin toxicity

paclitaxel: Decreased doxorubicin clearance
phenobarbital: Possibly increased doxorubicin excretion
progesterone: Possibly enhanced doxorubicin-induced neutropenia
and thrombocytopenia
streptozocin: Possibly inhibited hepatic metabolism of doxorubicin
trastuzumab: Possibly increased incidence and severity of cardiac
dysfunction
vaccines, killed virus: Possibly decreased antibody response to vaccine
vaccines, live virus: Possibly increased adverse effects of vaccine, severe infection, and decreased antibody response to vaccine

Adverse Reactions

CNS: Chills, fever
CV: Arrhythmias, cardiomyopathy, cardiotoxicity
EENT: Conjunctivitis, esophagitis, stomatitis
GI: Diarrhea, GI ulceration or necrosis, nausea, vomiting
GU: Uric acid nephropathy, reddish urine
HEME: Anemia, leukopenia, myelosuppression, thrombocytopenia
SKIN: Alopecia; cellulitis; extravasation; hyperpigmentation of
soles, palms, or nails; erythematous streaking along vein used for
insertion; infusion site pain; recall postirradiation erythema; urti-
caria
Other: Hyperuricemia

Nursing Considerations

- **WARNING** Be aware that doxorubicin hydrochloride liposome should not be substituted for doxorubicin hydrochloride. These drugs are not interchangeable; severe adverse reactions may result.
- Be aware that doxorubicin should be administered only under
  the supervision of a qualified physician and that initial treatment usually takes place in a hospital.
- Follow facility protocols for preparation and handling of antineoplastic drugs and appropriate disposal of used equipment.
- Monitor liver and renal function tests and CBC, including
  hematocrit, platelet count, and WBC count with differential, before and periodically during therapy. Be aware that cardiac
  evaluation, including ECG, radionuclide angiography to determine ejection fraction, and echocardiography, will be performed
  before, during, and sometimes after doxorubicin therapy.
- Be aware that doxorubicin is available in various concentrations.
  Reconstitute doxorubicin with 0.9% sodium chloride injection to
  a final concentration of 2 mg/ml. Withdraw appropriate amount

of air from vial when preparing drug to prevent pressure build-up. Shake vial to allow contents to dissolve. Inspect solution for particles or discoloration before administration.

- Use most reconstituted solutions within 7 days if stored at room temperature and in normal room light, or within 15 days if refrigerated at 2° to 8° C (36° to 46° F) and protected from sunlight. However, consult manufacturer's recommendations because some preparations may be stable for a shorter period.
- Administer doxorubicin into a large vein by a free-flowing I.V. infusion of D_5W or NS over at least 3 minutes. Watch for red streaking along vein or facial flushing, which may indicate too-rapid administration.
- Wash your skin thoroughly with soap and water and irrigate your eyes if exposed to doxorubicin.
- Avoid contact with patient's urine or other body fluids—for example, by wearing latex gloves when caring for pediatric patients—for at least 5 days after each treatment.
- **WARNING** Monitor patient for signs of doxorubicin-induced cardiotoxicity, including cardiomyopathy and life-threatening heart failure, which may occur during therapy or months to years afterward. Patients with a history of prior mediastinal irradiation and young or elderly patients receiving concurrent cyclophosphamide therapy are at increased risk for developing cardiotoxicity at lower doses. Be prepared to administer digitalis preparations, diuretics, and afterload reducers such as ACE inhibitors if heart failure occurs.
- Monitor serum uric acid level before and during therapy, especially in patients with a history of gout or urate calculi. Expect antigout drug dosage to be adjusted if blood uric acid level is elevated from doxorubicin therapy. Oral hydration and allopurinol may be administered to prevent uric acid nephropathy.
- Monitor patients with a history of bone marrow depression, chickenpox (including recent exposure), and herpes zoster because they're at increased risk for severe generalized disease. Assess patients with leukopenia for signs of infection, including fever, chills, and cough.
- Be aware that adverse reactions can vary when doxorubicin is administered in combination therapy. Review information for all drugs administered as part of a specific regimen, including drug interactions and adverse effects.
- Assess I.V. insertion site for signs of extravasation, such as redness or pain. Tissue necrosis can occur because drug is a vesicant. (However, extravasation can be painless or can occur even

with blood return in I.V. line.) If extravasation occurs, immediately stop injection or infusion and apply ice. Then restart injection or infusion in another vein.

- Before reconstituting doxorubicin, store it at 15° to 30° C (59° to 86° F) and protect from light.

PATIENT TEACHING

- Instruct patient receiving doxorubicin to immediately report adverse reactions, such as unusual bruising or bleeding; black, tarry stools; blood in urine or stools; or pinpoint red spots on skin.
- Inform patient that urine may be red-tinged for 1 or 2 days after treatment.
- Stress the importance of keeping scheduled follow-up appointments and undergoing prescribed diagnostic tests, such as cardiac evaluation, especially to parents of pediatric patients, who are at increased risk for delayed cardiotoxicity, delayed growth, and temporary gonadal impairment.
- Caution patient to avoid sports and other activities that increase the risk of accidental injury. Also advise her to take measures to avoid infection, such as maintaining good oral hygiene (for example, by using soft-bristled toothbrush) and washing hands before touching eyes or nose.
- Advise patient with thrombocytopenia to avoid alcohol and aspirin to reduce the risk of GI bleeding.
- Advise patient not receive live or killed virus vaccines during therapy and for 3 months to 1 year after therapy is completed, unless approved by prescriber. Urge her to avoid people who have received such vaccines or to wear a protective mask when she's around them.
- Suggest that patient with stomatitis eat soft, bland foods served cold or at room temperature to decrease irritation.
- Inform patient that her hair should grow back after therapy but that the color and texture may be different.
- Advise female patient not to breast-feed during therapy.
- Urge both male and female patients to use two methods of birth control during therapy.

doxorubicin hydrochloride liposome
Caelyx (CAN), Doxil

Class and Category
Chemical: Anthracycline
Therapeutic: Antibiotic antineoplastic
Pregnancy category: D

Indications and Dosages

▶ *To treat Kaposi's sarcoma associated with AIDS*
I.V. INFUSION
Adults. 20 mg/m^2 over 30 min q 3 wk.
▶ *To treat refractory ovarian cancer*
I.V. INFUSION
Adults. 40 to 50 mg/m^2 infused at 1 mg/min initially to minimize risk of infusion reaction; then drug infused over 1 to 2 hr. Repeated q 4 wk.
DOSAGE ADJUSTMENT Dosage reduced by 50% when serum bilirubin level is 1.2 to 3 mg/dl and by 75% when serum bilirubin level is 3 mg/dl.

Mechanism of Action

May induce fragmentation of tumor cell DNA by inhibiting topo-isomerase II, an enzyme that usually acts to catalyze the breakage and reformation of DNA linkages. Antitumor activity and toxicity may be related to the formation of intracellular oxygen free radicals, which may lead to cell death after reaction with DNA, RNA, cell membranes, and proteins. Liposomal encapsulation may enhance doxorubicin accumulation in Kaposi's sarcoma (KS) lesions and allow passage through endothelial cell gaps present in lesions similar to those of KS.

Incompatibilities

Don't mix liposomal doxorubicin with diluents other than D$_5$W or with other drugs or bacteriostatic agents.

Contraindications

Breast-feeding women, hypersensitivity to doxorubicin hydrochloride or to liposomal components

Interactions

DRUGS

actinomycin D: Acute "recall" pneumonitis after local radiation therapy in children
blood-dyscrasia–causing drugs (such as cephalosporins and cisplatin): Increased leukopenic and thrombocytopenic effects of doxorubicin
bone marrow depressants (such as colchicine and methotrexate): Increased bone marrow depression
carbamazepine: Decreased blood carbamazepine level
cisplatin: Risk of leukemia
cyclophosphamide: Potentiated cyclophosphamide-induced hemorrhagic cystitis, increased risk of doxorubicin-induced cardiotoxicity

cyclosporine: Possibly decreased doxorubicin metabolism; increased risk of severe and prolonged hematologic toxicity, coma, and seizures

cytarabine: Possibly necrotizing colitis

dactinomycin, mitomycin, nifedipine, and other calcium channel blockers: Increased risk of doxorubicin-induced cardiotoxicity

digoxin: Decreased blood digoxin level

fosphenytoin, phenytoin: Possibly decreased blood phenytoin level

methotrexate and other hepatoxic drugs: Possibly impaired hepatic function, increased risk of doxorubicin toxicity

paclitaxel: Decreased doxorubicin clearance

phenobarbital: Possibly increased doxorubicin excretion

progesterone: Possibly enhanced doxorubicin-induced neutropenia and thrombocytopenia

streptozocin: Possibly inhibited hepatic metabolism of doxorubicin

trastuzumab: Possibly increased incidence and severity of cardiac dysfunction

vaccines, killed virus: Possibly decreased antibody response to vaccine

vaccines, live virus: Possibly increased adverse effects of vaccine, severe infection, and decreased antibody response to vaccine

Adverse Reactions

CNS: Anxiety, asthenia, chills, dizziness, fever, headache, insomnia

CV: Cardiotoxicity (dose-related or cumulative effect), chest pain

EENT: Conjunctivitis, mucous membrane disorder (changes in mouth or nose lining), oral candidiasis, pharyngitis, stomatitis, taste perversion

GI: Abdominal pain, anorexia, constipation, diarrhea, dysphagia, ileus, nausea, vomiting

GU: Reddish urine

HEME: Anemia, leukopenia, neutropenia, thrombocytopenia

MS: Back pain

RESP: Dyspnea, pneumonia

SKIN: Alopecia, injection site pain, jaundice, palmar-plantar erythrodysesthesia, rash, recall postirradiation erythema, pruritus

Other: Allergic reaction, infection, infusion reaction

Nursing Considerations

- **WARNING** Be aware that doxorubicin hydrochloride should not be substituted for doxorubicin hydrochloride liposome. These drugs are not interchangeable; severe adverse reactions may result.
- Be aware that liposomal doxorubicin should be administered only under the supervision of a qualified physician.

- Follow facility protocols for preparation and handling of antineoplastic drugs and appropriate disposal of used equipment.
- Monitor hepatic and renal function tests and CBC, including hematocrit, platelet count, and WBC count with differential, before and periodically during therapy. Be aware that cardiac evaluation, including ECG, radionuclide angiography to determine ejection fraction, and echocardiography, will be performed before, during, and sometimes after doxorubicin hydrochloride liposome therapy.
- Wear gloves and other protective garments (according to facility protocol) when working with this drug. Wash skin thoroughly with soap and water to remove drug if exposed.
- Dilute up to 90 mg of liposomal doxorubicin in 250 ml of D_5W. Inspect solution for particles before administration and discard if particles are present. Be aware that liposomal doxorubicin is a red, translucent solution.
- Use diluted solution within 24 hours if stored at 2° to 8° C (36° to 46° F). Administer without an in-line filter.
- Monitor patient for signs of an infusion reaction, such as flushing, dyspnea, facial edema, headache, chills, back pain, chest or throat tightness, and hypotension. Such a reaction may resolve if infusion rate is decreased; however, in most patients, it will resolve within several hours or a day after infusion is terminated.
- **WARNING** Monitor patient for drug-induced cardiotoxicity, including cardiomyopathy and life-threatening heart failure, which may occur during therapy or months to years afterward. Patients with a history of prior mediastinal irradiation, those who are receiving concurrent cyclophosphamide therapy, and those who have previously received anthracyclines or anthracenediones are at increased risk for developing cardiotoxicity at lower doses. Be prepared to administer digitalis preparations, diuretics, and afterload reducers such as ACE inhibitors if heart failure occurs.
- Monitor patient for stomatitis, signs of bone marrow depression, or palmar-plantar erythrodysesthesia (swelling, pain, erythema, and skin peeling of hands and feet); these adverse reactions may require dosage reduction or drug discontinuation.
- Monitor patients with a history of bone marrow depression, chickenpox (including recent exposure), and herpes zoster because they're at increased risk for severe generalized disease. Assess patients with leukopenia for signs of infection, including fever, chills, and cough.

- Assess I.V. insertion site for signs of extravasation, such as redness or pain. (However, extravasation can be painless.) If extravasation occurs, immediately stop injection or infusion and apply ice. Follow facility protocol, if available, for management of extravasation. Then restart injection or infusion in another vein.
- Before diluting liposomal doxorubicin, store it at 2° to 8° C (36° to 46° F). Drug may be frozen for up to 1 month.

PATIENT TEACHING
- Instruct patient receiving liposomal doxorubicin to immediately report adverse reactions, such as swelling, blisters, or burning of hands or feet; unusual bruising or bleeding; black, tarry stools; blood in urine or stools; or red pinpoint spots on the skin.
- Inform patient that urine may be red-tinged for 1 or 2 days after treatment.
- Stress the importance of keeping scheduled follow-up appointments and undergoing prescribed diagnostic tests, such as cardiac evaluation.
- Caution patient to avoid sports and other activities that increase the risk of accidental injury. Also advise her to take measures to avoid infection, such as maintaining good oral hygiene (for example, by using soft-bristled toothbrush) and washing hands before touching eyes or nose.
- Advise patient with thrombocytopenia to avoid alcohol and aspirin to reduce the risk of GI bleeding.
- Advise patient not to receive live or killed virus vaccines during therapy and for a period afterward, unless approved by prescriber. Urge her to avoid people who have received such vaccines or to wear a protective mask when she's around them.
- Advise patient with stomatitis to try eating soft, bland foods served cold or at room temperature to decrease irritation.
- Inform patient that her hair should grow back after treatment but that the color and texture may be different.
- Advise female patient not to breast-feed during therapy.
- Urge both male and female patients to use two methods of birth control during therapy.

doxycycline calcium
Vibramycin
doxycycline hyclate
(contains 100 or 200 mg of base per injection vial)
Alti-Doxycycline (CAN), Apo-Doxy (CAN), Doryx, Doxycin (CAN), Vibramycin, Vibra-Tabs

Class and Category
Chemical: Oxytetracycline derivative
Therapeutic: Antibiotic
Pregnancy category: D

Indications and Dosages

▶ *To treat cutaneous, GI, or inhalation anthrax*
I.V. INFUSION
Adults, adolescents, and children who weigh more than 45 kg (99 lb). 100 mg (base) q 12 hr for 60 days.
Children who weigh less than 45 kg. 2.2 mg (base)/kg q 12 hr for 60 days.

▶ *To treat endocervical, rectal, and urethral infections caused by*
Chlamydia trachomatis
I.V. INFUSION
Adults and children over age 8 who weigh more than 45 kg. 200 mg (base) q.d. or 100 mg (base) q 12 hr on day 1 and then 100 to 200 mg (base) q.d. or 50 to 100 mg (base) q 12 hr. *Maximum:* 300 mg (base)/day.
Children who weigh 45 kg or less. 4.4 mg (base)/kg q.d. or 2.2 mg (base)/kg q 12 hr on day 1 and then 2.2 to 4.4 mg (base)/kg q.d. or 1.1 to 2.2 mg (base)/kg q 12 hr.

▶ *To treat epididymo-orchitis caused by* C. trachomatis *or* Neisseria gonorrhoeae *or nongonococcal urethritis caused by* C. trachomatis
I.V. INFUSION
Adults and children over age 8 who weigh more than 45 kg. 200 mg (base) q.d. or 100 mg (base) q 12 hr on day 1 and then 100 to 200 mg (base) q.d. or 50 to 100 mg (base) q 12 hr. *Maximum:* 300 mg (base)/day.
Children who weigh 45 kg or less. 4.4 mg (base)/kg q.d. or 2.2 mg (base)/kg q 12 hr on day 1 and then 2.2 to 4.4 mg (base)/kg q.d. or 1.1 to 2.2 mg (base)/kg q 12 hr.

▶ *To treat early syphilis in penicillin-allergic patients*
I.V. INFUSION
Adults and children over age 8 who weigh more than 45 kg. 150 mg (base) q 12 hr for at least 10 days. *Maximum:* 300 mg (base)/day.
Children who weigh 45 kg or less. 4.4 mg (base)/kg q.d. or 2.2 mg (base)/kg q 12 hr on day 1 and then 2.2 to 4.4 mg (base)/kg q.d. or 1.1 to 2.2 mg (base)/kg q 12 hr.

▶ *To treat syphilis of more than 1 year's duration in penicillin-allergic patients*

I.V. INFUSION

Adults and children over age 8 who weigh more than 45 kg. 150 mg (base) q 12 hr for at least 10 days. *Maximum:* 300 mg (base)/day.

Children who weigh 45 kg or less. 4.4 mg (base)/kg q.d. or 2.2 mg (base)/kg q 12 hr on day 1 and then 2.2 to 4.4 mg (base)/kg q.d. or 1.1 to 2.2 mg (base)/kg q 12 hr.

▶ *To treat all other infections caused by susceptible organisms*

I.V. INFUSION

Adults and children over age 8 who weigh more than 45 kg. 200 mg (base) q.d. or 100 mg (base) q 12 hr on day 1 and then 100 to 200 mg (base) q.d. or 50 to 100 mg (base) q 12 hr. *Maximum:* 300 mg (base)/day.

Children who weigh 45 kg or less. 4.4 mg (base)/kg q.d. or 2.2 mg (base)/kg q 12 hr on day 1 and then 2.2 to 4.4 mg (base)/kg q.d. or 1.1 to 2.2 mg (base)/kg q 12 hr.

Mechanism of Action

Exerts a bacteriostatic effect against a wide variety of gram-positive and gram-negative organisms. Doxycycline is more lipophilic than other tetracyclines, which allows it to pass more easily through the bacterial lipid bilayer, where it binds reversibly to 30S ribosomal subunits. Bound doxycycline blocks the binding of aminoacyl transfer RNA to messenger RNA, thus inhibiting bacterial protein synthesis.

Contraindications

Hypersensitivity to any tetracycline

Interactions

DRUGS

barbiturates, carbamazepine, phenytoin: Increased clearance and decreased effects of doxycycline

digoxin: Increased bioavailability of digoxin, possibly leading to digitalis toxicity

oral anticoagulants: Possibly increased hypoprothrombinemic effects of these drugs

oral contraceptives: Decreased effectiveness of estrogen-containing oral contraceptives, increased risk of breakthrough bleeding

penicillins: Inhibited bactericidal action

Adverse Reactions

CNS: Paresthesia

CV: Phlebitis

EENT: Black "hairy" tongue, glossitis, hoarseness, oral candidiasis, pharyngitis, stomatitis, tooth discoloration

GI: Anorexia; bulky, loose stools; diarrhea; dysphagia; enterocolitis; hepatotoxicity; nausea; rectal candidiasis; vomiting

GU: Anogenital lesions, dark yellow or brown urine, elevated BUN level, vaginal candidiasis

HEME: Eosinophilia, hemolytic anemia, neutropenia, thrombocytopenia

SKIN: Dermatitis, photosensitivity, rash, urticaria

Other: Anaphylaxis, injection site phlebitis, superinfection

Nursing Considerations

- Avoid giving doxycycline to breast-feeding women because of the risk of enamel hypoplasia, inhibited linear skeletal growth, oral and vaginal candidiasis, photosensitivity reactions, and tooth discoloration in breast-feeding infant.
- Avoid giving drug to children younger than age 8 because it may cause permanent discoloration and enamel hypoplasia of developing teeth.
- Expect to adjust dosage for patients with hepatic disease to avoid drug accumulation.
- **WARNING** Don't give doxycycline by I.M. or S.C. route.
- Be aware that tetracyclines aren't routinely used to treat infections with gram-positive bacteria because many of these organisms are resistant. Tetracyclines aren't effective against viruses or fungi.
- Reconstitute doxycycline with 10 or 20 ml of sterile water for injection (or other diluent recommended by manufacturer, such as NS, D5W, or LR) for 100-mg or 200-mg vial, respectively. Further dilute 100-mg solution in 100 to 1,000 ml or 200-mg solution in 200 to 2,000 ml. Be aware that concentrations lower than 0.1 mg/ml or higher than 1 mg/ml are not recommended.
- Avoid rapid administration. Administration time can vary but is usually 1 to 4 hours.
- Observe patient frequently for injection site phlebitis, a common adverse effect of I.V. administration.
- Monitor liver enzyme levels to detect hepatotoxicity.
- Expect doxycycline to increase the risk of oral, rectal, or vaginal candidiasis—especially in elderly or debilitated patients and

those on prolonged therapy—by changing the normal balance of microbial flora.

• Be aware that storage time varies for reconstituted and diluted doxycycline solutions, depending on diluent used, storage temperature, exposure to light, and concentration. Consult package insert for manufacturer's recommendations. Before reconstituting doxycycline, store it at 15° to 30° C (59° to 86° F) and protect from light.

PATIENT TEACHING

• Instruct patient to report anorexia, diarrhea, upset stomach, nausea, or vomiting during doxycycline therapy.

• If patient is being treated for a sexually transmitted disease, explain that her partner may need treatment as well.

• Inform patient that her urine may become dark yellow or brown during doxycycline therapy.

• Instruct patient to avoid sun exposure and ultraviolet light during therapy.

• Advise patients who take an oral contraceptive to use an additional contraceptive method during therapy.

droperidol
Inapsine

Class and Category
Chemical: Butyrophenone derivative
Therapeutic: Anesthesia adjunct, antiemetic, sedative-hypnotic
Pregnancy category: C

Indications and Dosages
▶ *To provide anesthesia premedication*
I.V. OR I.M. INJECTION
Adults and adolescents. 2.5 to 5 mg I.M. 30 to 60 min before surgery.
Children. 0.075 to 0.15 mg/kg I.V. 30 to 60 min before surgery.
▶ *To induce anesthesia*
I.V. INJECTION
Adults and adolescents. *Initial:* 1.25 to 2.5 mg/9 to 11 kg (20 to 25 lb) or 0.1 to 0.14 mg/kg administered with general anesthesia. *Maintenance:* Additional 1.25 to 2.5 mg, as needed.
Children. 0.075 to 0.15 mg/kg administered with general anesthesia.

▶ *As adjunct to regional anesthesia*
I.V. OR I.M. INJECTION
Adults and adolescents. 2.5 to 5 mg.
▶ *To provide sedative-hypnotic effects for diagnostic procedures performed without anesthesia (conscious sedation)*
I.M. INJECTION
Adults and adolescents. 1.25 to 5 mg 30 to 60 min before procedure, followed by another 1.25 to 2.5 mg I.V., if indicated.
▶ *To prevent postoperative nausea and vomiting*
I.V. OR I.M. INJECTION
Adults and adolescents. 7 to 20 mcg/kg after procedure.
Children. 0.02 to 0.075 mg/kg after procedure.
DOSAGE ADJUSTMENT Initial dosage reduced for elderly patients because of increased risk of hypotension and excessive sedation.

Route	Onset	Peak	Duration
I.V., I.M.	3 to 10 min	In 30 min	2 to 4 hr

Mechanism of Action
Produces sedation by blocking postsynaptic dopamine receptors in the limbic system. Droperidol may reduce nausea by blocking dopamine receptors in the chemoreceptor trigger zone in the reticular formation of the medulla oblongata. It also may produce antiemetic effects by attaching to postsynaptic gamma-aminobutyric acid receptors in the chemoreceptor trigger zone.

Contraindications
Hypersensitivity to droperidol or its components

Interactions
DRUGS
amoxapine, haloperidol, loxapine, metoclopramide, metyrosine, molindone, olanzapine, phenothiazines, pimozide, rauwolfia alkaloids, risperidone, tacrine, thioxanthenes: Possibly increased risk of severe extrapyramidal reactions
anesthetics: Possibly hypotension and peripheral vasodilation
antihypertensives: Possibly orthostatic hypotension
bromocriptine, levodopa: Possibly inhibited actions of these drugs
CNS depressants: Additive CNS depression
epinephrine: Possibly paradoxical reduction of blood pressure
propofol: Possibly decreased antiemetic effect of both drugs

ACTIVITIES

alcohol use: Additive CNS depression

Adverse Reactions

CNS: Anxiety, drowsiness, dystonia, restlessness
CV: Hypertension, hypotension, sinus tachycardia
EENT: Fixed upward position of eyeballs, laryngospasm
MS: Spasms of tongue, face, neck, and back muscles
RESP: Bronchospasm

Nursing Considerations

• Monitor blood pressure frequently in patients with cardiac disease, who may not be able to compensate for droperidol's hypotensive effect.
• Assess patients with parkinsonism for worsening of condition, which may be an adverse effect of droperidol use.
• Monitor heart rate and ECG in patients with hypokalemia, hypomagnesemia, or preexisitng QT interval prolongation and in those with acute alcoholism because they're at increased risk for arrhythmias and, rarely, sudden death.
• Assess patients with pheochromocytoma for hypertension and tachycardia.
• Monitor patients with epilepsy, severe depression, parkinsonism, or impaired cardiovascular function for signs of exacerbation.
• Expect altered LOC to last for up to 12 hours after drug is given.
• If drug causes extrapyramidal reactions, such as restlessness, dystonia, and oculogyric crisis, expect to administer an anticholinergic, such as benztropine or diphenhydramine. Be sure to maintain a patent airway and oxygenation.
• If severe hypotension develops, expect to administer phenylephrine. If hypotension is related to hypovolemia, expect to administer fluids.
• Store drug at 15° to 30° C (59° to 86° F) and protect from light.

PATIENT TEACHING

• Instruct patient to ask for help with ambulation on first postoperative day because LOC may be altered for up to 12 hours.
• Caution patient to avoid drinking alcohol, taking CNS depressants, driving, and operating machinery for 24 hours after receiving droperidol.

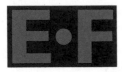

eflornithine hydrochloride
(alpha-difluoromethylornithine, DFMO)
Ornidyl

Class and Category
Chemical: Difluoromethylornithine
Therapeutic: Antiprotozoal
Pregnancy category: C

Indications and Dosages
▶ *To treat the meningoencephalitic stage of* Trypanosoma brucei gambiense *infection (sleeping sickness)*
I.V. INFUSION
Adults. 100 mg/kg given over at least 45 min q 6 hr for 14 days.

Route	Onset	Peak	Duration
I.V.	Unknown	4 to 6 hr	Unknown

Mechanism of Action
Inhibits the enzyme ornithine decarboxylase, which is needed for decarboxylation of ornithine. This process is the first step in polyamine synthesis, which is needed for protozoal cell division and differentiation.

Incompatibilities
Don't administer eflornithine with any other drug.

Contraindications
Hypersensitivity to eflornithine or its components

Interactions
DRUGS
other bone marrow depressants (such as chloramphenicol and doxorubicin): Possibly increased bone marrow depression
ototoxic drugs (such as aminoglycosides and NSAIDs): Increased risk of ototoxicity with long-term eflornithine therapy

Adverse Reactions

CNS: Asthenia, dizziness, headache, seizures
EENT: Hearing loss
GI: Abdominal pain, anorexia, diarrhea, vomiting
HEME: Anemia, eosinophilia, leukopenia, myelosuppression, thrombocytopenia
Other: Alopecia, facial edema

Nursing Considerations

• Monitor creatinine clearance of patients with impaired renal function, and plan to reduce eflornithine dosage, as prescribed, based on results.
• Before drug infusion, dilute eflornithine concentrate with sterile water for injection. Using strict aseptic technique, withdraw the contents of a 100-ml vial and inject 25 ml into each of four I.V. diluent bags that contain 100 ml of sterile water. The resulting solution contains 40 mg/ml of eflornithine (5,000 mg of eflornithine in 125 ml total volume).
• Store bags of diluted eflornithine at 4° C (39° F) to reduce the risk of contamination. Use diluted drug within 24 hours.
• Expect to monitor CBC, including platelet count, before treatment, twice weekly during treatment, and weekly after therapy stops until hematologic values return to baseline.
• Don't give other I.V. drugs while infusing eflornithine.
• Take infection-control and bleeding precautions because drug may cause myelosuppression. Adjust dosage or stop therapy as prescribed, based on severity.
• Take seizure precautions during therapy.
• Consult prescriber about the need for serial audiography, if appropriate, to detect hearing loss.
• Store undiluted vials at room temperature, and protect from freezing and light.

PATIENT TEACHING

• Stress the importance of keeping follow-up medical appointments because relapse may occur for up to 24 months after eflornithine treatment ends.
• Teach patient how to follow infection-control and bleeding precautions if myelosuppression occurs.
• Instruct patient to report adverse reactions to prescriber.
• Caution patient about the risk of seizures; advise him not to perform potentially hazardous activities during therapy.

enalaprilat
Vasotec I.V.

Class and Category
Chemical: Dicarbocyl-containing ACE inhibitor
Therapeutic: Antihypertensive
Pregnancy category: C (first trimester), D (later trimesters)

Indications and Dosages
▶ *To control hypertension*
I.V. INJECTION
Adults. 1.25 mg q 6 hr.
DOSAGE ADJUSTMENT Initial dose reduced to 0.625 mg for patients who have sodium and water depletion from diuretic therapy, are receiving diuretics, or have a creatinine clearance below 30 ml/min/1.73 m^2. If response is inadequate after 1 hr, dose of 0.625 mg is repeated and therapy continued at 1.25 mg q 6 hr.

Route	Onset	Peak	Duration
I.V.	15 min	1 to 4 hr	About 6 hr

Mechanism of Action
May reduce blood pressure by affecting the renin-angiotensin-aldosterone system. By inhibiting ACE, enalaprilat:
- prevents conversion of angiotensin I to angiotensin II, a potent vasoconstrictor that also stimulates the adrenal cortex to secrete aldosterone
- may inhibit renal and vascular production of angiotensin II
- decreases the serum angiotensin II level and increases serum renin activity, thereby decreasing aldosterone secretion and slightly increasing the serum potassium level and fluid loss
- decreases vascular tone and blood pressure
- inhibits aldosterone release, which reduces sodium and water reabsorption and increases their excretion, further reducing blood pressure.

Contraindications
History of angioedema from previous ACE inhibitor therapy; hypersensitivity to enalapril, enalaprilat, or their components

Interactions

DRUGS

allopurinol, bone marrow depressants (such as amphotericin B and methotrexate), procainamide, systemic corticosteroids: Possibly increased risk of fatal neutropenia or agranulocytosis

cyclosporine, potassium-sparing diuretics, potassium supplements: Increased risk of hyperkalemia

diuretics, other antihypertensives: Additive hypotensive effects

lithium: Increased blood lithium level and lithium toxicity

NSAIDs: Possibly reduced antihypertensive effects of enalapril and enalaprilat

sympathomimetics: Possibly reduced therapeutic effects of enalapril and enalaprilat

FOODS

potassium-containing salt substitutes: Increased risk of hyperkalemia

ACTIVITIES

alcohol use: Possibly additive hypotensive effect

Adverse Reactions

CNS: Ataxia, confusion, CVA, depression, dizziness, dream disturbances, fatigue, headache, insomnia, nervousness, peripheral neuropathy, somnolence, syncope, vertigo, weakness

CV: Angina, arrhythmias, cardiac arrest, hypotension, MI, orthostatic hypotension, palpitations, pulmonary embolism and infarction, Raynaud's phenomenon

EENT: Blurred vision, conjunctivitis, dry eyes and mouth, glossitis, hoarseness, lacrimation, loss of smell, pharyngitis, rhinorrhea, stomatitis, taste perversion, tinnitus

ENDO: Gynecomastia

GI: Abdominal pain, anorexia, constipation, diarrhea, hepatic failure, hepatitis, ileus, indigestion, melena, nausea, pancreatitis, vomiting

GU: Flank pain, impotence, oliguria, renal failure, UTI

MS: Muscle spasms

RESP: Asthma, bronchitis, bronchospasm, cough, dyspnea, pneumonia, pulmonary edema, pulmonary infiltrates, upper respiratory tract infection

SKIN: Alopecia, diaphoresis, erythema multiforme, exfoliative dermatitis, flushing, pemphigus, photosensitivity, pruritus, rash, Stevens-Johnson syndrome, toxic epidermal necrolysis, urticaria

Other: Anaphylaxis, angioedema, herpes zoster, hyperkalemia

Nursing Considerations

- Be aware that patients with impaired renal function may require a decreased dosage or less frequent doses of enalaprilat because of the risk of increased blood enalaprilat level and hyperkalemia. Monitor urinary protein level before and periodically during enalaprilat therapy.
- Administer enalaprilat undiluted, or dilute with up to 50 ml of D₅W, NS, D₅NS, or D₅LR. Use diluted enalaprilat within 24 hours if stored at room temperature. Administer each dose over at least 5 minutes.
- Measure blood pressure immediately after first dose and frequently for at least 2 hours thereafter. If hypotension requires a dosage reduction, monitor blood pressure frequently for 2 hours after reduced dose is administered and frequently for another hour after blood pressure has stabilized.
- Monitor blood pressure regularly during therapy. If patient develops hypotension, place him in supine position and expect to give I.V. NS or another volume expander, as prescribed.
- Monitor heart rate and rhythm. Expect to obtain repeated 12-lead ECG tracings.
- Monitor laboratory test results to check hepatic and renal function, leukocyte count, and serum potassium level.
- Monitor closely for angioedema of the face, lips, tongue, glottis, larynx, and limbs. If patient develops angioedema of the face and lips, stop drug and give an antihistamine, as prescribed, for symptoms. If tongue, glottis, or larynx is involved, assess for airway obstruction and prepare to give epinephrine 1:1,000 (0.3 to 0.5 ml) S.C. and maintain a patent airway.
- Closely assess for anaphylaxis in patients who receive dialysis with high-flux membranes, treatment with Hymenoptera venom, or LDL apheresis with dextran sulfate.
- Store drug between 15° and 30° C (59° and 86° F).

PATIENT TEACHING
- Inform patient that he may experience light-headedness and fainting, especially during first few days of enalaprilat therapy. Advise him to change position slowly and to avoid potentially hazardous activities until drug's CNS effects are known.
- Inform patient that diarrhea, excessive sweating, vomiting, and other conditions may cause dehydration, which can lead to dizziness, fainting, and very low blood pressure during therapy. Urge sufficient fluid intake to prevent dehydration and related

adverse reactions. Instruct patient to report severe or prolonged diarrhea or vomiting.
- Urge patient to immediately report angioedema and other adverse reactions, including persistent dry cough.
- Advise patient to consult prescriber before using salt substitutes, potassium supplements, or other drugs (including OTC drugs) while receiving enalaprilat.

epinephrine
(adrenaline)
Adrenalin, Ana-Guard
epinephrine hydrochloride
Adrenalin

Class and Category
Chemical: Catecholamine
Therapeutic: Antianaphylactic, bronchodilator, cardiac stimulant, vasopressor
Pregnancy category: C

Indications and Dosages
▶ *To treat anaphylaxis*
I.V. INFUSION
Adults and adolescents. 100 to 250 mcg given slowly.
▶ *To treat severe anaphylactic shock*
I.V. INFUSION
Adults. 1 mcg/min, titrated to 2 to 10 mcg/min for desired hemodynamic response.
▶ *To treat cardiac arrest*
I.V. INJECTION
Adults. 0.5 to 1 mg q 3 to 5 min during resuscitation.
Children. 10 mcg/kg, followed by 100 mcg/kg q 3 to 5 min, if needed. If two doses produce no response, subsequent doses are increased to 200 mcg/kg q 5 min.
Neonates. 10 to 30 mcg/kg q 3 to 5 min.

Route	Onset	Peak	Duration
I.V.	Rapid	Unknown	1 to 2 min

> ## Mechanism of Action
>
> Acts on alpha and beta receptors. This nonselective adrenergic agonist stimulates:
>
> - alpha$_1$ receptors, which constricts arteries and may decrease bronchial secretions
> - presynaptic alpha$_2$ receptors, which inhibits norepinephrine release by negative feedback
> - postsynaptic alpha$_2$ receptors, which constricts arteries
> - beta$_1$ receptors, which induces positive chronotropic and inotropic responses
> - beta$_2$ receptors, which dilates arteries, relaxes bronchial smooth muscles, increases glycogenolysis, and prevents mast cells from secreting histamine and other substances, thus reversing bronchoconstriction and edema.

Incompatibilities

Don't mix epinephrine with alkalies or oxidizing agents, including bromine, chlorine, chromates, iodine, metal salts (as from iron), nitrites, oxygen, and permanganates, because these substances can destroy epinephrine.

Contraindications

Cerebral arteriosclerosis, coronary insufficiency, counteraction of phenothiazine-induced hypotension, dilated cardiomyopathy, general anesthesia with halogenated hydrocarbons or cyclopropane, hypersensitivity to epinephrine or its components, labor, angle-closure glaucoma, organic brain damage, shock (nonanaphylactic)

Interactions

DRUGS

alpha-adrenergic blockers, drugs with alpha-adrenergic action, rapid-acting vasodilators: Blockage of epinephrine's alpha-adrenergic effect, possibly causing severe hypotension and tachycardia
beta blockers: Mutual inhibition of therapeutic effects, possibly severe hypertension and cerebral hemorrhage
digoxin, quinidine: Increased risk of arrhythmias
dihydroergotamine, ergoloid mesylates, ergonovine, ergotamine, methylergonovine, methysergide, oxytocin: Increased risk of vasoconstriction, causing gangrene, peripheral vascular ischemia, or severe hypertension
diuretics, other antihypertensives: Decreased antihypertensive effects
hydrocarbon inhalation anesthetics: Increased risk of severe atrial and ventricular arrhythmias

insulin, oral antidiabetic drugs: Decreased effects of these drugs
MAO inhibitors: Possibly increased vasopressor effect of epinephrine and hypertensive crisis
maprotiline, tricyclic antidepressants: Potentiated cardiovascular effects of epinephrine, possibly causing arrhythmias, hyperpyrexia, severe hypertension, or tachycardia
sympathomimetics: Additive CNS stimulation, increased cardiovascular effects of either drug
thyroid hormones: Increased effects of either drug
xanthines: Increased CNS stimulation, additive toxic effects

Adverse Reactions

CNS: Anxiety, chills, fever, dizziness, hallucinations, headache, insomnia, light-headedness, nervousness, restlessness, seizures, tremor, vertigo, weakness
CV: Arrhythmias; chest discomfort or pain; fast, irregular, or slow heartbeat; palpitations; severe hypertension
EENT: Blurred vision, miosis
GI: Nausea, vomiting
GU: Dysuria, urinary hesitancy, urine retention
MS: Muscle twitching, severe muscle spasms
RESP: Dyspnea
SKIN: Cold skin, diaphoresis, flushed or red face or skin, pallor
Other: Allergic reaction, hyperkalemia, hypokalemia, injection site pain and stinging

Nursing Considerations

- Dilute the 1:1,000 (1 mg/ml) solution of parenteral epinephrine to strength of 1:10,000, using sterile water for injection. Be aware that some preparations contain sulfites.
- Shake suspension thoroughly before withdrawing dose; refrigerate suspension between uses.
- Inspect epinephrine solution or suspension before use. Don't use if solution is pink or brown (which means that air has entered the vial) or contains particles. Discard unused portions.
- Be aware that epinephrine shouldn't be given by intra-arterial injection because marked vasoconstriction may cause gangrene.
- Monitor patients with angina or arrhythmias because epinephrine may exacerbate these conditions.
- Be aware that drug should be used cautiously in patients with asthma or emphysema and degenerative heart disease. Epinephrine's inotropic effect equals that of dopamine and dobutamine; its chronotropic effect exceeds that of both.

- Monitor elderly patients and those with cardiovascular disease (other than those listed above), hypertension, hyperthyroidism, prostatic hypertrophy, or psychoneurologic disorders for exacerbation of condition or increased adverse effects.
- Monitor for potassium imbalances. Initially, hyperkalemia occurs when hepatocytes release potassium. Hypokalemia may quickly follow as skeletal muscles take up potassium.
- Monitor patients with diabetes for increased blood glucose level, as ordered.
- Assess for decreased urine output, which could signal urine retention. Ask patient if he's experiencing urinary hesitancy.
- **WARNING** At least twice the peripheral I.V. dose of epinephrine may be given by endotracheal instillation if drug is used to treat cardiac arrest. Two dilutions are needed for this regimen; use great caution to avoid medication errors.
- Store drug between 15° and 25° C (59° and 77° F); protect from freezing and light.

PATIENT TEACHING
- Advise patient receiving epinephrine to report symptoms that don't improve or improve but then worsen.
- Advise patient to immediately report blurred vision, chest pain, difficulty breathing, a fast or irregular heartbeat, or increased sweating.

epoetin alfa
(EPO, erythropoietin alfa, recombinant erythropoietin, r-HuEPO)
Epogen, Eprex (CAN), Procrit

Class and Category
Chemical: 165–amino acid glycoprotein identical to human erythropoietin
Therapeutic: Antianemic
Pregnancy category: C

Indications and Dosages
▶ *To treat anemia from renal failure*
I.V. INJECTION
Adults and adolescents. *Initial:* 50 to 100 U/kg 3 times/wk; increased by 25 U/kg after 8 wk if hematocrit hasn't risen by 5 or 6 points and is still below desired range (30% to 36%). *Maintenance:* Dosage gradually decreased by 25 U/kg q 4 or more wk to

lowest dose that keeps hematocrit at 30% to 36%. *Maximum:* 300 U/kg 3 times/wk.

Children on dialysis. 50 U/kg 3 times/wk; increased after 8 wk if hematocrit hasn't risen by 5 or 6 points and is still below desired range of 30% to 36%. *Maintenance:* Dosage gradually decreased to lowest dose that keeps hematocrit at 30% to 36%.

▶ *To treat anemia in HIV-infected patients who take zidovudine*
I.V. INJECTION

Adults with serum erythropoietin level of 500 mU/ml or less who receive 4,200 mg or less of zidovudine/wk. *Initial:* 100 U/kg 3 times/wk; increased by 50 to 100 U/kg q 4 to 8 wk after 8 wk of therapy. *Maintenance:* Dosage gradually titrated to maintain desired response, based on such factors as variations in zidovudine dosage and occurrence of infection or inflammation. *Maximum:* 300 U/kg 3 times/wk.

DOSAGE ADJUSTMENT For patients being treated for anemia caused by renal failure, therapy is temporarily discontinued if hematocrit reaches or exceeds 36% and is resumed at a lower dose when hematocrit returns to desired range. For patients being treated for anemia related to zidovudine use, therapy is temporarily discontinued if hematocrit reaches or exceeds 40% and is resumed at a 25% lower dose when hematocrit returns to desired range.

Route	Onset	Peak	Duration
I.V.	In 2 to 6 wk	In 2 mo	About 2 wk

Mechanism of Action
Stimulates the release of reticulocytes from the bone marrow into the bloodstream, where they develop into mature RBCs.

Incompatibilities
Don't mix epoetin alfa with any other drug.

Contraindications
Hypersensitivity to human albumin or products made from mammal cells, uncontrolled hypertension

Interactions
DRUGS
antihypertensives: Increased blood pressure (to hypertensive level), especially when hematocrit rises rapidly

heparin: Increased heparin requirement in hemodialysis patients
iron supplements: Increased iron requirement and need for increased dose

Adverse Reactions

CNS: Dizziness, fatigue, headache, seizures
CV: Chest pain, edema, hypertension, tachycardia
GI: Diarrhea, nausea, vomiting
HEME: Polycythemia
MS: Bone pain, muscle weakness
RESP: Dyspnea
SKIN: Rash, urticaria
Other: Flulike symptoms, hyperkalemia, injection site pruritus or stinging

Nursing Considerations

- Be aware that certain conditions, such as aluminum intoxication, folic acid deficiency, hemolysis, infection, inflammation, iron deficiency, malignant neoplasm, osteitis (fibrosa cystica), and vitamin B_{12} deficiency, may decrease or delay patient's response to epoetin alfa.
- Don't shake vial during preparation to avoid denaturing glycoprotein and inactivating epoetin alfa.
- Discard unused portion of single-dose vial because it contains no preservatives. Discard unused portion of multidose vial after 21 days.
- **WARNING** Be aware that the multidose vial of epoetin contains benzyl alcohol, which can cause a fatal toxic syndrome in neonates and premature infants, characterized by CNS, respiratory, circulatory, and renal impairment and metabolic acidosis.
- Expect to increase heparin dose if patient receives hemodialysis because epoetin alfa can increase RBC volume, which may cause blood clots to form in the dialyzer, hemodialysis vascular access, or both.
- Expect to give an iron supplement (such as I.V. iron dextran), if needed, because iron requirements rise when erythropoiesis consumes existing iron stores.
- Monitor drug effectiveness by checking hematocrit, typically twice weekly, until it stabilizes at 30% to 36%. Thereafter, hematocrit can be monitored less frequently.

• Be aware that the risk of hypertensive or thrombotic complications increases if hematocrit rises by more than 4 points in 2 weeks.
• Monitor patient frequently for drug-induced increase in blood pressure. Patients with preexisting hypertension (even if controlled) or a history of cardiac disorders caused by hypertension are at increased risk for hypertension, which may lead to hypertensive encephalopathy.
• Monitor patients with vascular disease or a hematologic disorder (such as hypercoagulation, myelodysplastic syndrome, or sickle cell disease) for potential complications from increased blood viscosity and peripheral vascular resistance, such as pulmonary embolism or CVA. Monitor patients with porphyria for signs of an exacerbation, such as peripheral neuropathy, fever, skin lesions, and discolored urine.
• Take seizure precautions, especially in patients with a history of seizure disorders.
• Store drug at 2° to 8° C (36° to 46° F); don't freeze.

PATIENT TEACHING
• Inform patient that the risk of seizures is highest during the first 90 days of epoetin alfa therapy. Discourage him from engaging in potentially hazardous activities during this time.
• Stress the importance of keeping follow-up medical appointments and appointments for laboratory tests.
• Encourage patient to eat iron-rich foods.
• Review possible adverse effects, and urge patient to report chest pain, headache, hives, rapid heartbeat, rash, seizures, shortness of breath, weight gain, or swelling of hands, fingers, feet, ankles, lower legs, and face.

epoprostenol sodium
(PGI₂, PGX, prostacyclin)
Flolan

Class and Category
Chemical: Natural prostaglandin
Therapeutic: Antihypertensive, vasodilator
Pregnancy category: B

Indications and Dosages

▶ *To provide long-term treatment of primary pulmonary hypertension and pulmonary hypertension secondary to scleroderma spectrum of diseases*

I.V. INFUSION

Adults. *Initial:* 2 ng/kg/min, increased by 2 ng/kg/min q 15 min or longer until dose-limiting adverse reactions (such as abdominal, chest, or musculoskeletal pain; anxiety; bradycardia; dizziness; dyspnea; flushing; headache; hypotension; nausea; tachycardia; and vomiting) occur. *Maintenance:* Dosage started at 4 ng/kg/min less than maximum rate tolerated during initial titration. If maximum rate tolerated was less than 5 ng/kg/min, long-term infusion rate is started at 50% of maximum rate.

DOSAGE ADJUSTMENT Continuous infusion rate adjusted based on persistence, recurrence, or worsening of primary pulmonary hypertension and dose-related adverse reactions.

Mechanism of Action

Acts as a natural prostaglandin to directly relax vascular smooth muscles, resulting in arterial dilation and inhibition of platelet aggregation. These actions decrease pulmonary vascular resistance, increase cardiac index and oxygen delivery, and limit thrombus formation.

Incompatibilities

Don't mix epoprostenol with other parenteral solutions or drugs.

Contraindications

Hypersensitivity to epoprostenol or its components; long-term use in patients with heart failure caused by severe left ventricular systolic dysfunction; pulmonary edema that developed while establishing epoprostenol dosage

Interactions

DRUGS

anticoagulants, antiplatelet drugs, NSAIDs: Increased risk of bleeding
antihypertensives, diuretics, vasodilators: Decreased blood pressure
digoxin: Possibly increased digoxin bioavailability

Adverse Reactions

CNS: Anxiety, chills, confusion, dizziness, fever, headache, nervousness, paresthesia, syncope, weakness
CV: Bradycardia, chest pain, hypotension, tachycardia
GI: Abdominal pain, diarrhea, nausea, vomiting

HEME: Thrombocytopenia
MS: Arthralgia, jaw pain, myalgia
RESP: Dyspnea, hypoxia
SKIN: Flushing
Other: Flulike symptoms, injection site infection and pain, sepsis, weight gain or loss

Nursing Considerations

- Reconstitute epoprostenol only with sterile diluent that comes in package. Don't dilute reconstituted epoprostenol.
- To make 100 ml of reconstituted solution at 3,000 ng/ml, dissolve contents of 0.5-mg vial with 5 ml of diluent; withdraw 3 ml and add enough diluent to make 100 ml. To make 100 ml of solution at 5,000 ng/ml, dissolve contents of 0.5-mg vial with 5 ml of diluent; withdraw contents and add enough diluent to make 100 ml. To make 100 ml of solution at 10,000 ng/ml, dissolve contents of two 0.5-mg vials each with 5 ml of diluent; withdraw contents and add enough diluent to make 100 ml. To make 100 ml of solution at 15,000 ng/ml, dissolve contents of 1.5-mg vial with 5 ml of diluent; withdraw contents and add enough diluent to make 100 ml.
- Give continuous infusion through a central venous catheter. Use peripheral I.V. infusion only until central access is established.
- Use an ambulatory infusion pump that is small, lightweight, and able to deliver 2 ng/kg/minute. It should have alarms for occlusion, end of infusion, and low battery. Use a polyvinyl chloride, polypropylene, or glass reservoir. Keep a backup pump and infusion set nearby to minimize disruptions in delivery.
- Administer a single container of reconstituted solution at room temperature over 8 hours. For extended use at temperatures above 25° C (77° F), use a cold pouch with frozen gel packs to keep drug at 2° to 8°C (36° to 46° F) for 12 hours. Don't expose to direct sunlight.
- After a new infusion rate has been established, monitor closely for adverse reactions. Measure blood pressure each time with patient standing and supine. Also, monitor heart rate for several hours after dosage adjustment. Assess for signs of pulmonary edema, such as dyspnea, anxiety, and hemoptysis, which may be associated with veno-occlusive disease.
- During prolonged infusion, monitor for dose-related adverse reactions. If they occur, expect to decrease infusion rate by 2 ng/kg/minute every 15 minutes, as prescribed, until adverse reactions resolve.

- **WARNING** Avoid abrupt withdrawal or a sudden large reduction in infusion rate, which could cause rebound pulmonary hypertension (asthenia, dizziness, and dyspnea) or
  death.
- Expect lower dosage to be ordered for elderly patients, especially those with hepatic, renal, or cardiac impairment or other
  diseases and those who may receive other drugs that can interact with epoprostenol.
- Protect reconstituted drug from light, and refrigerate for no
  longer than 48 hours. Discard solution that has been frozen or
  that has been refrigerated for longer than 48 hours.
- Before reconstituting epoprostenol, store it and diluent at 15° to
  25° C (59° to 77° F); protect from freezing and light.

PATIENT TEACHING

- Inform patient that epoprostenol is infused continuously
  through a permanent indwelling central venous catheter by a
  small infusion pump.
- Stress that patient must commit to long-term therapy, possibly
  for years.
- Teach patient or caregiver how to reconstitute drug, administer
  it, and care for the permanent central venous catheter.
- Urge patient to maintain prescribed infusion rate and to consult
  prescriber before altering it.
- Caution patient that even brief interruptions in drug delivery
  may cause rapid worsening of symptoms.
- Instruct patient to notify prescriber if adverse reactions occur.
  Stress the importance of keeping follow-up appointments to assess for adverse reactions and evaluate his response to therapy.
- Make sure patient or caregiver has ready access to emergency
  phone numbers. Advise patient to carry medical identification
  documenting his use of epoprostenol and its purpose.
- Caution patient to avoid saunas, hot baths, and sunbathing,
  which can increase the risk of hypertension.

eptifibatide
Integrilin

Class and Category
Chemical: Cyclic heptapeptide
Therapeutic: Platelet aggregation inhibitor
Pregnancy category: B

Indications and Dosages

▶ *To treat unstable angina and non–Q-wave MI*
I.V. INFUSION
Adults. *Initial:* 180 mcg/kg over 1 to 2 min as soon as possible after diagnosis. *Maintenance:* 2 mcg/kg/min by continuous infusion beginning immediately after initial dose and continuing until discharge or coronary artery bypass grafting, up to 72 hr.
DOSAGE ADJUSTMENT For patients with serum creatinine level of 2 to 4 mg/dl, initial dosage reduced to 135 mcg/kg over 1 to 2 min and maintenance dosage to 0.5 mcg/kg/min by continuous infusion. Drug discontinued before coronary artery bypass graft surgery or if platelet count falls below 100,000/mm³.
▶ *To prevent thrombosis related to percutaneous transluminal coronary angioplasty (PTCA)*
I.V. INFUSION
Adults. *Initial:* 135 mcg/kg over 1 to 2 min immediately before procedure. *Maintenance:* 0.5 mcg/kg/min by continuous infusion beginning immediately after initial dose and continuing for 20 to 24 hr. *Maximum:* 96 hr of therapy.

Route	Onset	Peak	Duration
I.V.	Immediate	In 15 min	4 to 8 hr

Mechanism of Action
Reversibly inhibits platelet aggregation by preventing the binding of fibrinogen, von Willebrand factor, and other adhesive ligands to the platelet receptor glycoprotein IIb/IIIa on activated platelets. As a result, eptifibatide disrupts the final cross-linking stage of platelet aggregation—and thrombus formation.

Incompatibilities
Don't administer eptifibatide through the same I.V. line as furosemide.

Contraindications
Active bleeding or CVA during previous 30 days, bleeding diathesis, dependence on dialysis, history of hemorrhagic CVA, hypersensitivity to eptifibatide, major surgery during previous 4 weeks, serum creatinine level of 2 mg/dl or higher for 180-mcg/kg dose or 2-mcg/kg/min infusion, serum creatinine level of 4 mg/dl or higher for 135-mcg/kg dose or 0.5-mcg/kg/min infusion, severe uncontrolled hypertension (systolic pressure above 200 mm Hg,

diastolic pressure above 110 mm Hg), thrombocytopenia (platelet count below 100,000/mm^3)

Interactions
DRUGS
anticoagulants, clopidogrel, dipyridamole, NSAIDs, thrombolytics, ticlopidine: Additive pharmacologic effects, increased risk of bleeding
other platelet aggregation inhibitors (especially inhibitors of platelet receptor glycoprotein IIb/IIIa, such as abciximab): Increased risk of additive pharmacologic effects

Adverse Reactions
CNS: Intracranial hemorrhage
CV: Hypotension
GI: Hematemesis
GU: Hematuria
HEME: Bleeding, decreased hemoglobin level, thrombocytopenia
Other: Anaphylaxis

Nursing Considerations
- Expect to obtain hematocrit, platelet count, and hemoglobin and serum creatinine levels before starting eptifibatide therapy to detect abnormalities. Also expect to obtain baseline APTT and PT.
- Withdraw bolus dose of eptifibatide from a 10-ml (2-mg/ml) vial into a syringe.
- Using a vented I.V. infusion set, administer a continuous infusion directly from the 100-ml (0.75 mg/ml) vial. Be sure to center the spike in the circle on top of the vial stopper.
- Be aware that eptifibatide may be administered in same I.V. line as NS or D$_5$NS containing potassium at a concentration of 60 mEq/L. It may also be administered in same I.V. line as alteplase, atropine, dobutamine, heparin, lidocaine, meperidine, metoprolol, midazolam, morphine, nitroglycerin, or verapamil.
- Expect to maintain APTT between 50 and 70 seconds or according to facility protocol during therapy unless patient undergoes PTCA.
- If patient undergoes PTCA, expect to maintain his activated clotting time between 300 and 350 seconds during the procedure.
- During therapy, avoid arterial and venous punctures, I.M. injections, urinary catheter use, nasotracheal or nasogastric intubation, and use of noncompressible I.V. sites, such as subclavian and jugular veins.

- Expect to discontinue eptifibatide and heparin and monitor patient closely if platelet count falls below 100,000/mm^3.
- Plan to discontinue drug, as prescribed, if patient undergoes coronary artery bypass surgery.

PATIENT TEACHING

- Instruct patient to immediately report bleeding during eptifibatide therapy.
- Reassure patient that he'll be monitored closely throughout therapy.
- Advise patient to avoid activities that may lead to bruising and bleeding.

erythromycin gluceptate
(contains 500 or 1,000 mg of base per vial)
Ilotycin

erythromycin lactobionate
(contains 500 or 1,000 mg of base per vial)
Erythrocin

Class and Category
Chemical: Macrolide
Therapeutic: Antibiotic
Pregnancy category: B

Indications and Dosages
▶ *To treat mild to moderate upper respiratory tract infections caused by* Haemophilus influenzae, Streptococcus pneumoniae, *or* Streptococcus pyogenes *(group A beta-hemolytic streptococci)*
I.V. INFUSION
Adults. 250 to 500 mg (base) q 6 hr for 10 days.
Children. 250 to 500 mg (base) q.i.d. or 20 to 50 mg (base)/kg/day in divided doses for 10 days. *Maximum:* Adult dosage.
▶ *To treat lower respiratory tract infections caused by* S. pneumoniae *or* S. pyogenes *(group A beta-hemolytic streptococci)*
I.V. INFUSION
Adults. 250 to 500 mg (base) q 6 hr for 10 days.
Children. 250 to 500 mg (base) q.i.d. or 20 to 50 mg (base)/kg/day in divided doses for 10 days. *Maximum:* Adult dosage.
▶ *To treat respiratory tract infections caused by* Mycoplasma pneumoniae
I.V. INFUSION
Adults. 500 mg (base) q 6 hr for 5 to 10 days or, for severe infections, up to 3 wk.

▶ *To treat mild to moderate skin and soft-tissue infections caused by* S. pyogenes *or* Staphylococcus aureus
I.V. INFUSION
Adults. 250 mg (base) q 6 hr or 500 mg (base) q 12 hr for 10 days. *Maximum:* 4 g (base)/day.
Children. 250 to 500 mg (base) q.i.d. or 20 to 50 mg (base)/kg/day in divided doses for 10 days. *Maximum:* Adult dosage.

▶ *To treat pertussis (whooping cough) caused by* Bordetella pertussis
I.V. INFUSION
Children. 500 mg (base) q.i.d. or 40 to 50 mg (base)/kg/day in divided doses for 5 to 14 days.

▶ *To treat diphtheria*
I.V. INFUSION
Adults and children. 500 mg (base) q 6 hr for 10 days.

▶ *To treat erythrasma*
I.V. INFUSION
Adults and children. 250 mg (base) t.i.d. for 21 days.

▶ *To treat intestinal amebiasis*
I.V. INFUSION
Adults. 250 mg (base) q 6 hr for 10 to 14 days.
Children. 30 to 50 mg (base)/kg/day in divided doses for 10 to 14 days

▶ *To treat pelvic inflammatory disease caused by* Neisseria gonorrhoeae
I.V. INFUSION
Adults. 500 mg (base) q 6 hr for 3 days and then 250 mg (base) q 6 hr for 7 days.

▶ *To treat newborn conjunctivitis*
I.V. INFUSION
Neonates. 50 mg (base)/kg/day in four divided doses for 14 days.

▶ *To treat pneumonia in neonates*
I.V. INFUSION
Neonates. 50 mg (base)/kg/day in divided doses for 21 days.

▶ *To treat Legionnaires' disease*
I.V. INFUSION
Adults. 1 to 4 g (base)/day in divided doses for 10 to 14 days.

▶ *To treat rheumatic fever*
I.V. INFUSION
Adults. 250 mg (base) q 12 hr.

▶ *To prevent bacterial endocarditis in patients with penicillin allergy who plan to undergo dental or upper respiratory tract surgery*
I.V. INFUSION
Adults. 1 g (base) given 1 to 2 hr before procedure and then 500 mg (base) 6 hr after initial dose.
Children. 20 mg (base)/kg given 2 hr before procedure and then 10 mg (base)/kg 6 hr after initial dose.
▶ *To treat listeriosis*
I.V. INFUSION
Adults. 250 mg (base) q 6 hr or 500 mg (base) q 12 hr. *Maximum:* 4 g (base)/day.

Mechanism of Action
Binds with the 50S ribosomal subunit of the 70S ribosome in many types of aerobic, anaerobic, gram-positive, and gram-negative bacteria. This action inhibits RNA-dependent protein synthesis in bacterial cells, causing them to die.

Contraindications
Astemizole, cisapride, or pimozide therapy; hypersensitivity to erythromycin, other macrolide antibiotics, or their components

Interactions
DRUGS
alfentanil: Decreased alfentanil clearance, prolonged alfentanil action
astemizole, cisapride, terfenadine: Increased risk of cardiotoxicity, torsades de pointes, ventricular tachycardia, and death
atorvastatin, lovastatin, pravastatin, simvastatin: Increased risk of rhabdomyolysis
carbamazepine, valproic acid: Possibly inhibited metabolism of these drugs, increasing their blood levels and risk of toxicity
chloramphenicol, lincomycin: Antagonized effects of these drugs
cyclosporine: Increased risk of nephrotoxicity
digoxin: Increased blood digoxin level and risk of digitalis toxicity
ergotamine: Decreased ergotamine metabolism, increased risk of vasospasm from ergotamine use
hepatotoxic drugs: Increased risk of hepatotoxicity
midazolam, triazolam: Increased pharmacologic effects of these drugs

oral contraceptives: Failed contraception, hepatotoxicity
ototoxic drugs: Increased risk of ototoxicity if patient with impaired renal function receives high doses of erythromycin
penicillins: Interference with bactericidal effects of penicillins
warfarin: Prolonged PT and risk of hemorrhage, especially in elderly patients
xanthines (except dyphylline): Increased serum theophylline level and risk of theophylline toxicity
ACTIVITIES
alcohol use: Alcohol level increased by 40%

Adverse Reactions

CNS: Fatigue, fever, malaise, weakness
CV: Cardiotoxicity (especially prolonged QT interval and torsades de pointes)
EENT: Hearing loss, oral candidiasis
GI: Abdominal cramps and pain, diarrhea, hepatotoxicity, nausea, vomiting
GU: Vaginal candidiasis
SKIN: Erythema, jaundice, pruritus, rash
Other: Fluid overload, injection site inflammation and phlebitis

Nursing Considerations

- Expect to obtain body fluid or tissue specimen for culture and sensitivity tests before administering first dose of erythromycin.
- Reconstitute by adding at least 10 ml of preservative-free sterile water for injection to each 500-mg vial or at least 20 ml of diluent to each 1-g vial. After initial drug reconstitution, erythromycin gluceptate can be stored for 7 days if refrigerated; erythromycin lactobionate solutions (50 mg/ml) remain stable for 24 hours at room temperature and for 14 days if refrigerated.
- For prolonged infusion of erythromycin gluceptate, expect to infuse a buffered solution up to 24 hours after dilution.
- For intermittent infusion of erythromycin gluceptate, dilute the dose if needed in 100 to 250 ml of NS or D₅W and administer slowly over 20 to 60 minutes.
- Further dilute erythromycin gluceptate solution, if needed, to 1 g/L in NS or D₅W injection for slow, continuous infusion. Diluted solution remains potent for 7 days if refrigerated.

- Further dilute erythromycin lactobionate solution, if needed, to 1 to 5 mg/ml in NS, LR, or other electrolyte solution for slow, continuous infusion. For intermittent infusion, dilute to a maximum concentration of 5 mg/ml and administer over 20 to 60 minutes. Diluted solution remains potent for 14 days if refrigerated and for 24 hours at room temperature.
- Be aware that erythromycin lactobionate infusions prepared in piggyback infusion bottles remain potent for 30 days if frozen, 24 hours if refrigerated, or 8 hours at room temperature. Don't store infusions prepared in the ADD-vantage system.
- **WARNING** Don't use diluent that contains benzyl alcohol if administering erythromycin to a neonate or premature infant. It may cause a fatal toxic syndrome characterized by CNS, respiratory, circulatory, and renal impairment and metabolic acidosis.
- Monitor QT interval periodically, especially in patients receiving high doses of erythromycin who have a history of prolonged QT interval or cardiac arrhythmias, because these patients are at high risk for arrhythmias or torsades de pointes.
- Periodically monitor liver function test results to detect signs of hepatotoxicity, which is most common with erythromycin estolate use. Signs typically appear within 2 weeks after continuous therapy starts and resolve when therapy stops.
- Assess hearing regularly, especially in elderly patients and those who receive 4 g or more/day or have hepatic or renal disease. Hearing impairment begins 36 hours to 8 days after initiation of treatment and usually starts to improve 1 to 14 days after therapy stops.
- Assess patient for signs of fluid overload, such as acute dyspnea and crackles.
- Before reconstituting erythromycin gluceptate or lactobionate, store drug at 15° to 30° C (59° to 86° F).

PATIENT TEACHING
- Advise patient to report symptoms that worsen or fail to improve after a few days of erythromycin therapy.
- Instruct patient to promptly report allergic reactions, such as rash and itching; hearing changes; or signs and symptoms of hepatic dysfunction, such as fever, yellow eyes or skin, or nausea and vomiting.

esmolol hydrochloride

Brevibloc

Class and Category

Chemical: Beta blocker
Therapeutic: Antiarrhythmic, antihypertensive
Pregnancy category: C

Indications and Dosages

▶ *To treat supraventricular tachycardia*

I.V. INFUSION

Adults. *Loading:* 500 mcg/kg over 1 min. *Maintenance:* If response to loading dose is adequate after 5 min, 50 mcg/kg/min infused for 4 min. If response is inadequate after 5 min, another 500 mcg/kg may be given over 1 min, followed by 100 mcg/kg/min for 4 min. Sequence repeated, as needed, until adequate response occurs, increasing maintenance dosage by 50 mcg/kg/min at each step. *Maximum:* 200 mcg/kg/min for 48 hr.

Children. 50 mcg/kg/min, titrated q 10 min up to 300 mcg/kg/min.

▶ *To treat intraoperative and postoperative tachycardia and hypertension*

I.V. INFUSION

Adults. *Initial:* 250 to 500 mcg/kg over 1 min. *Maintenance:* 50 mcg/kg/min infused over 4 min. If response is inadequate after 5 min, another 250 to 500 mcg/kg may be given over 1 min, followed by 100 mcg/kg/min for 4 min. Sequence repeated, as needed, up to 4 times, increasing by 50 mcg/kg/min each time. *Maximum:* 200 mcg/kg/min for 48 hr.

DOSAGE ADJUSTMENT Subsequent loading doses omitted, increments decreased to 25 mcg/kg/min, and titration intervals increased to 10 min as heart rate approaches desired level or if blood pressure decreases too much.

Route	Onset	Peak	Duration
I.V.	Immediate	Unknown	10 to 20 min

Mechanism of Action

Inhibits stimulation of beta$_1$ receptors primarily in the heart, which decreases cardiac excitability, cardiac output, and myocardial oxygen demand. Esmolol also decreases renin release from the kidneys, which helps reduce blood pressure.

Incompatibilities
Don't mix esmolol with 5% sodium bicarbonate injection.

Contraindications
Cardiogenic shock, hypersensitivity to beta blockers, overt heart failure, second- or third-degree heart block, sinus bradycardia

Interactions
DRUGS

antihypertensives: Possibly hypotension

digoxin: Increased blood digoxin level

insulin, oral antidiabetic drugs: Possibly masking of signs and symptoms of hypoglycemia caused by these drugs

MAO inhibitors: Possibly severe hypertension if esmolol is administered within 14 days of discontinuing MAO inhibitor therapy

neuromuscular blockers: Possibly potentiated and prolonged action of these drugs

phenytoin: Possibly increased cardiac depression

reserpine and other catecholamine-depleting drugs: Possibly bradycardia and hypotension

sympathomimetics, xanthine derivatives: Possibly inhibited therapeutic effects of both drugs, decreased theophylline clearance

Adverse Reactions
CNS: Anxiety, confusion, depression, dizziness, drowsiness, fatigue, fever, headache, syncope

CV: Bradycardia, chest pain, decreased peripheral circulation, heart block, hypotension

GI: Nausea, vomiting

RESP: Dyspnea, wheezing

SKIN: Diaphoresis, flushing, pallor

Other: Infusion site pain, redness, and swelling

Nursing Considerations
- Be aware that esmolol is not administered for intraoperative or postoperative hypertension that results mainly from vasoconstriction caused by hypothermia.
- Expect to give lowest possible dose to patients with allergies, asthma, bronchitis, or emphysema. If bronchospasm occurs, expect to discontinue infusion immediately and give a beta$_2$-stimulating drug, as ordered.
- **WARNING** Examine esmolol label closely to verify that you're using the correct concentration; concentrations of 10 mg/ml (100 mg/10-ml vial) and 250 mg/ml (2,500 mg/10-ml

vial) are available. The 250-mg/ml concentration is *not* for direct I.V. injection.

- Before using drug, inspect it for particles or discoloration.
- Don't give 250-mg/ml (2,500-mg/10 ml) concentration by direct I.V. push. Dilute it to a 10-mg/ml infusion by first removing 20 ml from 500 ml of a compatible I.V. solution, such as D₅W or D₅NS, and then adding 5 g of esmolol to the solution.
- Use diluted solution within 24 hours if stored at room temperature.
- Use a 100-mg vial (prediluted to 10 mg/ml) to give loading dose. For a 70-kg (154-lb) patient, loading dose for 500 mcg/kg/minute would be 3.5 ml.
- Monitor blood pressure and heart rate frequently during therapy. Keep in mind that hypotension can occur at any dose but usually is dose-related. Hypotension typically reverses within 30 minutes after dose is decreased or infusion is stopped.
- Monitor for signs of increased adverse reactions in patients with supraventricular arrhythmias, decreased cardiac output, hypotension, or other symptoms of hemodynamic compromise and in those who are taking drugs that decrease peripheral resistance or myocardial filling, contractility, or impulse generation.
- Also monitor for signs of increased adverse reactions in patients with impaired renal function, especially those with end-stage renal disease, because drug is excreted by the kidneys.
- Inspect infusion site regularly for evidence of thrombophlebitis (pain, redness, or swelling at site). Infusions of 20-mg/ml concentration are more likely to cause serious vein irritation than those of 10-mg/ml concentration. Extravasation of 20-mg/ml concentration may cause a serious local reaction and, possibly, skin necrosis. Don't infuse more than 10 mg/ml into a small vein or through a butterfly catheter.
- Before diluting drug, store it at 15° to 30° C (59° to 86° F). Avoid elevated temperatures.

PATIENT TEACHING

- Urge patient receiving esmolol to report adverse reactions immediately.
- Reassure patient that his blood pressure, heart rate, and response to therapy will be monitored throughout esmolol therapy.

estrogens (conjugated)

Premarin

Class and Category

Chemical: Estrogen derivative, steroid hormone
Therapeutic: Ovarian hormone replacement
Pregnancy category: X

Indications and Dosages

▶ *To treat dysfunctional uterine bleeding*

I.V. INFUSION

Adults. 25 mg, repeated in 6 to 12 hr if needed.

Mechanism of Action

Increase the rate of DNA and RNA synthesis in the cells of female reproductive organs, hypothalamus, pituitary glands, and other target organs. In the hypothalamus, estrogens reduce the release of gonadotropin-releasing hormone, which decreases pituitary release of follicle-stimulating hormone and luteinizing hormone. In women, these hormones are required for normal genitourinary and other essential body functions. At the cellular level, estrogens increase cervical secretions, cause endometrial cell proliferation, and increase uterine tone.

Incompatibilities

Don't combine estrogens with acid solutions, ascorbic acid, or protein hydrolysate because they're incompatible.

Contraindications

Abnormal or undiagnosed vaginal bleeding; breast, endometrial, or estrogen-dependent cancer; hypersensitivity to conjugated estrogens or their components; pregnancy; thromboembolic disorders

Interactions

DRUGS

aminocaproic acid: Possibly increased hypercoagulability caused by aminocaproic acid

barbiturates, carbamazepine, hydantoins, rifabutin, rifampin: Possibly reduced activity of estrogen and medroxyprogesterone

bromocriptine: Possibly interference with bromocriptine's therapeutic effects

calcium: Possibly increased calcium absorption

corticosteroids: Increased therapeutic and toxic effects of corticosteroids

cyclosporine: Increased risk of hepatotoxicity and nephrotoxicity

didanosine, lamivudine, zalcitabine: Possibly pancreatitis

hepatotoxic drugs (such as isoniazid): Increased risk of hepatitis and hepatotoxicity

oral antidiabetic drugs: Decreased therapeutic effects of these drugs

somatrem, somatropin: Possibly accelerated epiphyseal maturation

tamoxifen: Possibly interference with tamoxifen's therapeutic effects

warfarin: Decreased anticoagulant effect

ACTIVITIES

smoking: Increased risk of CVA, pulmonary embolism, thrombophlebitis, and transient ischemic attack

Adverse Reactions

CNS: CVA, depression, dizziness, headache, migraine headache

CV: MI, peripheral edema, pulmonary embolism, thromboembolism, thrombophlebitis

EENT: Intolerance of contact lenses

ENDO: Breast enlargement, pain, tenderness, or tumors; gynecomastia; hyperglycemia

GI: Abdominal cramps or pain, anorexia, constipation, diarrhea, gallbladder obstruction, hepatitis, increased appetite, nausea, pancreatitis, vomiting

GU: Amenorrhea, breakthrough bleeding, cervical erosion, clear vaginal discharge, dysmenorrhea, increased libido (females), prolonged or heavy menstrual bleeding, vaginal candidiasis

SKIN: Acne, alopecia, hirsutism, jaundice, melasma, oily skin, purpura, rash, seborrhea, urticaria

Other: Folic acid deficiency, hypercalcemia (in metastatic bone disease), weight gain or loss

Nursing Considerations

- Reconstitute conjugated estrogen by slowly adding NS, dextrose, or invert sugar solution and gently mixing; don't shake vigorously. Use within a few hours or store for up to 60 days at 2° to 8° C (36° to 46° F). Discard if solution is discolored or contains precipitate.
- Administer estrogen slowly because rapid administration may cause perineal or vaginal burning.
- Assess for peripheral edema, a sign of fluid retention.

- Evaluate patient's fluid intake and output, checking for positive fluid balance.
- Assess for signs of depression, such as changes in mental status, affect, and mood.
- Monitor serum calcium level to detect severe hypercalcemia in patients with bone metastasis from breast cancer.
- Expect to discontinue drug during periods of immobilization, 4 weeks before elective surgery, and if jaundice develops.
- Before reconstituting drug, store it at 2° to 8° C (36° to 46° F).

PATIENT TEACHING
- Urge patient receiving estrogen to immediately report breakthrough bleeding.
- Advise patient to eat solid foods to relieve nausea, if necessary.
- Instruct patient to perform a monthly breast self-examination and to comply with all prescribed follow-up examinations, especially endometrial tests, because natural and synthetic estrogens increase the risk of breast and endometrial cancer.
- Encourage patient to stay active to reduce the risk of thrombophlebitis.

ethacrynate sodium
Edecrin

Class and Category
Chemical: Ketone derivative of anyloxyacetic acid
Therapeutic: Diuretic
Pregnancy category: B

Indications and Dosages
▶ *To promote diuresis in heart failure; hepatic cirrhosis; renal disease; ascites of short duration caused by cancer, idiopathic edema, or lymphedema; and edema in children (excluding infants with congenital heart disease or nephrotic syndrome)*

I.V. INFUSION
Adults. *Initial:* 50 mg or 0.5 to 1 mg/kg. Dose repeated in 2 to 4 hr, if needed, then q 4 to 6 hr based on patient response. In an emergency, dose repeated q 1 hr, if needed. *Maximum:* 100 mg as a single dose.

Route	Onset	Peak	Duration
I.V.	5 min	15 to 30 min	2 hr

Mechanism of Action

Probably inhibits the sulfhydryl-catalyzed enzyme systems that cause sodium and chloride resorption in the proximal and distal tubules and the ascending limb of the loop of Henle. These inhibitory effects increase urinary excretion of sodium, chloride, and water, causing profound diuresis. The drug also increases the excretion of potassium, hydrogen, calcium, magnesium, bicarbonate, ammonium, and phosphate.

Incompatibilities

Don't mix or infuse ethacrynate sodium with whole blood or its derivatives.

Contraindications

Anuria; hypersensitivity to ethacrynate sodium, ethacrynic acid, sulfonylureas, or their components; infancy; severe diarrhea

Interactions

DRUGS

ACE inhibitors, antihypertensives: Possibly hypotension

aminoglycosides: Increased risk of ototoxicity

amiodarone: Increased risk of arrhythmias

amphotericin B: Increased risk of electrolyte imbalances, nephrotoxicity, and ototoxicity

anticoagulants, thrombolytics: Possibly potentiated anticoagulation and risk of hemorrhage

corticosteroids: Increased risk of gastric hemorrhage

digoxin: Increased risk of digitalis toxicity

insulin, oral antidiabetic drugs: Possibly increased blood glucose level and decreased therapeutic effects of these drugs

lithium: Increased risk of lithium toxicity

neuromuscular blockers: Possibly increased neuromuscular blockade

NSAIDs: Possibly decreased effects of ethacrynate sodium

sympathomimetics: Possibly interference with hypotensive effects of ethacrynate sodium

ACTIVITIES

alcohol use: Possibly potentiated hypotensive and diuretic effects of ethacrynate sodium

Adverse Reactions

CNS: Confusion, fatigue, headache, malaise, nervousness

CV: Orthostatic hypotension

EENT: Blurred vision, hearing loss, ototoxicity (ringing or buzzing in ears), sensation of fullness in ears, yellow vision

ENDO: Hyperglycemia, hypoglycemia
GI: Abdominal pain, anorexia, diarrhea, dysphagia, GI bleeding, nausea, vomiting
GU: Hematuria, interstitial nephritis, polyuria
HEME: Agranulocytosis, severe neutropenia, thrombocytopenia
SKIN: Rash
Other: Hyperuricemia, hypochloremic alkalosis, hypokalemia, hypomagnesemia, hyponatremia, hypovolemia, infusion site irritation and pain

Nursing Considerations

- Dilute ethacrynate sodium with D$_5$W or NS for I.V. infusion. Discard unused portion after 24 hours. Don't use diluted solution that is cloudy or opalescent. Infuse slowly over 30 minutes.
- Weigh patient daily and assess for signs of electrolyte imbalance and dehydration. Monitor blood pressure and fluid intake and output, and check laboratory test results. Be aware that elderly patients may be more sensitive to drug's effects. Notify prescriber about significant changes, which may require dosage reduction or temporary drug discontinuation.
- If patient develops hypokalemia, administer replacement potassium, as ordered.
- **WARNING** Monitor hepatic function test results in patients with advanced hepatic cirrhosis, especially those with a history of electrolyte imbalance or hepatic encephalopathy, because drug may lead to life-threatening hepatic coma.
- Monitor blood glucose level frequently, especially if patient has diabetes mellitus, because drug may cause hyperglycemia or hypoglycemia.
- Notify prescriber if patient experiences hearing loss, vertigo, or ringing, buzzing, or sense of fullness in his ears. Drug may need to be discontinued.
- Store drug between 15° and 30° C (59° and 86° F).

PATIENT TEACHING

- Instruct patient to immediately report diarrhea; buzzing, fullness, or ringing in ears; hearing loss; severe nausea; vertigo; or vomiting because ethacrynate sodium therapy may need to be discontinued.
- Advise patient to change position slowly to minimize effects of orthostatic hypotension, especially if he takes an antihypertensive.
- Caution patient not to drink alcohol, stand for prolonged periods, or exercise during hot weather because these activities may exacerbate orthostatic hypotension.

- Unless contraindicated, urge patient to eat more high-potassium foods and to take a potassium supplement, if prescribed, to prevent hypokalemia.
- Inform diabetic patient that his blood glucose level will be checked frequently to detect alterations.

etidronate disodium
Didronel

Class and Category
Chemical: Bisphosphonate
Therapeutic: Antihypercalcemic, bone resorption inhibitor
Pregnancy category: C

Indications and Dosages
▶ *To treat moderate to severe hypercalcemia caused by cancer*
I.V. INFUSION
Adults. *Initial:* 7.5 mg/kg/day infused over at least 2 hr for 3 to 7 successive days. Oral etidronate therapy may begin at 20 mg/kg/day for 30 days on the day after last infusion.
DOSAGE ADJUSTMENT Dosage reduced if patient has renal impairment. Drug not administered if serum creatinine level exceeds 5 mg/dl.

Mechanism of Action
Inhibits the abnormal bone resorption that may occur with cancer and reduces the amount of calcium that enters the blood from resorbed bone.

Contraindications
Hypersensitivity to etidronate, other bisphosphonates, or their components; severe renal impairment

Interactions
None known for I.V. form.

Adverse Reactions
EENT: Altered taste, metallic taste
GI: Diarrhea, elevated liver function test results, nausea
GU: Nephrotoxicity
MS: Bone fractures
SKIN: Pruritus, rash, urticaria
Other: Allergic reaction, angioedema, hypocalcemia

Nursing Considerations
- Dilute etidronate in at least 250 ml of NS or D$_5$W. Store diluted solution at room temperature for up to 48 hours. Administer slowly over at least 2 hours.
- **WARNING** Monitor for hypocalcemia if patient receives drug for longer than 3 days.
- Expect to hydrate patients with normal renal function with NS to increase urine output; also expect to administer diuretics to increase the rate of calcium excretion.
- Monitor elderly patients for signs of overhydration, such as peripheral edema and dyspnea. Avoid overhydration in patients with heart failure.
- Expect to continue etidronate therapy for up to 90 days if serum calcium level remains within acceptable range.
- Before diluting drug, store it at 15° to 30° C (59° to 86° F). Don't freeze.

PATIENT TEACHING
- Instruct patient receiving etidronate to immediately report signs of an allergic reaction, such as a rash, hives, difficulty swallowing, or swollen hands, feet, lower legs, or face.

etoposide
Toposar, VePesid
etoposide phosphate
Etopophos

Class and Category
Chemical: Podophyllotoxin derivative
Therapeutic: Antineoplastic
Pregnancy category: D

Indications and Dosages
▶ *To treat germ cell testicular cancer*
I.V. INFUSION
Adults. 50 to 100 mg (base)/m^2 q.d. for 5 days to 100 mg/m^2 on days 1, 3, and 5. Course repeated q 3 to 4 wk.
▶ *To treat small-cell lung cancer*
I.V. INFUSION
Adults. 35 mg (base)/m^2 q.d. for 4 days to 50 mg/m^2 q.d. for 5 days. Course repeated q 3 to 4 wk.

> ## Mechanism of Action
> Appears to act at the premitotic stage of cell division to inhibit DNA synthesis by blocking topoisomerase II, an enzyme responsible for uncoiling and repairing damaged DNA. Etoposide is cell-cycle dependent and cell-cycle–phase specific, exerting maximum effect on the S and G_2 phases of cell division.

Contraindications

Hypersensitivity to etoposide, etoposide phosphate, or their components

Interactions

DRUGS

blood-dyscrasia–causing drugs (such as cephalosporins and sulfasalazine): Increased risk of leukopenia and thrombocytopenia

bone marrow depressants (such as carboplatin and lomustine): Possibly additive bone marrow depression

cyclosporine: Possibly increased blood etoposide level and increased risk of adverse reactions

phosphatase activity inhibitors (such as levamisole): Possibly inhibition of etoposide phosphate

vaccines, killed virus: Possibly decreased antibody response to vaccine

vaccines, live virus: Possibly decreased antibody response to vaccine, increased adverse effects of vaccine, and severe infection

Adverse Reactions

CNS: CNS toxicity, neurotoxicity
CV: Hypotension, thrombophlebitis
EENT: Stomatitis
GI: Anorexia, diarrhea, hepatotoxicity, nausea, vomiting
HEME: Anemia, leukopenia, myelosuppression (dose-related), thrombocytopenia
SKIN: Alopecia, phlebitis, pruritus, rash
Other: Anaphylaxis-like reaction, metabolic acidosis

Nursing Considerations

- Follow facility protocols for preparation and handling of antineoplastic drugs and for appropriate disposal of used equipment.
- Monitor CBC, including hematocrit, platelet count, and WBC with differential, before and intermittently during etoposide therapy.
- Be aware that adverse reactions can vary when etoposide is administered in combination therapy. Review information for all

drugs administered as part of a specific regimen, including drug interactions and adverse effects.

* Anticipate dosage adjustment in patients with impaired renal or hepatic function because they may experience decreased hepatic clearance or elimination of etoposide.
* Dilute etoposide injection with D$_5$W or NS to a concentration of 0.2 to 0.4 mg/ml (200 to 400 mcg/ml). Be aware that a precipitate may form if concentration exceeds 0.4 mg/ml. Use 0.2-mg/ml concentration within 96 hours and 0.4-mg/ml concentration within 24 hours when stored at 25° C (77° F) under normal fluorescent light. Be aware that cracking and leaking of container has been observed when *undiluted* etoposide is placed in a plastic container made of ABS (acrylonitrile, butadiene, and styrene).
* Reconstitute etoposide phosphate for injection using 5 or 10 ml of sterile water for injection, 5% dextrose injection, 0.9% sodium chloride injection, bacteriostatic water for injection with benzyl alcohol, or bacteriostatic sodium chloride for injection with benzyl alcohol to a concentration of 20 mg/ml or 10 mg/ml, respectively. Drug may be administered as reconstituted or further diluted with D$_5$W or NS to a final concentration as low as 0.1 mg/ml. Use reconstituted or diluted solution within 24 hours when stored at 20° to 25° C (68° to 77° F) or 2° to 8° C (36° to 46° F). Allow refrigerated solution to warm to room temperature before use.
* Administer an antiemetic, as prescribed, before administering etoposide to minimize nausea and vomiting.
* Inspect patient's mouth for signs of stomatitis before administering each dose.
* Infuse etoposide slowly, over 30 to 60 minutes, to prevent hypotension. Administer etoposide phosphate for injection over 5 to 10 minutes.
* **WARNING** Monitor patient for hypotension, which can result from too-rapid infusion. If hypotension occurs, stop infusion and notify prescriber immediately. Expect to administer fluids and other supportive treatment and then resume etoposide infusion at a slower rate.
* If etoposide solution comes in contact with your skin or mucosa, wash it off thoroughly with warm water.
* Monitor serum albumin level, as ordered. Patients with low serum albumin concentrations are at increased risk for drug-related toxicity.

- **WARNING** Monitor for hypersensitivity reactions, such as rash, pruritus, wheezing, and dysphagia from laryngeal edema. If such reactions occur, discontinue infusion and notify prescriber immediately. If anaphylaxis occurs, administer epinephrine, antihistamines, and corticosteroids, as prescribed.
- Monitor patients who have or have recently been exposed to chicken pox or who have herpes zoster for signs and symptoms of severe, generalized disease.
- Be aware that patients who are receiving concurrent or consecutive radiation therapy are at risk for additive bone marrow depression.
- If patient develops thrombocytopenia, implement protective precautions according to facility policy.
- Assess for signs of infection, such as fever, if patient develops leukopenia. Expect to obtain appropriate specimens for culture and sensitivity testing.
- Before diluting etoposide injection, store it at a controlled room temperature. Store etoposide phosphate for injection at 2° to 8° C (36° to 46° F); don't freeze.

PATIENT TEACHING

- Advise patient to have dental work completed before beginning etoposide treatment, if possible, or to defer such work until blood counts return to normal because etoposide can delay healing and cause gingival bleeding. Teach patient proper oral hygiene, and advise him to use a soft-bristled toothbrush.
- Advise patient to immediately report GI upset.
- Instruct patient who develops bone marrow depression to avoid people with infections. Advise him to report fever, chills, cough, hoarseness, lower back or side pain, or painful or difficult urination because these signs and symptoms may signal an infection.
- Advise patient to immediately report unusual bleeding or bruising, black or tarry stools, blood in urine or stool, or red pinpoint spots on skin.
- Stress the importance of avoiding accidental cuts from sharp objects, such as razor blades or fingernail clippers, because excessive bleeding or infection may occur.
- Caution patient to avoid contact sports and other activities that put him at risk for bruising or injury.

- Instruct patient to avoid touching his eyes or inside of his nose unless he washes his hands immediately beforehand.
- Advise patient with stomatitis to eat bland, soft foods served cold or at room temperature to decrease irritation.
- Advise patient to use contraception to avoid pregnancy during etoposide therapy and to notify prescriber immediately if pregnancy occurs.
- Stress the importance of complying with the dosage regimen and keeping follow-up medical appointments and appointments for laboratory tests.
- Caution patient to avoid receiving immunizations unless approved by prescriber. Instruct him to avoid people who have recently received vaccines or to wear a protective mask over his nose and mouth when in their presence.

famotidine
Pepcid

Class and Category
Chemical: Thiazole derivative
Therapeutic: Antiulcer agent, gastric acid secretion inhibitor
Pregnancy category: B

Indications and Dosages
▶ *To provide short-term treatment of active duodenal ulcer*
I.V. INFUSION OR INJECTION
Adults and adolescents over age 16. 20 mg q 12 hr, infused over 15 to 30 min or injected over at least 2 min.
Children ages 1 to 16. *Initial:* 0.25 mg/kg q 12 hr, infused over 15 to 30 min or injected over at least 2 min. *Maximum:* 40 mg/day.
▶ *To provide short-term treatment of active, benign gastric ulcer*
I.V. INFUSION OR INJECTION
Adults and adolescents over age 16. 20 mg q 12 hr.
Children ages 1 to 16. *Initial:* 0.25 mg/kg q 12 hr. *Maximum:* 40 mg/day.
▶ *To treat gastroesophageal reflux disease*
I.V. INFUSION OR INJECTION
Children ages 1 to 16. *Initial:* 0.25 mg/kg q 12 hr. *Maximum:* 40 mg/day.

▶ *To treat gastric hypersecretory conditions, such as Zollinger-Ellison syndrome*
I.V. INFUSION OR INJECTION
Adults and adolescents. 20 mg q 12 hr.
DOSAGE ADJUSTMENT Dosage reduced or dosing interval increased to q 36 to 48 hr if needed in patients with creatinine clearance of less than 50 ml/min/1.73 m^2.

Route	Onset	Peak	Duration
I.V.	In 30 min	0.5 to 3 hr	10 to 12 hr

Mechanism of Action

In normal digestion, parietal cells in the gastric epithelium secrete hydrogen (H$^+$) ions, which combine with chloride ions (Cl$^-$) to form hydrochloric acid (HCl), as shown top right. However, HCl can inflame, ulcerate, and perforate the gastric and intestinal mucosa that's normally protected by mucus. Famotidine, an H$_2$-receptor antagonist, reduces HCl formation by preventing histamine from binding with H$_2$ receptors on the surface of parietal cells, as shown bottom right. By doing so, the drug helps prevent peptic ulcers from forming and helps heal existing ones.

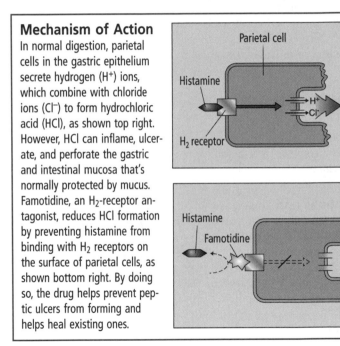

Contraindications

Hypersensitivity to famotidine, other H$_2$-receptor antagonists, or their components

Interactions

DRUGS
antacids, sucralfate: Possibly decreased absorption of famotidine
bone marrow depressants: Increased risk of blood dyscrasias
itraconazole, ketoconazole: Possibly decreased absorption of these drugs

ACTIVITIES

alcohol use: Possibly increased blood alcohol level

Adverse Reactions

CNS: Asthenia, dizziness, fatigue, fever, headache, insomnia, mental or mood changes

CV: Arrhythmias, palpitations

EENT: Dry mouth, laryngeal edema, tinnitus

GI: Abdominal pain, anorexia, constipation, diarrhea, hepatitis, nausea, vomiting

HEME: Agranulocytosis, aplastic anemia, leukopenia, neutropenia, pancytopenia, thrombocytopenia

MS: Arthralgia

RESP: Bronchospasm, dyspnea, wheezing

SKIN: Alopecia, dry skin, erythema multiforme, exfoliative dermatitis, jaundice, pruritus, rash, Stevens-Johnson syndrome, toxic epidermal necrolysis, urticaria

Other: Anaphylaxis, angioedema, facial edema, hyperuricemia

Nursing Considerations

- Dilute famotidine with NS or other solution to 5 to 10 ml; give I.V. injection slowly, over at least 2 minutes. Alternatively, dilute in 100 ml of D_5W and infuse over 15 to 30 minutes, or infuse premixed injection (20 mg/50 ml NS) over 15 to 30 minutes.

- Monitor patients with impaired renal function for increased CNS adverse reactions, such as dizziness, insomnia, and mental or mood changes.

- **WARNING** Be aware that some famotidine preparations contain benzyl alcohol, which can cause a fatal toxic syndrome in neonates and premature infants, characterized by CNS, respiratory, circulatory, and renal impairment and metabolic acidosis.

- Before diluting famotidine, store it at 2° to 8° C (36° to 46° F); don't freeze.

PATIENT TEACHING

- Caution patient to avoid smoking and drinking alcoholic beverages, coffee, and cola during famotidine therapy because these activities irritate the stomach and can delay ulcer healing.

fenoldopam mesylate

Corlopam

Class and Category

Chemical: Dopamine agonist
Therapeutic: Antihypertensive
Pregnancy category: B

Indications and Dosages

▶ *To treat severe hypertension when rapid, but quickly reversible, emergency reduction of blood pressure is clinically indicated, including malignant hypertension with deteriorating end-organ function*

I.V. INFUSION

Adults. *Initial:* 0.025 to 0.3 mcg/kg/min, individualized according to patient weight and desired effect. *Usual:* 0.01 to 1.6 mcg/kg/min. *Maximum:* 1.6 mcg/kg/min for up to 48 hr.

Route	Onset	Peak	Duration
I.V.	Rapid	Unknown	Unknown

Mechanism of Action

Stimulates dopamine D_1–like postsynaptic receptors, which mediate renal and mesenteric vasodilation. This vasodilating activity lowers blood pressure and total peripheral resistance while increasing renal blood flow.

Contraindications

Hypersensitivity to fenoldopam or its components

Interactions

DRUGS

antihypertensives: Additive hypotensive effect
dopamine antagonists, metoclopramide: Possibly decreased effects of fenoldopam

Adverse Reactions

CNS: Anxiety, headache, light-headedness
CV: Hypotension, ST- and T-wave changes, tachycardia
EENT: Increased intraocular pressure
GI: Abdominal pain, nausea
SKIN: Diaphoresis, flushing
Other: Hypokalemia, injection site pain

Nursing Considerations

- Reconstitute by adding 40 mg of fenoldopam (4 ml of concentrate) to 1,000 ml of NS or D₅W, or 20 mg of fenoldopam (2 ml of concentrate) to 500 ml of NS or D₅W, or 10 mg of fenoldopam (1 ml of concentrate) to 250 ml of NS or D₅W to produce a final fenoldopam concentration of 40 mcg/ml.
- Don't use solution if it contains particles or is cloudy. Discard any diluted solution that is not used within 24 hours.
- Infuse drug through a mechanical infusion pump for proper control of infusion rate.
- Expect to titrate dosage in increments of 0.05 to 0.1 mcg/kg/minute, as prescribed.
- Expect to monitor heart rate and blood pressure every 15 minutes during fenoldopam therapy because most of drug's effect on blood pressure occurs within 15 minutes of any dosage change.
- Be aware that patient may be started on oral antihypertensive therapy, as prescribed, any time after blood pressure is stable during fenoldopam infusion.
- **WARNING** Assess for signs of increased myocardial oxygen demand, especially in patients with heart failure or a history of angina, because fenoldopam may produce a rapid decline in blood pressure, resulting in symptomatic hypotension and a dose-dependent increase in heart rate.
- Monitor serum potassium level because fenoldopam decreases serum potassium concentrations, which may cause hypokalemia, exacerbate arrhythmias, or precipitate conduction abnormalities, especially in patients with cardiac disease.
- Monitor patients with glaucoma or increased intraocular pressure for changes in vision because fenoldopam causes a dose-dependent increase in intraocular pressure.
- Be alert for an allergic or anaphylactic reaction to sodium metabisulfite, a component of fenoldopam injection, especially in patients with asthma.
- Before diluting fenoldopam, store it at 2° to 30° C (36° to 86° F).

PATIENT TEACHING

- Inform patient that she'll be switched from fenoldopam to an oral antihypertensive once her blood pressure is controlled.
- Instruct patient to expect frequent monitoring of vital signs.

fentanyl citrate
Sublimaze

Class, Category, and Schedule
Chemical: Opioid, phenylpiperidine derivative
Therapeutic: Anesthesia adjunct
Pregnancy category: C
Controlled substance: Schedule II

Indications and Dosages
▶ *As adjunct to regional anesthesia*
I.V. INJECTION
Adults. 0.05 to 0.1 mg (fentanyl base) by slow I.V. over 1 to 2 min.

Route	Onset	Peak	Duration
I.V.	1 to 2 min	3 to 5 min	30 to 60 min

Mechanism of Action
Binds to opioid receptor sites in the CNS, altering the perception of, and emotional response to, pain by inhibiting the ascending pain pathways. Fentanyl also may alter neurotransmitter release from afferent nerves that are responsive to painful stimuli. The drug also produces respiratory depression by acting directly on respiratory centers in the brain stem.

Contraindications
Asthma; hypersensitivity to fentanyl, alfentanil, or sufentanil; hypersensitivity to narcotics; myasthenia gravis; significant respiratory depression; upper airway obstruction

Interactions
DRUGS
antihypertensives, diuretics: Possibly potentiated hypotension
benzodiazepines: Possibly reduced fentanyl dose required for anesthesia induction
buprenorphine: Possibly decreased therapeutic effects of buprenorphine
CNS depressants: Possibly increased CNS and respiratory depression and hypotension
MAO inhibitors: Possibly unpredictable, even fatal, effects if taken within 14 days of fentanyl
metoclopramide: Possibly antagonized effect of metoclopramide on gastric motility

nalbuphine, pentazocine: Possibly antagonized analgesic, respiratory depressant, and CNS depressant effects of fentanyl; possibly additive hypotensive and CNS and respiratory depressant effects of both drugs
naloxone: Antagonized analgesic, hypotensive, CNS, and respiratory depressant effects of fentanyl
naltrexone: Possibly blocked therapeutic effects of fentanyl
neuromuscular blockers: Possibly prevention or reversal of fentanyl-induced muscle rigidity
ACTIVITIES
alcohol use: Increased CNS and respiratory depression and hypotension

Adverse Reactions

CNS: Chills, confusion, depression, dizziness, drowsiness, light-headedness, paradoxical stimulation, seizures, syncope
CV: Arrhythmias, asystole, bradycardia, circulatory depression, hypertension, hypotension, tachycardia
EENT: Laryngospasm, vision changes
GI: Abdominal pain, constipation, nausea, vomiting
GU: Urinary hesitancy, urine retention
MS: Muscle rigidity or twitching
RESP: Apnea, bronchospasm, depressed cough reflex, dyspnea, respiratory arrest or depression
SKIN: Pruritus, rash, urticaria
Other: Drug tolerance, physical or psychological dependence (with long-term use)

Nursing Considerations

• Be aware that fentanyl should be administered by individuals who are experienced in using I.V. anesthetics and managing respiratory effects. Make sure that emergency equipment and an opioid antagonist are readily available.
• Be aware that 100 mcg of fentanyl is equivalent in potency to 10 mg of morphine.
• Expect dosage to be decreased for patients with a history of hypothyroidism because they're at increased risk for respiratory and CNS depression.
• Monitor patient closely—especially blood pressure and respiratory rate—during and after fentanyl administration. Prolonged observation is warranted if patient received multiple or high doses.

- **WARNING** Expect respiratory depressant effects to last longer than analgesic effects. Also be prepared for residual drug to potentiate the effects of subsequent doses. Residual drug can be detected for at least 6 hours after I.V. dose and 17 hours after dose of other forms.
- **WARNING** Assess for signs of overdose, such as cardiopulmonary arrest, hypoventilation, pupil constriction, respiratory and CNS depression, seizures, and shock. Provide verbal and physical stimulation, as needed, and give naloxone (possibly in repeated doses), as prescribed. Be prepared to assist with endotracheal intubation and mechanical ventilation and to provide fluids.
- Be aware that patients with a history of cardiac bradyarrhythmias may experience an exacerbation of this condition. Patients with cardiac disorders that lead to compromised cardiac reserve are also at risk for severe bradycardia and decreased blood pressure, especially if they received a rapid induction dose.
- Assess patients with a history of head injury, preexisting increased ICP, or intracranial lesions for signs of increased respiratory depression or further elevation of ICP.
- Be aware that elimination of fentanyl may be delayed in patients with impaired renal function.
- Store drug at 15° to 30° C (59° to 86° F); protect from freezing and light.

PATIENT TEACHING
- Instruct patient to avoid alcohol and other CNS depressants during fentanyl therapy unless prescribed.

filgrastim
(granulocyte colony-stimulating factor, rG-CSF)
Neupogen

Class and Category
Chemical: Granulocyte colony-stimulating factor
Therapeutic: Antineutropenic, hematopoietic stimulator
Pregnancy category: C

Indications and Dosages
▶ *To prevent infection after myelosuppressive chemotherapy*
I.V. INFUSION
Adults. 5 mcg/kg q.d. over 15 to 30 min. Increased, if needed, by 5 mcg/kg with each chemotherapy cycle.

▶ *To reduce the duration of neutropenia after bone marrow transplantation*
I.V. INFUSION
Adults. 10 mcg/kg q.d. over 4 hr or as a continuous infusion over 24 hr.
S.C. INFUSION
Adults. 10 mcg/kg as a continuous infusion over 24 hr.
▶ *To enhance peripheral blood progenitor cell collection in autologous hematopoietic stem cell transplantation*
S.C. INFUSION OR INJECTION
Adults. 10 mcg/kg as continuous infusion over 24 hr or as a single injection, beginning 4 days before first leukapheresis and continuing until last day of leukapheresis.
DOSAGE ADJUSTMENT Dosage reduced for patients whose absolute neutrophil count remains above 10,000/mm^3.

Route	Onset	Peak	Duration
I.V.	In 5 min	Unknown	Unknown

Mechanism of Action

Is pharmacologically identical to human granulocyte colony-stimulating factor, an endogenous hormone synthesized by monocytes, endothelial cells, and fibroblasts. Filgrastim induces the formation of neutrophil progenitor cells by binding directly to receptors on the surface of granulocytes, which then divide and differentiate. It also potentiates the effects of mature neutrophils, which reduces fever and the risk of infection raised by severe neutropenia.

Incompatibilities

Don't mix filgrastim in vial or syringe with NS because precipitate will form.

Contraindications

Hypersensitivity to filgrastim, its components, or proteins derived from *Escherichia coli*

Interactions

DRUGS
lithium: Increased neutrophil production

Adverse Reactions

CNS: Fever, headache
CV: Transient supraventricular tachycardia, vasculitis

GI: Splenomegaly
HEME: Leukocytosis
MS: Arthralgia; bone pain; myalgia; pain in arms, legs, lower back, or pelvis
SKIN: Pruritus, rash, Sweet's syndrome (sores on skin)
Other: Anaphylaxis, injection site pain and redness

Nursing Considerations

- Warm filgrastim to room temperature before injection. Discard drug if stored longer than 6 hours at room temperature or 24 hours in refrigerator.
- Withdraw only one dose from a vial; don't repuncture the vial.
- Don't shake the solution.
- For continuous infusion, dilute in D_5W (not NS) to produce less than 15 mcg/ml.
- If patient is receiving chemotherapy, administer filgrastim over 15 to 30 minutes. Don't administer within 24 hours of cytotoxic chemotherapy or within 12 hours of radiation therapy.
- Monitor for signs of an allergic reaction, such as difficulty breathing or rash. If such a reaction occurs, discontinue infusion and notify prescriber at once. If anaphylaxis occurs, administer antihistamine, epinephrine, corticosteroid, and bronchodilator as prescribed.
- Monitor CBC, hematocrit, and platelet count two or three times weekly, as appropriate.
- Inform prescriber and expect to discontinue drug if leukocytosis occurs or if absolute neutrophil count consistently exceeds 10,000/mm³.
- Anticipate decreased response to drug if patient has received extensive radiation therapy or long-term chemotherapy.
- As prescribed, administer nonopioid analgesics for mild to moderate bone pain and opioid analgesics for severe bone pain.
- Before using drug, store it at 2° to 8° C (36° to 46° F); don't freeze.

PATIENT TEACHING

- Advise patient to immediately report possibly serious adverse reactions, such as difficulty breathing, rash, or chest tightness, during filgrastim therapy. Also instruct her to report signs of a possible infection, such as fever, rash, or chills.
- If patient can self-administer filgrastim, teach her how to prepare, administer, and store it. Caution her not to reuse needle,

syringe, or vial. Provide her with puncture-resistant container for needle and syringe disposal.
* Stress the importance of returning for follow-up laboratory tests.

fluconazole
Diflucan

Class and Category
Chemical: Triazole derivative
Therapeutic: Antifungal
Pregnancy category: C

Indications and Dosages
▶ *To treat oral and esophageal candidiasis*
I.V. INJECTION
Adults and adolescents. 200 mg on day 1, followed by 100 mg q.d. for at least 2 (oral) or 3 (esophageal) wk after symptoms resolve.
Children. 3 mg/kg q.d. for at least 2 (oral) or 3 (esophageal) wk and then for 2 wk after esophageal symptoms resolve.
▶ *To treat systemic candidiasis*
I.V. INJECTION
Adults and adolescents. 400 mg on day 1, followed by 200 mg q.d. for at least 4 wk and then for 2 wk after symptoms resolve.
▶ *To treat cryptococcal meningitis*
I.V. INJECTION
Adults and adolescents. 400 mg q.d. until patient responds to treatment, then 200 to 400 mg q.d. for 10 to 12 wk after CSF culture is negative. *Maintenance:* 200 mg q.d. to suppress relapse.
Children. 6 to 12 mg/kg/day for 10 to 12 wk after CSF culture is negative.
▶ *To prevent candidiasis after bone marrow transplantation*
I.V. INJECTION
Adults and adolescents. 400 mg q.d. starting several days before procedure if severe neutropenia is expected and continued for 7 days after absolute neutrophil count exceeds 1,000/mm^3.
DOSAGE ADJUSTMENT Dosage reduced for patients with hepatic or renal impairment. Dosage reduced by 50% for patients with creatinine clearance of 11 to 50 ml/min/1.73 m^2.

Mechanism of Action

Damages fungal cells by interfering with a cytochrome P-450 enzyme needed to convert lanosterol to ergosterol, an essential part of the fungal cell membrane. Decreased ergosterol synthesis causes increased cell permeability, which allows cell contents to leak. Fluconazole also may inhibit endogenous respiration, interact with membrane phospholipids, inhibit transformation of yeasts to mycelial forms, inhibit purine uptake, and impair triglyceride and phospholipid biosynthesis.

Incompatibilities

Don't add fluconazole to I.V. bag that contains any other drug.

Contraindications

Hypersensitivity to fluconazole or its components

Interactions

DRUGS

astemizole, terfenadine: Increased blood levels of these drugs
cimetidine: Decreased blood fluconazole level
cyclosporine: Increased blood cyclosporine level
glipizide, glyburide, tolbutamide: Increased risk of hypoglycemia
hydrochlorothiazide: Increased blood fluconazole level from decreased excretion
isoniazid, rifampin: Decreased fluconazole effects
nonsedating antihistamines: Increased blood antihistamine level, increased risk of cardiotoxicity
oral anticoagulants: Increased anticoagulant effects
phenytoin: Increased blood phenytoin level
rifabutin: Increased blood rifabutin level
theophylline: Increased blood theophylline level
zidovudine: Increased blood zidovudine level

Adverse Reactions

CNS: Chills, dizziness, drowsiness, fever, headache, seizures
GI: Abdominal pain, anorexia, constipation, diarrhea, hepatic failure, nausea, vomiting
HEME: Agranulocytosis, leukopenia, thrombocytopenia
SKIN: Exfoliative dermatitis, photosensitivity, rash

Nursing Considerations

- Expect to obtain BUN and serum creatinine levels as well as culture and sensitivity and liver function test results before administering first dose of fluconazole.

- Discard I.V. solution that is cloudy or contains precipitate. Don't infuse more than 200 mg/hour or add supplemental drugs to infusion.
- Monitor hepatic and renal function periodically during therapy, and notify prescriber if you detect signs of dysfunction.
- Assess for rash every 8 hours during therapy, and notify prescriber if rash occurs.
- If patient receives an oral anticoagulant, monitor coagulation test results and assess for bleeding.
- Monitor for symptoms of overdose, such as hallucinations and paranoia. If they occur, provide supportive treatment, gastric lavage and, possibly, hemodialysis, which can reduce blood fluconazole level by half after about 3 hours.
- If patient is undergoing hemodialysis, administer daily dose of fluconazole after hemodialysis to avoid decreased blood fluconazole level.
- Store drug at 15° to 30° C (59° to 86° F); don't freeze.

PATIENT TEACHING
- Advise patient who takes an oral antidiabetic drug that her blood glucose level will be monitored frequently during fluconazole therapy because of the increased risk of hypoglycemia.
- Advise breast-feeding patient to consult prescriber about possibly discontinuing breast-feeding during fluconazole therapy.

flumazenil

Anexate (CAN), Romazicon

Class and Category

Chemical: Imidazobenzodiazepine derivative
Therapeutic: Benzodiazepine antidote
Pregnancy category: C

Indications and Dosages

▶ *To reverse sedation from benzodiazepine therapy*
I.V. INJECTION
Adults. 0.2 mg, repeated after 45 to 60 sec if response is inadequate and then repeated q 1 min, if needed. If sedation recurs, regimen may be repeated q 20 min up to maximum dose. *Maximum:* 1 mg over 5 min or 3 mg in 1-hr period.

▶ *To reverse benzodiazepine toxicity or suspected overdose*
I.V. INJECTION
Adults. 0.2 mg, followed by 0.3 mg 30 to 60 sec later if response is inadequate and then 0.5 mg repeated q 1 min. If sedation recurs, regimen is repeated q 20 min. *Maximum:* 3 mg in 1-hr period.
I.V. INFUSION
Adults. *Usual:* 0.1 to 0.4 mg/hr, titrated to desired level of arousal.

Route	Onset	Peak	Duration
I.V.	1 to 2 min	6 to 10 min	Variable

Mechanism of Action
Antagonizes the CNS effects of benzodiazepines by competing for their binding sites.

Contraindications
Evidence of tricyclic antidepressant overdose; hypersensitivity to flumazenil, benzodiazepines, or their components; use of benzodiazepine to control ICP, status epilepticus, or a potentially life-threatening condition

Interactions
DRUGS
benzodiazepines: Benzodiazepine withdrawal symptoms, including seizures
tetracyclic or tricyclic antidepressants (overdose): High risk of seizures
FOODS
all foods: Flumazenil clearance increased by 50% if food is ingested during I.V. administration

Adverse Reactions
CNS: Agitation, anxiety, ataxia, confusion, dizziness, drowsiness, emotional lability, fatigue, headache, hypoesthesia, insomnia, paresthesia, resedation, seizures, tremor, vertigo
CV: Hot flashes, hypertension, palpitations
EENT: Blurred vision, diplopia, dry mouth
GI: Nausea, vomiting
RESP: Dyspnea, hyperventilation, hypoventilation
SKIN: Diaphoresis, flushing, rash
Other: Injection site pain and thrombophlebitis

Nursing Considerations

- Before using flumazenil, make sure that emergency drugs and equipment are readily available. Be prepared to assist with seizure management, especially when flumazenil is being used to reverse long-term or high-dose benzodiazepine use or to treat a mixed overdose in which one of the drugs ingested may increase the risk of seizures.
- Give flumazenil undiluted or diluted in a syringe with D₅W, NS, or LR. Administer over 15 to 30 seconds directly into tubing of a free-flowing, compatible I.V. solution. Use a large vein, if possible, to minimize pain at site. Avoid extravasation because drug may irritate tissue.
- Discard prepared syringes if not used within 24 hours.
- Be aware that drug may cause signs of benzodiazepine withdrawal in drug-dependent patient. Also, abrupt awakening from benzodiazepine overdose can cause agitation, dysphoria, and increased adverse reactions.
- Be aware that benzodiazepine reversal may cause a panic attack in patient with a history of these episodes. Expect to adjust dosage carefully.
- Assess for increased stress or anxiety from benzodiazepine withdrawal, especially in patients with cardiac disease, because blood pressure may rise as a result.
- Monitor for signs of resedation and hypoventilation for at least 2 hours after giving flumazenil because drug has a short half-life. Be aware that patient shouldn't be discharged until the risk of resedation has resolved.
- Store drug at 15° to 30° C (59° to 86° F).

PATIENT TEACHING

- Caution patient to avoid alcohol and OTC drugs for 10 to 24 hours after flumazenil administration.
- Advise patient to avoid potentially hazardous activities for 18 to 24 hours after discharge.
- Inform patient and family that agitation, emotional lability, and panic attack (if patient has a history of such episodes) can follow flumazenil administration. Instruct them to watch for depression, difficulty breathing, flushing, hyperventilation, insomnia, palpitations, and tremor.

fluorouracil
(5-FU)
Adrucil

Class and Category
Chemical: Pyrimidine analogue antimetabolite
Therapeutic: Antineoplastic
Pregnancy category: D

Indications and Dosages
▶ *To treat colorectal, breast, gastric, or pancreatic cancer*
I.V. INFUSION
Adults and adolescents. *Initial:* 7 to 12 mg/kg q.d. for 4 days; then after 3 days if no toxicity has occurred, 7 to 10 mg/kg q 3 days for a total course of 2 wk. Alternatively, 12 mg/kg q.d. for 4 days; then after 1 day if no toxicity has occurred, 6 mg/kg q.o.d. for 4 or 5 doses (days 6, 8, 10, and 12) for a total course of 12 days. *Maintenance:* 7 to 12 mg/kg q 7 to 10 days or 300 to 500 mg/m^2 q.d. for 4 to 5 days, repeated monthly. *Maximum adult dose:* 800 mg q.d. (400 mg q.d. for poor-risk patients).
Adults and adolescents who have not received a loading dose. 15 mg/kg or 500 to 600 mg/m^2 q wk.
DOSAGE ADJUSTMENT For poor-risk patients, dosage adjusted to 3 to 6 mg/kg q.d. for 3 days; then after 1 day if no toxicity occurs, 3 mg/kg q.o.d. for 3 doses. Dosage may also be adjusted for patients who have previously received cytotoxic drug therapy with alkylating agents or high-dose pelvic radiation and for patients with impaired renal or hepatic function.

Mechanism of Action
Inhibits the formation of thymidylate from uracil, which interferes with DNA synthesis and, to a lesser extent, RNA formation. This may create a thymine deficiency, which provokes unbalanced cell growth and death, most markedly in cells that grow rapidly and take up fluorouracil at a rapid rate. Fluorouracil is cell-cycle–phase specific; it's active during the S phase of cell division.

Contraindications
Bone marrow depression, hypersensitivity to fluorouracil, major surgery within 1 month before fluorouracil administration, poor nutritional status, potentially serious infection

Interactions

DRUGS

blood-dyscrasia–causing drugs (such as cephalosporins and sulfasalazine): Increased risk of leukopenia and thrombocytopenia
bone marrow depressants (such as carboplatin and lomustine): Possibly additive bone marrow depression
cimetidine: Possibly increased peak concentrations of fluorouracil
leucovorin: Possibly increased therapeutic and toxic fluorouracil effects
vaccines, killed virus: Possibly decreased antibody response to vaccine
vaccines, live virus: Possibly decreased antibody response to vaccine, increased adverse effects of vaccine, and severe infection
warfarin and other coumarin-derived anticoagulants: Increased anticoagulant effect

Adverse Reactions

CNS: Acute cerebellar syndrome, confusion, disorientation, euphoria, headache, weakness
CV: Angina, myocardial ischemia, thrombophlebitis
EENT: Nystagmus, stomatitis
GI: Anorexia, diarrhea, esophogopharyngitis, GI ulceration, nausea, vomiting
HEME: Agranulocytosis, anemia, bone marrow depression, leukopenia, pancytopenia, thrombocytopenia
RESP: Pneumopathy
SKIN: Alopecia, dry skin and fissuring, maculopapular rash, palmar-plantar erythrodysesthesia syndrome, pruritus
Other: Anaphylaxis, infection

Nursing Considerations

• Follow facility protocols for preparation and handling of antineoplastic drugs and for appropriate disposal of used equipment.
• Be aware that fluorouracil should be administered only under the supervision of a qualifed physician. Expect patient to be hospitalized at least during the first course of therapy.
• Be aware that estimated lean body mass (dry weight) may be used to calculate dosage for obese patients and for those with weight gain secondary to abnormal fluid retention, ascites, or edema. Maximum fluorouracil daily dose for any patient should not exceed 800 mg.
• Monitor CBC, including hematocrit, platelet count, and WBC with differential, and liver function tests, including bilirubin and LDH values, before and intermittently during fluorouracil

therapy, as ordered. Inspect patient's mouth for stomatitis before each dose.

• **WARNING** Be aware that adverse reactions can vary when fluorouracil is administered in combination therapy and that some reactions, such as severe diarrhea with dehydration and electrolyte imbalances, may be life-threatening. Review information for all drugs given as part of a specific regimen, including drug interactions and adverse effects. Expect increased patient evaluation and dosage adjustments based on combination used and incidence and severity of adverse reactions.

• Dilute fluorouracil with D_5W or NS. If using the 50-ml vial, don't use a syringe or needle to avoid leakage and contamination; instead, use a sterile dispensing device or a transfer set that accepts a syringe hub. Use proper aseptic technique under a laminar flow hood. Use diluted solution within 8 hours.

• Be aware that slight discoloration doesn't affect drug's potency or safety.

• **WARNING** Be aware that fluorouracil should not be administered intrathecally because of the increased risk of neurotoxicity.

• Infuse fluorouracil slowly, over 2 to 24 hours, to reduce the risk of toxicity. However, be aware that rapid injection (over 1 to 2 minutes) may be more effective.

• **WARNING** Because of fluorouracil's extremely toxic effects, expect to discontinue infusion if patient develops any of the following adverse reactions: diarrhea, esophagopharyngitis (heartburn with potential for sloughing and ulceration), GI bleeding or ulceration, hemorrhage (from any site), intractable vomiting, marked leukopenia or rapidly falling leukocyte count, stomatitis, or thrombocytopenia. Expect to restart infusion at a lower dose when adverse reactions subside.

• Monitor patients who have, or have recently been exposed to, chicken pox or who have herpes zoster for signs and symptoms of severe, generalized disease.

• Assess for signs of infection, such as fever, if patient develops leukopenia. Expect to obtain appropriate specimens for culture and sensitivity testing.

• **WARNING** Be aware that myocardial ischemia can occur several hours after a dose (even later doses). Continue to assess patient for signs of ischemia throughout the course of treatment.

• Be aware that patients who are receiving concurrent or consecutive radiation therapy are at risk for additive bone marrow depression.

• Assess patient for signs of palmar-plantar erythrodysesthesia syndrome (also known as hand-foot syndrome), characterized by tingling of hands and feet, followed by pain, erythema, and swelling. Expect symptoms to subside 5 to 7 days after interruption of therapy.

• Store drug at 15° to 30° C (59° to 86° F); protect from freezing and light. Heat solution to 60° C (140° F) and shake vigorously to dissolve precipitates formed at low temperatures. Allow solution to cool to body temperature before use.

PATIENT TEACHING

• Advise patient to have dental work completed before beginning fluorouracil treatment, if possible, or to defer such work until blood counts return to normal because drug can delay healing and cause gingival bleeding. Teach patient proper oral hygiene, and advise her to use a soft-bristled toothbrush.

• Instruct patient who develops bone marrow depression to avoid persons with infections. Advise her to report fever, chills, cough, hoarseness, lower back or side pain, or painful or difficult urination because these signs and symptoms may signal an infection.

• Advise patient to immediately report unusual bleeding or bruising, black or tarry stools, blood in urine or stool, or red pinpoint spots on skin.

• Stress the importance of avoiding accidental cuts from sharp objects, such as razor blades or fingernail clippers, because excessive bleeding or infection may occur.

• Urge patient to avoid contact sports or other activities that put her at risk for bruising or injury.

• Instruct patient to avoid touching her eyes or inside of her nose unless she washes her hands immediately beforehand.

• Advise patient to use contraception to avoid pregnancy during therapy and to notify prescriber immediately if pregnancy occurs.

• Advise patient with stomatitis to eat bland, soft foods served cold or at room temperature to decrease irritation.

• Stress the importance of complying with the dosage regimen and of keeping follow-up medical appointments and appointments for laboratory tests.

• Caution patient to avoid receiving immunizations unless approved by prescriber. Instruct her to avoid people who have recently received vaccines or to wear a protective mask over her nose and mouth when in their presence.

folic acid
(vitamin B₉)

Folvite

Class and Category

Chemical: Water-soluble B-complex vitamin
Therapeutic: Nutritional supplement
Pregnancy category: A

Indications and Dosages

▶ *To prevent deficiency based on U.S. and Canadian recommended daily allowances*

I.V INFUSION

Adults and children age 11 and older. Dosage individualized based on patient need and given as part of total parenteral nutrition solution.

▶ *To treat deficiency*

I.V. INFUSION

Adults and children age 11 and older. 0.25 to 1 mg q.d. until hematologic response occurs.

Mechanism of Action

Acts as a catalyst for normal production of RBCs, helping to prevent megaloblastic anemia, and helps maintain normal homocysteine levels. After being converted to tetrahydrofolic acid in the intestines, folic acid promotes synthesis of several enzymes, including purine and thymidylates; metabolism of amino acids, including glycine and methionine; and metabolism of histidine—all of which are essential for normal cell structure and growth.

Contraindications

Hypersensitivity to folic acid or its components

Interactions

DRUGS

analgesics, carbamazepine, estrogens (including oral contraceptives), phenobarbital, primidone: Possibly increased folic acid requirements

hydantoin anticonvulsants: Possibly decreased effectiveness of these drugs, possibly increased folic acid requirements
methotrexate, pyrimethamine, triamterene, trimethoprim: Possibly decreased effectiveness of folic acid
sulfasalazine: Possibly decreased folic acid absorption

Adverse Reactions

Other: Allergic reaction (bronchospasm, erythema, fever, malaise, rash, pruritus)

Nursing Considerations

- **WARNING** Don't administer injection form of folic acid containing benzyl alcohol to neonates or premature infants because they may develop a fatal toxic syndrome characterized by CNS, respiratory, circulatory, and renal impairment and metabolic acidosis.
- Be aware that although folic acid will correct hematologic disorders associated with pernicious anemia, neurologic problems will progressively worsen.
- Store drug at 15° to 30° C (59° to 86° F); protect from freezing and light.

PATIENT TEACHING
- Inform patient that folic acid supplements are not a substitute for proper diet. Teach her that the best sources of dietary folic acid are green vegetables, potatoes, cereals, and organ meats. Recommend that she eat raw green vegetables because cooking destroys up to 90% of folic acid found in food.
- Explain to patients with pernicious anemia that folic acid won't affect the neurologic symptoms associated with the disease.

foscarnet sodium

Foscavir

Class and Category

Chemical: Organic pyrophosphate analogue
Therapeutic: Antiviral
Pregnancy category: C

Indications and Dosages

▶ *To treat cytomegalovirus retinitis*
I.V. INFUSION
Adults. *Induction:* 90 mg/kg over 1 1/2 to 2 hr q 12 hr, or 60 mg/kg over 1 hr q 8 hr, for 14 to 21 days. *Maintenance:* 90 to 120 mg/kg over 2 hr q.d.

DOSAGE ADJUSTMENT To achieve induction dose equivalent of 90 mg/kg q 12 hr in patients with impaired renal function, dosage reduced as follows: for creatinine clearance greater than 1 to 1.4 ml/min/kg, 70 mg/kg q 12 hr; for creatinine clearance greater than 0.8 to 1 ml/min/kg, 50 mg/kg q 12 hr; for creatinine clearance greater than 0.6 to 0.8 ml/min/kg, 80 mg/kg q 24 hr; for creatinine clearance greater than 0.5 to 0.6 ml/min/kg, 60 mg/kg q 24 hr; for creatinine clearance greater than or equal to 0.4 to 0.5 ml/min/kg, 50 mg/kg q 24 hr; and for creatinine clearance less than 0.4 ml/min/kg, use not recommended.

To achieve induction dose equivalent of 60 mg/kg q 8 hr in patients with impaired renal function, dosage reduced as follows: for creatinine clearance greater than 1 to 1.4 ml/min/kg, 45 mg/kg q 8 hr; for creatinine clearance greater than 0.8 to 1 m/min/kg, 50 mg/kg q 12 hr; for creatinine clearance greater than 0.6 to 0.8 ml/min/kg, 40 mg/kg q 12 hr; for creatinine clearance greater than 0.5 to 0.6 ml/min/kg, 60 mg/kg q 24 hr; for creatinine clearance greater than or equal to 0.4 to 0.5 ml/min/kg, 50 mg/kg q 24 hr; and for creatinine clearance less than 0.4 ml/min/kg, use not recommended.

DOSAGE ADJUSTMENT For patients with impaired renal function who are receiving 90-mg/kg/day maintenance dose, dosage reduced as follows: for creatinine clearance greater than 1 to 1.4 ml/min/kg, 70 mg/kg q.d.; for creatinine clearance greater than 0.8 to 1 ml/min/kg, 50 mg/kg q.d.; for creatinine clearance greater than 0.6 to 0.8 ml/min/kg, 80 mg/kg q 48 hr; for creatinine clearance greater than 0.5 to 0.6 ml/min/kg, 60 mg/kg q 48 hr; for creatinine clearance greater than or equal to 0.4 to 0.5 ml/min/kg, 50 mg/kg q 48 hr; and for creatinine clearance less than 0.4 ml/min/kg, use not recommended.

For patients with impaired renal function who are receiving 120-mg/kg/day maintenance dose, dosage reduced as follows: for creatinine clearance greater than 1 to 1.4 ml/min/kg, 90 mg/kg q day; for creatinine clearance greater than 0.8 to 1 ml/min/kg, 65 mg/kg q day; for creatinine clearance greater than 0.6 to 0.8 ml/min/kg, 105 mg/kg q 48 hr; for creatinine clearance greater than 0.5 to 0.6 ml/min/kg, 80 mg/kg q 48 hr; for creatinine clearance greater than or equal to 0.4 to 0.5 ml/min/kg, 65 mg/kg q 48 hr; and for creatinine clearance less than 0.4 ml/min/kg, use not recommended.

▶ *To treat acyclovir-resistant mucocutaneous herpes simplex*
I.V. INFUSION
Adults. 40 mg/kg over 1 hr q 8 or 12 hr for 14 to 21 days or until healed.

DOSAGE ADJUSTMENT For patients with impaired renal function who are receiving 40-mg/kg dose q 8 hr, dosage reduced as follows: for creatinine clearance greater than 1 to 1.4 ml/min/kg, 30 mg/kg q 8 hr; for creatinine clearance greater than 0.8 to 1 ml/min/kg, 35 mg/kg q 12 hr; for creatinine clearance greater than 0.6 to 0.8 ml/min/kg, 25 mg/kg q 12 hr; for creatinine clearance greater than 0.5 to 0.6 ml/min/kg, 40 mg/kg q 24 hr; for creatinine clearance greater than or equal to 0.4 to 0.5 ml/min/kg, 35 mg/kg q 24 hr; and for creatinine clearance less than 0.4 ml/min/kg, use not recommended.

For patients with impaired renal function who are receiving 40-mg/kg dose q 12 hr, dosage reduced as follows: for creatinine clearance greater than 1 to 1.4 ml/min/kg, 30 mg/kg q 12 hr; for creatinine clearance greater than 0.8 to 1 ml/min/kg, 20 mg/kg q 12 hr; for creatinine clearance greater than 0.6 to 0.8 ml/min/kg, 35 mg/kg q 24 hr; for creatinine clearance greater than 0.5 to 0.6 ml/min/kg, 25 mg/kg q 24 hr; for creatinine clearance greater than or equal to 0.4 to 0.5 ml/min/kg, 20 mg/kg q 24 hr; and for creatinine clearance less than 0.4 ml/min/kg, use not recommended.

Mechanism of Action
Inhibits replication of herpes simplex virus types 1 and 2, Epstein-Barr virus, cytomegalovirus, human herpes virus 6, and varicella-zoster virus by selectively inhibiting the pyrophosphate-binding site of viral DNA polymerase, an enzyme used in the viral DNA replication process. Viral replication resumes when drug therapy ceases.

Incompatibilities
Don't mix foscarnet through the same I.V. line or concurrently through the same catheter as any other solution or drug. Foscarnet is incompatible with solutions containing calcium, 30% dextrose solution, or LR. To avoid precipitation, don't mix foscarnet with acyclovir, amphotericin B, co-trimoxazole, dobutamine, droperidol, ganciclovir, haloperidol, pentamidine, trimetrexate, or vancomycin. To avoid gas production, don't mix foscarnet with diazepam, digoxin, lorazepam, midazolam, or promethazine hy-

drochloride. To avoid cloudiness or color change, don't mix foscarnet with diphenhydramine, leucovorin, or prochlorperazine.

Contraindications

Clinically significant hypersensitivity to foscarnet sodium

Interactions

DRUGS

aminoglycosides, amphotericin B, cidofovir, and other nephrotoxic drugs: Increased risk of nephrotoxicity

pentamidine (I.V.): Hypocalcemia, hypomagnesemia, and nephrotoxicity

ritonavir, saquinavir: Abnormal renal function

zidovudine: Possibly increased risk of anemia

Adverse Reactions

CNS: Headache, neurotoxicity (including dizziness, paresthesia, seizures)

CV: Phlebitis

EENT: Mouth or throat ulcers

GI: Abdominal pain, anorexia, diarrhea, nausea, vomiting

GU: Elevated serum creatinine level, genital ulcers, nephrotoxicity

HEME: Anemia, granulocytopenia, leukopenia

Other: Hypocalcemia, hypophosphatemia, hyperphosphatemia, hypomagnesemia, hypokalemia

Nursing Considerations

- Expect to hydrate patient with $1/2$ to 1 L of NS or D_5W, as ordered, before first dose of foscarnet and with each subsequent dose to avoid nephrotoxicity.
- Prepare peripheral infusion by diluting with an equal amount of D_5W or NS, which will result in a concentration of 12 mg/ml. Use diluted drug within 24 hours, and discard any unused portion. Infuse undiluted foscarnet (24 mg/ml) by central line to prevent venous irritation.
- Administer 60-mg/kg doses over at least 1 hour and higher doses over at least 2 hours.
- **WARNING** Always administer foscarnet at a steady rate using an infusion pump; rapid infusion may result in increased blood level of foscarnet, which can lead to acute hypocalcemia or another toxicity.
- Monitor serum electrolyte levels, especially calcium, magnesium, phosphate, and potassium, 2 to 3 times a week during induction and weekly during maintenance therapy, as ordered. Be

aware that patient may have decreased ionized calcium level even if serum calcium level seems to be normal. Assess patient for signs of hypocalcemia, such as perioral tingling, numbness, and paresthesia. Be aware that electrolyte abnormalities can cause severe effects, such as arrhythmias, seizures, and tetany.

• Obtain baseline BUN and serum creatinine levels; then monitor these levels 2 to 3 times a week during induction therapy and at least once a week during maintenance therapy, as ordered. Assess input and output of patients who are dehydrated, are using other nephrotoxic drugs, or have preexisting impaired renal function because foscarnet increases the risk of nephrotoxicity. Monitor elderly patients, who are more likely to have decreased renal function.

• Monitor CBC periodically during foscarnet therapy, especially in patients with preexisting anemia, because foscarnet may decrease hemoglobin concentration.

• Store drug at 15° to 30° C (59° to 86° F); don't freeze. Discard drug if it becomes frozen because a precipitate will form.

PATIENT TEACHING

• Advise patient receiving foscarnet to immediately report signs of hypocalcemia, such as tingling around mouth or numbness of arms or legs, as well as other adverse reactions, such as changes in urination pattern or increased eye pain.

• Stress the importance of keeping follow-up medical appointments and appointments for laboratory tests.

• Inform patient that retinitis may continue to progress and vision loss may occur during treatment. Encourage her to undergo follow-up ophthalmic examinations, even after she has completed treatment.

fosphenytoin sodium
Cerebyx

Class and Category
Chemical: Hydantoin derivative
Therapeutic: Anticonvulsant
Pregnancy category: D

Indications and Dosages
▶ *To treat status epilepticus*
I.V. INFUSION
Adults and adolescents. *Initial:* 15 to 20 mg of phenytoin equivalent (PE)/kg at 100 to 150 PE/min. *Maintenance:* 4 to 6 mg

PE/kg/day in divided doses b.i.d. to q.i.d. *Maximum:* 30 mg PE/kg as total loading dose.

Children. *Initial:* 15 to 20 mg PE/kg given at up to 3 mg PE/kg/min. *Maintenance:* 4 to 6 mg PE/kg/day in divided doses b.i.d. to q.i.d.

▶ *To prevent or treat seizures during and after neurosurgery*

I.V. INFUSION

Adults and adolescents. *Initial:* 10 to 20 mg PE/kg, not to exceed 150 mg PE/min. *Maintenance:* 4 to 6 mg PE/kg/day in divided doses b.i.d. to q.i.d. *Maximum:* 30 mg PE/kg as total loading dose.

Mechanism of Action

Is converted from fosphenytoin (a prodrug) to phenytoin, which limits the spread of seizure activity and the start of new seizures. Phenytoin does so by regulating voltage-dependent sodium and calcium channels in neurons, inhibiting calcium movement across neuronal membranes, and enhancing the sodium-potassium–adenosine triphosphatase activity in neurons and glial cells. These actions may stem from phenytoin's ability to slow the recovery rate of inactivated sodium channels.

Contraindications

Hypersensitivity to fosphenytoin, phenytoin, other hydantoins, or their components

Interactions

DRUGS

acetaminophen (long-term use): Increased risk of hepatotoxicity
acyclovir: Decreased blood phenytoin level, loss of seizure control
alfentanil: Increased clearance and decreased effectiveness of alfentanil
amiodarone, fluoxetine: Possibly increased blood phenytoin level and risk of toxicity
antacids: Possibly decreased phenytoin effectiveness
antineoplastics: Increased phenytoin metabolism
beta blockers: Increased myocardial depression
bupropion, clozapine, loxapine, MAO inhibitors, maprotiline, phenothiazines, pimozide, thioxanthenes: Possibly lowered seizure threshold and decreased therapeutic effects of phenytoin, possibly intensified CNS depressant effects of these drugs
calcium: Possibly impaired phenytoin absorption

calcium channel blockers: Possibly increased blood phenytoin level
carbamazepine: Decreased blood carbamazepine level, possibly increased blood phenytoin level and risk of toxicity
chloramphenicol, cimetidine, disulfiram, isoniazid, methylphenidate, metronidazole, phenylbutazone, ranitidine, salicylates, sulfonamides, trimethoprim: Possibly impaired metabolism of these drugs, increased risk of phenytoin toxicity
CNS depressants: Possibly increased CNS depression
corticosteroids, cyclosporine, digoxin, disopyramide, doxycycline, furosemide, levodopa, mexiletine, quinidine: Decreased therapeutic effects of these drugs
diazoxide: Possibly decreased therapeutic effects of both drugs
dopamine: Possibly sudden hypotension or cardiac arrest after I.V. fosphenytoin administration
estrogen- and progestin-containing contraceptives: Possibly breakthrough bleeding and decreased contraceptive effectiveness
estrogens, progestins: Decreased therapeutic effects, increased blood phenytoin level
felbamate: Possibly impaired metabolism and increased blood level of phenytoin
fluconazole, itraconazole, ketoconazole, miconazole: Increased blood phenytoin level
folic acid: Increased phenytoin metabolism, decreased seizure control
haloperidol: Possibly lowered seizure threshold and decreased therapeutic effects of fosphenytoin; possibly decreased blood haloperidol level
insulin, oral antidiabetic drugs: Possibly increased blood glucose level and decreased therapeutic effects of these drugs
lamotrigine: Possibly decreased therapeutic effects of lamotrigine
lidocaine: Possibly decreased blood lidocaine level, increased myocardial depression
lithium: Increased risk of lithium toxicity
methadone: Possibly increased methadone metabolism, leading to withdrawal symptoms
molindone: Possibly lowered seizure threshold, impaired absorption, and decreased therapeutic effects of phenytoin
omeprazole: Possibly increased blood phenytoin level
oral anticoagulants: Possibly impaired metabolism of these drugs and increased risk of phenytoin toxicity; possibly increased anticoagulant effects initially and then decreased effects with prolonged therapy

rifampin: Possibly decreased therapeutic effects of phenytoin
streptozocin: Possibly decreased therapeutic effects of streptozocin
sucralfate: Possibly decreased phenytoin absorption
tricyclic antidepressants: Possibly lowered seizure threshold and decreased therapeutic effects of phenytoin; possibly decreased blood antidepressant level
valproic acid: Decreased blood phenytoin level, increased blood valproic acid level
vitamin D analogues: Decreased vitamin D analogue activity
xanthines: Possibly inhibited phenytoin absorption and increased clearance of xanthines
zaleplon: Increased clearance and decreased effectiveness of zaleplon
ACTIVITIES
alcohol use: Possibly decreased phenytoin effectiveness

Adverse Reactions

CNS: Agitation, amnesia, asthenia, ataxia, cerebral edema, chills, coma, confusion, CVA, delusions, depression, dizziness, emotional lability, encephalitis, encephalopathy, extrapyramidal reactions, fever, headache, hemiplegia, hostility, hypoesthesia, lack of coordination, malaise, meningitis, nervousness, neurosis, paralysis, personality disorder, positive Babinski's sign, seizures, somnolence, speech disorders, stupor, subdural hematoma, syncope, transient paresthesia, tremor, vertigo
CV: Atrial flutter, bradycardia, bundle-branch block, cardiac arrest, cardiomegaly, edema, heart failure, hypertension, hypotension, orthostatic hypotension, palpitations, PVCs, shock, tachycardia, thrombophlebitis
EENT: Amblyopia, conjunctivitis, diplopia, dry mouth, earache, epistaxis, eye pain, gingival hyperplasia, hearing loss, hyperacusis, increased salivation, loss of taste, mydriasis, nystagmus, pharyngitis, photophobia, rhinitis, sinusitis, taste perversion, tinnitus, tongue swelling, visual field defects
ENDO: Diabetes insipidus, hyperglycemia, ketosis
GI: Anorexia, constipation, diarrhea, dysphagia, elevated liver function test results, flatulence, gastritis, GI bleeding, hepatic necrosis, hepatitis, ileus, indigestion, nausea, vomiting
GU: Albuminuria, dysuria, incontinence, oliguria, polyuria, renal failure, urine retention, vaginal candidiasis
HEME: Anemia, easy bruising, leukopenia, thrombocytopenia
MS: Arthralgia, back pain, leg cramps, muscle twitching, myalgia, myasthenia, myoclonus, myopathy

RESP: Apnea, asthma, atelectasis, bronchitis, dyspnea, hemopty-sis, hyperventilation, hypoxia, increased cough, increased sputum production, pneumonia, pneumothorax
SKIN: Contact dermatitis, diaphoresis, maculopapular or pustular rash, nodules, photosensitivity, skin discoloration, Stevens-Johnson syndrome, transient pruritus, urticaria
Other: Cachexia, cryptococcosis, dehydration, facial edema, flu-like symptoms, hyperkalemia, hypokalemia, hypophosphatemia, infection, injection site reaction, lymphadenopathy, sepsis

Nursing Considerations

- **WARNING** Express the dosage, concentration, and infusion rate of fosphenytoin in PE units. Misreading an order or a label could result in a massive overdose.
- Dilute drug in D5W or NS to 1.5 to 25 mg PE/ml. Use within 8 hours if stored at room temperature or within 24 hours if re-frigerated.
- Inspect parenteral solution before administration. Discard solu-tion that contains particles or is discolored.
- Be aware that drug is also administered by I.M. injection for maintenance doses. I.M. injection shouldn't be given for status epilepticus because I.V. route allows faster onset and peak.
- Keep in mind that I.V. fosphenytoin administration doesn't re-quire use of a filter, as does phenytoin administration.
- Don't administer fosphenytoin solution at a rate exceeding 150 mg PE/minute because of the risk of hypotension. For a 50-kg (110-lb) patient, infusion typically takes 5 to 7 minutes. Be aware that I.V. fosphenytoin may be administered more rap-idly than I.V. phenytoin.
- Follow loading dose with maintenance dosage of oral or par-enteral phenytoin or parenteral fosphenytoin, as prescribed.
- As prescribed, give an I.V. benzodiazepine (such as lorazepam or diazepam) with fosphenytoin; otherwise, drug's full antiepileptic effect won't be immediate.
- Monitor ECG, blood pressure, and respiratory function during fosphenytoin infusion and for 10 to 20 minutes afterward.
- Expect to obtain blood fosphenytoin (phenytoin) level 2 hours after infusion. Therapeutic level generally ranges from 10 to 20 mcg/ml; steady state may be reached after several days to sev-eral weeks.
- Be aware that fosphenytoin may be substituted for oral pheny-toin sodium at same total daily dose and frequency. If pre-

scribed, give daily amount in two or more divided doses to maintain seizure control.

- When switching between phenytoin and fosphenytoin, remember that small differences in phenytoin bioavailability can lead to significant changes in blood phenytoin level and an increased risk of toxicity.
- If drug causes transient, infusion-related paresthesia and pruritus, decrease dosage or discontinue infusion, as ordered.
- Monitor CBC for thrombocytopenia or leukopenia—signs of hematologic toxicity. Also monitor serum albumin level and results of renal and liver function tests.
- Anticipate increased frequency and severity of adverse reactions after I.V. administration in patients with hepatic or renal impairment or hypoalbuminemia.
- Discontinue drug, as ordered, if patient develops signs of hypersensitivity—such as acute hepatotoxicity (hepatic necrosis and hepatitis), fever, lymphadenopathy, and skin reactions—during first 2 months of therapy.
- Monitor blood phenytoin level to detect early signs of toxicity, such as diplopia, nausea, confusion, slurred speech, and vomiting. Expect to reduce dosage or stop drug if such signs occur.
- **WARNING** Monitor for seizures because phenytoin is excitatory at toxic levels.
- **WARNING** If patient has bradycardia or heart block rhythm, notify prescriber and expect to withhold drug because severe CV reactions and death have occurred.
- Expect to provide vitamin D supplement if patient has inadequate dietary intake and is receiving long-term anticonvulsant treatment.
- Document type, onset, and characteristics of seizures as well as response to treatment.
- Before diluting fosphenytoin, store it at 2° to 8° C (36° to 46° F); don't freeze.

PATIENT TEACHING
- Inform patient that fosphenytoin typically is used for short-term treatment.
- Instruct patient to immediately report bothersome symptoms, especially rash and swollen glands.
- Because gingival hyperplasia may develop during long-term therapy, emphasize the importance of good oral hygiene and gum massage.
- Urge patient to consume an adequate amount of vitamin D–rich foods.

furosemide

Lasix, Lasix Special (CAN), Uritol (CAN)

Class and Category

Chemical: Sulfonamide
Therapeutic: Antihypertensive, diuretic
Pregnancy category: C

Indications and Dosages

▶ *To reduce edema caused by cirrhosis, heart failure, and renal disease, including nephrotic syndrome*

I.V. INFUSION OR INJECTION

Adults. 20 to 40 mg as a single dose, increased by 20 mg q 2 hr until desired response occurs.

Children. 1 mg/kg as a single dose, increased by 1 mg/kg q 2 hr until desired response occurs. *Maximum:* 6 mg/kg/dose.

DOSAGE ADJUSTMENT Initial single dose limited to 20 mg for elderly patients.

▶ *To manage mild to moderate hypertension, as adjunct to treat acute pulmonary edema and hypertensive crisis*

I.V. INFUSION OR INJECTION

Adults with normal renal function. 40 to 80 mg as a single dose over several min.

Adults with acute renal failure or pulmonary edema. 100 to 200 mg as a single dose over several minutes.

DOSAGE ADJUSTMENT For patients with acute pulmonary edema without hypertensive crisis, dosage reduced to 40 mg, followed by 80 mg 1 hr later if therapeutic response doesn't occur.

Route	Onset	Peak	Duration
I.V.	5 min	In 30 min	2 hr

Mechanism of Action

Inhibits sodium and water reabsorption in the loop of Henle and increases urine formation. As the body's plasma volume decreases, aldosterone production increases, which promotes sodium reabsorption and the loss of potassium and hydrogen ions. Furosemide also increases the excretion of calcium, magnesium, bicarbonate, ammonium, and phosphate. By reducing intracellular and extracellular fluid volume, the drug reduces blood pressure and decreases cardiac output. Over time, cardiac output returns to normal.

Incompatibilities
Don't mix furosemide (a milky, buffered alkaline solution) with highly acidic solutions.

Contraindications
Anuria unresponsive to furosemide; hypersensitivity to furosemide, sulfonamides, or their components

Interactions
DRUGS
ACE inhibitors: Possibly first-dose hypotension
aminoglycosides, cisplatin: Increased risk of ototoxicity
amiodarone: Increased risk of arrhythmias from hypokalemia
chloral hydrate: Possibly diaphoresis, hot flashes, and hypertension
digoxin: Increased risk of digitalis toxicity related to hypokalemia
insulin, oral antidiabetic drugs: Increased blood glucose level
lithium: Increased risk of lithium toxicity
NSAIDs: Possibly decreased diuresis
phenytoin, probenecid: Possibly decreased therapeutic effects of furosemide
propranolol: Possibly increased blood propranolol level
thiazide diuretics: Possibly profound diuresis and electrolyte imbalance
ACTIVITIES
alcohol use: Possibly increased hypotensive and diuretic effects of furosemide

Adverse Reactions
CNS: Dizziness, fever, headache, paresthesia, restlessness, vertigo, weakness
CV: Orthostatic hypotension, shock, thromboembolism, thrombophlebitis
EENT: Blurred vision, ototoxicity, stomatitis, tinnitus, transient hearing loss (rapid I.V. injection), yellow vision
ENDO: Hyperglycemia
GI: Abdominal cramps, anorexia, constipation, diarrhea, indigestion, nausea, pancreatitis, vomiting
GU: Bladder spasms, glycosuria
HEME: Agranulocytosis (rare), anemia, aplastic anemia (rare), azotemia, hemolytic anemia, leukopenia, thrombocytopenia
MS: Muscle spasms
SKIN: Erythema multiforme, exfoliative dermatitis, jaundice, photosensitivity, pruritus, purpura, rash, urticaria

Other: Allergic reaction (interstitial nephritis, necrotizing vasculitis, systemic vasculitis), dehydration, hyperuricemia, hypochloremia, hypokalemia, hyponatremia, hypovolemia

Nursing Considerations

- Obtain patient's weight before and periodically during furosemide therapy to monitor fluid loss.
- For once-a-day dosing, give drug in the morning so patient's sleep won't be interrupted by increased need to urinate.
- Prepare drug for infusion with NS, LR, or D_5W. Use within 24 hours.
- Administer drug slowly over 1 to 2 minutes to prevent ototoxicity. Expect to administer high doses by controlled I.V. infusion at a rate not exceeding 4 mg/minute.
- Expect patient to have periodic hearing tests during prolonged or high-dose I.V. therapy.
- Monitor blood pressure and hepatic and renal function as well as BUN, blood glucose, and serum creatinine, electrolyte, and uric acid levels, as appropriate.
- Be aware that elderly patients are more susceptible to drug's hypotensive and electrolyte-altering effects and thus are at greater risk for shock and thromboembolism.
- **WARNING** Be aware that furosemide use in patients with advanced hepatic cirrhosis, especially those who also have a history of electrolyte imbalance or hepatic encephalopathy, may lead to lethal hepatic coma. Assess patient with cirrhosis for signs of deteriorating hepatic function, such as confusion, decreasing mental alertness, lethargy, and asterixis.
- If patient is at high risk for hypokalemia, give potassium supplements along with furosemide, as prescribed.
- Expect to discontinue furosemide at maximum dosage if oliguria persists for longer than 24 hours.
- Be aware that furosemide may worsen left ventricular hypertrophy and adversely affect glucose tolerance and lipid metabolism.
- Notify prescriber if patient experiences hearing loss, vertigo, or ringing, buzzing, or sense of fullness in her ears. Drug may need to be discontinued.
- Store drug at 15° to 30° C (59° to 86° F); protect from freezing and light.

PATIENT TEACHING

- Advise patient receiving furosemide to change position slowly to minimize effects of orthostatic hypotension, and to take furosemide with food or milk to reduce GI distress.

- Caution patient against drinking alcoholic beverages, standing for prolonged periods, and exercising in hot weather because these actions increase the hypotensive effect of furosemide.
- Emphasize the importance of controlling weight and diet, especially of limiting sodium intake.
- Unless contraindicated, urge patient to eat more high-potassium foods and to take a potassium supplement, if prescribed, to prevent hypokalemia.
- Instruct patient to keep follow-up appointments with prescriber to monitor progress. Urge her to report persistent, severe nausea, vomiting, and diarrhea because these reactions may cause dehydration.
- Inform diabetic patient that her blood glucose level will be checked frequently.

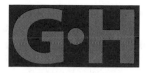

ganciclovir sodium

Cytovene (CAN), Cytovene-IV

Class and Category

Chemical: Acyclic guanosine analogue
Therapeutic: Antiviral
Pregnancy category: C

Indications and Dosages

▶ *To treat cytomegalovirus (CMV) retinitis in immunocompromised patients, including patients with AIDS*

I.V. INFUSION

Adults and adolescents. *Induction:* 5 mg/kg over at least 1 hr q 12 hr for 14 to 21 days. *Maintenance:* 5 mg/kg over at least 1 hr q.d. for 7 days a week, or 6 mg/kg over at least 1 hr q.d. for 5 days a week.

▶ *To prevent CMV disease in transplant recipients at risk for it*

I.V. INFUSION

Adults and adolescents. *Induction:* 5 mg/kg over at least 1 hr q 12 hr for 7 to 14 days. *Maintenance:* 5 mg/kg over at least 1 hr q.d. for 7 days a week or 6 mg/kg over at least 1 hr q.d. for 5 days a week.

DOSAGE ADJUSTMENT For patients with impaired renal function, dosage reduced as follows: for creatinine clearance of 50 to 69 ml/min/1.73 m^2, induction and maintenance dosages reduced to 2.5 mg/kg q 12 hr; for creatinine clearance of 25 to 49 ml/min/1.73 m^2, induction dosage reduced to 2.5 mg/kg q 24 hr and maintenance dosage reduced to 1.25 mg/kg q 24 hr; for creatinine clearance of 10 to 24 ml/min/1.73 m^2, induction dosage reduced to 1.25 mg/kg q 24 hr and maintenance dosage reduced to 0.625 mg/kg q 24 hr; and for creatinine clearance of less than 10 ml/min/1.73 m^2, induction dosage reduced to 1.25 mg/kg three times a week after dialysis and maintenance dosage reduced to 0.625 mg/kg three times a week after dialysis.

Incompatibilities

Don't mix ganciclovir with bacteriostatic water for injection containing parabens because a precipitate may form.

Mechanism of Action

Inhibits replication of CMV. Infected cells take up ganciclovir, which is then converted by cellular enzymes to ganciclovir triphosphate. Ganciclovir triphosphate is incorporated into the DNA chain and inhibits viral DNA polymerase, an enzyme used in the viral DNA replication process. This inhibits DNA synthesis by suppressing the ability of the DNA chain to elongate, which is part of the cellular replication process. Uninfected cells also take up ganciclovir and produce low levels of ganciclovir triphosphate, but the drug inhibits viral DNA polymerase more effectively than it inhibits cellular polymerase.

Contraindications

Hypersensitivity to ganciclovir or acyclovir

Interactions

DRUGS

blood-dyscrasia–causing drugs (such as cephalosporins and sulfasalazine), bone marrow depressants (such as carboplatin and lomustine): Possibly additive bone marrow depression

didanosine: Increased blood didanosine level, possibly increased blood ganciclovir level

imipenem and cilastatin: Possible risk of generalized seizures

nephrotoxic drugs (such as amphotericin B, cyclosporine, and tacrolimus): Possibly increased serum creatinine level, increased risk of impaired renal function, decreased ganciclovir elimination, and increased risk of ganciclovir toxicity

probenecid: Possibly decreased ganciclovir elimination and increased risk of ganciclovir toxicity

zidovudine: Possibly hematologic toxicity

Adverse Reactions

CNS: Fever, mental and mood changes, nervousness, neuropathy, tremors

GI: Abdominal pain, anorexia, diarrhea, elevated liver function test results, nausea, vomiting

HEME: Anemia, granulocytopenia, leukopenia, neutropenia, thrombocytopenia

SKIN: Rash

Other: Infusion site pain

Nursing Considerations

- Monitor CBC and platelet count before initiating ganciclovir therapy, every 2 days during induction, and at least once a week thereafter. Expect to perform daily neutrophil and platelet counts in patients undergoing hemodialysis, patients with neutrophil counts less than 1,000/mm^3 at beginning of treatment, and patients who have had leukopenia during previous treatment with ganciclovir or other nucleoside analogues.

- Be aware that ganciclovir shouldn't be given to patient with neutrophil count of less than 500/mm^3 or platelet count of less than 25,000/mm^3.

- Be aware that ganciclovir shares some mutagenic and carcinogenic properties of antineoplastics. Follow facility protocols for preparation and handling of such drugs and for appropriate disposal of used equipment.

- **WARNING Avoid inhaling, ingesting, or coming in direct contact with ganciclovir. If ganciclovir solution comes in contact with your skin or mucosa, wash it off thoroughly with soap and water. If drug comes in contact with your eye, irrigate it thoroughly with plain water.**

- To reconstitute ganciclovir, add 10 ml of sterile water for injection to 500-mg vial to yield a concentration of 50 mg/ml. Don't use bacteriostatic water for injection containing parabens to reconstitute ganciclovir because a precipitate may form. Shake vial until solution is clear. Store at room temperature and use within 12 hours.

- Further dilute reconstituted ganciclovir, typically with 100 ml of NS, D$_5$W, LR, or Ringer's solution, to a final concentration of 10 mg/ml or less. Refrigerate if not administered immediately. Use within 24 hours.

- Infuse ganciclovir at a constant rate, over at least 1 hour, through a central or peripheral line. Ensure that patient is adequately hydrated, as ordered.

- Expect to administer no more than 1.25 mg/kg/24 hours if patient receives hemodialysis. Administer ganciclovir dose after hemodialysis to prevent decreased plasma ganciclovir level.

- Be aware that reinduction treatment may be ordered if CMV retinitis progresses while patient is on maintenance therapy.

- Monitor renal and liver function tests, as ordered. Anticipate a dosage adjustment or increased dosing intervals if renal function test results are elevated.

- Observe patient for fever, chills, pharyngitis, tiredness or weakness, or unusual bleeding or ecchymosis. Be aware that granulocytopenia typically occurs during the first week of treatment but may occur at any time.
- Be aware that patients receiving concurrent radiation therapy are at risk for additive bone marrow depression.
- Store unopened vials below 40° C (104° F).

PATIENT TEACHING
- Inform patient that ganciclovir is not a cure for CMV retinitis and that the disease may progress during or after treatment. Explain that maintenance therapy is used to help prevent relapse.
- Advise patient to contact prescriber immediately if he notices unusual bleeding or bruising, black or tarry stools, blood in urine or stool, or red pinpoint spots on skin.
- Teach patient proper oral hygiene and encourage him to use a soft-bristled toothbrush because ganciclovir can delay healing, increase the risk of infection, and cause gingival bleeding. Advise patient to check with prescriber before undergoing any dental work.
- Stress the importance of avoiding accidental cuts from sharp objects, such as razors or fingernail clippers, because excessive bleeding or infection may occur.
- Teach patient about the need for contraception during ganciclovir treatment because drug has caused birth defects in animals. Advise female patients to use effective contraceptive method during treatment and male patients to use barrier protection during treatment and for 90 days afterward. Inform patient that ganciclovir may cause infertility.
- Stress the importance of keeping follow-up appointments, including those for ophthalmic examinations, which may be scheduled weekly during induction and every 4 weeks during maintenance therapy.

gatifloxacin
Tequin

Class and Category
Chemical: Fluoroquinolone
Therapeutic: Antibiotic
Pregnancy category: C

Indications and Dosages

▶ *To treat acute bacterial exacerbations of chronic bronchitis caused by* Haemophilus influenzae, H. parainfluenzae, Moraxella catarrhalis, Staphylococcus aureus, or Streptococcus pneumoniae; *complicated UTIs caused by* Escherichia coli, Klebsiella pneumoniae, *or* Proteus mirabilis; *and acute pyelonephritis caused by* E. coli

I.V. INFUSION

Adults. 400 mg q.d. for 7 to 10 days.

▶ *To treat acute sinusitis caused by* H. influenzae *or* S. pneumoniae

I.V. INFUSION

Adults. 400 mg q.d. for 10 days.

▶ *To treat community-acquired pneumonia caused by* Chlamydia pneumoniae, H. influenzae, H. parainfluenzae, Legionella pneumophila, M. catarrhalis, Mycoplasma pneumoniae, S. aureus, *or* S. pneumoniae

I.V. INFUSION

Adults. 400 mg q.d. for 7 to 14 days.

▶ *To treat uncomplicated cystitis caused by* E. coli, K. pneumoniae, *or* P. mirabilis

I.V. INFUSION

Adults. 400 mg as a single dose or 200 mg q.d. for 3 days.

▶ *To treat uncomplicated urethral gonorrhea in men, and cervical and acute rectal gonorrhea in women caused by* Neisseria gonorrhoeae

I.V. INFUSION

Adults. 400 mg as a single dose.

DOSAGE ADJUSTMENT For patients with creatinine clearance of less than 40 ml/min/1.73 m^2 and those receiving hemodialysis or continuous peritoneal dialysis, initial dose of 400 mg is followed by reduced dosage of 200 mg q.d., as prescribed. No dosage adjustment is required for single-dose treatments or for treatment of uncomplicated cystitis.

Mechanism of Action

Interferes with bacterial cell replication by inhibiting the bacterial enzyme DNA gyrase, which is essential for replication, transcription, and repair of bacterial DNA. Gatifloxacin also inhibits topoisomerase IV, an enzyme involved in the partitioning of chromosomal DNA during bacterial cell division.

Incompatibilities

Don't add other drugs to gatifloxacin injection or infuse gatifloxacin through same I.V. line as other drugs.

Contraindications

Hypersensitivity to gatifloxacin, other fluoroquinolones, or their components

Interactions

DRUGS

digoxin: Possibly increased blood digoxin level
oral antidiabetic drugs: Possibly altered glucose control
probenecid: Increased blood level and sustained half-life of gatifloxacin

Adverse Reactions

CNS: Chills, dizziness, fever, headache, insomnia, nightmares, paresthesia, tremor, vertigo
CV: Chest pain, palpitations, peripheral edema, vasodilation
EENT: Abnormal vision, glossitis, mouth ulcers, oral candidiasis, pharyngitis, stomatitis, taste perversion, tinnitus
GI: Abdominal pain, constipation, diarrhea, indigestion, nausea, vomiting
GU: Dysuria, hematuria, vaginitis
MS: Back pain, tendinitis, tendon rupture
RESP: Dyspnea
SKIN: Diaphoresis, rash
Other: Infusion site inflammation

Nursing Considerations

- Dilute gatifloxacin concentrate for infusion with an appropriate amount of a compatible solution, such as D_5W, NS, 0.45NS, D_5LR, 5% sodium bicarbonate, Plasma-Lyte 56 and D_5W, or sterile water for injection, to yield a final concentration of 2 mg/ml. Use solutions prepared with 5% sodium bicarbonate immediately, as prescribed. No further dilution is needed when using premixed flexible bags. Don't use an I.V. line with series connections to decrease the risk of air embolism.
- Inspect I.V. solution before infusion. Use only if solution remains clear and light yellow or greenish yellow. Discard if particulate matter is present.
- Be aware that premixed solutions should not be frozen. Diluted 2-mg/ml solutions may be stored for 14 days at 20° to 26° C (68° to 77° F) or 2° to 8° C (36° to 46° F). Diluted solutions may also be frozen for up to 6 months at −25° to −10° C (−13° to 14° F). Thaw at controlled room temperature.
- Infuse I.V. solution over 60 minutes, using an infusion pump to avoid too-rapid or bolus administration.

- **WARNING** Be aware that gatifloxacin may cause prolonged QTc interval, leading to an increased risk of ventricular arrhythmias in susceptible patients, especially those with hypokalemia and those taking quinidine, procainamide, amiodarone, or sotalol.
- Monitor for signs and symptoms of digoxin toxicity, such as arrhythmias, vision disturbances, and altered mental status, because gatifloxacin may increase blood digoxin level.
- Monitor patient for nightmares and insomnia because gatifloxacin may cause excessive CNS stimulation. If patient develops these symptoms, notify prescriber immediately and expect to discontinue drug.
- Keep in mind that use of any fluoroquinolone may increase patient's risk of tendon rupture.
- Before diluting gatifloxacin (premixed or concentrate), store it at controlled room temperature.

PATIENT TEACHING
- Instruct patient receiving gatifloxacin to immediately report signs of an allergic reaction, such as rash.
- Advise patient to immediately report tendon pain, inflammation, or rupture because drug may need to be discontinued.
- Inform diabetic patient taking oral antidiabetic drugs that his blood glucose level will be checked frequently.

gentamicin sulfate

Cidomycin (CAN), Garamycin, G-Mycin, Jenamicin

Class and Category

Chemical: Aminoglycoside derived from *Micromonospora purpurea*
Therapeutic: Antibiotic
Pregnancy category: D

Indications and Dosages

▶ *To treat serious bacterial infections caused by aerobic gram-negative organisms and some gram-positive organisms, including* Citrobacter *species,* Enterobacter *species,* Escherichia coli, Klebsiella *species,* Proteus *species,* Pseudomonas aeruginosa, Serratia *species,* Staphylococcus aureus, *and many strains of* Streptococcus *species*

I.V. INFUSION
Adults and adolescents. 1 to 1.7 mg/kg q 8 hr for 7 to 10 days.
Children. 2 to 2.5 mg/kg q 8 hr for 7 to 10 days.
Infants. 2.5 mg/kg q 8 to 16 hr for 7 to 10 days.

Premature or full-term neonates up to age 1 week. 2.5 mg/ kg q 12 to 24 hr for 7 to 10 days.

▶ *To treat uncomplicated UTIs*

I.V. INFUSION

Adults and adolescents who weigh 60 kg (132 lb) or more. 160 mg q.d. or 80 mg q 12 hr.

Adults and adolescents who weigh less than 60 kg. 3 mg/kg q.d. or 1.5 mg/kg q 12 hr.

DOSAGE ADJUSTMENT Supplemental dose of 1 to 1.7 mg/ kg (2 to 2.5 mg/kg for children) given after hemodialysis, based on severity of infection.

Mechanism of Action

Binds to negatively charged sites on the outer cell membrane of bacteria, thereby disrupting the membrane's integrity. Gentamicin also binds to bacterial ribosomal subunits and inhibits protein synthesis. Both actions lead to cell death.

Incompatibilities

Don't administer gentamicin through same I.V. line as other drugs, especially beta-lactam antibiotics (penicillins and cephalosporins), because substantial mutual inactivation may occur. Give drugs through separate sites.

Contraindications

Hypersensitivity to gentamicin or its components, hypersensitivity or serious toxic reaction to other aminoglycosides

Interactions

DRUGS

aminoglycosides (concurrent use of two or more): Decreased bacterial uptake of each drug, increased risk of ototoxicity and nephrotoxicity

cephalosporins, enflurane, methoxyflurane, vancomycin: Increased risk of nephrotoxicity

loop diuretics: Increased risk of ototoxicity and nephrotoxicity

neuromuscular blockers: Prolonged respiratory depression, increased neuromuscular blockade

penicillins: Inactivation of gentamicin by certain penicillins, increased risk of nephrotoxicity

Adverse Reactions

CNS: Acute organic mental syndrome, confusion, depression, fever, headache, increased protein in cerebrospinal fluid, lethargy, myasthenia gravis–like syndrome, neurotoxicity (dizziness, hearing loss, tinnitus, vertigo), peripheral neuropathy or encephalopathy (muscle twitching, numbness, seizures, skin tingling), pseudotumor cerebri
CV: Hypertension, hypotension, palpitations
EENT: Blurred vision, increased salivation, laryngeal edema, ototoxicity, stomatitis, vision changes
GI: Anorexia, nausea, splenomegaly, transient hepatomegaly, vomiting
GU: Nephrotoxicity
HEME: Anemia, eosinophilia, granulocytopenia, increased or decreased reticulocyte count, leukopenia, thrombocytopenia
MS: Arthralgia, leg cramps
RESP: Pulmonary fibrosis, respiratory depression
SKIN: Alopecia, generalized burning sensation, pruritus, purpura, rash, urticaria
Other: Anaphylaxis, injection site pain, superinfection, weight loss

Nursing Considerations

- Before gentamicin therapy begins, expect to obtain a body fluid or tissue specimen for culture and sensitivity testing, as ordered.
- Dilute each dose with 50 to 200 ml of NS or D₅W to yield no more than 1 mg/ml. Be aware that no further dilution is needed if premixed flexible bags are used. Don't use an I.V. line with series connections when administering drug from a premixed flexible container to decrease the risk of air embolism. Don't administer if solution is discolored or contains precipitate. Administer slowly over 30 to 60 minutes.
- Expect to adjust dosage based on peak and trough blood drug levels drawn after third maintenance dose, as prescribed.
- Don't give gentamicin to pregnant women because drug can cause hearing loss in fetus.
- **WARNING** Be alert for allergic reactions—including anaphylaxis and, possibly, life-threatening asthmatic episodes—because some forms of drug contain sodium bisulfite.
- Assess for signs of other infections because gentamicin may cause overgrowth of nonsusceptible organisms.
- Be aware that premature infants, neonates, elderly patients, patients with impaired renal function, and dehydrated patients are at increased risk for nephrotoxicity.

- Be aware that premixed form contains 19.6 mEq of sodium per 50 ml. Take this into consideration if patient is on a sodium-restricted diet.
- Be aware that infants with botulism and patients with myasthenia gravis or Parkinson's disease may experience increased muscle weakness.
- Be aware that patients with impairment of cranial nerve VIII are at increased risk for ototoxicity or vestibular toxicity.
- Store vial at 15° to 30° C (59° to 86° F); store flexible bag at 2° to 30° C (36° to 86° F). Don't freeze gentamicin.

PATIENT TEACHING
- Stress the importance of completing the full course of gentamicin therapy.
- Instruct patient to immediately report adverse reactions, such as hearing loss, to avoid permanent effects.
- Emphasize the importance of keeping follow-up appointments and having diagnostic tests, such as audiometric tests and renal function tests, if ordered.

glucagon

Glucagon Diagnostic Kit, Glucagon Emergency Kit

Class and Category

Chemical: Synthetic hormone
Therapeutic: Antihypoglycemic, diagnostic aid adjunct
Pregnancy category: B

Indications and Dosages

▶ *To provide emergency treatment of severe hypoglycemia*
I.V. INJECTION
Adults and children who weigh more than 20 kg (44 lb).
1 mg, repeated in 15 min, if needed.
Children who weigh 20 kg or less. 0.5 mg, or 0.02 to 0.03 mg/kg, repeated in 15 min, if needed.
▶ *To provide diagnostic assistance by inhibiting bowel peristalsis in radiologic examination of GI tract*
I.V. INJECTION
Adults. 0.25 to 2 mg before procedure. Dose, route, and timing vary with segment of GI tract examined and length of procedure.

Route	Onset	Peak	Duration
I.V.	5 to 20 min*†	Unknown	90 min*‡

Mechanism of Action

Increases production of adenylate cyclase, which catalyzes the conversion of adenosine triphosphate to cAMP, a process that in turn activates phosphorylase. Phosphorylase promotes the breakdown of glycogen to glucose (glycogenolysis) in the liver. As a result, the blood glucose level increases and GI smooth muscles relax.

Incompatibilities

Don't mix glucagon with sodium chloride or solutions that have a pH of 3.0 to 9.5; use with dextrose solutions instead.

Contraindications

Hypersensitivity to glucagon or its components, pheochromocytoma

Interactions

DRUGS

oral anticoagulants: Possibly interference with anticoagulant metabolism, increasing anticoagulant effects

Adverse Reactions

CV: Hypotension (with hypersensitivity reaction), tachycardia
GI: Nausea, vomiting
RESP: Bronchospasm, respiratory distress
SKIN: Urticaria
Other: Allergic reaction

Nursing Considerations

- Rouse patient as quickly as possible because prolonged hypoglycemia can cause cerebral damage. Confirm low blood glucose level by performing a rapid blood glucose test.
- Reconstitute 1-mg vial of glucagon with 1 ml of diluent or 10-mg vial with 10 ml of diluent. Don't give more than 1 mg/ml. Dilute large doses with sterile water for injection. Swirl gently to mix. Use immediately after reconstitution.
- Before injecting glucagon, place unconscious patient on his side to prevent aspiration of vomitus when he regains consciousness.

---

* For antihypoglycemic action.
† 45 sec to 1 min for smooth-muscle relaxation.
‡ 9 to 25 min for smooth-muscle relaxation.

- Administer by slow I.V. injection to decrease the risk of adverse reactions, such as tachycardia and vomiting.
- If patient doesn't respond to glucagon, expect to administer I.V. dextrose.
- When patient has regained consciousness, give him oral carbohydrates to restore hepatic glycogen stores and prevent secondary hypoglycemia.
- Monitor blood glucose level during hypoglycemic episode and every hour for 3 to 4 hours, or as ordered, after patient regains consciousness.
- Keep in mind that glucagon isn't effective in patients with depleted hepatic glycogen stores caused by such conditions as adrenal insufficiency, chronic hypoglycemia, and starvation.
- Before reconstituting glucagon, store it at 15° to 30° C (59° to 86° F).

PATIENT TEACHING
- Instruct patient to monitor his blood glucose level, especially when signs of hypoglycemia occur.
- Teach patient and family members how to recognize signs of hypoglycemia and when to notify prescriber.
- Advise patient to carry candy or other simple sugars with him to treat early hypoglycemia.
- Emphasize the importance of a consistent diet, regular exercise, and proper use of insulin or an oral antidiabetic drug.
- Make sure unstable diabetic patients and family members know how to give glucagon subcutaneously in case of hypoglycemia. Instruct family members to keep patient on his side and give him a carbohydrate when he awakens. Advise against giving fluids by mouth until patient is fully conscious.
- Instruct patient and family members to call for emergency medical assistance after glucagon treatment, especially if patient can't ingest oral glucose or if he's taking the sulfonylurea chlorpropamide, to decrease the risk of secondary hypoglycemia.

glycopyrrolate
Robinul, Robinul Forte

Class and Category
Chemical: Quaternary ammonium compound
Therapeutic: Antiarrhythmic, anticholinergic, cholinergic adjunct
Pregnancy category: B

Indications and Dosages

▶ *To treat peptic ulcer disease*
I.V. INJECTION
Adults and adolescents. 0.1 to 0.2 mg q 4 hr, p.r.n. *Maximum:* 4 doses/day.

▶ *To counteract intraoperative and anesthesia-induced arrhythmias*
I.V. INJECTION
Adults and adolescents. 0.1 mg, repeated q 2 to 3 min, if needed.
Children over age 2. 0.0044 mg/kg, repeated q 2 to 3 min, if needed. *Maximum:* 0.1 mg as a single dose.

▶ *As cholinergic adjunct in curariform block*
I.V. INJECTION
Adults and children over age 2. 0.2 mg glycopyrrolate for each 1 mg of neostigmine or each 5 mg of pyridostigmine when given together.

Route	Onset	Peak	Duration
I.V.	1 min	Unknown	2 to 3 hr*

Mechanism of Action

Inhibits acetylcholine's action on postganglionic muscarinic receptors throughout the body. Depending on the receptors' location, glycopyrrolate produces various effects, such as:

• reducing the volume and acidity of gastric secretions
• inhibiting vagal stimulation of the heart
• relaxing smooth muscle in the GI and GU tracts.

Incompatibilities

Don't mix glycopyrrolate with alkaline drugs or solutions that have a pH over 6.0 because drug stability may be affected. A pH over 6.0 may occur if glycopyrrolate is mixed with dexamethasone sodium phosphate or LR solution. Gas or precipitate may form if glycopyrrolate is mixed in same syringe as chloramphenicol, diazepam, dimenhydrinate, methohexital sodium, pentobarbital sodium, secobarbital sodium, sodium bicarbonate, or thiopental sodium.

---

* For vagal blocking effect.

Contraindications

Angle-closure glaucoma, asthma, hemorrhage with hemodynamic instability, hepatic disease, hypersensitivity to anticholinergics, ileus, intestinal atony, myasthenia gravis, obstructive GI or urinary disorders, toxic megacolon, ulcerative colitis

Interactions

DRUGS

anticholinergics, tricyclic antidepressants: Possibly increased anticholinergic effects

antimyasthenics: Possibly reduced intestinal motility

atenolol: Possibly potentiated effects of atenolol

calcium- or magnesium-containing antacids, carbonic anhydrase inhibitors, citrates, sodium bicarbonate: Possibly reduced excretion and increased therapeutic and adverse effects of glycopyrrolate

cyclopropane: Possibly ventricular arrhythmias

digoxin: Possibly potentiated digoxin effects

haloperidol, phenothiazines: Possibly decreased effectiveness of these drugs

ketoconazole: Possibly decreased ketoconazole absorption

metoclopramide: Possibly antagonized effects of metoclopramide

opioid analgesics: Possibly severe constipation, urine retention, and ileus

potassium chloride: Possibly increased severity of potassium chloride–induced gastric lesions

Adverse Reactions

CNS: Confusion, dizziness, drowsiness, headache, insomnia, nervousness, weakness

CV: Bradycardia (with low doses), palpitations, tachycardia (with high doses)

EENT: Blurred vision, cycloplegia, dry mouth, increased intraocular pressure, loss of taste, mydriasis, nasal congestion, photophobia, taste perversion

GI: Abdominal distention, constipation, dysphagia, nausea, vomiting

GU: Impotence, urinary hesitancy, urine retention

RESP: Dyspnea

SKIN: Decreased sweating (possibly leading to heat exhaustion), flushing, urticaria

Nursing Considerations

• Administer glycopyrrolate by direct injection without diluting. Or inject into tubing of a compatible I.V. solution unless it contains an alkaline drug or sodium bicarbonate.

- Be aware that glycopyrrolate can be mixed or administered with various solutions and drugs, including D_5W, $D_{10}W$, D_5NS, $D_{10}NS$, meperidine injection, morphine sulfate, fentanyl and droperidol injection, hydroxyzine injection, neostigmine injection, and pyridostigmine injection.
- **WARNING** Check all doses carefully because even a slight overdose can lead to toxicity.
- Perform continuous cardiac monitoring, as ordered, to assess for arrhythmias during drug administration.
- Monitor patients with arrhythmias, bradycardia, heart failure, hypertension, hyperthyroidism, or tachycardia for exacerbations of these conditions caused by glycopyrrolate's anticholinergic effects. Monitor blood pressure in patients with toxemia from pregnancy because they're at risk for aggravated hypertension.
- Monitor urine output and be alert for urine retention, especially in patients with autonomic neuropathy.
- To prevent overheating caused by decreased sweating, adjust the room temperature and make sure patient is well hydrated.
- Be aware that elderly patients and patients with impaired renal function are at increased risk for adverse reactions.
- Be aware that infants, patients with Down syndrome, and children with brain damage or spastic paralysis may be more sensitive to drug's effects.
- Store drug at 15° to 30° C (59° to 86° F).

PATIENT TEACHING
- Instruct patient to consult prescriber before taking any OTC drugs during glycopyrrolate therapy.
- Caution patient about possible drowsiness and dizziness. Advise him to avoid potentially hazardous activities until drug's CNS effects are known.
- Suggest that he use sugarless hard candy, ice, or saliva substitute to relieve dry mouth.
- Instruct patient to avoid exertion and hot environments because he's prone to heat exhaustion while taking glycopyrrolate.
- Urge patient to maintain hydration by drinking at least 8 glasses of water daily, unless contraindicated.
- Instruct patient to notify prescriber if he experiences abdominal distention, difficulty breathing, difficulty urinating, eye pain, irregular heartbeat or palpitations, sensitivity to light, or severe constipation.
- Advise patient to wear sunglasses in bright light.

- Inform male patient that reversible impotence may occur during therapy.
- If urinary hesitancy occurs, advise patient to void before taking each dose.

granisetron hydrochloride
Kytril

Class and Category
Chemical: Carbazole
Therapeutic: Antiemetic
Pregnancy category: B

Indications and Dosages
▶ *To prevent nausea and vomiting caused by chemotherapy*
I.V. INFUSION
Adults and adolescents. 10 mcg/kg diluted and infused over 5 min, starting 30 min before chemotherapy; or 10 mcg/kg undiluted and infused over 30 sec, starting 30 min before chemotherapy.

Mechanism of Action
Has a high affinity for serotonin-releasing 5-hydroxytryptamine$_3$ receptors along vagal nerve endings in the intestines. Because of this affinity, granisetron prevents the nausea and vomiting that usually result when serotonin is released by damaged enterochromaffin cells.

Incompatibilities
Don't mix granisetron in same solution as other drugs.

Contraindications
Hypersensitivity to granisetron or its components

Interactions
DRUGS
allopurinol, barbiturates and other cytochrome-P450 hepatic enzyme inducers, hepatic enzyme inhibitors: Possibly altered clearance and half-life of granisetron

Adverse Reactions
CNS: Asthenia, chills, CNS stimulation, drowsiness, fever, headache, insomnia, somnolence, syncope

CV: Arrhythmias, chest pain, hypertension
EENT: Taste perversion
GI: Abdominal pain, anorexia, constipation, diarrhea, elevated liver function test results, nausea, vomiting
HEME: Anemia, leukopenia, thrombocytopenia
RESP: Dyspnea
SKIN: Alopecia, pruritus, rash, urticaria

Nursing Considerations

- **WARNING** Read the label carefully to prevent a potential drug overdose. Granisetron is available in concentrations of 1 mg/ml, but dosage is expressed in micrograms (mcg).
- Dilute granisetron with NS or D_5W to a total volume of 20 to 50 ml. Mixture may be stored for up to 24 hours. Use only on days when chemotherapy is given.
- **WARNING** Be aware that patients with a hypersensitivity to ondansetron may also be hypersensitive to granisetron.
- Provide mouth care and sugarless hard candy to help alleviate nausea.
- Monitor liver function test results for elevations.
- Review CBC results for reduced WBC, RBC, and platelet counts.
- Store drug at 2° to 30° C (36° to 86° F); protect from freezing and light.

PATIENT TEACHING
- Inform patient that granisetron is given before chemotherapy to help prevent nausea.
- Advise patient to report constipation, difficulty breathing, fever, rash, severe diarrhea, or severe headache. Also caution him about possible drowsiness.
- Suggest that patient use sugarless hard candy to help alleviate nausea.

heparin calcium
Calcilean (CAN), Calciparine

heparin sodium
Hepalean (CAN), Heparin Leo (CAN), Heparin Lock Flush, Liquaemin

Class and Category
Chemical: Glycosaminoglycan
Therapeutic: Anticoagulant
Pregnancy category: C

Indications and Dosages

▶ *To prevent and treat deep vein thrombosis and pulmonary embolism, to treat peripheral arterial embolism, and to prevent thromboembolism before and after cardioversion of chronic atrial fibrillation*

I.V. INFUSION OR INJECTION

Adults. *Loading:* 35 to 70 U/kg or 5,000 U by injection. Then 20,000 to 40,000 U infused over 24 hours.

Children. *Loading:* 50 U/kg by injection. Then 100 U/kg infused q 4 hr or 20,000 U/m^2 infused over 24 hours.

I.V. INJECTION

Adults. *Initial:* 10,000 U. *Maintenance:* 5,000 to 10,000 U q 4 to 6 hr.

Children. *Initial:* 50 U/kg. *Maintenance:* 100 U/kg/dose q 4 hr.

I.V. OR S.C. INJECTION

Adults. *Loading:* 5,000 U I.V., then 10,000 to 20,000 U S.C. *Maintenance:* 8,000 to 10,000 U S.C. q 8 hr or 15,000 to 20,000 U S.C. q 12 hr.

▶ *To diagnose and treat disseminated intravascular coagulation (DIC)*

I.V. INFUSION OR INJECTION

Adults. 50 to 100 U/kg q 4 hr. Drug may be discontinued if no improvement occurs in 4 to 8 hours.

Children. 25 to 50 U/kg q 4 hr. Drug may be discontinued if no improvement occurs in 4 to 8 hours.

▶ *To prevent clots in patients undergoing open-heart and vascular surgery*

I.V. INFUSION OR INJECTION

Adults. 300 U/kg for procedures that last less than 60 min; 400 U/kg for procedures that last longer than 60 min. *Minimum:* 150 U/kg.

Children. 300 U/kg for procedures that last less than 60 min. Then dosage is based on coagulation test results. *Minimum:* 150 U/kg.

▶ *To maintain heparin lock patency*

I.V. INJECTION

Adults. 10 to 100 U/ml heparin flush solution (enough to fill device) after each use of device.

Route	Onset	Peak	Duration
I.V.	Immediate	Minutes	Unknown
S.C.	In 20 to 60 min	Unknown	Unknown

Mechanism of Action
Binds with antithrombin III, enhancing antithrombin III's inactivation of the coagulation enzymes thrombin (factor IIa) and factors Xa and XIa. At low doses, heparin inhibits factor Xa and prevents the conversion of prothrombin to thrombin. Thrombin is necessary for the conversion of fibrinogen to fibrin; without fibrin, clots can't form. At high doses, heparin inactivates thrombin, preventing fibrin formation and existing clot extension.

Incompatibilities
Don't mix heparin with any other drug unless you have an order to do so and have checked with pharmacist. Heparin is incompatible with many drugs and solutions, especially ones that contain a phosphate buffer, sodium bicarbonate, or sodium oxalate.

Contraindications
Hypersensitivity to heparin or its components; severe thrombocytopenia; uncontrolled bleeding, except in DIC

Interactions
DRUGS
antihistamines, digoxin, nicotine, tetracyclines: Decreased anticoagulant effect of heparin
aspirin, NSAIDs, platelet aggregation inhibitors, sulfinpyrazone: Increased platelet inhibition and risk of bleeding
cefamandole, cefoperazone, cefotetan, methimazole, plicamycin, propylthiouracil, valproic acid: Possibly hypoprothrombinemia and increased risk of bleeding
chloroquine, hydroxychloroquine: Possibly thrombocytopenia and increased risk of hemorrhage
ethacrynic acid, glucocorticoids, salicylates: Increased risk of bleeding and GI ulceration and hemorrhage
nitroglycerin: Possibly decreased anticoagulant effect of heparin
probenecid: Possibly increased anticoagulant effect of heparin
thrombolytics: Increased risk of hemorrhage
ACTIVITIES
smoking: Decreased anticoagulant effect of heparin

Adverse Reactions
CNS: Chills, dizziness, fever, headache, peripheral neuropathy
CV: Chest pain
EENT: Epistaxis, gingival bleeding, rhinitis
GI: Abdominal distention and pain, hematemesis, melena, nausea, vomiting

GU: Hematuria, hypermenorrhea
HEME: Easy bruising, excessive bleeding from wounds, thrombo-cytopenia
MS: Back pain, myalgia, osteoporosis
RESP: Dyspnea, wheezing
SKIN: Alopecia, cyanosis, petechiae, pruritus, urticaria
Other: Anaphylaxis

Nursing Considerations

- **WARNING** Administer heparin only by I.V. or S.C. route; I.M. injection causes hematoma, irritation, and pain.
- Avoid injecting any drugs by I.M. route during heparin therapy to decrease the risk of bleeding and hematoma.
- **WARNING** Don't administer heparin that contains benzyl alcohol to neonates or premature infants because they may develop a fatal toxic syndrome characterized by CNS, respiratory, circulatory, and renal impairment and metabolic acidosis.
- To prepare heparin for continuous infusion, invert container at least six times to prevent drug from pooling. Don't use solution if it's discolored.
- Expect to obtain APTT after 8 hours of continuous I.V. therapy. Use the arm opposite the infusion site.
- For intermittent I.V. therapy, expect to adjust dose based on co-agulation test results performed 30 minutes earlier. Therapeutic range is typically 1.5 to 2.5 times the control.
- Administer S.C. heparin into the anterior abdominal wall, above the iliac crest, and 5 cm (2") or more away from the umbilicus. To minimize subcutaneous tissue trauma, lift adipose tissue away from deep tissues; don't aspirate for blood before injecting drug; don't move needle while injecting drug; and don't massage the injection site before or after injection. Keep in mind that you can apply gentle pressure to the site after you withdraw the needle.
- Alternate injection sites, and observe for signs of bleeding and hematoma formation.
- Take safety precautions to prevent bleeding, such as having patient use a soft-bristled toothbrush and an electric razor.
- Monitor blood test results and observe for signs of bleeding, such as ecchymosis, epistaxis, hematemesis, hematuria, melena, and petechiae. Be aware that menstruating women, alcoholics,

patients with a GI ulcer, and those with impaired renal or hepatic function are at increased risk for bleeding or hemorrhage. Hypertensive patients are at increased risk for cerebral hemorrhage.

- Monitor for signs and symptoms of an allergic reaction, such as wheezing, rash, and itching, especially in patients with a history of asthma or allergies.
- Make sure all health care providers know that patient is receiving heparin.
- Keep protamine sulfate on hand to use as an antidote for heparin. Be aware that each milligram of protamine sulfate neutralizes 100 U of heparin.
- Be aware that prescriber may order oral anticoagulants before discontinuing heparin to avoid increased coagulation caused by heparin withdrawal. Heparin may be discontinued when full therapeutic effect of oral anticoagulant is achieved.
- Know that women over age 60 have the highest risk of hemorrhage during therapy.
- Store drug at 15° to 30° C (59° to 86° F); don't freeze.

PATIENT TEACHING

- Explain that heparin can't be taken orally.
- Inform patient about the increased risk of bleeding; urge her to avoid injuries and to use a soft-bristled toothbrush and an electric razor.
- Advise patient to avoid drugs that interact with heparin, such as aspirin and ibuprofen.
- Instruct patient and family to watch for and report abdominal or lower back pain, black stools, bleeding gums, bloody urine, excessive menstrual bleeding, nosebleeds, and severe headaches.
- Inform patient that temporary hair loss may occur.
- Advise patient to wear or carry appropriate medical identification.

hydralazine hydrochloride
Apresoline (CAN)

Class and Category
Chemical: Phthalazine derivative
Therapeutic: Antihypertensive, vasodilator
Pregnancy category: C

Indications and Dosages

▶ *To manage severe essential hypertension when drug can't be taken orally or when need to reduce blood pressure is urgent*

I.V. INJECTION

Adults. 5 to 40 mg, repeated as needed.

Children. 1.7 to 3.5 mg/kg/day in divided doses q 4 to 6 hr, as needed.

Incompatibilities

Don't mix hydralazine in I.V. infusion solutions.

Route	Onset	Peak	Duration
I.V.	5 to 20 min	10 to 80 min	2 to 6 hr

Mechanism of Action

May act in a manner that resembles organic nitrates and sodium nitroprusside, except that hydralazine is selective for arteries. This drug:

• exerts a direct vasodilating effect on vascular smooth muscle
• interferes with calcium movement in vascular smooth muscle by altering cellular calcium metabolism
• dilates arteries rather than veins, which minimizes orthostatic hypotension and increases cardiac output and cerebral blood flow
• causes a reflex autonomic response that increases heart rate, cardiac output, and left ventricular ejection fraction
• has a positive inotropic effect on the heart.

Contraindications

Coronary artery disease, hypersensitivity to hydralazine or its components, mitral valve disease

Interactions

DRUGS

beta blockers: Increased effects of both drugs

diazoxide, MAO inhibitors, other antihypertensives: Risk of severe hypotension

epinephrine: Possibly decreased vasopressor effect of epinephrine

NSAIDs: Decreased hydralazine effects

sympathomimetics: Possibly decreased antihypertensive effect of hydralazine

Adverse Reactions

CNS: Chills, fever, headache, peripheral neuritis
CV: Angina, edema, orthostatic hypotension, palpitations, tachycardia
EENT: Lacrimation, nasal congestion
GI: Anorexia, constipation, diarrhea, nausea, vomiting
RESP: Dyspnea
SKIN: Blisters, flushing, pruritus, rash, urticaria
Other: Lupuslike symptoms (especially with high doses), lymphadenopathy

Nursing Considerations

- Monitor CBC, lupus erythematosus cell preparation, and ANA titer before hydralazine therapy and periodically, as appropriate, during long-term treatment.
- Use drug immediately after opening ampule.
- Anticipate that drug may change color in solution. Consult pharmacist if color change occurs.
- Be aware that hydralazine also may undergo color changes when exposed to a metal filter.
- Monitor blood pressure and pulse rate regularly and weigh patient daily during therapy.
- Check blood pressure with patient in lying, sitting, and standing positions, and watch for signs of orthostatic hypotension. Expect orthostatic hypotension to be most common in the morning, during hot weather, and with exercise.
- WARNING Expect to discontinue drug immediately if patient experiences lupuslike symptoms, such as arthralgia, fever, myalgia, pharyngitis, and splenomegaly.
- Expect prescriber to withdraw drug gradually to avoid a rapid increase in blood pressure.
- Before opening ampule, store it at 15° to 30° C (59° to 86° F); don't freeze.
- Expect to treat peripheral neuritis with pyridoxine.

PATIENT TEACHING

- Advise patient to change position slowly, especially in the morning, while receiving hydralazine. Caution her that hot showers may increase hypotension.
- Instruct patient to immediately report fever, aching muscles and joints, and sore throat.
- Urge patient to report numbness and tingling in the limbs, which may require treatment with another drug.

hydrocortisone sodium phosphate
Hydrocortone Phosphate
hydrocortisone sodium succinate
A-hydroCort, Solu-Cortef

Class and Category
Chemical: Glucocorticoid
Therapeutic: Adrenocorticoid replacement, anti-inflammatory
Pregnancy category: Not rated

Indications and Dosages
▶ *To treat severe inflammation or acute adrenal insufficiency*
I.V. INFUSION OR INJECTION (HYDROCORTISONE SODIUM PHOS-
PHATE)
Adults. 15 to 240 mg/day as a single dose or in divided doses.
Usual: One-half to one-third of the oral dose.
DOSAGE ADJUSTMENT Dosage increased to more than
240 mg/day if needed to treat acute disease.
I.V. INFUSION OR INJECTION (HYDROCORTISONE SODIUM SUCCINATE)
Adults. 100 to 500 mg q 2, 4, or 6 hr.

Route	Onset	Peak	Duration
I.V. (phosphate, succinate)	Rapid	Unknown	Unknown

Mechanism of Action
Binds to intracellular glucocorticoid receptors and suppresses the inflammatory and immune responses by:
- inhibiting neutrophil and monocyte accumulation at the inflammation site
  and suppressing their phagocytic and bactericidal activity
- stabilizing lysosomal membranes
- suppressing the antigen response of macrophages and helper T cells
- inhibiting the synthesis of cellular mediators of the inflammatory response,
  such as cytokines, interleukins, and prostaglandins.

Contraindications
Hypersensitivity to hydrocortisone or its components, recent vaccination with live-virus vaccine, systemic fungal infection

Interactions
DRUGS
acetaminophen: Increased risk of hepatotoxicity
amphotericin B, carbonic anhydrase inhibitors: Possibly severe hypokalemia

anabolic steroids, androgens: Increased risk of edema and severe acne
anticholinergics: Possibly increased intraocular pressure
anticoagulants, thrombolytics: Increased risk of GI ulceration and hemorrhage, possibly decreased therapeutic effects of these drugs
asparaginase: Increased risk of hyperglycemia and toxicity
aspirin, NSAIDs: Increased risk of GI distress and bleeding
digoxin: Possibly hypokalemia-induced arrhythmias and digitalis toxicity
ephedrine, phenobarbital, phenytoin, rifampin: Decreased blood hydrocortisone level
estrogens, oral contraceptives: Possibly increased therapeutic and toxic effects of hydrocortisone
isoniazid: Possibly decreased therapeutic effects of isoniazid
mexiletine: Possibly decreased blood mexiletine level
neuromuscular blockers: Possibly increased neuromuscular blockade, causing respiratory depression or apnea
potassium-depleting drugs (such as thiazide diuretics): Possibly severe hypokalemia
potassium supplements: Possibly decreased effects of these supplements
salicylates: Possibly decreased effectiveness and blood level of salicylates
somatrem, somatropin: Possibly decreased therapeutic effects of these drugs
streptozocin: Increased risk of hyperglycemia
vaccines: Decreased antibody response and increased risk of neurologic complications
ACTIVITIES
alcohol use: Increased risk of GI distress and bleeding

Adverse Reactions

CNS: Ataxia, behavioral changes, depression, dizziness, euphoria, fatigue, headache, increased ICP with papilledema, insomnia, malaise, mood changes, paresthesia, seizures, steroid psychosis, syncope, vertigo
CV: Arrhythmias (from hypokalemia), fat embolism, heart failure, hypertension, hypotension, thromboembolism, thrombophlebitis
EENT: Exophthalmos, glaucoma, increased intraocular pressure, nystagmus, posterior subcapsular cataracts
ENDO: Adrenal insufficiency during stress, cushingoid symptoms (buffalo hump, central obesity, moon face, supraclavicular fat pad enlargement), diabetes mellitus, growth suppression in children, hyperglycemia, negative nitrogen balance from protein catabolism

GI: Abdominal distention, hiccups, increased appetite, nausea, pancreatitis, peptic ulcer, ulcerative esophagitis, vomiting

GU: Amenorrhea, glycosuria, menstrual irregularities, perineal burning or tingling

HEME: Easy bruising, leukocytosis

MS: Arthralgia; aseptic necrosis of femoral and humeral heads; compression fractures; muscle atrophy, twitching, or weakness; myalgia; osteoporosis; spontaneous fractures; steroid myopathy; tendon rupture

SKIN: Acne; altered skin pigmentation; diaphoresis; erythema; hirsutism; necrotizing vasculitis; petechiae; purpura; rash; scarring; sterile abscess; striae; subcutaneous fat atrophy; thin, fragile skin; urticaria

Other: Anaphylaxis, hypocalcemia, hypokalemia, hypokalemic alkalosis, impaired wound healing, masking of signs of infection, metabolic alkalosis, suppressed skin test reaction, weight gain

Nursing Considerations

- Be aware that systemic hydrocortisone shouldn't be given to immunocompromised patients, such as those with fungal and other infections, including amebiasis, hepatitis B, tuberculosis, vaccinia, and varicella.
- **WARNING** Don't administer hydrocortisone that contains benzyl alcohol to neonates or premature infants because they may develop a fatal toxic syndrome characterized by CNS, respiratory, circulatory, and renal impairment and metabolic acidosis.
- Give daily dose of hydrocortisone in the morning to mimic the normal peak in adrenocortical secretion of corticosteroids.
- Don't give acetate injectable suspension by I.V. route. This form is used for intra-articular, intralesional, and soft-tissue injections.
- Give hydrocortisone sodium succinate as a direct I.V. injection over 30 seconds to several minutes, or as an intermittent or continuous infusion. For infusion, dilute to 1 mg/ml or less with D_5W, NS, or D_5NS. Use reconstituted hydrocortisone sodium succinate within 3 days. Protect reconstituted solution from light, and discard if not clear.
- **WARNING** Avoid rapid administration of high doses of hydrocortisone, which may cause anaphylaxis, angioedema, seizures, and possibly sudden death. Maintain ECG monitoring, as prescribed, and have emergency equipment and drugs readily available.

- Dilute hydrocortisone sodium phosphate with D$_5$W or NS, and use diluted solution within 24 hours.
- Be aware that high-dose therapy shouldn't be given for longer than 48 hours. Be alert for depression or psychotic episodes during high-dose therapy.
- Regularly monitor weight, blood pressure, and serum electrolyte levels during therapy.
- Expect hydrocortisone to exacerbate infections or mask their signs and symptoms.
- Monitor blood glucose level in diabetic patients, and increase insulin or oral antidiabetic drug dosage, as prescribed.
- Know that elderly patients are at high risk for osteoporosis during long-term therapy.
- Anticipate the possibility of acute adrenal insufficiency with stress, such as emotional upset, fever, surgery, and trauma. Increase hydrocortisone dosage, as prescribed.
- **WARNING** Avoid withdrawing drug suddenly after long-term therapy because adrenal crisis can result. Expect to reduce dosage gradually, as prescribed, and to monitor patient's response.
- Store hydrocortisone at 15° to 30° C (59° to 86° F); don't freeze.

PATIENT TEACHING
- Instruct patient receiving hydrocortisone to report early signs of adrenal insufficiency: anorexia, difficulty breathing, dizziness, fainting, fatigue, joint pain, muscle weakness, and nausea.
- Inform patient that she may bruise easily.
- Advise patient on long-term therapy to have periodic ophthalmic examinations and to carry or wear medical identification.

hydromorphone hydrochloride
(dihydromorphinone)
Dilaudid, Dilaudid-HP

Class, Category, and Schedule
Chemical: Phenanthrene derivative, semisynthetic opioid derivative
Therapeutic: Opioid analgesic
Pregnancy category: C
Controlled substance: Schedule II

Indications and Dosages
▶ *To relieve moderate to severe pain*
I.V. INJECTION
Adults. 1 mg q 3 hr, p.r.n.

Route	Onset	Peak	Duration
I.V.	10 to 15 min	15 to 30 min	2 to 3 hr

Mechanism of Action

May bind with opioid receptors in the spinal cord and higher levels in the CNS. In this way, hydromorphone is believed to stimulate mu and kappa receptors, thus altering the perception of, and emotional response to, pain.

Contraindications

Acute asthma; hypersensitivity to hydromorphone, other opioid analgesics, or their components; increased ICP; severe respiratory depression; upper respiratory tract obstruction

Interactions

DRUGS

anticholinergics: Increased risk of ileus, severe constipation, or urine retention

antihypertensives, diuretics, guanadrel, guanethidine, mecamylamine: Increased risk of orthostatic hypotension

barbiturate anesthetics: Increased sedative effect of hydromorphone

belladonna alkaloids, difenoxin and atropine, diphenoxylate and atropine, kaolin pectin, loperamide, paregoric: Increased risk of CNS depression and severe constipation

buprenorphine, butorphanol, dezocine, nalbuphine, pentazocine: Possibly potentiated or suppressed symptoms of spontaneous narcotic withdrawal

CNS depressants, other opioid analgesics: Additive CNS depression and hypotension

hydroxyzine: Increased analgesia, CNS depression, and hypotension

metoclopramide: Decreased effect of metoclopramide on GI motility

naloxone: Possibly withdrawal symptoms in physically dependent patients

naltrexone: Possibly prolonged respiratory depression or cardiac arrest

neuromuscular blockers: Additive CNS depression

ACTIVITIES

alcohol use: Increased CNS depression

Adverse Reactions

CNS: Anxiety, confusion, dizziness, drowsiness, euphoria, hallucinations, headache, nervousness, restlessness, sedation, somnolence, tremor, weakness

CV: Hypertension, orthostatic hypotension, palpitations, tachycardia
EENT: Blurred vision, diplopia, dry mouth, laryngeal edema, laryngospasm, nystagmus, tinnitus
GI: Abdominal cramps, anorexia, biliary tract spasm, constipation, hepatotoxicity, nausea, vomiting
GU: Dysuria, urine retention
RESP: Dyspnea, respiratory depression, wheezing
SKIN: Diaphoresis, flushing
Other: Injection site pain, redness, and swelling; physical and psychological dependence

Nursing Considerations

- To improve analgesic action, give hydromorphone before pain becomes intense.
- Instruct patient to lie down during hydromorphone administration and for a period afterward to lessen dizziness, light-headedness, nausea, and vomiting.
- **WARNING** Administer hydromorphone slowly over several minutes. Rapid administration may cause serious adverse reactions, including anaphylaxis, severe respiratory depression, hypotension, peripheral circulatory collapse, and cardiac arrest. Make sure emergency equipment and drugs are available.
- Administer hydromorphone by direct injection over at least 2 minutes. For infusion, mix drug with D_5W, NS, or Ringer's solution.
- Monitor for respiratory depression, especially in patients who are having an acute asthma attack and those with chronic respiratory disease. Children, elderly patients, and debilitated or seriously ill patients are at increased risk for respiratory depression. Keep resuscitation equipment and naloxone nearby.
- Monitor for signs of drug-induced CNS depression or increased CSF pressure, such as altered LOC, restlessness, and irritability, in patients with a head injury, intracranial lesions, or other conditions that could cause these effects. Patients who are taking, or have recently taken, drugs that cause CNS depression are also more susceptible to these effects. Take appropriate safety precautions.
- Be aware that hydromorphone may induce or exacerbate arrhythmias or seizures in patients with a history of these conditions and may mask symptoms of acute abdominal conditions.
- Be aware that patients with a history of drug abuse (including acute alcoholism), emotional instability, or suicidal ideation or attempts are at increased risk for opioid abuse.

- Assess for constipation.
- Monitor for signs of physical dependence or abuse.
- Anticipate that drug may mask or worsen gallbladder pain.
- Store drug at 15° to 30° C (59° to 86° F); protect from freezing and light.

PATIENT TEACHING
- Instruct patient receiving hydromorphone to report constipation, difficulty breathing, severe nausea, or vomiting.
- Inform patient that drug may cause drowsiness and sedation. Advise her to avoid potentially hazardous activities until drug's CNS effects are known.
- Advise patient to change position slowly to minimize effects of orthostatic hypotension.
- To prevent constipation, encourage patient to consume plenty of fluids and high-fiber foods, if not contraindicated by another condition.
- Instruct patient to report pain before it becomes severe.
- Caution patient to avoid alcohol and OTC drugs during therapy, unless prescriber approves.

hyoscyamine sulfate

Levsin

Class and Category

Chemical: Belladonna alkaloid, tertiary amine
Therapeutic: Antimuscarinic, antispasmodic
Pregnancy category: C

Indications and Dosages

▶ *To treat peptic ulcers and GI tract disorders caused by spasm*

I.V. INJECTION

Adults and adolescents. 0.25 to 0.5 mg q 4 to 6 hr.
Children. Dosage individualized by weight.

▶ *To control salivation and excessive secretions during surgical procedures*

I. V. INJECTION

Adults and adolescents. 0.5 mg 30 to 60 min before procedure.

Route	Onset	Peak	Duration
I.V.	2 to 3 min	15 to 30 min	4 hr

Mechanism of Action

Competitively inhibits acetylcholine at autonomic postganglionic cholinergic receptors. Because the most sensitive receptors are in the salivary, bronchial, and sweat glands, hyoscyamine acts mainly to reduce salivary, bronchial, and sweat gland secretions. It also causes GI smooth muscle to contract and decreases gastric secretion and GI motility. In addition, hyoscyamine causes the bladder detrusor muscle to contract; reduces nasal and oropharyngeal secretions; and decreases airway resistance from relaxation of smooth muscle in the bronchi and bronchioles.

Contraindications

Acute hemorrhage and hemodynamic instability; angle-closure glaucoma; hepatic disease; hypersensitivity to hyoscyamine, other anticholinergics, or their components; ileus; intestinal atony; myasthenia gravis; myocardial ischemia; obstructive GI disease; obstructive uropathy; renal disease; severe ulcerative colitis; tachycardia; toxic megacolon

Interactions

DRUGS

anticholinergics: Possibly increased anticholingeric effects
calcium- and magnesium-containing antacids, carbonic anhydrase inhibitors, citrates, sodium bicarbonate, urinary alkalinizers: Possibly potentiated therapeutic and adverse effects of hyoscyamine
haloperidol: Possibly decreased therapeutic effects of haloperidol
ketoconazole: Possibly reduced ketoconazole absorption
metoclopramide: Possibly antagonized therapeutic effects of metoclopramide
opioid analgesics: Increased risk of severe constipation and ileus

Adverse Reactions

CNS: Drowsiness, insomnia
EENT: Blurred vision; dry mouth, nose, and throat; photophobia
ENDO: Decreased lactation
GI: Constipation
GU: Impotence, urine retention
SKIN: Decreased sweating
Other: Heatstroke, injection site redness and urticaria

Nursing Considerations

• Give hyoscyamine 30 to 60 minutes before meals and at bedtime. Give bedtime dose at least 2 hours after last meal.

- **WARNING** Expect an increased risk of drug-induced heat-stroke in hot or humid weather because hyoscyamine decreases sweating.
- **WARNING** Be aware that lower doses may paradoxically decrease the heart rate and that higher doses affect nicotinic receptors in autonomic ganglia, causing delirium, disorientation, hallucinations, and restlessness.
- Monitor patients with the following conditions for exacerbations caused by drug's anticholinergic effects: arrhythmias, coronary artery disease, heart failure, hiatal hernia with reflux esophagitis, hypertension, hyperthyroidism, or tachycardia. Also monitor blood pressure in patients with toxemia from pregnancy because they're at risk for aggravated hypertension.
- Monitor urine output, and be alert for urine retention, especially in patients with autonomic neuropathy.
- Be aware that infants, patients with Down syndrome, and children with brain damage or spastic paralysis may be more sensitive to drug's effects.
- Be aware that elderly patients and patients with impaired renal function are at increased risk for adverse reactions.
- Store drug at 15° to 30° C (59° to 86° F); don't freeze.

PATIENT TEACHING
- Instruct patient to void before receiving each dose of hyoscyamine and to report trouble urinating during hyoscyamine therapy.
- Inform patient that drug may cause drowsiness. Advise her to avoid potentially hazardous activities until drug's CNS effects are known.
- If patient reports dry mouth, suggest using sugarless hard candy or gum.
- Inform male patient that drug may cause impotence. If it occurs, suggest that he discuss it with prescriber.
- Advise patient to avoid exposure to high temperatures and to increase fluid intake, unless contraindicated.

ibutilide fumarate

Corvert

Class and Category

Chemical: Methanesulfonanilide derivative
Therapeutic: Class III antiarrhythmic
Pregnancy category: C

Indications and Dosages

▶ *To rapidly convert recent-onset atrial flutter or fibrillation to sinus rhythm*

I.V. INFUSION

Adults who weigh 60 kg (132 lb) or more. 1 mg over 10 min. Repeated 10 min after first dose is finished if arrhythmia persists.
Adults who weigh less than 60 kg. 0.01 mg/kg over 10 min. Repeated 10 min after first dose is finished if arrhythmia persists.
DOSAGE ADJUSTMENT Infusion discontinued if arrhythmia is terminated or if sustained or nonsustained ventricular tachycardia or prolonged QT or QTc interval develops.

Mechanism of Action

May promote sodium movement through slow inward sodium channels in myocardial cell membranes. Ibutilide also may inhibit a component of potassium channels in myocardial cell membranes involved in cardiac repolarization. These actions prolong the cardiac action potential by delaying repolarization and increasing atrial and ventricular refractoriness. As a result, the sinus rate slows and AV conduction is delayed.

Contraindications

Hypersensitivity to ibutilide or its components

Interactions

DRUGS

amiodarone, astemizole, disopyramide, maprotiline, phenothiazines, procainamide, quinidine, sotalol, tricyclic antidepressants: Possibly prolonged QT interval, leading to increased risk of proarrhythmias

Adverse Reactions

CNS: Headache, syncope
CV: AV block, bradycardia, bundle-branch block, heart failure, hypertension, hypotension, idioventricular rhythm, orthostatic hypotension, palpitations, prolonged QT interval, sinus and supraventricular tachycardia, supraventricular arrhythmias, ventricular arrhythmias, ventricular tachycardia (sustained and non-sustained)
GI: Nausea
GU: Renal failure

Nursing Considerations

- Before administering ibutilide, check serum electrolyte levels and expect to correct abnormalities, as prescribed. Be especially alert for hypokalemia and hypomagnesemia, which can lead to arrhythmias.
- Give drug undiluted, or dilute it in 50 ml of NS or D_5W. Add contents of 10-ml vial (0.1 mg/ml) to 50 ml of solution to obtain 0.017 mg/ml. Use polyvinyl chloride plastic bags or polyolefin bags for ibutilide admixtures. Administer within 24 hours (48 hours if refrigerated).
- Infuse drug slowly over 10 minutes.
- As ordered, monitor cardiac rhythm continuously during drug infusion and for at least 4 hours afterward—longer if arrhythmias appear or if patient has abnormal hepatic function. Observe for ventricular ectopy.
- **WARNING** Be aware that ibutilide use is not recommended for patients with a history of prolonged QT interval or torsades de pointes. Also be aware that patients with bradycardia, heart failure, or a history of low left ventricular ejection fraction are at increased risk for torsades de pointes and those with a history of chronic atrial fibrillation are at increased risk for recurrence after conversion to sinus rhythm.
- Before preparing ibutilide, store it at 20° to 25° C (68° to 77° F).
- Make sure that a defibrillator and drugs to treat sustained ventricular tachycardia are available during therapy and when monitoring patient after therapy.

PATIENT TEACHING

- Inform patient that ibutilide will be administered by I.V. infusion and that his heart rhythm will be monitored continuously during the infusion.

- Ask patient to report chest pain, faintness, numbness, tingling, palpitations, and shortness of breath.
- Advise patient to keep follow-up appointments to monitor heart rhythm.

imipenem and cilastatin sodium

Primaxin (CAN), Primaxin ADD-Vantage, Primaxin IV

Class and Category

Chemical: Thienamycin derivative (imipenem), heptenoic acid derivative (cilastatin sodium)
Therapeutic: Antibiotic
Pregnancy category: C

Indications and Dosages

▶ *To treat severe or life-threatening bacterial infections (including endocarditis, pneumonia, and septicemia as well as bone, joint, intra-abdominal, skin, and soft-tissue infections) caused by gram-positive anaerobic organisms, such as most staphylococci and streptococci and some enterococci (including* Enterococcus faecalis*); most strains of Entero-bacteriaceae (including* Citrobacter *species,* Enterobacter *species,* Escherichia coli, Klebsiella *species,* Morganella morganii, Proteus mirabilis, Providencia stuartii, and* Serratia marcescens*); and many gram-negative aerobic and anaerobic species (including* Bacteroides *species,* Campylobacter *species,* Clostridium *species,* Haemophilus influenzae, Legionella *species,* Neisseria gonorrhoeae, and* Pseudomonas aeruginosa*)*

I.V. INFUSION (DOSAGES BASED ON IMIPENEM CONTENT)

Adults and adolescents. 500 mg q 6 hr to 1,000 mg q 6 to 8 hr. *Maximum:* 50 mg/kg or 4 g/day, whichever is lower.

Children age 3 months and older. 15 to 25 mg/kg q 6 hr. *Maximum:* 2,000 to 4,000 mg/day.

Infants ages 4 weeks to 3 months who weigh 1,500 g (3 lb, 3 oz) or more. 25 mg/kg q 6 hr. *Maximum:* 2,000 to 4,000 mg/day.

Neonates ages 1 to 4 weeks who weigh 1,500 g or more. 25 mg/kg q 8 hr. *Maximum:* 2,000 to 4,000 mg/day.

Neonates under age 1 week who weigh 1,500 g or more. 25 mg/kg q 12 hr. *Maximum:* 2,000 to 4,000 mg/day.

▶ *To treat moderate infections caused by the organisms listed above*

I.V. INFUSION (DOSAGES BASED ON IMIPENEM CONTENT)

Adults and adolescents. 500 mg q 6 to 8 hr up to 1,000 mg q 8 hr. *Maximum:* 50 mg/kg or 4 g/day, whichever is lower.

Children age 3 months and older. 15 to 25 mg/kg q 6 hr. *Maximum:* 2,000 to 4,000 mg/day.

Infants ages 4 weeks to 3 months who weigh 1,500 g or more. 25 mg/kg q 6 hr. *Maximum:* 2,000 to 4,000 mg/day.

Neonates ages 1 to 4 weeks who weigh 1,500 g or more. 25 mg/kg q 8 hr. *Maximum:* 2,000 to 4,000 mg/day.

Neonates under age 1 week who weigh 1,500 g or more. 25 mg/kg q 12 hr. *Maximum:* 2,000 to 4,000 mg/day.

▶ *To treat mild infections caused by the organisms listed above*
I.V. INFUSION (DOSAGES BASED ON IMIPENEM CONTENT)

Adults and adolescents. 250 to 500 mg q 6 hr. *Maximum:* 50 mg/kg or 4 g/day, whichever is lower.

Children age 3 months and older. 15 to 25 mg/kg q 6 hr. *Maximum:* 2,000 (for fully susceptible organisms) to 4,000 (for moderately susceptible organisms) mg/day.

Infants ages 4 weeks to 3 months who weigh 1,500 g or more. 25 mg/kg q 6 hr. *Maximum:* 2,000 to 4,000 mg/day.

Neonates ages 1 to 4 weeks who weigh 1,500 g or more. 25 mg/kg q 8 hr. *Maximum:* 2,000 to 4,000 mg/day.

Neonates under age 1 week who weigh 1,500 g or more. 25 mg/kg q 12 hr. *Maximum:* 2,000 to 4,000 mg/day.

▶ *To treat uncomplicated UTIs caused by the organisms listed above*
I.V. INFUSION (DOSAGES BASED ON IMIPENEM CONTENT)

Adults and adolescents. 250 mg q 6 hr. *Maximum:* 50 mg/kg or 4 g/day, whichever is lower.

▶ *To treat complicated UTIs caused by the organisms listed above*
I.V. INFUSION (DOSAGES BASED ON IMIPENEM CONTENT)

Adults and adolescents. 500 mg q 6 hr. *Maximum:* 50 mg/kg or 4 g/day, whichever is lower.

DOSAGE ADJUSTMENT Dosage reduced based on creatinine clearance for patients with impaired renal function.

Mechanism of Action

Produces two related actions. During bacterial cell wall synthesis, imipenem selectively binds to penicillin-binding proteins that are responsible for cell wall formation. This action causes bacterial cells to rapidly lyse and die. Cilastatin sodium inhibits imipenem's breakdown in the kidneys, thus maintaining a high imipenem level in the urinary tract.

Incompatibilities
Don't administer imipenem and cilastatin through same I.V. line as beta-lactam antibiotics or aminoglycosides.

Contraindications
Hypersensitivity to imipenem, its components, or other beta-lactam antibiotics; meningitis

Interactions
DRUGS

cyclosporine: Increased adverse CNS effects of both drugs
ganciclovir: Increased risk of seizures
probenecid: Slightly increased blood level and half-life of imipenem

Adverse Reactions
CNS: Confusion, dizziness, fever, seizures, somnolence, tremor, weakness
CV: Hypotension
EENT: Glossitis, oral candidiasis
GI: Diarrhea, nausea, pseudomembranous colitis, vomiting
RESP: Wheezing
SKIN: Diaphoresis, pruritus, rash, urticaria
Other: Anaphylaxis, infusion site thrombophlebitis

Nursing Considerations
• Obtain body fluid and tissue specimens for culture and sensitivity testing, as ordered, before giving first dose of imipenem and cilastatin. Expect to start therapy before test results are available.
• Add about 10 ml of diluent to each 250- or 500-mg vial and shake well. Transfer this reconstituted drug to at least 100 ml of prescribed I.V. solution. After the transfer, add another 10 ml of diluent to each vial, shake, and then transfer to infusion container. Shake infusion container until clear. To reconstitute piggyback bottles, add 100 ml of diluent to each 250- or 500-mg infusion bottle, and shake well.
• Administer reconstituted drug within 4 to 10 hours (24 to 48 hours if refrigerated), depending on diluent used. Color may range from clear to yellow; don't administer solution that contains particles.
• Infuse 500-mg or smaller dose over 20 to 30 minutes and 750- to 1,000-mg dose over 40 to 60 minutes.
• **WARNING** Avoid rapid administration, which may result in an infusion rate reaction characterized by dizziness, nausea, vomiting, diaphoresis, and tiredness.

- Expect increased risk of imipenem-induced seizures in patients with brain lesions, head trauma, or history of CNS disorders and in those receiving more than 2 g of drug daily.
- Assess for signs and symptoms of allergic reaction and bacterial or fungal superinfection.
- Before reconstituting imipenem and cilastatin, store it below 30° C (86° F); don't freeze.

PATIENT TEACHING

- Instruct patient receiving imipenem and cilastatin to immediately report severe diarrhea. Inform him that yogurt and buttermilk can help maintain intestinal flora and decrease diarrhea. Advise him not to take any antidiarrheals withhout first checking with prescriber.
- Review with patient other possibly serious adverse reactions, such as difficulty breathing, rash, and hives, and tell him to report any that occur.
- Instruct patient to report discomfort at I.V. insertion site.

immune globulin intravenous (human)
(IGIV, immune serum globulin, ISG, IVIG)
Gamimune N 5%, Gamimune N 5% S/D, Gamimune N 10%, Gamimune N 10% S/D, Gammagard S/D, Gammagard S/D 0.5 g, Gammar-P IV, Iveegam, Polygam S/D, Sandoglobulin, Venoglobulin-I, Venoglobulin-S 5%, Venoglobulin-S 10%

Class and Category
Chemical: Polyvalent antibody
Therapeutic: Antibacterial, anti–Kawasaki disease agent, antipolyneuropathy agent, antiviral, immunizing agent, platelet count stimulator
Pregnancy category: C

Indications and Dosages
▶ *To treat primary immunodeficiency*
I.V. INFUSION
Adults and adolescents. 200 to 400 mg/kg q mo. If response is inadequate, dosing frequency increased to twice monthly.
▶ *To treat idiopathic thrombocytopenic purpura (ITP)*
I.V. INFUSION
Adults and adolescents. 400 mg/kg/day for 2 to 5 consecutive days. If response is inadequate, additional 400 to 1,000 mg/kg given q several wk as needed.

DOSAGE ADJUSTMENT In acute ITP of childhood, I.V. therapy may be discontinued after 2nd day of 5-day course if initial platelet count response is adequate (30,000 to 50,000/mm³). In chronic ITP, an additional I.V. infusion may be prescribed if platelet count falls below 30,000/mm³ or if patient develops significant bleeding.

▶ *As adjunct to treat Kawasaki disease*
I.V. INFUSION
Adults and adolescents. 2 g/kg as a single dose.

▶ *As adjunct to treat bacterial infections secondary to B-cell chronic lymphocytic leukemia*
I.V. INFUSION
Adults and adolescents. 400 mg/kg q 3 to 4 wk.

▶ *To prevent bacterial infection in children with HIV who are immunosuppressed*
I.V. INFUSION (GAMIMUNE N 5% OR 10%)
Children. 400 mg/kg q.d. every 28 days.

Route	Onset	Peak	Duration
I.V.	Unknown	Unknown	21 to 28 days

Mechanism of Action
Releases antibody-specific globulins to produce an antibody-antigen reaction that results in bacterial lysis and facilitates bacterial phagocytosis. In treatment of ITP, immune globulin blocks iron receptors on macrophages to increase immunoglobulin action. Immune globulin also increases cytokine production and improves B-cell immune function by regulating T-cell and macrophage activity. Newly formed antigen-antibody complexes produce split complement components that cause bacterial lysis.

In Kawasaki disease and bacterial infections secondary to B-cell chronic lymphocytic leukemia, immune globulin neutralizes bacterial and viral toxins that harm the immune and inflammatory responses.

Incompatibilities
Don't mix immune globulin with any other drugs or with any I.V. solutions other than D₅W or diluent supplied by manufacturer because effects of doing so are unknown.

Contraindications
Hypersensitivity to immune globulin (human) or its components, IgA deficiency in patients with known antibody to IgA

Interactions

DRUGS

vaccines, live virus: Possibly decreased response to vaccine

Adverse Reactions

CNS: Faintness, fatigue, headache, light-headedness, malaise
CV: Tachycardia
GI: Nausea, vomiting
MS: Arthralgia; back, chest, or hip pain; myalgia
RESP: Dyspnea, wheezing
SKIN: Cyanosis
Other: Anaphylaxis; infusion site pain, rash, or urticaria

Nursing Considerations

- Before administering immune globulin, monitor patient's fluid volume and BUN and serum creatinine levels, as ordered, to determine if patient is at risk for acute renal failure. Those at increased risk include patients with existing renal insufficiency, diabetes mellitus, volume depletion, sepsis, or paraproteinemia; those taking concomitant nephrotoxic drugs; and those over age 65. Expect drug to be discontinued if renal function deteriorates.
- Consult manufacturer's guidelines to determine appropriate flow rate for initiating immune globulin infusion. Expect to increase flow rate after 15 to 30 minutes, according to guidelines.
- To reconstitute drug, follow manufacturer's guidelines and use only diluent recommended by manufacturer. Don't shake solution; excessive shaking causes foaming. If product or diluent is cold, expect drug to take up to 20 minutes to dissolve.
- If drug is reconstituted outside of sterile laminar airflow conditions, administer it immediately and discard any unused portions.
- **WARNING** Monitor for an acute inflammatory reaction in patients who have never received immune globulin therapy before, in those whose last treatment was more than 8 weeks before, and in those whose initial infusion rate exceeded 1 ml/minute. Within 30 minutes to 1 hour after beginning of infusion, assess for chills, fever, facial flushing, feeling of tightness in chest, dizziness, nausea and vomiting, diaphoresis, and hypotension. Notify prescriber immediately if such symptoms occur, and be prepared to stop infusion until symptoms have subsided.
- **WARNING** After immune globulin administration, monitor patient closely for aseptic meningitis. Notify prescriber if patient develops drowsiness, fever, nausea and vomiting, nuchal

rigidity, photophobia, painful eye movements, or severe headache.
- Assess severely ill patients with impaired cardiac function for cardiac complications, such as hypertension or heart failure.
- Monitor blood glucose level periodically in patients with diabetes mellitus because they may experience a transient increase.
- Be aware that immune globulin intravenous is made from human plasma and therefore may contain infectious agents, such as viruses. However, the risk that such a virus will be transmitted through the infusion has been reduced by screening of blood donors for prior exposure to certain viruses, testing of donated blood for presence of certain viral infections, and inactivation or removal of certain viruses from the product.
- Store drug at 2° to 8° C (36° to 46° F); don't freeze.

PATIENT TEACHING
- Instruct patient to immediately report any symptoms he experiences after receiving immune globulin.
- Inform patient that he'll need to postpone any vaccinations containing a live virus for up to 11 months after receiving immune globulin because drug may delay or inhibit his response to vaccine.

inamrinone lactate
(amrinone lactate)
Inocor

Class and Category
Chemical: Bipyridine derivative
Therapeutic: Cardiac inotrope
Pregnancy category: C

Indications and Dosages
▶ *To treat heart failure in patients who haven't responded sufficiently to digoxin, diuretics, or vasodilators*
I.V. INFUSION
Adults. *Initial:* 0.75 mg/kg by bolus administered over 2 to 3 min and repeated after 30 min, if needed. *Maintenance:* 5 to 10 mcg/kg/min by infusion. *Maximum:* 10 mg/kg/day.

Route	Onset	Peak	Duration
I.V.	2 to 5 min	In 10 min	30 min to 2 hr

Mechanism of Action

Inhibits phosphodiesterase enzymes that normally degrade myocardial cAMP. This action increases intracellular levels of cAMP, which regulates intracellular and extracellular calcium balance. An increased intracellular cAMP level enhances the influx of calcium into the cell, thereby increasing the force of myocardial contractions. Inamrinone also acts directly on peripheral vascular smooth-muscle cells, causing relaxation and dilation. This action reduces preload and afterload.

Incompatibilities

Don't administer inamrinone through same I.V. line as furosemide to prevent precipitate formation. Don't dilute inamrinone in solution that contains dextrose because a chemical interaction occurs over 24 hours.

Contraindications

Hypersensitivity to inamrinone, bisulfites, or their components; severe aortic or pulmonary valvular disease

Interactions

DRUGS

disopyramide: Possibly severe hypotension

Adverse Reactions

CNS: Fever
CV: Chest pain, hypotension, pericarditis, supraventricular tachycardia, ventricular arrhythmias
GI: Abdominal pain, anorexia, elevated liver function test results, hepatotoxicity, nausea, vomiting
HEME: Elevated erythrocyte sedimentation rate, thrombocytopenia (especially with high-dose or long-term treatment)
MS: Myositis
RESP: Hypoxemia, pleuritis
SKIN: Jaundice
Other: Infusion site burning

Nursing Considerations

• **WARNING** Be aware that inamrinone may increase the risk of ventricular arrhythmias in patients with atrial flutter or fibrillation. To minimize this risk, expect to pretreat such patients with digoxin.

- Administer inamrinone undiluted or diluted in NS or 0.45NS to a concentration of 1 to 3 mg/ml, as prescribed. Use diluted solution within 24 hours. Don't use if solution is discolored or contains particles.
- **WARNING** Monitor vital signs regularly. If blood pressure falls significantly, slow or stop inamrinone infusion and notify prescriber.
- Monitor weight, cardiac index, central venous pressure, pulmonary artery wedge pressure, and fluid intake and output as appropriate to assess effectiveness of therapy.
- **WARNING** Assess frequently for signs of thrombocytopenia, such as bruising or bleeding and altered platelet count. If signs appear, expect to decrease inamrinone dose or discontinue drug.
- Store drug at 15° to 30° C (59° to 86° F) and protect from light.

PATIENT TEACHING
- Instruct patient to report dizziness, which may indicate hypotension, or signs of an allergic reaction, such as a rash, facial swelling, or difficulty breathing or swallowing.

indomethacin sodium trihydrate
Indocid PDA (CAN), Indocin I.V.

Class and Category
Chemical: Indoleacetic acid derivative
Therapeutic: Antigout agent, anti-inflammatory, antirheumatic
Pregnancy category: Not rated

Indications and Dosages
▶ *To treat hemodynamically significant patent ductus arteriosus in premature infants who weigh 500 to 1,750 g (1 to 3.9 lb)*
I.V. INJECTION
Infants over age 7 days. *Initial:* 200 mcg/kg (0.2 mg/kg) over 5 to 10 sec; 1 or 2 additional doses of 250 mcg/kg (0.25 mg/kg) given at 12- to 24-hr intervals, if needed.
Neonates ages 2 to 7 days. *Initial:* 200 mcg/kg (0.2 mg/kg) over 5 to 10 sec; 1 or 2 additional doses of 200 mcg/kg (0.2 mg/kg) given at 12- to 24-hr intervals, if needed.
Neonates under age 48 hours. *Initial:* 200 mcg/kg (0.2 mg/kg) over 5 to 10 sec; 1 or 2 additional doses of 100 mcg/kg (0.1 mg/kg) given at 12- to 24-hr intervals, if needed.

Mechanism of Action

May inhibit the synthesis of E-series prostaglandins, which are thought to maintain the patency of the ductus arteriosus. By inhibiting prostaglandin synthesis, indomethacin promotes closure of a persistent patent ductus arteriosus.

Incompatibilities

Don't mix reconstituted indomethacin sodium with I.V. infusion solutions.

Contraindications

Allergy or hypersensitivity to aspirin, indomethacin, iodides, other NSAIDs, or their components; coagulation defects; active bleeding (especially intracranial hemorrhage or GI bleeding); coagulation defects; congenital heart disease requiring a patent ductus arteriosus to ensure adequate pulmonary or systemic blood flow; necrotizing enterocolitis (diagnosed or suspected); significantly impaired renal function; untreated infection (diagnosed or suspected); thrombocytopenia

Interactions

DRUGS

acetaminophen: Increased risk of adverse renal effects (with long-term use of both drugs)

aminoglycosides: Increased risk of aminoglycoside toxicity

aspirin, other NSAIDs: Increased risk of adverse GI effects and non-GI bleeding

bone marrow depressants: Possibly increased leukopenic or thrombocytopenic effects of these drugs

cefamandole, cefoperazone, cefotetan: Increased risk of hypoprothrombinemia and bleeding

colchicine, platelet aggregation inhibitors: Increased risk of GI bleeding, hemorrhage, and ulcers

corticosteroids, potassium supplements: Increased risk of adverse GI effects

cyclosporine: Increased risk of nephrotoxicity from both drugs, increased blood cyclosporine level

diflunisal: Increased blood indomethacin level and risk of GI bleeding

digoxin: Increased blood digoxin level and risk of digitalis toxicity

diuretics (loop, potassium-sparing, and thiazide): Decreased diuretic and antihypertensive effects *gold compounds, lithium, methotrexate, and other nephrotoxic drugs:* Increased risk of adverse renal effects

heparin, oral anticoagulants, thrombolytics: Increased anticoagulant effects and risk of hemorrhage

plicamycin, valproic acid: Increased risk of hypoprothrombinemia and GI bleeding, hemorrhage, and ulcers

Adverse Reactions

CNS: Intracranial hemorrhage

CV: Bradycardia, fluid retention, pulmonary hypertension

ENDO: Hypoglycemia

GI: Abdominal distention, GI bleeding, hepatic dysfunction, ileus (transient), intestinal perforation, vomiting

GU: Oliguria, renal dysfunction

HEME: Unusual bleeding or bruising

Other: Hyperkalemia, hyponatremia

Nursing Considerations

- To reconstitute indomethacin, add 1 to 2 ml of preservative-free sodium chloride for injection or preservative-free sterile water to vial. A solution made with 1 ml of diluent contains 100 mcg (0.1 mg) of indomethacin/0.1 ml. A solution made with 2 ml of diluent contains 50 mcg (0.05 mg) of indomethacin/0.1 ml. Use solution immediately because it contains no preservatives. Discard unused portion.
- Be aware that scheduled doses may be withheld if infant or neonate has anuria or a significant decrease in urine output (less than 0.6 ml/kg/hr).
- Avoid extravasation to protect surrounding tissue.
- Anticipate a second course (another three doses) of indomethacin if patent ductus arteriosus fails to close or reopens. After two courses, surgery may be performed.
- Because indomethacin causes sodium retention, monitor weight and blood pressure, especially if patient has hypertension.
- Be alert for signs of GI bleeding and ulceration, which can occur without warning.
- **WARNING** Be aware that drug's anti-inflammatory action may mask signs of infection.

PATIENT TEACHING

- Urge parents to immediately report bloody or black, tarry stools; fever; itching; rash; or swelling in arms or legs.

infliximab

Remicade

Class and Category

Chemical: Monoclonal antibody
Therapeutic: Anti-inflammatory
Pregnancy category: C

Indications and Dosages

▶ *To manage moderate to severe Crohn's disease*

I.V. INFUSION

Adults. 5 mg/kg over 2 hr.

DOSAGE ADJUSTMENT For patients with fistulizing Crohn's disease, 5-mg/kg infusion repeated 2 and 6 wk after first infusion.

▶ *To treat signs and symptoms and inhibit progression of structural damage in patients with moderate to severe active rheumatoid arthritis in combination with methotrexate therapy when patient hasn't responded to methotrexate alone*

I.V. INFUSION

Adults. 3 mg/kg over at least 2 hr; repeated 2 wk and 6 wk after initial infusion and then q 8 wk.

DOSAGE ADJUSTMENT For patients with an incomplete response, dosage may be increased to 10 mg/kg, or frequency may be increased to q 4 wk.

Mechanism of Action

Binds with cytokine tumor necrosis factor alpha (TNF alpha), thus preventing it from binding with its receptors. As a result, TNF alpha can't induce proinflammatory cytokines (such as interleukins) and increase endothelial permeability (a change that normally enhances leukocyte migration). These actions lead to reduced infiltration of inflammatory cells into inflamed areas of the intestine and joints.

Incompatibilities

Don't infuse infliximab in same I.V. line with other drugs or through plasticized polyvinyl chloride infusion equipment or devices.

Contraindications

Hypersensitivity to infliximab, murine proteins, or their components

Interactions

None known.

Adverse Reactions

CNS: Chills, dizziness, fatigue, fever, headache, syncope
CV: Chest pain, hypertension, hypotension
EENT: Oral candidiasis, pharyngitis, rhinitis, sinusitis
GI: Abdominal hernia, abdominal pain; cholecystitis; diarrhea; intestinal obstruction, perforation, or stenosis; nausea; splenic infarction; splenomegaly; vomiting
GU: Kidney infarction, ureteral obstruction, UTI, vaginal candidiasis, vaginitis
HEME: Thrombocytopenia
MS: Back pain, myalgia
RESP: Bronchitis, cough, dyspnea, pneumonia, upper respiratory tract infection, wheezing
SKIN: Facial flushing, pruritus, rash, urticaria
Other: Lupuslike symptoms, lymphoma

Nursing Considerations

- To reconstitute infliximab, use a 21G (or smaller) needle to add 10 ml of sterile water for injection to each vial of drug. Swirl gently to mix; don't shake. Be aware that solution may foam and be clear or light yellow.
- Withdraw a volume equal to amount of reconstituted drug from a 250-ml glass bottle or a polypropylene or polyolefin infusion bag of NS. Then add the reconstituted infliximab to the bottle to dilute it to 250 ml. Use within 3 hours.
- Administer infliximab infusion over at least 2 hours, using a polyethylene-lined infusion set with an in-line, sterile, nonpyrogenic, low-protein-binding filter that is 1.2 microns or less in pore size. Don't reuse infusion set.
- Be prepared to stop infusion if a hypersensitivity reaction occurs. Keep acetaminophen, antihistamines, corticosteroids, and epinephrine on hand for immediate use. A reaction may occur 2 hours to 12 days after infusion.
- Assess for signs of infection, especially if patient receives immunosuppressant therapy or has a chronic infection. Upper res-

piratory tract infections and UTIs are most common, but sepsis and fatal infections have occurred.
- Before using infliximab, store it at 2° to 8° C (36° to 46° F); don't freeze.

PATIENT TEACHING
- Explain that infliximab won't cure Crohn's disease but can promote remission by decreasing inflammation.
- Inform patient that drug can be given only by I.V. route and should take effect within 1 to 2 weeks.
- Urge patient to report signs of infection, such as burning with urination, cough, and sore throat, as well as signs of an infusion reaction, such as chest pain, chills, dyspnea, facial flushing, fever, itching, headache, and rash. Inform him that an infusion reaction may occur up to 12 days after he receives the drug.

insulin injection, regular
Regular Iletin II, Regular Insulin
insulin human injection, regular
Humulin R, Novolin ge Toronto (CAN), Novolin R
insulin human injection, buffered regular
Velosulin BR

Class and Category
Chemical: Polypeptide hormone
Therapeutic: Antidiabetic
Pregnancy category: B

Indications and Dosages
▶ *To treat diabetic ketoacidosis*
I.V. INJECTION OR INFUSION
Adults and adolescents. Loading dose of 0.15 USP Insulin Unit/kg, followed by 0.1 USP Insulin Unit/kg/hr by continuous infusion.

Route	Onset	Peak	Duration
I.V.*	10 to 30 min	15 to 30 min	30 to 60 min

Contraindications
Hypersensitivity to specific insulin preparation (animal or human)

*Individual responses vary.

Mechanism of Action

Controls the storage and metabolism of carbohydrates, proteins, and fats that bind to receptor sites on cellular plasma membranes, especially in the liver, muscle, and adipose tissues. In hyperglycemia, the body lacks sufficient insulin or is unable to use insulin to transport glucose through the cellular membranes. When this occurs, the body uses proteins and fats for energy. The liver produces excess ketone bodies, which accumulate in the blood; metabolic acidosis develops, resulting in diabetic ketoacidosis.

Insulin stimulates carbohydrate metabolism in skeletal and cardiac muscle and adipose tissue by facilitating transport of glucose into these cells. It also increases conversion of glucose to glycogen in the liver and suppresses hepatic glucose output.

Interactions

DRUGS

ACE inhibitors, anabolic steroids (such as stanozolol and oxandrolone), androgens, antidiabetic drugs, bromocriptine, clofibrate, ketoconazole, lithium, mebendazole, pyridoxine, sulfonamides, theophylline: Increased risk of hypoglycemia

beta blockers (systemic and oral), guanethidine, MAO inhibitors (such as furazolidone), procarbazine: Possibly hyperglycemia or hypoglycemia and masking of hypoglycemic adverse effects

calcium channel blockers, clonidine, corticosteroids, danazole, dextrothyroxine, diazoxide (parenteral), epinephrine, estrogen, glucagon, growth hormone, heparin, loop and thiazide diuretics, morphine, oral contraceptives (containing estrogen and progestin), phenytoin, sulfinpyrazone, thyroid hormones: Possibly hyperglycemia

carbonic anhydrase inhibitors (such as acetazolamide), sulfonylureas: Possibly increased hypoglycemic response

chloroquine, quinidine, quinine: Increased risk of hypoglycemia, increased blood insulin level

NSAIDs, salicylates (large doses): Increased hypoglycemic effect

octreotide: Possibly hyperglycemia or hypoglycemia

pentamidine: Possibly hyperglycemia, hypoglycemia, or hypoinsulinemia

tetracycline: Increased tissue sensitivity to insulin

ACTIVITIES

alcohol use: Increased hypoglycemic effect of insulin, increased risk of prolonged hypoglycemia

marijuana use, smoking: Possibly hyperglycemia

Adverse Reactions

CV: Edema
ENDO: Hypoglycemia
Other: Allergic reaction, weight gain

Nursing Considerations

- **WARNING** Be aware that the 100-USP unit concentration of regular insulin is the only type of insulin that should be used for I.V. infusion.
- Monitor patient's blood glucose level frequently, as ordered, before starting insulin infusion and at least hourly, as ordered, during the infusion.
- Don't use cloudy or viscous regular insulin. Use only clear, colorless solutions. In addition, use only syringes specifically calibrated to measure 100–USP unit concentrations when preparing for infusion.
- Be aware that insulin can be adsorbed to glass and plastic I.V. infusion containers and I.V. tubing. To minimize adsorption, allow 50 ml of diluted solution to run through the infusion apparatus before use and wait 30 minutes to administer a prepared solution. Follow facility protocols for preparing and administering insulin I.V. infusions.
- Monitor urine ketone and glucose levels, as ordered. Expect *urine* glucose levels to return to normal more slowly than *blood* glucose levels.
- Be aware that patients with impaired renal or hepatic function may require an increase or decrease in insulin dosage.
- Monitor blood pH and serum electrolyte levels, particularly potassium, sodium chloride, and phosphate, as ordered. After initially experiencing hyperkalemia due to decreased pH, patient may develop hypokalemia as potassium reenters cells with insulin administration.
- Expect to decrease infusion rate when blood glucose level is 300 mg/dl or less. Expect a separate infusion of D_5W to be ordered when blood glucose level is 250 mg/dl.
- Assess patient for signs and symptoms of hypoglycemia, including anxiety, behavioral changes, blurred vision, cold sweats, confusion, cool skin, decreased concentration, headache, hunger, nausea, nervousness, nightmares, restless sleep, pallor, shakiness, slurred speech, tachycardia, tiredness, and weakness. Severe hypoglycemia may also cause coma or seizures.

- Anticipate an appropriate S.C. or I.M. dose of insulin to be ordered 30 minutes before discontinuation of insulin infusion.
- Store regular insulin at 2° to 8° C (36° to 46° F); protect from freezing and sunlight.

PATIENT TEACHING
- Advise patient receiving insulin infusion to immediately report signs of abnormal blood glucose level, including anxiety, tachycardia, blurred vision, and tremors.
- Review with patient events that may trigger a change in insulin requirements, including fever, infection, injury, psychological or physical stress, surgery, and medical conditions affecting food intake or absorption, such as vomiting and diarrhea.
- Stress the importance of keeping follow-up appointments, of administering insulin as prescribed, and of self-monitoring blood glucose level.
- Refer patient to an outpatient diabetes education program, if needed, for additional information and support.

interferon alfa-2b, recombinant
Intron A

Class and Category
Chemical: Cytokine
Therapeutic: Antineoplastic, immunomodulator
Pregnancy category: C

Indications and Dosages
▶ *To treat malignant melanoma*
I.V. INFUSION, S.C. INJECTION
Adults. *Initial:* 20 million IU/m^2 I.V. for 5 consecutive days/wk for 4 wk. *Maintenance:* 10 million IU/m^2 S.C. 3 times/week for 48 wk.

Mechanism of Action
Believed to exert a cytostatic effect, reducing the rate of cell proliferation by delaying RNA and protein production. This delay induces cells to enter a resting stage. Interferon alfa-2b also increases the action of human natural killer cells, which have the ability to lyse certain tumor cells and normal targets. In addition, the drug selectively increases the number of cytotoxic T-cells, thereby affecting tumor growth, and increases phagocytic activity of macrophages.

Contraindications

Hypersensitivity to interferon alfa or its components

Interactions

DRUGS

barbiturates and other CNS depressants: Possibly increased CNS depression

blood-dyscrasia–causing drugs (such as cephalosporins and sulfasalazine): Increased risk of leukopenia and thrombocytopenia

bone marrow depressants (such as carboplatin and lomustine): Possibly increased bone marrow depression

theophylline: Risk of decreased theophylline clearance and increased blood theophylline level

vaccines, killed virus: Possibly decreased antibody response to vaccine

vaccines, live virus: Possibly decreased antibody response to vaccine, increased adverse effects of vaccine, and severe infection

ACTIVITIES

alcohol use: Increased risk of CNS depression

Adverse Reactions

CNS: Dizziness, fatigue, neurotoxicity, peripheral neuropathy
CV: Cardiotoxicity, hypotension
EENT: Altered taste, blurred vision, dry mouth, stomatitis
GI: Anorexia, diarrhea, hepatotoxicity, nausea, vomiting
HEME: Anemia, leukopenia, neutropenia, thrombocytopenia
MS: Leg cramps
SKIN: Alopecia, diaphoresis, dry skin, pruritus, rash
Other: Flulike symptoms, weight loss

Nursing Considerations

- **WARNING** Be aware that recombinant interferon alfa-2b is *not* interchangeable with other interferon preparations, including interferon alfa-2a, -n1, and -n3. Don't use interferon alfa-2b solution for injection for I.V. treatment of malignant melanoma; use the recombinant powder for injection.
- Monitor liver function tests, hematocrit, hemoglobin, platelet count, and total and differential leukocyte count before and periodically during therapy.
- Obtain an ECG before and during therapy, as ordered, in patients with a history of cardiac disease or advanced malignant melanoma.
- Anticipate the need to hydrate patient before therapy. Monitor blood pressure during therapy to detect hypotensive changes.

- Reconstitute interferon with appropriate amount of bacteriostatic water for injection provided by manufacturer. Agitate gently to dissolve. Expect liquid to be clear and colorless to light yellow. Use within 1 month if stored between 2° and 8° C (36° and 46° F).
- Be aware that patients receiving concurrent or consecutive radiation therapy and those who have received previous cytotoxic drug therapy are at risk for additive bone marrow depression. Expect prescriber to decrease dosage.
- If patient develops thrombocytopenia, implement protective precautions according to facility policy.
- Monitor patients with severe renal disease for exacerbation caused by fever and dehydrating effects of interferon alfa-2b. Monitor patients with cardiac disease (including recent MI), diabetes mellitus prone to ketoacidosis, or pulmonary disease for exacerbations of these conditions caused by interferon-induced fever and chills.
- Monitor patients with herpes zoster or recent or current chicken pox (including recent exposure) for signs and symptoms of severe generalized disease.
- Assess patients with a history of autoimmune disease for exacerbation of condition.
- Be aware that elderly patients may be more prone to drug's adverse effects because of underlying CNS, cardiac, or renal disease.
- Be aware that patients with a history of compromised CNS function, severe psychiatric conditions, or seizure disorders are at risk for severe CNS adverse reactions. Neuropsychiatric follow-up may be ordered, especially for patients receiving high doses of drug.
- Administer acetaminophen, as ordered, to prevent or treat flu-like symptoms, such as fever or headache.
- Be aware that interferon alfa-2b is also given S.C. in combination with ribavirin for treatment of chronic hepatitis. Consult manufacturer's insert for specific information, including contraindications, adverse reactions, and nursing considerations, relating to combination therapy.
- Store drug at 2° to 8° C (36° to 46° F).

PATIENT TEACHING
- Advise patient to avoid potentially hazardous activities until interferon alfa-2b's CNS effects are known.
- Instruct patient to avoid alcohol and CNS depressants during therapy.

- Advise patient to contact prescriber immediately if he notices unusual bleeding or bruising, black or tarry stools, blood in urine or stools, or red pinpoint spots on skin.
- Instruct patient to avoid touching his eyes or inside of nose unless he washes hands immediately beforehand.
- Urge patient to avoid people with infection if he develops bone marrow depression. Advise him to contact prescriber if he experiences fever, chills, cough, hoarseness, lower back or side pain, or painful or difficult urination because these signs and symptoms may signal an infection.
- Teach patient proper oral hygiene, and advise him to use a soft-bristled toothbrush because drug can delay healing, increase the risk of infection, and cause gingival bleeding. Advise patient to check with prescriber before undergoing any dental work.
- Stress the importance of avoiding accidental cuts from sharp objects, such as razors and fingernail clippers, because excessive bleeding or infection may occur. Also, caution patient to avoid contact sports and other activities that increase the risk of injury.
- If patient will self-administer interferon alpha-2b, teach him and his caregiver the proper administration technique, including bedtime administration to decrease effect of fatigue on daily activities.
- Caution patient and caregiver not to reuse needles or syringes, and teach them how to properly dispose of needles and syringes in puncture-resistant containers.
- Stress the importance of complying with the dosage regimen and of keeping follow-up medical appointments and appointments for laboratory tests.

irinotecan hydrochloride

Camptosar

Class and Category

Chemical: Synthetic camptothecin derivative
Therapeutic: Antineoplastic
Pregnancy category: D

Indications and Dosages

▶ *To treat colorectal cancer*

I.V. INFUSION

Adults receiving drug as a single agent. 125 mg/m^2 over 90 min q wk for 4 wk, followed by 2-wk rest period, then subsequent courses. Alternatively, 240 to 350 mg/m^2 over 90 min q 3 wk. *Maximum:* 150 mg/m^2/wk.

DOSAGE ADJUSTMENT Dosage is highly individualized, ranging from 50 to 150 mg/m^2, and may be adjusted in increments—typically of 25 to 50 mg/m^2. Doses may even be omitted, based on severity of adverse reactions, according to the National Cancer Institute's (NCI) Common Toxicity Criteria. (See *Selected Common Toxicity Criteria* in the appendices.) Expect initial dose to be decreased to 100 mg/m^2 or less for patients over age 65 with impaired hepatic function *and* a history of pelvic or abdominal irradiation.

Adults receiving drug in combination with fluorouracil and leucovorin. If administering fluorouracil-leucovorin boluses, 125 mg/m^2 over 90 minutes on days 1, 8, 15, and 22, with next course beginning on day 43. Alternatively, if administering fluorouracil-leucovorin infusions, 180 mg/m^2 over 90 minutes on days 1, 15, and 29, with next course beginning on day 43. *Maximum:* 125 mg/m^2/wk.

DOSAGE ADJUSTMENT Dosage reduced or doses omitted based on severity of adverse reactions, according to NCI's Common Toxicity Criteria.

Mechanism of Action

Inhibits the activity of topoisomerase I, an enzyme that allows single-strand breaks in the double-stranded DNA chain. Single-strand breaks during DNA replication, recombination, and repair decrease the torsional strain of the DNA configuration. Irinotrecan and its metabolite, SN-38, bind to the topoisomerase I complex and prevent religation of the single-strand breaks, which normally takes place after the DNA has relaxed. This action halts DNA replication, resulting in DNA damage and, eventually, in cell death.

Incompatibilities

Don't refrigerate irinotecan diluted with NS because a precipitate may form. Don't mix irinotecan with any other drugs.

Contraindications

Hypersensitivity to irinotecan

Interactions

DRUGS

blood-dyscrasia–causing drugs (such as cephalosporins and sulfasalazine): Increased risk of leukopenia and thrombocytopenia

bone marrow depressants (such as carboplatin and lomustine): Possibly additive bone marrow depression

corticosteroids, cyclosporine, and other immunosuppressive drugs: Increased risk of infection

dexamethasone: Possibly hyperglycemia, increased risk of lymphocytopenia

laxatives: Increased risk of severe diarrhea

vaccine, killed virus: Possibly decreased antibody response to vaccine

vaccine, live virus: Possibly decreased antibody response to vaccine, increased adverse effects of vaccine, and severe infection

Adverse Reactions

CNS: Asthenia, chills, fever, headache

CV: Bradycardia, edema, vasodilation (flushing)

EENT: Rhinitis, stomatitis

GI: Abdominal cramps or pain, abdominal distention, anorexia, bloating, constipation, diarrhea, indigestion, nausea, vomiting

HEME: Anemia, leukopenia, neutropenia, thrombocytopenia

RESP: Cough, dyspnea, upper respiratory tract infection

SKIN: Alopecia, diaphoresis, rash

Other: Allergic reaction, anaphylaxis, dehydration, infection (minor), weight loss

Nursing Considerations

- Be aware that irinotecan should be administered only under the supervision of a qualified physician and in a setting where appropriate diagnostic and treatment facilities are available.
- Expect to obtain hemoglobin level and leukocyte and platelet counts before beginning each course of therapy and periodically thereafter. Expect dosage to be adjusted if test results reveal hematologic toxicity—for example, a granulocyte count less than $1,500/mm^3$ or a platelet count less than $100,000/mm^3$.
- Follow facility policy for handling antineoplastic drugs and for appropriate disposal of used equipment. If irinotecan solution comes in contact with your skin, wash if off thoroughly with soap and water. If drug comes in contact with mucous membranes, irrigate the area thoroughly with water.
- Dilute irinotecan with D_5W (preferred) or NS to a concentration of 0.12 to 2.8 mg/ml. Discard unused portion in single-use vials (2 ml and 5 ml).
- Because drug contains no preservatives, use solutions prepared with D_5W within 6 hours if stored at controlled room temper-

ature or within 24 hours if refrigerated at 2° to 8° C (36° to 46° F).

- Don't refrigerate solutions diluted with NS because a precipitate will form. Use solutions prepared with NS within 6 hours if stored at room temperature.

- Be aware that adverse reactions can vary when irinotecan is administered in combination therapy. Review information for all drugs administered as part of a specific regimen, including drug interactions and adverse effects. Expect dosage to be adjusted based on type of combination therapy used and on incidence and severity of adverse reactions.

- Assess patient's GI status frequently for signs of diarrhea, which may occur immediately after a dose of irinotecan or more than 24 hours afterward. Expect prescriber to order loperamide at first sign of diarrhea or increased frequency of bowel movements.

- Monitor liver function test results periodically, as prescribed, to identify signs of hepatic function impairment or worsening impairment.

- Monitor patients with herpes zoster or recent or current chicken pox (including recent exposure) for signs and symptoms of severe generalized disease.

- Assess for signs of infection, such as fever, if patient develops leukopenia. Expect to obtain appropriate specimens for culture and sensitivity testing. Be aware that patients with a preexisting infection may experience impaired recovery.

- Be aware that patients receiving concurrent or consecutive radiation therapy and those with preexisting bone marrow depression are at risk for increased bone marrow depression.

- If extravasation occurs, stop the infusion, flush the area with sterile water, and apply ice. Then restart the infusion in another vein.

- Monitor patients with drug-induced vomiting and diarrhea for signs of dehydration, such as decreased urine output, poor skin turgor, dry and furrowed tongue, and dry mucous membranes. Patients taking diuretics are at increased risk and may have diuretic withheld if vomiting or diarrhea occurs.

- Store drug at 15° to 30° C (59° to 86° F); protect from freezing and light.

PATIENT TEACHING

- Advise patient to have dental work completed before irinotecan treatment begins, if possible, or to defer such work until blood counts return to normal because drug can delay healing and cause gingival bleeding. Teach patient proper oral hygiene, and suggest that he use a toothbrush with soft bristles.
- Instruct patient to immediately report nausea, vomiting, or diarrhea during irinotecan therapy. Advise him to avoid foods that may irritate the GI system, including high-fiber foods (bran, whole grain breads, and raw fruits and vegetables) and fatty, spicy, or fried foods.
- Advise patient to report burning or other signs of extravasation, such as redness, at I.V. insertion site.
- Encourage patient to drink fluids as prescribed. Urge him to avoid alcohol and caffeinated beverages, such as coffee and cola, which can exacerbate dehydration.
- If patient develops thrombocytopenia, implement protective precautions according to facility policy.
- Urge patient to avoid people with infection if he develops bone marrow depression. Advise him to contact prescriber if he experiences fever, chills, cough, hoarseness, lower back or side pain, or painful or difficult urination because these signs and symptoms may signal an infection.
- Advise patient to contact prescriber immediately if he notices unusual bleeding or bruising, black or tarry stools, blood in urine or stools, or red pinpoint spots on skin.
- Instruct patient to avoid touching his eyes or inside of nose unless he washes hands immediately beforehand.
- Stress the importance of avoiding accidental cuts from sharp objects, such as razors or nail clippers, because excessive bleeding or infection may occur. Also, caution patient to avoid contact sports and other activities that increase the risk of injury.
- Caution patient to avoid receiving immunizations unless approved by prescriber. Instruct him to avoid people who have recently received vaccines or to wear a protective mask that covers his nose and mouth when he's around them.
- Advise patient with stomatitis to eat bland, soft foods served cold or at room temperature to decrease irritation.
- Stress the importance of complying with the dosage regimen and of keeping follow-up medical appointments and appointments for laboratory tests.

iron dextran
(contains 50 mg of elemental iron per milliliter)
DexFerrum, DexIron (CAN), InFeD

Class and Category
Chemical: Iron salt, mineral
Therapeutic: Antianemic
Pregnancy category: C

Indications and Dosages
▶ *To treat iron deficiency anemia*
I.V. INFUSION
Adults and children who weigh over 15 kg (33 lb). Dose
(ml) = 0.0442 (desired hemoglobin − observed hemoglobin) ×
lean body weight (in kg) + (0.26 × lean body weight). Alternatively, consult dosage table in package insert. *Maximum:* 2 ml
(100 mg)/day.
**Children over age 4 months who weigh 5 to 15 kg (11 to
33 lb).** Dose (ml) = 0.0442 (desired hemoglobin − observed hemoglobin) × weight (kg) + (0.26 × weight). Alternatively, consult dosage table in package insert. *Maximum:* 1 ml (50 mg)/day.
▶ *To replace iron lost in blood loss*
I.V. INFUSION
Adults. Replacement iron (mg) = ml of blood loss × hematocrit.

Mechanism of Action
Restores hemoglobin and replenishes iron stores. Iron, an essential component of hemoglobin, myoglobin, and several enzymes (including cytochromes, catalase, and peroxidase), is needed for catecholamine metabolism and normal neutrophil function. In iron dextran therapy, iron binds to available protein parts after the drug has been split into iron and dextran by cells of the reticuloendothelial system. The bound iron forms hemosiderin or ferritin, physiologic forms of iron, and transferrin, which replenish hemoglobin and depleted iron stores. Dextran is metabolized or excreted.

Incompatibilities
Don't mix iron dextran with blood for transfusion, other drugs,
or parenteral nutrition solutions for I.V. infusion.

Contraindications
Anemia other than iron deficiency, hypersensitivity to iron dextran or its components

Interactions
None known.

Adverse Reactions
CNS: Chills, disorientation, dizziness, fever, headache, malaise, paresthesia, seizures, syncope, unconsciousness, weakness
CV: Arrhythmias, bradycardia, chest pain, shock, hypotension, hypertension, tachycardia
EENT: Altered taste
GI: Abdominal pain, diarrhea, nausea, vomiting
GU: Hematuria
HEME: Leukocytosis
MS: Arthralgia, arthritis, backache, myalgia, rhabdomyolysis
RESP: Bronchospasm, dyspnea, respiratory arrest, wheezing
SKIN: Cyanosis, diaphoresis, rash, pruritus, purpura, urticaria
Other: Anaphylaxis, infusion site phlebitis

Nursing Considerations
- Expect oral iron therapy to be discontinued before iron dextran therapy is initiated. Iron dextran is administered only when oral therapy is not feasible; it also may be administered by I.M. injection.
- Expect to monitor hemoglobin, hematocrit, serum ferritin, and transferrin saturation, as ordered, before, during, and after iron dextran therapy.
- **WARNING** Before initiating therapy, administer a test dose of 0.5 ml of iron dextran gradually over 30 seconds, as prescribed, and monitor closely for an anaphylactic reaction.
- Wait 1 to 2 hours before administering the remainder of the dose. Infuse undiluted iron dextran slowly, at a rate not to exceed 1 ml/minute (50 mg/minute).
- **WARNING** Monitor patient closely for signs and symptoms of anaphylaxis, such as severe hypotension, loss of consciousness, collapse, dyspnea, and seizures, during and after infusion. Patients with a history of asthma or known allergies are at increased risk for anaphylaxis and, possibly, death. Institute emergency resuscitation measures as needed, including epinephrine administration, as prescribed.
- **WARNING** Assess blood pressure frequently after drug administration because hypotension is a common adverse effect that may be related to infusion rate; avoid rapid infusion.

- Be aware that patient may exhibit adverse reactions, including arthralgia, backache, chills, and vomiting, 1 to 2 days after drug therapy. Symptoms should resolve within 3 to 4 days.
- Assess patients with a history of rheumatoid arthritis for exacerbation of joint pain and swelling.
- Monitor patients with preexisting cardiovascular disease for an exacerbation due to drug's adverse effects.
- Assess patient for iron overload, characterized by sedation, decreased activity, pale eyes, and bleeding in GI tract and lungs.
- Store iron dextran at 15° to 30° C (59° to 86° F).

PATIENT TEACHING

- Instruct patient to immediately report signs of an adverse reaction, such as shortness of breath, wheezing, or rash, during iron dextran therapy.
- Advise patient not to take any oral iron preparations without first consulting prescriber.
- Inform patient that symptoms of iron deficiency may include decreased stamina, learning problems, shortness of breath, and fatigue. During periods of anemia, encourage patient to plan periods of activity and rest in order to avoid excessive fatigue.
- Stress the importance of following dosage regimen and of keeping follow-up medical appointments and appointments for laboratory tests.

iron sucrose

(contains 100 mg of elemental iron per 5 ml)
Venofer

Class and Category

Chemical: Iron salt, mineral
Therapeutic: Antianemic
Pregnancy category: B

Indications and Dosages

▶ *To treat iron deficiency anemia in hemodialysis patients receiving erythropoietin*

I.V. INFUSION OR INJECTION

Adults. *Initial:* 100 mg of elemental iron during dialysis. *Usual:* 100 mg of elemental iron q wk to 3 times/wk to a total dose of 1,000 mg. Dosage repeated as needed to maintain target levels of hemoglobin and hematocrit and acceptable blood iron levels. *Maximum:* 100 mg/dose.

Mechanism of Action

Acts to replenish iron stores lost during dialysis because of increased erythropoiesis and insufficient absorption of iron from the GI tract. Iron is an essential component of hemoglobin, myoglobin, and several enzymes (including cytochromes, catalase, and peroxidase), and is needed for catecholamine metabolism and normal neutrophil function. Iron sucrose injection also normalizes RBC production by binding with hemoglobin or being stored as ferritin in reticuloendothelial cells of the liver, spleen, and bone marrow.

Incompatibilities

Don't mix iron sucrose with other drugs or parenteral nutrition solutions for I.V. infusion.

Contraindications

Anemia other than iron deficiency, hypersensitivity to iron salts or their components, iron overload

Interactions

DRUGS

chloramphenicol: Possibly decreased effectiveness of iron sucrose
oral iron preparations: Possibly reduced absorption of oral iron supplements

Adverse Reactions

CNS: Dizziness, fever, headache, malaise
CV: Chest pain, hypertension, hypotension
GI: Abdominal pain, diarrhea, elevated liver function test results, nausea, vomiting
MS: Leg cramps, muscle weakness, myalgia
RESP: Cough, dyspnea, pneumonia
SKIN: Pruritus
Other: Anaphylaxis, fluid overload, infusion or injection site redness

Nursing Considerations

• Expect to monitor hemoglobin, hematocrit, serum ferritin, and transferrin saturation, as ordered, before, during, and after iron sucrose therapy. Make sure that serum iron levels are tested 48 hours after last dose. Notify prescriber and expect to discontinue therapy if blood iron levels are normal or elevated, to prevent iron toxicity.

- To reconstitute iron sucrose injection for infusion, dilute 100 mg of elemental iron in a maximum of 100 ml of NS immediately before infusion. Infuse over at least 15 minutes. Discard any unused diluted solution.
- Administer drug directly into a dialysis line by slow I.V. injection or by infusion at a rate of 20 mg/minute, not to exceed 100 mg per injection.
- **WARNING** Monitor closely for signs and symptoms of anaphylaxis, such as severe hypotension, loss of consciousness, collapse, dyspnea, or seizures, during and after drug administration. Institute emergency resuscitation measures as needed.
- **WARNING** Assess blood pressure frequently after drug administration because hypotension is a common adverse reaction that may be related to infusion rate or total cumulative dose; avoid rapid infusion.
- Assess patient for iron overload, characterized by sedation, decreased activity, pale eyes, and bleeding in GI tract and lungs.
- Store drug at controlled room temperature.

PATIENT TEACHING
- Advise patient not to take any oral iron preparations during iron sucrose therapy without first consulting prescriber.
- Inform patient that symptoms of iron deficiency may include decreased stamina, learning problems, shortness of breath, and fatigue.

isoproterenol hydrochloride
Isuprel

Class and Category
Chemical: Catecholamine
Therapeutic: Antiarrhythmic, bronchodilator
Pregnancy category: C

Indications and Dosages
▶ *To manage bronchospasm during anesthesia*
I.V. INJECTION
Adults. 0.01 to 0.02 mg, repeated p.r.n.
▶ *To treat bradycardia with significant hemodynamic change, such as third-degree heart block or prolonged QT interval*
I.V. INFUSION
Adults. *Initial:* 2 mcg/min, titrated according to heart rate, as ordered. *Maximum:* 10 mcg/min.

Route °	Onset	Peak	Duration
I.V.	In 5 min*	Unknown	10 min†

Mechanism of Action

Stimulates beta$_1$ receptors in the myocardium and cardiac conduction system, resulting in positive inotropic and chronotropic effects. Isoproterenol also shortens the AV conduction time and refractory period in patients with AV block. This action increases the ventricular rate and halts bradycardia and associated syncope.

In addition, isoproterenol attaches to beta$_2$ receptors on bronchial cell membranes. This action stimulates the intracellular enzyme adenylate cyclase to convert adenosine triphosphate to cAMP. An increased intracellular level of cAMP relaxes bronchial smooth-muscle cells, stabilizes mast cells, and inhibits histamine release.

Contraindications

Angina pectoris, heart block or tachycardia from digitalis toxicity, hypersensitivity to isoproterenol or its components (such as sulfite in some preparations), tachyarrhythmias, ventricular arrhythmias that require inotropic therapy

Interactions

DRUGS

alpha blockers, other drugs with alpha-blocking effects: Possibly decreased peripheral vasoconstricting and hypertensive effects of isoproterenol

astemizole, cisapride, drugs that prolong QTc interval, terfenadine: Possibly prolonged QTc interval

beta blockers (ophthalmic): Decreased effects of isoproterenol, increased risk of bronchospasm, wheezing, decreased pulmonary function, and respiratory failure

beta blockers (systemic): Increased risk of bronchospasm, decreased effects of both drugs

digoxin: Increased risk of arrhythmias, hypokalemia, and digitalis toxicity

diuretics, other antihypertensives: Possibly decreased antihypertensive effects

---

* For treatment of bradycardia; unknown for treatment of bronchospasm.
† For treatment of bradycardia; 1 to 2 hr for treatment of bronchospasm.

ergot alkaloids: Increased vasoconstriction and vasopressor effects
hydrocarbon inhalation anesthetics: Increased risk of atrial and ventricular arrhythmias
MAO inhibitors: Intensified and extended cardiac stimulation and vasopressor effects
quinidine, other drugs that affect myocardial reaction to sympathomimetics: Increased risk of arrhythmias
theophylline: Increased risk of cardiotoxicity, decreased blood theophylline level
thyroid hormones: Increased effects of both drugs, increased risk of coronary insufficiency in patients with coronary artery disease
tricyclic antidepressants: Increased vasopressor response, increased risk of prolonged QTc interval and arrhythmias

Adverse Reactions
CNS: Dizziness, headache, insomnia, nervousness, syncope, tremor, weakness
CV: Adams-Stokes syndrome, angina, arrhythmias, bradycardia, hypertension, hypotension, palpitations, tachycardia, ventricular arrhythmias
EENT: Blurred vision, oropharyngeal edema
ENDO: Hyperglycemia
GI: Nausea, vomiting
MS: Muscle spasms and twitching
RESP: Bronchospasm, dyspnea, wheezing
SKIN: Diaphoresis, erythema multiforme, pallor, pruritus, rash, Stevens-Johnson syndrome, urticaria
Other: Angioedema, hypokalemia

Nursing Considerations
- Expect to give lowest possible dose of isoproterenol for shortest possible time to minimize tolerance.
- Don't administer drug if it is pink or brown or contains precipitate.
- Inspect label carefully to verify correct concentration. Concentrations range from 0.02 mg/ml (1:50,000) to 0.2 mg/ml (1:5,000).
- Administer infusion through large vein, and monitor for signs of extravasation.
- Monitor blood pressure, cardiac rhythm, central venous pressure, and urine output during administration. Adjust infusion rate to response, as ordered.
- Notify prescriber immediately if heart rate increases significantly or exceeds 110 beats/minute during infusion.

- Know that drug may increase pulse pressure and cause hypotension. Expect to reduce infusion slowly to decrease the risk of hypotension.
- **WARNING** Be aware that isoproterenol markedly increases the risk of arrhythmias. If an arrhythmia occurs, expect to give a cardioselective beta blocker, such as atenolol, as prescribed.
- Be aware that isoproterenol isn't used regularly to treat asthma, decreased cardiac output, hypotension, or shock because it increases the risk of arrhythmias, hypotension, and ischemia.
- **WARNING** If isoproterenol aggravates a ventilation-perfusion problem, expect patient's blood oxygen level to fall even as his breathing seems to improve.
- Consult manufacturer's guidelines for storage information. Recommended temperature varies with form used.

PATIENT TEACHING
- Instruct patient receiving isoproterenol to report chest pain, difficulty breathing, dizziness, hyperglycemic symptoms (such as abdominal cramps, lethargy, nausea, and vomiting), insomnia, irregular heartbeat, palpitations, tremor, and weakness.

itraconazole
Sporanox

Class and Category
Chemical: Triazole derivative
Therapeutic: Antifungal
Pregnancy category: C

Indications and Dosages
▶ *To treat pulmonary and extrapulmonary blastomycosis, histoplasmosis, and refractory aspergillosis*
I.V. INFUSION
Adults and adolescents. 200 mg infused over 1 hr q 12 hr for 4 doses, then 200 mg q.d. Drug changed to P.O. form within 14 days and therapy continued for at least 3 mo.
DOSAGE ADJUSTMENT In life-threatening situations, loading dose adjusted to 200 mg P.O. or I.V. t.i.d. for 3 days. I.V. itraconazole shouldn't be used in patients with creatinine clearance of less than 30 ml/min/1.73 m^2.

▶ *To treat blastomycosis caused by* Blastomyces dermatitidis *and histoplasmosis caused by* Histoplasma capsulatum

CAPSULES

Adults and adolescents. *Initial:* 200 mg q.d., increased by 100 mg/day, if needed; dosage greater than 200 mg given in divided doses b.i.d. *Maximum:* 400 mg/day.

▶ *To treat aspergillosis that is unresponsive to amphotericin B*

CAPSULES

Adults and adolescents. 200 to 400 mg/day; dosage greater than 200 mg/day given in divided doses b.i.d.

Mechanism of Action

Inhibits the synthesis of ergosterol, an essential component of fungal cell membranes, by binding with a cytochrome P-450 enzyme necessary to convert lanosterol to ergosterol. The lack of ergosterol results in increased cellular permeability and leakage of cell contents. Itraconazole also may lead to fungal cell death by inhibiting fungal respiration under aerobic conditions.

Incompatibilities

Don't administer itraconazole through same I.V. line as other drugs. Don't mix I.V. itraconazole with D_5W or solutions that contain LR.

Contraindications

Concurrent therapy with astemizole, cisapride, HMG-CoA inhibitors (lovastatin and simvastatin), oral midazolam, pimozide, quinidine, terfenadine, or triazolam; hypersensitivity to itraconazole or its components

Interactions

DRUGS

antacids, anticholinergics, H_2-receptor antagonists, omeprazole, sucralfate: Possibly decreased itraconazole absorption (with oral form)

astemizole, terfenadine: Possibly increased blood levels of these drugs and risk of life-threatening arrhythmias and death

buspirone: Elevated blood buspirone level and increased risk of adverse effects

busulfan, docetaxel, vinca alkaloids: Possibly decreased blood levels of these drugs

calcium channel blockers: Possibly inhibited metabolism of these drugs *carbamazepine, phenobarbital:* Possibly decreased blood itraconazole level

cisapride: Possibly inhibited cisapride metabolism, which may lead to life-threatening CV complications as well as sudden death

clarithromycin: Possibly increased blood clarithromycin level

cyclosporine: Possibly increased blood cyclosporine level

didanosine: Possibly decreased therapeutic effects of itraconazole (with oral form)

digoxin: Possibly increased blood digoxin level and risk of digitalis toxicity

indinavir, ritonavir, saquinavir: Possibly increased blood levels of these drugs; possibly increased blood itraconazole level (indinavir, ritonavir)

isoniazid, rifabutin, rifampin, rifapentine: Decreased blood itraconazole level, possibly increased blood rifabutin level

lovastatin, simvastatin: Increased blood levels of these drugs, possibly rhabdomyolysis

oral antidiabetic drugs: Risk of hypoglycemia

oral midazolam, triazolam: Elevated blood levels and possibly prolonged sedative effects of these drugs

phenytoin: Possibly increased blood phenytoin level and decreased blood itraconazole level

pimozide, quinidine: Possibly life-threatening CV complications, including ventricular arrhythmias and death

tacrolimus: Increased blood tacrolimus level

warfarin: Increased anticoagulant effect of warfarin

Adverse Reactions

CNS: Chills, dizziness, drowsiness, fatigue, fever, headache, vertigo
CV: Hypertension
GI: Abdominal pain, anorexia, constipation, diarrhea, elevated liver function test results, flatulence, hepatotoxicity, hyperbilirubinemia, indigestion, nausea, vomiting
RESP: Cough, dyspnea
SKIN: Diaphoresis, pruritus, rash
Other: Hypokalemia

Nursing Considerations

- Be aware that I.V. itraconazole is for infusion only. Don't administer by bolus.
- **WARNING** Keep in mind that itraconazole is a potent inhibitor of the cytochrome P-450 3A4 (CYP3A4) isoenzyme system, which may increase blood levels of drugs metabolized by this system. Patients using such drugs as astemizole and

cisapride concomitantly with itraconazole or other CYP3A4 inhibitors have experienced life-threatening cardiovascular complications, such as prolonged QT interval, torsades de pointes, and ventricular tachycardia, as well as sudden death.

- Infuse each I.V. dose over 1 hour.
- Administer itraconazole capsules with a meal to ensure maximal absorption. However, don't administer oral solution with food.
- Keep in mind that patients with AIDS may have hypochlorhydria, which reduces drug absorption. Expect to administer higher doses of itraconazole to such patients.
- Monitor liver function test results in patients with impaired hepatic function and those who have experienced hepatotoxicity with other drugs.
- Assess for rash every 8 hours during therapy; notify prescriber if rash occurs.
- If patient also receives warfarin, monitor PT and assess for signs and symptoms of bleeding.
- If patient also receives digoxin, monitor blood digoxin level as appropriate to detect toxic level, and assess patient for signs and symptoms of digitalis toxicity, such as nausea and yellow vision.
- Store at or below 25° C (77° F); protect from freezing and light.

PATIENT TEACHING
- Advise patient receiving itraconazole to immediately report abdominal pain, diarrhea, headache, nausea, rash, or vomiting.
- Instruct patient to report signs of liver problems, such as abdominal pain, dark urine, fatigue, loss of appetite, pale stools, weakness, or yellow eyes or skin.
- Instruct patient to take itraconazole capsules with a meal.
- Advise patient to complete entire course of therapy, even if he feels better.
- If patient also takes an oral antidiabetic drug, instruct him to monitor his blood glucose level frequently because of the increased risk of hypoglycemia.
- Advise patient to avoid taking antacids with oral itraconazole.
- Advise patient to notify prescriber immediately of changes in other drugs, such as new drugs and dosage changes.
- Instruct patient to take a missed dose as soon as he remembers, unless it's within 4 hours of the next dose. Caution against double-dosing.
- Advise breast-feeding patient to consult prescriber about continuing breast-feeding during itraconazole therapy.

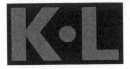

kanamycin sulfate
Kantrex

Class and Category
Chemical: Aminoglycoside
Therapeutic: Antibiotic
Pregnancy category: D

Indications and Dosages
▶ *To treat infections caused by gram-negative organisms (including* Acinetobacter *species,* Enterobacter aerogenes, Escherichia coli, Haemophilus influenzae, Klebsiella pneumoniae, Neisseria *species,* Proteus *species,* Providencia *species,* Salmonella *species,* Serratia marcescens, Shigella *species, and* Yersinia *species) and gram-positive organisms (including* Staphylococcus aureus and Staphylococcus epidermidis*)*

I.V. INFUSION
Adults and children. 5 mg/kg q 8 hr or 7.5 mg/kg q 12 hr for 7 to 10 days. *Maximum:* 1.5 g/day.

DOSAGE ADJUSTMENT For elderly patients and those with renal failure, dosage reduced and blood kanamycin level and renal function test results monitored.

Route	Onset	Peak	Duration
I.V.	Rapid	Unknown	Unknown

Mechanism of Action
Binds to negatively charged sites on bacterial outer cell membranes, which disrupts cell membrane integrity. Kanamycin also binds to bacterial ribosomal subunits and inhibits protein synthesis; these actions lead to cell death.

Contraindications
Hypersensitivity to kanamycin, other aminoglycosides, or their components

Incompatibilities
Don't mix kanamycin in same syringe or administer through same I.V. line as other antibiotics.

Interactions
DRUGS
cephalosporins, vancomycin: Increased risk of nephrotoxicity
digoxin, loop diuretics: Increased ototoxic and nephrotoxic effects of kanamycin
general anesthetics, neuromuscular blockers: Increased risk of neuromuscular blockade
penicillins: Inactivation of kanamycin or synergistic effects

Adverse Reactions
CNS: Ataxia, dizziness, headache
EENT: Hearing loss
GI: Diarrhea
GU: Elevated BUN and serum creatinine levels, oliguria, proteinuria
MS: Muscle paralysis
RESP: Apnea
SKIN: Injection site irritation or pain, rash, pruritus, urticaria

Nursing Considerations
- Obtain body fluid or tissue specimen for culture and sensitivity testing before kanamycin therapy begins, as indicated. Therapy may begin before test results are available.
- Dilute 500-mg vial with 100 to 200 ml of NS or D_5W, or 1-g vial with 200 to 400 ml of NS or D_5W, and infuse over 30 to 60 minutes. Adjust amount of diluent proportionately for pediatric doses. Be aware that vial contents may darken during storage but that this won't affect potency.
- Keep patient well hydrated before and during therapy.
- Monitor blood kanamycin level periodically during therapy, as appropriate.
- Be aware that prolonged treatment increases the risk of ototoxicity and nephrotoxicity. Monitor hearing and renal function if therapy lasts longer than 10 days.
- Store drug at 15° to 30° C (59° to 86° F); don't freeze.

PATIENT TEACHING
- Advise patient to report dizziness, hearing loss, and severe diarrhea or headache during kanamycin therapy.
- Explain the need to receive kanamycin at prescribed intervals around the clock until patient completes full course of therapy.

ketorolac tromethamine
Toradol

Class and Category
Chemical: Acetic acid derivative
Therapeutic: Analgesic, anti-inflammatory
Pregnancy category: C

Indications and Dosages
▶ *To treat moderate to severe pain*
I.V. INJECTION
Adults ages 16 to 64. *Initial:* 30 mg as a single dose or 30 mg q 6 hr p.r.n. *Maximum:* 120 mg/day for no longer than 5 days.
DOSAGE ADJUSTMENT For patients who weigh less than 50 kg, elderly patients, and patients with impaired renal function, initial dose reduced to 15 mg, followed by oral ketorolac if needed; or 15 mg q 6 hr p.r.n., up to maximum of 60 mg/day for no longer than 5 days.

Route	Onset	Peak	Duration
I.V.	30 to 60 min	1 to 2 hr	4 to 6 hr

Mechanism of Action
Blocks the activity of cyclooxygenase, the enzyme needed to synthesize prostaglandins. Prostaglandins mediate the inflammatory response and cause local vasodilation, swelling, and pain. They also promote pain transmission from the periphery to the spinal cord. By blocking cyclooxygenase and inhibiting prostaglandins, this NSAID reduces inflammatory symptoms and relieves pain.

Contraindications
Advanced renal impairment or risk of renal impairment due to volume depletion; before or during surgery if hemostasis is critical; breast-feeding; cerebrovascular bleeding; concurrent use of aspirin or other salicylates, other NSAIDs, or probenecid; hemophilia or other bleeding problems, including coagulation or platelet function disorders; hemorrhagic diathesis; history of GI bleeding, GI perforation, or peptic ulcer disease; hypersensitivity to ketorolac tromethamine, aspirin, other NSAIDs, or their components; incomplete hemostasis; labor and delivery

Interactions

DRUGS

ACE inhibitors: Increased risk of renal function impairment

acetaminophen, gold compounds: Increased risk of adverse renal effects

amphotericin, penicillamine, and other nephrotoxic drugs: Increased risk or severity of adverse renal effects

antihypertensives, diuretics: Possibly reduced effects of these drugs

aspirin and other salicylates, other NSAIDs: Additive toxicity

cefamandole, cefoperazone, cefotetan: Possibly hypoprothrombinemia

corticosteroids, potassium supplements: Increased risk of gastric ulceration or hemorrhage

furosemide: Decreased effects of furosemide

heparin, oral anticoagulants, platelet aggregation inhibitors, thrombolytics: Increased risk of GI bleeding

lithium: Possibly increased blood lithium level and increased risk of lithium toxicity

methotrexate: Possibly methotrexate toxicity

plicamycin, valproic acid: Possibly hypoprothrombinemia and increased risk of bleeding

probenecid: Decreased elimination of ketorolac, increased risk of adverse effects

ACTIVITIES

alcohol use: Increased risk of adverse GI effects

Adverse Reactions

CNS: Dizziness, drowsiness, headache

CV: Edema, fluid retention, hypertension

EENT: Stomatitis

GI: Abdominal pain; bloating; constipation; diarrhea; flatulence; GI bleeding, perforation, or ulceration; hepatic failure; indigestion; nausea; vomiting

SKIN: Diaphoresis, pruritus, rash

Other: Anaphylaxis, injection site pain, unusual weight gain

Nursing Considerations

- Read ketorolac label carefully. Don't use I.M. form for I.V. administration. Be aware that ketorolac is not for intrathecal or epidural use.
- Administer drug over at least 15 seconds.
- Notify prescriber if pain relief is inadequate or if breakthrough pain occurs between doses because supplemental doses of an opioid analgesic may be required.

- **WARNING** Monitor liver function test results for possible elevations. If elevated levels persist or worsen, notify prescriber and expect to discontinue drug, as ordered, to prevent hepatic impairment.
- **WARNING** Monitor patients with a history of peripheral edema, heart failure, or hypertension for adequate fluid balance because drug can promote fluid retention and exacerbate these conditions. Assess for dyspnea, edema, unexplained rapid weight gain, and decreased activity tolerance. Notify prescriber if such symptoms develop.
- Be aware that maximum duration of ketorolac therapy (including oral and I.M. forms) is 5 days.
- Store drug at 15° to 30° C (59° to 86° F), and protect from light.

PATIENT TEACHING
- Advise patient to avoid taking acetaminophen, aspirin, other salicylates, and other NSAIDs while receiving ketorolac unless prescriber approves.
- Caution patient to avoid potentially hazardous activities until drug's CNS effects are known.
- Urge patient to avoid alcohol during ketorolac therapy because of increased risk of adverse GI effects.
- Encourage patient to have dental procedures performed before starting drug therapy because of increased risk of bleeding.
- Teach patient proper oral hygiene measures, and encourage him to use a soft-bristled toothbrush during ketorolac therapy.

labetalol hydrochloride
Normodyne, Trandate

Class and Category
Chemical: Benzamine derivative
Therapeutic: Antihypertensive
Pregnancy category: C

Indications and Dosages
▶ *To manage severe hypertension and treat hypertensive emergencies*
I. V. INFUSION
Adults. 200 mg diluted in 160 ml of D$_5$W and infused at 2 mg/min until desired response occurs.
I.V. INJECTION
Adults. 20 mg given over 2 min; additional doses given in increments of 40 to 80 mg q 10 min as indicated until desired response occurs. *Maximum:* 300 mg.

Route	Onset	Peak	Duration
I.V.	2 to 5 min	5 to 15 min	2 to 4 hr

Mechanism of Action

Selectively blocks alpha$_1$ and beta$_2$ receptors in vascular smooth muscle and beta$_1$ receptors in the heart. These actions reduce peripheral vascular resistance and blood pressure. Potent beta blockade prevents reflex tachycardia, which commonly occurs when alpha blockers reduce the resting heart rate, cardiac output, or stroke volume.

Incompatibilities

Don't dilute labetalol in sodium bicarbonate solution or administer through same I.V. line as alkaline drugs, such as furosemide; doing so may cause a white precipitate to form.

Contraindications

Asthma, cardiogenic shock, heart failure, hypersensitivity to labetalol or its components, second- or third-degree heart block, severe bradycardia

Interactions

DRUGS

allergen immunotherapy, allergenic extracts for skin testing: Increased risk of serious systemic reaction or anaphylaxis

calcium channel blockers, clonidine, diazoxide, guanabenz, reserpine: Possibly hypotension

cimetidine: Possibly increased labetalol effects

estrogens, NSAIDs: Possibly reduced antihypertensive effect of labetalol

general anesthetics: Increased risk of hypotension and myocardial depression

insulin, oral antidiabetic drugs: Increased risk of hyperglycemia

nitroglycerin: Possibly hypertension

phenoxybenzamine, phentolamine: Possibly additive alpha$_1$-blocking effects

sympathomimetics with alpha- and beta-adrenergic effects (such as pseudoephedrine): Possibly hypertension, excessive bradycardia, or heart block

xanthines (aminophylline and theophylline): Possibly decreased therapeutic effects of both drugs

FOODS
all food: Increased blood labetalol level
ACTIVITIES
alcohol use: Increased labetalol effects

Adverse Reactions

CNS: Anxiety, confusion, depression, dizziness, drowsiness, fatigue, paresthesia, syncope, vertigo, weakness, yawning
CV: Bradycardia, chest pain, edema, heart block, heart failure, hypotension, orthostatic hypotension, ventricular arrhythmias
EENT: Nasal congestion, taste perversion
GI: Elevated liver function test results, hepatic necrosis, hepatitis, indigestion, nausea, vomiting
GU: Ejaculation failure, impotence
RESP: Dyspnea, wheezing
SKIN: Jaundice, pruritus, rash, scalp tingling

Nursing Considerations

- Dilute labetalol to a final concentration of 1 or 3 mg/ml. Administer infusion by infusion pump or another method that allows precise measurement.
- During labetalol administration, monitor blood pressure according to facility policy, usually every 5 minutes for 30 minutes, then every 30 minutes for 2 hours, and then every hour for 6 hours. Monitor ECG as ordered.
- Keep patient in supine position for 3 hours after I.V. administration.
- **WARNING** Be aware that labetalol masks common signs of shock.
- Monitor blood glucose level in diabetic patient because labetalol may conceal symptoms of hypoglycemia such as tachycardia.
- Expect to discontinue drug if patient's liver function test results are elevated. Monitor closely for signs of hepatotoxicity, such as jaundice and flulike symptoms.
- Monitor for signs of heart failure, such as dyspnea and crackles. Expect to administer a digitalis glycoside, a diuretic, or both at first sign of heart failure. If heart failure continues, expect to discontinue labetalol gradually, if possible.
- Monitor patients who are concurrently receiving other drugs with antihypertensive effects. Expect labetalol dosage to be adjusted if patient experiences adverse reactions, such as hypotension or bradycardia, or if prescriber adds or discontinues another drug.

- Store drug at 2° to 30° C (36° to 86° F); protect from freezing and light.

PATIENT TEACHING

- Advise patient to report confusion, difficulty breathing, rash, slow pulse, and swelling in arms or legs during labetalol therapy.
- Suggest that patient rise slowly and avoid sudden position changes to minimize effects of orthostatic hypotension.
- Inform diabetic patient that her blood glucose level will be monitored frequently; instruct her to report signs of hypoglycemia.
- Inform patient that transient scalp tingling may occur during early phase of treatment.

lepirudin
Refludan

Class and Category
Chemical: Yeast-derived recombinant form of hirudin
Therapeutic: Anticoagulant
Pregnancy category: B

Indications and Dosages
▶ *To prevent thromboembolic complications in patients with heparin-induced thrombocytopenia and associated thromboembolic disease*

I.V. INFUSION AND INJECTION

Adults. *Initial:* 0.4 mg/kg, but no more than 44 mg, given by bolus over 15 to 20 sec, followed by continuous infusion of 0.15 mg/kg/hr for 2 to 10 days or longer, as indicated. *Maximum:* 0.21 mg/kg/hr.

DOSAGE ADJUSTMENT For patients with renal insufficiency, bolus dose decreased to 0.2 mg/kg and infusion rate adjusted as follows: for creatinine clearance of 45 to 60 ml/min/1.73 m^2, 50% of standard infusion rate; for creatinine clearance of 30 to 44 ml/min/1.73 m^2, 30% of standard infusion rate; for creatinine clearance of 15 to 29 ml/min/1.73 m^2, 15% of standard infusion rate; for creatinine clearance of less than 15 ml/min/1.73 m^2, drug probably discontinued.

Route	Onset	Peak	Duration
I.V.	Immediate	Unknown	Unknown

Mechanism of Action

Forms a tight bond with thrombin, neutralizing this enzyme's actions, even when the enzyme is trapped within clots. One molecule of lepirudin binds with one molecule of thrombin. Thrombin causes fibrinogen to convert to fibrin, which is essential for clot formation.

Incompatibilities

Don't mix lepirudin in same I.V. line with other drugs.

Contraindications

Hypersensitivity to lepirudin or other hirudins

Interactions

DRUGS

oral anticoagulants, platelet aggregation inhibitors, thrombolytics: Increased risk of bleeding complications and enhanced effects of lepirudin

Adverse Reactions

CNS: Chills, fever, intracranial hemorrhage
CV: Heart failure
EENT: Epistaxis
GI: GI or rectal bleeding, hepatic dysfunction
GU: Hematuria, vaginal bleeding
HEME: Anemia, easy bruising, hematoma
RESP: Hemoptysis, pneumonia
SKIN: Excessive bleeding from wounds, rash, pruritus, urticaria
Other: Injection site bleeding, sepsis

Nursing Considerations

- Monitor BUN level and creatinine clearance, as ordered, before initiating lepirudin therapy. Expect dosage adjustment if creatinine clearance falls below 60 ml/min/1.73 m^2.
- Be aware that patients with heparin-induced thrombocytopenia have a low platelet count, which can lead to severe bleeding and even death. Lepirudin prevents clotting without further reducing platelet count.
- Be aware that lepirudin should be used cautiously in patients with conditions that increase the risk of bleeding, such as an anomaly of vessels or organs; bacterial endocarditis; hemorrhagic diathesis; recent CVA; recent intracerebral surgery or

other neuraxial procedures; recent major bleeding, major surgery, organ biopsy, or puncture of large blood vessel; severe renal function impairment; or severe uncontrolled hypertension.

• To reconstitute drug, mix it with NS or sterile water for injection. Warm solution to room temperature before administering.

• For I.V. bolus, reconstitute 50 mg with 1 ml of sterile water for injection or sodium chloride for injection. Then further dilute by withdrawing reconstituted solution into a 10-ml syringe and adding enough sterile water for injection, sodium chloride for injection, or D_5W to produce a total volume of 10 ml, or 5 mg of lepirudin/ml. Administer prescribed dose immediately, over 15 to 20 seconds.

• For I.V. infusion, reconstitute 2 vials of drug and transfer to infusion bag that contains 250 or 500 ml of NS or D_5W. Concentration will be 0.4 or 0.2 mg/ml. Use within 24 hours.

• Expect to obtain APTT before intiating therapy, 4 hours after starting infusion, and then daily (more often for patients with hepatic or renal impairment).

• Adjust infusion rate as prescribed, according to patient's APTT ratio, which is APTT divided by a control value. Target APTT ratio during treatment is 1.5 to 2.5.

• Stop infusion for 2 hours, as ordered, if APTT is above target range. Expect to decrease infusion rate by one-half when restarting. If APTT is below target range, expect to increase rate in 20% increments and recheck APTT in 4 hours.

• Avoid I.M. injections or needle sticks during therapy to minimize the risk of hematoma.

• Observe I.M. injection sites, I.V. infusion sites, and wounds for bleeding.

• Monitor for ecchymoses on arms and legs, epistaxis, hematemesis, hematuria, melena, and vaginal bleeding.

• Store unopened vials at 2° to 25° C (36° to 77° F).

PATIENT TEACHING

• Instruct patient to report unusual or unexpected bleeding, such as blood in urine, easy bruising, nosebleeds, tarry stools, and vaginal bleeding, during lepirudin therapy.

• Advise patient to avoid bumping arms and legs because of the risk of bruising.

• Instruct patient to use an electric razor and a soft-bristled toothbrush to minimize risk of bleeding.

levofloxacin

Levaquin

Class and Category

Chemical: Fluoroquinolone
Therapeutic: Antibiotic
Pregnancy category: C

Indications and Dosages

▶ *To treat acute maxillary sinusitis caused by* Haemophilus influenzae, Moraxella catarrhalis, *or* Streptococcus pneumoniae
I.V. INFUSION
Adults. 500 mg q.d. for 10 to 14 days.

▶ *To treat acute exacerbations of chronic bacterial bronchitis caused by*
H. influenzae, H. parainfluenzae, M. catarrhalis, S. pneumoniae,
or Staphylococcus aureus
I.V. INFUSION
Adults. 500 mg q.d. for 7 days.

▶ *To treat community-acquired pneumonia caused by* Chlamydia
pneumoniae, H. influenzae, H. parainfluenzae, Klebsiella
pneumoniae, Legionella pneumophila, M. catarrhalis, Mycoplasma pneumoniae, S. aureus, *or* S. pneumoniae
I.V. INFUSION
Adults. 500 mg q.d. for 7 to 14 days.

▶ *To treat uncomplicated UTIs caused by* Escherichia coli, K. pneumoniae, *or* Staphylococcus saprophyticus
I.V. INFUSION
Adults. 250 mg q.d. for 3 days.

▶ *To treat complicated UTIs and acute pyelonephritis caused by* E. coli
I.V. INFUSION
Adults. 250 mg q.d. for 10 days.

▶ *To treat mild to moderate skin and soft-tissue infections caused by*
S. aureus *or* Streptococcus pyogenes
I.V. INFUSION
Adults. 500 mg q.d. for 7 to 10 days.

▶ *To treat complicated skin and skin-structure infections caused by*
methicillin-sensitive S. aureus, Enterococcus faecalis, S. pyogenes,
or Proteus mirabilis
I.V. INFUSION
Adults. 750 mg q.d. for 7 to 14 days.
DOSAGE ADJUSTMENT For patients with impaired renal
function, dosage reduced as follows: for complicated UTIs in
patients with creatinine clearance of 10 to 19 ml/min/1.73 m^2,

250 mg initially and then maintenance dosage of 250 mg q 48 hr. For complicated skin and skin-structure infections in patients with creatinine clearance of 20 to 49 ml/min/1.73 m², 750 mg initially and then maintenance dosage of 750 mg q 48 hr; with creatinine clearance of 10 to 19 ml/min/1.73 m², 750 mg initially and then maintenance dosage of 500 mg q 48 hr. For all other indications, in patients with creatinine clearance of 50 to 80 ml/min/1.73 m², 500 mg initially and then maintenance dosage of 500 mg q 24 hr; with creatinine clearance of 20 to 49 ml/min/1.73 m², 500 mg initially and then maintenance dosage of 250 mg q 24 hr; with creatinine clearance of 10 to 19 ml/min/1.73 m², 500 mg initially and then maintenance dosage of 250 mg q 48 hr.

Mechanism of Action
Interferes with bacterial cell replication by inhibiting the bacterial enzyme DNA gyrase, which is essential for replication and repair of bacterial DNA.

Contraindications
Hypersensitivity to levofloxacin, other fluoroquinolones, or their components

Interactions
DRUGS
antineoplastics: Decreased blood levofloxacin level
cimetidine: Increased blood levofloxacin level
cyclosporine: Increased risk of nephrotoxicity
NSAIDs: Possibly increased CNS stimulation and risk of seizures
oral anticoagulants: Increased anticoagulant effects and risk of bleeding
oral antidiabetic drugs: Possibly hyperglycemia or hypoglycemia
theophylline: Increased blood theophylline level and risk of toxicity

Adverse Reactions
CNS: Anxiety, dizziness, headache, nervousness, seizures, sleep disturbance
EENT: Taste perversion
ENDO: Hypoglycemia, hyperglycemia
GI: Abdominal pain, anorexia, constipation, diarrhea, flatulence, indigestion, nausea, pseudomembranous colitis, vomiting
GU: Crystalluria, vaginal candidiasis
HEME: Eosinophilia, hemolytic anemia

MS: Back pain, tendon rupture
SKIN: Photosensitivity, pruritus, rash, urticaria
Other: Anaphylaxis

Nursing Considerations

- Expect to obtain culture and sensitivity test results before levofloxacin treatment begins.
- Monitor renal function test results before and during levofloxacin treatment, as ordered, especially in patients with impaired renal function.
- To prepare a 250-mg dose, withdraw 10 ml from a 500-mg/20 ml vial and dilute with 40 ml of diluent recommended by manufacturer, such as NS, D$_5$W, D$_5$NS, or D$_5$LR; to prepare a 500-mg dose, withdraw 20 ml from a 500-mg/20 ml vial and dilute with 80 ml of diluent; to prepare a 750-mg dose, withdraw 30 ml from a 500-mg/20 ml vial and dilute with 120 ml of diluent. Infuse a 250- or 500-mg dose over at least 60 minutes; infuse a 750-mg dose over at least 90 minutes. Be aware that too-rapid administration can result in hypotension.
- Be aware that a premixed form of levofloxacin in flexible containers is also available. To prevent air embolism, don't administer this form through an I.V. line with series connections.
- Ensure that patient is well hydrated during treatment to prevent crystalluria.
- Frequently monitor blood glucose level of diabetic patient who uses an oral antidiabetic drug because these drugs may interact with levofloxacin, causing hyperglycemia or hypoglycemia.
- Monitor for seizures, especially in patients with CNS disorders that may lower the seizure threshold, such as epilepsy and severe cerebral arteriosclerosis.
- Monitor patient for nightmares and insomnia because levofloxacin can cause excessive CNS stimulation. If such reactions occur, notify prescriber at once and expect to discontinue drug.

PATIENT TEACHING

- Advise patient to increase fluid intake during levofloxacin therapy.
- Instruct patient to immediately report signs of an allergic reaction, such as a rash or difficulty breathing.
- Instruct patient to immediately report tendon pain and inflammation.
- Advise patient to avoid excessive sunlight and to wear sunscreen because of increased risk of photosensitivity.

• Inform diabetic patient that her blood glucose level will be monitored frequently; instruct her to report signs of hypoglycemia.

levorphanol tartrate
Levo-Dromoran

Class, Category, and Schedule
Chemical: Morphinan derivative
Therapeutic: Opioid analgesic
Pregnancy category: Not rated
Controlled substance: Schedule II

Indications and Dosages
▶ *To relieve moderate to severe pain*
I.V. INJECTION
Adults. Up to 1 mg q 3 to 6 hr, p.r.n. *Maximum:* 8 mg/day for non-opioid-dependent patients.

Route	Onset	Peak	Duration
I.V.	Unknown	In 20 min	4 to 5 hr

Mechanism of Action
Decreases intracellular cAMP level by inhibiting adenylate cyclase, which regulates the release of pain neurotransmitters, such as substance P, gamma-aminobutyric acid, dopamine, acetylcholine, and noradrenaline. Levorphanol also stimulates mu and kappa opioid receptors, altering the perception of pain and, possibly, the emotional response to it.

Incompatibilities
Don't mix levorphanol tartrate with solutions that contain aminophylline, ammonium chloride, amobarbital sodium, chlorothiazide sodium, heparin sodium, methicillin sodium, nitrofurantoin sodium, novobiacin sodium, pentobarbital sodium, perphenazine, phenobarbital sodium, phenytoin, secobarbital sodium, sodium bicarbonate, sodium iodide, sulfadiazine sodium, sulfisoxazole diethanolamine, or thiopental sodium.

Contraindications
Acute alcoholism, acute or severe asthma, anoxia, hypersensitivity to levorphanol tartrate or its components, increased ICP, respiratory depression, upper airway obstruction

Interactions

DRUGS

alfentanil, CNS depressants, fentanyl, sufentanil: Possibly increased CNS and respiratory depression and hypotension

anticholinergics: Increased risk of severe constipation

antidiarrheals (such as difenoxin and atropine, kaolin, and loperamide): Possibly severe constipation and increased CNS depression

antihypertensives: Increased risk of hypotension

buprenorphine: Possibly decreased therapeutic effects of levorphanol and increased risk of respiratory depression

hydroxyzine: Increased risk of CNS depression and hypotension

metoclopramide: Possibly antagonized effects of metoclopramide

naloxone, naltrexone: Decreased therapeutic effects of levorphanol

neuromuscular blockers: Increased risk of prolonged CNS and respiratory depression

ACTIVITIES

alcohol use: Possibly increased CNS and respiratory depression and hypotension

Adverse Reactions

CNS: Amnesia, coma, confusion, delusions, depression, dizziness, drowsiness, dyskinesia, hypokinesia, insomnia, nervousness, personality disorder, seizures

CV: Bradycardia, cardiac arrest, hypotension, orthostatic hypotension, palpitations, shock, tachycardia

EENT: Abnormal vision, diplopia, dry mouth

GI: Abdominal pain, biliary tract spasm, constipation, hepatic failure, indigestion, nausea, vomiting

GU: Dysuria, urine retention

RESP: Apnea, hyperventilation

SKIN: Cyanosis, pruritus, rash, urticaria

Other: Injection site pain, redness, and swelling; physical and psychological dependence

Nursing Considerations

- **WARNING** Be aware that levorphanol may be habit-forming and that patients with a history of drug abuse (including acute alcoholism), emotional instability, or suicidal ideation or attempts are at increased risk for opioid abuse.
- **WARNING** Administer levorphanol slowly, over several minutes, because rapid administration of other opioid analgesics has caused anaphylaxis, severe respiratory depression, hypotension, peripheral circulatory collapse, and cardiac arrest. Keep emergency equipment and drugs nearby.

- Assess respiratory status closely, especially in patients having an acute asthma attack and those with adrenal insufficiency, chronic respiratory disease, hypothyroidism, myxedema, severe hepatic or renal impairment, or conditions that increase CSF pressure, because drug causes respiratory depression. Elderly, extremely ill, or debilitated patients and patients who have recently taken, or are currently taking, drugs with respiratory depressant effects are also more sensitive to levorphanol's effects.
- Monitor supine and standing blood pressure periodically, and notify prescriber of orthostatic hypotension.
- Carefully assess for adverse reactions in elderly patients because they're especially sensitive to levorphanol and at increased risk for constipation.
- Monitor for signs of drug-induced CNS depression or increased CSF pressure, such as altered LOC, restlessness, and irritability, in patients with a coma, head injury, intracranial lesions, or other conditions that could cause these effects. Patients who are taking, or have recently taken, drugs that depress the CNS are also more susceptible to these effects.
- Be aware that opioids such as levorphanol may induce or exacerbate arrhythmias or seizures in patients with a history of these conditions or may mask symptoms of acute abdominal conditions.
- Because levorphanol is metabolized in the liver, monitor patients with hepatic impairment and those taking drugs that decrease hepatic clearance for signs of increased sedation.
- Monitor patients with prostatic hypertrophy, renal function impairment, or urethral stricture and those who have recently undergone urinary tract surgery for signs of urine retention, such as difficulty voiding or feeling that bladder isn't empty after voiding, peripheral edema, or weight gain. Impaired renal function can affect excretion of levorphanol, causing increased effects.
- Monitor patients with biliary tract disease for biliary colic (pain in upper midline area that may radiate to the back and right shoulder), which may be caused by drug-induced increase in intracholedochal pressure.
- Because levorphanol's effects on the heart aren't known, expect limited use of this drug in patients with acute MI, ventricular dysfunction, or coronary insufficiency.
- Store drug between 15° and 30° C (59° and 86° F); don't freeze.

PATIENT TEACHING
• Instruct patient to lie down during levorphanol administration and for a period afterward to lessen drug's hypotensive effects (dizziness, light-headedness) and other adverse effects, such as nausea and vomiting.
• Advise patient to avoid potentially hazardous activities until drug's CNS effects are known.
• Instruct patient to avoid alcoholic beverages while taking levorphanol.
• Direct patient to change position slowly to minimize effects of orthostatic hypotension.
• Advise patient to report constipation, nausea, or vomiting.
• Suggest that patient relieve dry mouth with sugarless candy or gum or ice chips.

levothyroxine sodium
(L-thyroxine sodium, T₄, thyroxine sodium)
Levothroid, Synthroid

Class and Category
Chemical: Synthetic thyroxine (T_4)
Therapeutic: Thyroid hormone replacement
Pregnancy category: A

Indications and Dosages
▶ *To treat severe hypothyroidism*
I.V. INJECTION
Adults. 50 to 100 mcg q.d. until therapeutic blood level is reached.
Children. 75% of usual P.O. dose q.d. until therapeutic blood level is reached.
▶ *To treat myxedema coma*
I.V. INJECTION
Adults. 200 to 500 mcg on day 1. If no significant improvement, 100 to 300 mcg on day 2. Daily dose continued as prescribed until therapeutic blood level is reached and P.O. administration is tolerated.
Children. 75% of usual P.O. dose q.d. until therapeutic blood level is reached and P.O. administration is tolerated.

Route	Onset	Peak	Duration
I.V.	6 to 8 hr	24 hr	Unknown

Mechanism of Action

Replaces endogenous thyroid hormone, which may exert its physiologic effects by controlling DNA transcription and protein synthesis. Levothyroxine exhibits all of the following actions of endogenous thyroid hormone:

- increases energy expenditure
- accelerates the rate of cellular oxidation, which stimulates body tissue growth, maturation, and metabolism
- regulates differentiation and proliferation of stem cells
- aids in myelination of nerves and development of synaptic processes in the nervous system
- regulates growth
- decreases blood and hepatic cholesterol concentrations
- enhances carbohydrate and protein metabolism, increasing gluconeogenesis and protein synthesis.

Contraindications

Acute MI (unless caused or complicated by hyperthyroidism), hypersensitivity to levothyroxine or its components, uncorrected adrenal insufficiency, untreated thyrotoxicosis

Interactions

DRUGS

adrenocorticoids: Possibly need for adrenocorticoid dosage adjustments as thyroid status changes

beta blockers: Possibly impaired action of beta blockers and decreased conversion of T_4 to triiodothyronine (T_3)

digoxin: Reduced therapeutic effects of digoxin

estrogen, phenylbutazone, phenytoin: Reduced binding of levothyroxine to protein, possibly requiring increased levothyroxine dosage

ketamine: Possibly hypertension and tachycardia

maprotiline: Increased risk of arrhythmias

oral anticoagulants: Altered anticoagulant activity, possibly need for anticoagulant dosage adjustment

sympathomimetics: Increased risk of coronary insufficiency in patients with coronary artery disease

tricyclic antidepressants: Increased therapeutic and toxic effects of both drugs

Adverse Reactions

CNS: Insomnia
ENDO: Hyperthyroidism (with overdose)
SKIN: Alopecia (transient), rash, urticaria

Nursing Considerations
- Expect to give levothyroxine I.V. if patient can't take tablets. Be aware that drug shouldn't be given S.C.
- Reconstitute drug by adding 5 ml of NS.
- Monitor PT of patient receiving anticoagulants; she may require a dosage adjustment.
- Monitor blood glucose level of diabetic patient. Prescriber may reduce antidiabetic drug dosage as thyroid hormone level enters therapeutic range. Be aware that levothyroxine use can lead to uncontrolled diabetes mellitus, requiring increased dosage of insulin or oral antidiabetic drug.
- Monitor patients with a history of cardiovascular disease for signs of ischemia or tachyarrhythmias. If such signs occur, notify prescriber and expect levothyroxine dosage adjustment.
- Expect patient to undergo regular thyroid function tests during levothyroxine therapy.
- Store drug at 15° to 30° C (59° to 86° F).

PATIENT TEACHING
- Inform patient that levothyroxine replaces a hormone that is normally produced by the thyroid gland and that drug usually is taken for life.
- Instruct patient to report signs of hyperthyroidism, such as diarrhea, excessive sweating, heat intolerance, insomnia, palpitations, and weight loss, during levothyroxine therapy.
- Inform patient with diabetes that her blood glucose level will be monitored frequently to assess the need for antidiabetic drug dosage adjustment.

lidocaine hydrochloride
(lignocaine hydrochloride)
Xylocaine, Xylocard (CAN)

Class and Category
Chemical: Aminoacyamide
Therapeutic: Class IB antiarrhythmic
Pregnancy category: B

Indications and Dosages
▶ *To treat ventricular tachycardia or ventricular fibrillation*
I.V. INFUSION AND INJECTION
Adults. *Loading:* 50 to 100 mg (or 1 to 1.5 mg/kg), administered at 25 to 50 mg/min. If desired response isn't achieved after 5 to

10 min, second dose of 25 to 50 mg (or 0.5 to 0.75 mg/kg) is given q 5 to 10 min until maximum loading dose (300 mg in 1 hr) has been given. *Maintenance:* 20 to 50 mcg/kg/min (1 to 4 mg/min) by continuous infusion. Smaller bolus dose repeated 15 to 20 min after start of infusion if needed to maintain therapeutic blood level. *Maximum:* 300 mg (or 3 mg/kg) over 1 hr.
Children. *Loading:* 1 mg/kg. *Maintenance:* 30 mcg/kg/min by continuous infusion. *Maximum:* 3 mg/kg.
DOSAGE ADJUSTMENT For elderly patients receiving lidocaine to treat arrhythmias and for patients with acute hepatitis or decompensated cirrhosis, loading dose and continuous infusion rate reduced by 50%.

Route	Onset	Peak	Duration
I.V.	45 to 90 sec	Immediate	10 to 20 min

Mechanism of Action
Combines with fast sodium channels in myocardial cell membranes, which inhibits sodium influx into cells and decreases ventricular depolarization, automaticity, and excitability during diastole.

Contraindications
Adams-Stokes syndrome; hypersensitivity to lidocaine, amide anesthetics, or their components; severe heart block (without artificial pacemaker); Wolff-Parkinson-White syndrome

Interactions
DRUGS
beta blockers, cimetidine: Increased blood lidocaine level and risk of toxicity
MAO inhibitors, tricyclic antidepressants: Risk of severe, prolonged hypertension
mexiletine, tocainide: Additive cardiac effects
neuromuscular blockers: Possibly increased neuromuscular blockade
phenytoin, procainamide: Increased cardiac depression

Adverse Reactions
CNS: Anxiety, confusion, difficulty speaking, dizziness, hallucinations, lethargy, paresthesia, seizures
CV: Bradycardia, cardiac arrest, hypotension, new or worsening arrhythmias

EENT: Blurred vision, diplopia, tinnitus
GI: Nausea
MS: Muscle twitching
RESP: Respiratory arrest or depression
Other: Allergic reaction; injection site burning, irritation, stinging, swelling, or tenderness

Nursing Considerations

- Carefully check prefilled lidocaine syringes before using. Use only syringes labeled "FOR CARDIAC ARRHYTHMIAS."
- Check label to verify that you're using a lidocaine preparation that does *not* contain preservatives or other drugs. Dilute drug with D5W, typically to a final concentration of 1 or 2 mg/ml. Consult manufacturer's guidelines for alternative dilution information. Include final concentration on label. Administer drug using an infusion pump or another device that allows precise measurement.
- Observe for respiratory depression after bolus injection and during I.V. infusion of lidocaine.
- Keep life-support equipment and vasopressors nearby during administration in case respiratory depression or other reactions occur.
- Titrate dosage, as prescribed, to minimum amount needed to prevent arrhythmias.
- During administration, place patient on cardiac monitor, as ordered, and closely observe her at all times. Monitor for worsening arrhythmias, widening QRS complex, and prolonged PR interval—possible signs of drug toxicity.
- Monitor blood lidocaine level, as ordered. Check for therapeutic level of 2 to 5 mcg/ml.
- If signs of toxicity, such as dizziness, occur, notify prescriber and expect to discontinue or slow infusion.
- Monitor vital signs as well as BUN and serum creatinine and electrolyte levels during and after therapy.
- Store drug at 15° to 30° C (59° to 86° F).

PATIENT TEACHING

- Advise patient who receives lidocaine to report difficulty speaking, dizziness, injection site pain, nausea, numbness or tingling, or vision changes.

lincomycin hydrochloride

Lincocin

Class and Category

Chemical: Lincosamide
Therapeutic: Bacteriostatic or bactericidal antibiotic
Pregnancy category: C

Indications and Dosages

▶ *To treat serious respiratory, skin, and soft-tissue infections caused by susceptible strains of streptococci, pneumococci, and staphylococci*

I.V. INFUSION

Adults. 600 mg to 1 g q 8 to 12 hr. *Maximum:* 8 g/day in divided doses for life-threatening infection.

Children over age 1 month. 10 to 20 mg/kg/day in divided doses q 8 to 12 hr, depending on severity of infection.

DOSAGE ADJUSTMENT Dosage reduced by 25% to 30% in patients with severely impaired renal function.

Mechanism of Action

Inhibits protein synthesis in susceptible bacteria by binding to the 50S sub-unit of bacterial ribosomes and preventing peptide bond formation, thus causing bacterial cells to die.

Incompatibilities

Don't administer lincomycin with novobiocin or kanamycin.

Contraindications

Hypersensitivity to lincomycin or clindamycin

Interactions

DRUGS

antimyasthenic drugs: Possibly antagonized effects of antimyasthenic drug

chloramphenicol, clindamycin, erythromycin: Possibly blocked access of lincomycin to its site of action

hydrocarbon inhalation anesthetics, neuromuscular blockers: Increased neuromuscular blockade, possibly severe respiratory depression

opioid analgesics: Increased risk of prolonged or increased respiratory depression

Adverse Reactions

CNS: Fever, vertigo
CV: Cardiac arrest and hypotension (with rapid administration)
EENT: Glossitis, stomatitis, tinnitus
GI: Abdominal cramps, colitis, diarrhea, nausea, pseudomembranous colitis, rectal candidiasis, vomiting
GU: Vaginal candidiasis
HEME: Agranulocytosis, eosinophilia, leukopenia, neutropenia, thrombocytopenic purpura
SKIN: Erythema multiforme, rash, Stevens-Johnson syndrome, urticaria
Other: Anaphylaxis, angioedema, superinfection

Nursing Considerations

• Expect to obtain a specimen for culture and sensitivity testing before administering first dose of lincomycin.
• **WARNING** Be aware that some preparations of lincomycin contain benzyl alcohol, which can cause a fatal toxic syndrome in neonates or premature infants, characterized by CNS, respiratory, circulatory, and renal impairment and metabolic acidosis. Because lincomycin has appeared in breast milk, breast-feeding patient may be required to discontinue drug or stop breast-feeding.
• Dilute 600-mg dose in at least 100 ml of D_5W, $D_{10}W$, NS, D_5NS, or other compatible diluent identified on manufacturer's insert. Dilute higher doses with 100 ml of a compatible diluent for each gram being administered—for example, you'd dilute a 3-g dose in at least 300 ml of diluent. Use diluted solution within 24 hours if stored at room temperature.
• **WARNING** Administer lincomycin over at least 1 hour for each gram being administered. For example, you'd infuse 1 g over 1 hour and 3 g over 3 hours. Too-rapid infusion may result in cardiac arrest or hypotension.
• **WARNING** Monitor for a hypersensitivity reaction, such as rash, pruritus, wheezing, and dysphagia due to laryngeal edema. If such reactions occur, discontinue infusion and notify prescriber immediately. If anaphylaxis occurs, administer epinephrine, antihistamines, oxygen, and corticosteroids, as prescribed. Be aware that patients with a history of asthma or significant allergies are at increased risk for a hypersensitivity reaction.
• Observe patient for signs of superinfection, such as vaginal itching and sore mouth.

- Monitor patient for signs of pseudomembranous colitis, such as watery, loose stools. Patients with a history of GI disease, particularly colitis or regional enteritis, are at increased risk for colitis. Be aware that antibiotic-related diarrhea may be more severe and less well tolerated in elderly patients. Expect to discontinue lincomycin if diarrhea occurs.
- Monitor results of liver and renal function tests, CBC, and platelet counts periodically during lincomycin therapy.
- Before diluting drug, store it at a controlled room temperature of 20° to 25° C (68° to 77° F).

PATIENT TEACHING
- Review with patient possibly serious adverse reactions associated with lincomycin use, such as difficulty breathing, rash, and chest tightness, and tell him to report any that occur.
- Inform him that yogurt or buttermilk can help maintain intestinal flora and may decrease the risk of diarrhea.
- Stress the importance of following dosage regimen and keeping follow-up medical appointments and appointments for laboratory tests.

linezolid

Zyvox

Class and Category

Chemical: Oxazolidinone
Therapeutic: Antibiotic
Pregnancy category: C

Indications and Dosages

▶ *To treat vancomycin-resistant* Enterococcus faecium *infections, including bacteremia*
I.V. INFUSION
Adults. 600 mg q 12 hr for 14 to 28 days.
▶ *To treat nosocomial pneumonia caused by* Staphylococcus aureus *(methicillin-susceptible and -resistant strains) or* Streptococcus pneumoniae *(penicillin-susceptible strains only) and community-acquired pneumonia, including accompanying bacteremia caused by* S. aureus *(methicillin-susceptible strains only) or* S. pneumoniae *(penicillin-susceptible strains only)*
I.V. INFUSION
Adults. 600 mg q 12 hr for 10 to 14 days.

▶ *To treat complicated skin and soft-tissue infections caused by* S. aureus *(methicillin-susceptible and -resistant strains),* Streptococcus pyogenes, *or* Streptococcus agalactiae

I.V. INFUSION

Adults. 600 mg q 12 hr for 10 to 14 days.

Mechanism of Action

Linezolid inhibits bacterial protein synthesis by interfering with the translation of ribonucleic acid (RNA) to protein. In bacteria, protein synthesis begins with the binding of one 30S ribosomal subunit and one 50S ribosomal subunit to a messenger RNA (mRNA) molecule to form a 70S initiation complex. The 50S ribosomal subunit consists of 23S ribosomal RNA (rRNA) and other ribosomal subunits. Then the process of translation begins.

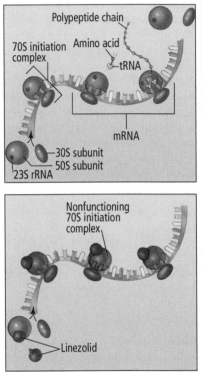

In translation, transfer RNA (tRNA) attaches to the 50S subunit and brings specific amino acids into place. As the tRNA and amino acids fall into place, they are joined by peptide bonds and elongate to form a polypeptide chain, as shown top right. This chain eventually combines with other polypeptide chains to form a complete protein molecule. After translation is complete, the ribosomal subunits fall away and are ready to combine with more mRNA to start the translation process again.

Linezolid binds to a site on the bacterial 23S rRNA of the 50S subunit. This action prevents the formation of a functional 70S initiation complex, an essential component of the bacterial translation process. Without proper protein production, as shown bottom right, susceptible bacteria can't multiply. Linezolid is bacteriostatic against staphylococci and enterococci and bactericidal against most streptococci.

Incompatibilities

Don't add other drugs to linezolid solution. Don't infuse linezolid in the same I.V. line as amphotericin B, chlorpromazine hydrochloride, co-trimoxazole, diazepam, erythromycin lactobionate, pentamidine isethionate, or phenytoin sodium because these drugs are physically incompatible. Don't infuse linezolid with ceftriaxone sodium because these drugs are chemically incompatible.

Contraindications

Hypersensitivity to linezolid or its components

Interactions

DRUGS

adrenergics (including pseudoephedrine and propanolamine): Enhanced vasopressor response of adrenergics, resulting in increased blood pressure

serotonergics: Possibly serotonin syndrome

FOODS

tyramine-containing foods and beverages: Possibly hypertension

Adverse Reactions

CNS: Dizziness, fever, headache, insomnia

CV: Hypertension

EENT: Oral candidiasis, tongue discoloration

GI: Abdominal pain, constipation, diarrhea, indigestion, nausea, pseudomembranous colitis, vomiting

GU: Vaginal candidiasis

HEME: Myelosuppression (anemia, leukopenia, pancytopenia, thrombocytopenia)

SKIN: Pruritus, rash

Nursing Considerations

- Obtain body tissue and fluid specimens for culture and sensitivity tests, as ordered, before giving first dose of linezolid. Be prepared to begin drug therapy before test results are known.
- Keep I.V. bags in overwrap until ready to use.
- If I.V. line is used to administer other drugs, be sure to flush line before and after administering linezolid.
- Infuse I.V. solution over 30 to 120 minutes with D5W, NS, or LR. To prevent air embolism, don't use an I.V. line with series connections.
- **WARNING** Monitor CBC weekly, as ordered, to detect signs of myelosuppression (such as thrombocytopenia), especially in patients who require more than 2 weeks of therapy, those with preexisting myelosuppression, those who are concomitantly

receiving drugs that suppress bone marrow, and those with chronic infection who have received previous or concomitant antibiotic therapy. Expect to discontinue linezolid if patient develops or experiences worsening of myelosuppression.

- Monitor bowel elimination pattern daily. Assess for signs of secondary infection, including oral candidiasis and profuse, watery diarrhea.
- Be aware that linezolid is a reversible nonselective MAO inhibitor and therefore has the potential to react with adrenergics and serotonergics.
- Store drug at controlled room temperature (25° C [77° F]); don't freeze.

PATIENT TEACHING
- Instruct patient to immediately report severe diarrhea because linezolid may need to be discontinued.
- Inform patient that entire course of linezolid therapy must be completed.
- Advise patient not to take OTC cold remedies without consulting prescriber because drugs containing pseudoephedrine or propanolamine may cause or worsen hypertension.
- Instruct patient to avoid foods and beverages containing large amounts of tyramine, including aged cheese, fermented or air-dried meats, sauerkraut, soy sauce, tap beers, red wines, and protein-rich foods that have been stored for long periods or poorly refrigerated.

liothyronine sodium
(L-triiodothyronine, sodium L-triiodothyronine, T₃, thyronine sodium)
Triostat

Class and Category
Chemical: Synthetic triiodothyronine (T_3)
Therapeutic: Thyroid hormone replacement
Pregnancy category: A

Indications and Dosages
▶ *To treat myxedema coma or premyxedema coma (severe hypothyroidism)*
I.V. INJECTION
Adults. *Initial:* 25 to 50 mcg; repeated q 4 to 12 hr, depending on patient's response.

DOSAGE ADJUSTMENT Initial dose decreased to 10 to 20 mcg for patients with known or suspected cardiovascular disease who are being treated for myxedema coma.

Route	Onset	Peak	Duration
I.V.	2 to 4 hr	2 days	Unknown

Mechanism of Action

Replaces endogenous thyroid hormone, which may exert its physiologic effects by controlling DNA transcription and protein synthesis. Liothyronine exhibits all of the following actions of endogenous thyroid hormone:

- increases energy expenditure
- accelerates the rate of cellular oxidation, which stimulates body tissue growth, maturation, and metabolism
- regulates differentiation and proliferation of stem cells
- aids in myelination of nerves and development of synaptic processes in the nervous system
- regulates growth
- decreases blood and hepatic cholesterol concentrations
- enhances carbohydrate and protein metabolism, increasing gluconeogenesis and protein synthesis.

Contraindications

Acute MI (unless caused or complicated by hypothyroidism), hypersensitivity to liothyronine or its components, uncorrected adrenal insufficiency, untreated thyrotoxicosis

Interactions
DRUGS

adrenocorticoids: Possibly need for adrenocorticoid dosage adjustments as thyroid status changes
beta blockers: Possibly impaired action of beta blockers
cholestyramine, colestipol: Decreased liothyronine absorption
digoxin: Reduced therapeutic effects of digoxin
estrogen, phenylbutazone, phenytoin: Reduced binding of liothyronine to protein, possibly requiring increased liothyronine dosage
insulin, oral antidiabetic drugs: Possibly uncontrolled diabetes mellitus, requiring increased dosage of insulin or oral antidiabetic drug
ketamine: Possibly hypertension and tachycardia
maprotiline: Increased risk of arrhythmias
oral anticoagulants: Altered anticoagulant activity, possibly need for anticoagulant dosage adjustment

sympathomimetics: Increased risk of coronary insufficiency in patients with coronary artery disease

theophylline: Decreased theophylline clearance

tricyclic antidepressants: Increased therapeutic and toxic effects of both drugs

Adverse Reactions

CNS: Insomnia

ENDO: Hyperthyroidism (with overdose)

SKIN: Alopecia (transient), rash, urticaria

Nursing Considerations

- Be aware that liothyronine is used most often when rapid-onset or rapidly reversible thyroid hormone replacement is needed.
- Give I.V. injections more than 4 hours but less than 12 hours apart.
- Evaluate response to therapy by monitoring pulse rate and blood pressure.
- Expect patient to undergo regular thyroid function tests during liothyronine therapy.
- Monitor PT of patient receiving anticoagulants; she may require a dosage adjustment.
- Monitor patients with a history of cardiovascular disease for signs of ischemia or tachyarrhythmias. If such signs occur, notify prescriber and expect to adjust liothyronine dosage.
- Frequently monitor blood glucose level of diabetic patient. Prescriber may reduce antidiabetic drug dosage as thyroid hormone level enters therapeutic range.
- Expect oral thyroid hormone replacement therapy to be initiated or resumed as soon as possible. Expect to discontinue infusion gradually if patient is switched to levothyroxine tablets because of levothyroxine's delayed onset of action.
- Be aware that patients with myxedema coma may also be prescribed corticosteroids; those with pituitary myxedema may also receive adrenocortical hormone replacement before or at beginning of liothyronine therapy; and those with primary myxedema may receive adrenocortical hormone replacement to prevent adrenocortical insufficiency and shock.
- Store drug at 2° to 8° C (36° to 46° F).

PATIENT TEACHING

- Advise patient receiving liothyronine to report signs of hyperthyroidism, such as chest pain, excessive sweating, heat intolerance, increased pulse rate, nervousness, and palpitations.

- Inform diabetic patient that her blood glucose level will be monitored frequently because antidiabetic drug dosage may need to be reduced.
- Inform patient of need for periodic blood tests to monitor drug's effectiveness.

lorazepam
Ativan

Class, Category, and Schedule
Chemical: Benzodiazepine
Therapeutic: Amnestic, antianxiety, anticonvulsant, sedative
Pregnancy category: D
Controlled substance: Schedule IV

Indications and Dosages
▶ *To provide preoperative sedation*
I.V. INJECTION
Adults and adolescents. 0.044 mg/kg or 2 mg, whichever is less, given 2 hr before procedure. *Maximum:* 0.05 mg/kg or total of 4 mg.
▶ *To treat status epilepticus*
I.V. INJECTION
Adults and adolescents. *Initial:* 4 mg at a rate of 2 mg/min; repeated in 10 to 15 min if seizures don't subside. *Maximum:* 8 mg/24 hr.

Route	Onset	Peak	Duration
I.V.	5 min	Unknown	12 to 24 hr

Mechanism of Action
May potentiate the effects of gamma-aminobutyric acid (GABA) and other inhibitory neurotransmitters by binding to specific benzodiazepine receptors in the limbic and cortical areas of the CNS. GABA inhibits excitatory stimulation, which helps control emotional behavior. The limbic system contains a highly dense area of benzodiazepine receptors, which may explain the drug's antianxiety effects. Also, lorazepam hyperpolarizes neuronal cells, thereby interfering with their ability to generate seizures.

Incompatibilities
Don't mix I.V. lorazepam in same syringe as buprenorphine.

Contraindications

Acute angle-closure glaucoma, hypersensitivity to lorazepam or its components, intra-arterial administration, psychosis

Interactions

DRUGS

CNS depressants: Additive CNS depression

digoxin: Possibly increased blood digoxin level and risk of digitalis toxicity

fentanyl: Possibly decreased therapeutic effects of fentanyl

probenecid: Possibly increased therapeutic and adverse effects of lorazepam

ACTIVITIES

alcohol use: Increased CNS depression

Adverse Reactions

CNS: Amnesia, anxiety, ataxia, confusion, delusions, depression, dizziness, drowsiness, euphoria, headache, hypokinesia, irritability, malaise, nervousness, slurred speech, tremor

CV: Chest pain, palpitations, tachycardia

EENT: Blurred vision, dry mouth, increased salivation, photophobia

GI: Abdominal pain, constipation, diarrhea, nausea, thirst, vomiting

GU: Libido changes

SKIN: Diaphoresis

Other: Injection site phlebitis, physical and psychological dependence, withdrawal symptoms

Nursing Considerations

- Use extreme caution when giving lorazepam to elderly patients because it can cause hypoventilation.
- Dilute drug with equal amount of sterile water for injection, sodium chloride for injection, or D_5W. Discard solution if you observe particles or discoloration. Give diluted drug slowly, at a rate not to exceed 2 mg/minute.
- Monitor respirations every 5 to 15 minutes, and keep emergency resuscitation equipment readily available.
- Because abrupt drug discontinuation increases the risk of withdrawal symptoms, expect to taper dosage gradually, especially in epileptic patients.
- Store drug at 2° to 8° C (36° to 46° F); protect from freezing and light.

PATIENT TEACHING
- Instruct patient to report excessive drowsiness and nausea during lorazepam therapy.
- Advise patient to avoid potentially hazardous activities until drug's CNS effects are known.
- Urge patient to avoid alcohol because it increases drug's CNS depressant effects.

magnesium chloride
(contains 200 mg of elemental magnesium per 1 ml of injection)
Chloromag
magnesium sulfate
(contains 100 to 500 mg of elemental magnesium per 1 ml of injection and 1 to 5 g of elemental magnesium per 10 ml of injection)

Class and Category
Chemical: Cation, electrolyte
Therapeutic: Antiarrhythmic, anticonvulsant, electrolyte replacement
Pregnancy category: A

Indications and Dosages
▶ *To treat severe hypomagnesemia*
I.V. INFUSION (MAGNESIUM CHLORIDE)
Adults. 4 g diluted in 250 ml of D$_5$W and infused at a rate not to exceed 3 ml/min. *Maximum:* 40 g/day.
I.V. INFUSION (MAGNESIUM SULFATE)
Adults and adolescents. 5 g diluted in 1 L of I.V. solution and infused over 3 hr.
▶ *To provide supplemental magnesium in total parenteral nutrition*
I.V. INFUSION (MAGNESIUM SULFATE)
Adults. 1 to 3 g/day.
Children. 0.25 to 1.25 g/day.
DOSAGE ADJUSTMENT Adult dosage may be increased to 6 g/day for certain conditions, such as short-bowel syndrome.
▶ *To prevent and control seizures in preeclampsia or eclampsia as well as seizures caused by epilepsy, glomerulonephritis, or hypothyroidism*
I.V. INFUSION OR INJECTION (MAGNESIUM SULFATE)
Adults. Loading: 4 g diluted in 250 ml of compatible solution and infused over 30 min. *Maintenance:* 1 to 2 g/hr by continuous infusion.

Route	Onset	Peak	Duration
I.V. *	Immediate	Unknown	About 30 min

* For anticonvulsant effect.

Mechanism of Action

Assists all enzymes involved in phosphate transfer reactions that use ATP. Magnesium is required for normal function of the ATP-dependent sodium-potassium pump in muscle membranes. It may effectively treat digitalis glycoside–induced arrhythmias because correction of hypomagnesemia improves the sodium-potassium pump's ability to distribute potassium into intracellular spaces and because magnesium decreases calcium uptake and potassium outflow through myocardial cell membranes.

As an anticonvulsant, magnesium depresses the CNS and blocks peripheral neuromuscular impulse transmission by decreasing the amount of available acetylcholine.

Incompatibilities

Don't combine magnesium sulfate with alkali carbonates or bicarbonates, alkali hydroxides, arsenates, calcium, clindamycin phosphate, dobutamine, fat emulsions, heavy metals, hydrocortisone sodium succinate, phosphates, polymyxin B, procaine hydrochloride, salicylates, sodium bicarbonate, strontium, and tartrates.

Contraindications

Hypersensitivity to magnesium salts or any component of magnesium-containing preparations
For magnesium chloride: Coma, heart disease, renal impairment
For magnesium sulfate: Heart block, MI, preeclampsia 2 hours or less before delivery

Interactions

DRUGS
amphotericin B, cisplatin, cyclosporine, gentamicin: Possibly magnesium wasting and need for magnesium dosage adjustment
calcium salts (I.V.): Possibly neutralization of magnesium sulfate's effects
CNS depressants: Possibly increased CNS depression
digoxin: Possibly heart block and conduction changes, especially when calcium salts are also administered
diuretics (loop or thiazide): Possibly hypomagnesemia
misoprostol: Increased misoprostol-induced diarrhea
neuromuscular blockers: Possibly increased neuromuscular blockade
nifedipine: Possibly increased hypotensive effects when taken with magnesium sulfate
potassium-sparing diuretics: Increased risk of hypermagnesemia

streptomycin, tetracycline, tobramycin: Possibly decreased therapeutic effectiveness of these drugs
FOODS
high-glucose intake: Increased urinary excretion of magnesium
ACTIVITIES
alcohol use: Increased urinary excretion of magnesium

Adverse Reactions

CNS: Decreased reflexes, dizziness, syncope
CV: Arrhythmias, hypotension
GI: Vomiting
MS: Muscle cramps
RESP: Dyspnea, respiratory depression or paralysis
SKIN: Diaphoresis
Other: Allergic reaction, hypermagnesemia, magnesium toxicity

Nursing Considerations

- **WARNING** Observe for early signs of hypermagnesemia: bradycardia, diminished deep tendon reflexes, diplopia, dyspnea, flushing, hypotension, nausea, slurred speech, vomiting, and weakness. Notify prescriber immediately if patient displays any of these signs.
- **WARNING** Be aware that magnesium may precipitate myasthenic crisis by decreasing patient's sensitivity to acetylcholine.
- Frequently assess cardiac status of patient taking drugs that lower heart rate, such as beta blockers, because magnesium may aggravate symptoms of heart block.
- **WARNING** Be aware that magnesium chloride for injection contains the preservative benzyl alcohol, which may cause a fatal toxic syndrome in neonates and premature infants, characterized by CNS, respiratory, circulatory, and renal impairment and metabolic acidosis.
- Monitor serum electrolyte levels in patients with renal insufficiency because they're at risk for magnesium toxicity.
- Be aware that magnesium salts aren't intended for long-term use.
- Store drug at 15° to 30° C (59° to 86° F); don't freeze.
PATIENT TEACHING
- Instruct patient to report signs of hypermagnesemia, such as shortness of breath, flushing, dizziness, and nausea.
- Inform patient that magnesium supplements used to replace electrolytes can cause diarrhea.

mannitol

Osmitrol, Resectisol

Class and Category

Chemical: Hexahydroxy alcohol
Therapeutic: Antiglaucoma agent, diagnostic agent, osmotic diuretic
Pregnancy category: B

Indications and Dosages

▶ *To reduce ICP or intraocular pressure*
I.V. INFUSION
Adults and adolescents. 0.25 to 2 g/kg as 15% to 25% solution given over 30 to 60 min. If used before eye surgery, 1.5 to 2 g/kg 60 to 90 min before procedure. *Maximum:* 6 g/kg/day.
DOSAGE ADJUSTMENT For small or debilitated patients, dosage reduced to 0.5 g/kg.

▶ *To diagnose oliguria or inadequate renal function*
I.V. INFUSION
Adults and adolescents. 200 mg/kg or 12.5 g as 15% to 20% solution given over 3 to 5 min. Second dose given only if patient fails to excrete 30 to 50 ml of urine in 2 to 3 hr. Drug discontinued if no response after second dose. Alternatively, 100 ml of 20% solution diluted in 180 ml of NS (forming 280 ml of 7.2% solution) and infused at 20 ml/min; followed by measurement of urine output. *Maximum:* 6 g/kg/day.

▶ *To prevent oliguria or acute renal failure*
I.V. INFUSION
Adults and adolescents. 50 to 100 g as 5% to 25% solution. *Maximum:* 6 g/kg/day.

▶ *To treat oliguria*
I.V. INFUSION
Adults and adolescents. 50 to 100 g as 15% to 25% solution given over 90 min to several hr. *Maximum:* 6 g/kg/day.

▶ *To promote diuresis in drug toxicity*
I.V. INFUSION
Adults and adolescents. *Loading:* 25 g. *Maintenance:* Up to 200 g as 5% to 25% solution given continuously to maintain urine output of 100 to 500 ml/hr with positive fluid balance of 1 to 2 L. *Maximum:* 6 g/kg/day.

▶ *To promote diuresis in hemolytic transfusion reaction*
I.V. INFUSION
Adults. 20 g given over 5 min and repeated if needed. *Maximum:* 6 g/kg/day.

Route	Onset	Peak	Duration
I.V.*	1 to 3 hr	Unknown	Up to 8 hr
I.V.†	30 to 60 min	Unknown	4 to 8 hr
I.V.‡	In 15 min	Unknown	3 to 8 hr

Mechanism of Action

Elevates plasma osmolality, causing water to flow from tissues, such as the brain and eyes, and from CSF, into extracellular fluid, thereby decreasing intracranial and intraocular pressure.

As an osmotic diuretic, mannitol increases the osmolarity of glomerular filtrate, which decreases water reabsorption. This leads to increased excretion of water, sodium, chloride, and toxic substances.

Incompatibilities

Don't administer mannitol through same I.V. line as blood or blood products.

Contraindications

Active intracranial bleeding (except during craniotomy), anuria, hepatic failure, hypersensitivity to mannitol or its components, pulmonary edema, severe dehydration, severe heart failure, severe pulmonary congestion, severe renal insufficiency

Interactions

DRUGS

digoxin: Increased risk of digitalis toxicity from hypokalemia
diuretics: Possibly increased therapeutic effects of mannitol

Adverse Reactions

CNS: Chills, dizziness, fever, headache, seizures
CV: Chest pain, heart failure, hypertension, tachycardia, thrombophlebitis
EENT: Blurred vision, dry mouth, rhinitis
GI: Diarrhea, nausea, thirst, vomiting
GU: Polyuria, urine retention
RESP: Pulmonary edema
SKIN: Extravasation with edema and tissue necrosis, rash, urticaria
Other: Dehydration, hyperkalemia, hypernatremia, hypervolemia, hypokalemia, hyponatremia (dilutional), metabolic acidosis, water intoxication

---

* To produce diuresis.
† To decrease intraocular pressure.
‡ To decrease ICP.

Nursing Considerations

- If crystals form in mannitol solution exposed to low temperature, place solution in hot-water bath to redissolve crystals.
- Use a 5-micron in-line filter when administering drug solution of 15% or greater.
- Use contents of container immediately. Discard unused portions.
- Expect to administer a test dose if patient has severe oliguria or a risk of impaired renal function. Prepare a test dose of 200 mg/kg as a 15% to 25% solution, and administer over 3 to 5 minutes, as prescribed. Alternatively, 6 g/m² as a 15% to 25% solution may be prescribed for children.
- During I.V. infusion of mannitol, monitor vital signs, central venous pressure, and fluid intake and output every hour. Measure urine output with indwelling urinary catheter, as appropriate.
- Expect to discontinue infusion, as prescribed, if patient exhibits signs of worsening heart failure, renal failure, or pulmonary congestion.
- Check weight and monitor BUN and serum creatinine electrolyte levels daily.
- Evaluate I.V. site frequently for signs of extravasation, such as edema, which can lead to necrosis.
- Provide frequent mouth care to relieve thirst and dry mouth.
- Store drug at 15° to 30° C (59° to 86° F); don't freeze.

PATIENT TEACHING
- Inform patient that he may experience dry mouth and thirst during mannitol therapy.
- Instruct patient to report chest pain, difficulty breathing, or pain at I.V. site.

meperidine hydrochloride
(pethidine hydrochloride)
Demerol

Class, Category, and Schedule
Chemical: Phenylpiperidine derivative opioid
Therapeutic: Opioid analgesic
Pregnancy category: Not rated
Controlled substance: Schedule II

Indications and Dosages
▶ *To provide preoperative sedation*
I.V. INJECTION
Adults. 15 to 35 mg/hr, p.r.n.

▶ *As adjunct to anesthesia*
I.V. INFUSION OR INJECTION

Adults. Individualized. Repeated slow injections of 10-mg/ml solution or continuous infusion of dilute solution (1 mg/ml) titrated as needed.

DOSAGE ADJUSTMENT For patients with creatinine clearance of 10 to 50 ml/min/1.73 m^2, dosage decreased by 25%; with creatinine clearance of less than 10 ml/min/1.73 m^2, dosage decreased by 50%.

Route	Onset	Peak	Duration
I.V.	1 min	5 to 7 min	2 to 4 hr

Mechanism of Action
Binds with opioid receptors in the spinal cord and higher levels of the CNS, which alters the perception of, and emotional response to, pain.

Incompatibilities
Don't mix meperidine in same syringe with aminophylline, barbiturates, heparin, iodides, methicillin, morphine sulfate, phenytoin, sodium bicarbonate, sulfadiazine, or sulfisoxazole.

Contraindications
Acute asthma; hypersensitivity to meperidine, narcotics, or their components; increased ICP; severe respiratory depression; upper respiratory tract obstruction; use within 14 days of MAO inhibitor therapy

Interactions
DRUGS

alfentanil, CNS depressants, fentanyl, sufentanil: Increased risk of CNS and respiratory depression and hypotension
amphetamines, MAO inhibitors: Risk of increased CNS excitation or depression with possibly fatal reactions
anticholinergics: Increased risk of severe constipation
antidiarrheals (such as loperamide and difenoxin and atropine): Increased risk of severe constipation and increased CNS depression
antihypertensives: Increased risk of hypotension
buprenorphine: Possibly decreased therapeutic effects of meperidine and increased risk of respiratory depression
hydroxyzine: Increased risk of CNS depression and hypotension

metoclopramide: Possibly decreased effects of metoclopramide
naloxone, naltrexone: Decreased pharmacologic effects of meperidine
neuromuscular blockers: Increased risk of prolonged respiratory and
CNS depression
oral anticoagulants: Possibly increased anticoagulant effect and risk
of bleeding
ACTIVITIES
alcohol use: Possibly increased CNS and respiratory depression and
hypotension

Adverse Reactions

CNS: Confusion, depression, dizziness, drowsiness, euphoria,
headache, increased ICP, lack of coordination, malaise, nervous-
ness, nightmares, restlessness, seizures, syncope, tremor
CV: Hypotension, orthostatic hypotension, tachycardia
EENT: Blurred vision, diplopia, dry mouth
GI: Abdominal cramps or pain, anorexia, constipation, ileus, nau-
sea, vomiting
GU: Dysuria, urinary frequency, urine retention
RESP: Dyspnea, respiratory arrest or depression, wheezing
SKIN: Diaphoresis, flushing, pruritus, rash, urticaria
Other: Injection site pain, redness, and swelling; physical and
psychological dependence

Nursing Considerations

- Instruct patient to lie down during meperidine administration
  to minimize dizziness, light-headedness, nausea, and vomiting.
- Give slowly by direct injection or as a slow continuous infusion.
  Mix with D_5W, NS, or Ringer's or LR solution.
- Keep naloxone available when giving meperidine.
- Monitor respiratory and cardiovascular status during treatment.
  Notify prescriber immediately and expect to discontinue drug if
  respiratory rate falls below 12 breaths/minute or if respiratory
  depth decreases. Be aware that patients with a history of hypothyroidism are at increased risk for respiratory and prolonged
  CNS depression. Patients having an acute asthma attack; elderly,
  debilitated, or severely ill patients; and those with chronic respiratory disease are at increased risk for respiratory depression.
- Monitor bowel function to detect constipation, and assess the
  need for stool softeners.
- Be aware that meperidine may induce or exacerbate arrhythmias or seizures in patients with a history of these conditions
  and may mask symptoms of acute abdominal conditions.

- Assess urine output; decreasing output may signal urine retention. Patients with prostatic hypertrophy, obstructive urethral stricture, or recent UTI are at increased risk.
- Be aware that patients with renal or hepatic impairment are at increased risk for adverse reactions because drug is metabolized in the liver and excreted by kidneys.
- Assess for signs of physical dependence and abuse.
- Expect withdrawal symptoms to occur if drug is abruptly withdrawn after long-term use.
- Store drug at 15° to 30° C (59° to 86° F); protect from freezing and light.

PATIENT TEACHING
- Advise patient to avoid potentially hazardous activities until meperidine's CNS effects are known. Caution ambulatory patient to take extra precautions because of the risk of drowsiness.
- Instruct patient to report constipation, severe nausea, and shortness of breath.
- Instruct patient to prevent postoperative atelectasis by turning, coughing, and deep-breathing.
- Urge patient to avoid alcohol, sedatives, and tranquilizers during meperidine therapy.

mephentermine sulfate
Wyamine

Class and Category
Chemical: Sympathomimetic amine
Therapeutic: Vasopressor
Pregnancy category: C

Indications and Dosages
▶ *To treat hypotension secondary to spinal anesthesia*
I.V. INJECTION
Adults. 30 to 45 mg (15 mg for obstetrical patients); may be repeated as needed to maintain blood pressure.
I.V. INFUSION
Adults. Dosage individualized based on patient response to therapy. Average dose is 1 to 5 mg/min.

Route	Onset	Peak	Duration
I.V.	Almost immediate	Unknown	15 to 30 min

Mechanism of Action

Stimulates alpha-adrenergic receptors directly and indirectly, resulting in positive inotropic and chronotropic effects. Indirect stimulation occurs by the release of norepinephrine from its storage sites in the heart and other tissues. By enhancing cardiac contraction, mephentermine improves cardiac output, thereby increasing blood pressure. Increased peripheral resistance from peripheral vasoconstriction may also contribute to increased blood pressure. Mephentermine can affect the heart rate but the change is variable, based on vagal tone. It may also stimulate beta-adrenergic receptors.

Contraindications

Hypersensitivity to mephentermine, phenothiazine-induced hypotension, use within 14 days of MAO inhibitor therapy

Interactions

DRUGS

alpha blockers, other drugs with alpha-blocking effects: Possibly decreased peripheral vasoconstrictive and hypertensive effects of mephentermine

beta blockers (ophthalmic): Decreased effects of mephentermine; increased risk of bronchospasm, wheezing, decreased pulmonary function, and respiratory failure

beta blockers (systemic): Increased risk of bronchospasm, decreased effects of both drugs

diuretics and other antihypertensives: Possibly reduced effectiveness of these drugs

doxapram: Possibly increased vasopressor effects of either drug

ergot alkaloids: Increased vasopressor effects

guanadrel, guanethidine, mecamylamine, methyldopa, reserpine: Possibly decreased effects of these drugs and increased risk of adverse effects

hydrocarbon inhalation anesthetics: Increased risk of atrial and ventricular arrhythmias

MAO inhibitors: Intensified and extended cardiac stimulation and vasopressor effects, possibly severe headache and hypertensive crisis

maprotiline, tricyclic antidepressants: Increased vasopressor response; increased risk of prolonged QTc interval, arrhythmias, hypertension, and hyperpyrexia

methylphenidate: Possibly increased vasopressor effect of mephentermine *nitrates:* Possibly reduced antianginal effects of nitrates and decreased vasopressor effect

other sympathomimetics (such as dopamine): Possibly increased cardiac effects and adverse reactions

oxytocin: Possibly severe hypertension

thyroid hormones: Increased effects of both drugs, increased risk of coronary insufficiency in patients with coronary artery disease

Adverse Reactions

CNS: Anxiety, dizziness, drowsiness, euphoria, headache, incoherence, nervousness, psychosis, restlessness, seizures, weakness

CV: Angina, arrhythmias (including bradycardia, tachycardia, and ventricular arrhythmias), hypertension, hypotension, palpitations, peripheral vasoconstriction

GI: Nausea, vomiting

RESP: Dyspnea

SKIN: Peripheral necrosis

Nursing Considerations

- Before administering mephentermine, expect to intervene, as ordered, to correct hemorrhage, hypovolemia, metabolic acidosis, or hypoxia.
- Discard vial if you observe discoloration or precipitate.
- Using D_5W or NS, prepare a 1-mg/ml concentration solution for infusion.
- Administer drug using an infusion pump to provide a controlled rate.
- Monitor blood pressure, cardiac rate and rhythm, central venous pressure (if appropriate), and urine output during administration. Adjust infusion rate according to patient response, as ordered. Be aware that patients with a history of cardiovascular disease (including hypertension) or hyperthyroidism and chronically ill patients are at increased risk for mephentermine's adverse cardiovascular effects.
- Assess patients with angle-closure glaucoma for signs of an exacerbation, such as eye pain or blurred vision.
- Assess circulation in patients with a history of occlusive vascular disease, such as atherosclerosis and Raynaud's disease, because mephentermine may cause decreased circulation and increase the risk of necrosis or gangrene. Inspect I.V. site periodically for signs of extravasation.
- **WARNING** Be aware that weeping, excitability, seizures, and hallucinations are some of the symptoms of mephenter-

mine overdose. Contact prescriber immediately if patient experiences such symptoms, and expect to provide supportive treatment.

- Be aware that mephentermine can increase contractions in pregnant women, especially during the third trimester. Expect drug to be prescribed only when benefits outweigh potential adverse effects.
- Store drug at 15° to 30° C (59° to 86° F); don't freeze.

PATIENT TEACHING

- Instruct patient receiving mephentermine to report adverse reactions, including chest pain, difficulty breathing, dizziness, irregular heartbeat, headache, and weakness.

meropenem

Merrem I.V.

Class and Category

Chemical: Carbapenem
Therapeutic: Antibiotic
Pregnancy category: B

Indications and Dosages

▶ *To treat complicated appendicitis and peritonitis caused by susceptible strains of alpha-hemolytic streptococci,* Bacteroides fragilis, B. thetaiotaomicron, Escherichia coli, Klebsiella pneumoniae, Peptostreptococcus *species, or* Pseudomonas aeruginosa

I.V. INFUSION OR INJECTION

Adults and children who weigh 50 kg (110 lb) or more. 1 g q 8 hr infused over 15 to 30 min or given as a bolus over 3 to 5 min.

Children over age 3 months who weigh less than 50 kg. 20 mg/kg q 8 hr infused over 15 to 30 min or given as a bolus over 3 to 5 min.

DOSAGE ADJUSTMENT For patients with creatinine clearance of 26 to 50 ml/min/1.73 m^2, dosage reduced to 1 g q 12 hr; with creatinine clearance of 10 to 25 ml/min/1.73 m^2, dosage reduced to 500 mg q 12 hr; with creatinine clearance of less than 10 ml/min/1.73 m^2, dosage reduced to 500 mg q 24 hr.

▶ *To treat bacterial meningitis caused by* Haemophilus influenzae, Neisseria meningitidis, *or* Streptococcus pneumoniae *in children*

I.V. INFUSION OR INJECTION

Children who weigh 50 kg or more. 2 g q 8 hr infused over 15 to 30 min or given as a bolus over 3 to 5 min.

Children over age 3 months who weigh less than 50 kg.
40 mg/kg q 8 hr infused over 15 to 30 min or given as a bolus
over 3 to 5 min. *Maximum:* 2 g q 8 hr.

Mechanism of Action
Penetrates cell walls of most gram-negative and gram-positive bacteria, inactivating penicillin-binding proteins. This action inhibits bacterial cell wall synthesis and causes cell death.

Incompatibilities
Don't mix meropenem in same solution as any other drugs.

Contraindications
Hypersensitivity to meropenem, other carbapenem drugs, beta lactams, or their components

Interactions
DRUGS
probenecid: Inhibited renal excretion of meropenem
valproic acid: Possibly decreased blood level and therapeutic effectiveness of valproic acid

Adverse Reactions
CNS: Headache, seizures
EENT: Epistaxis, glossitis, oral candidiasis
GI: Anorexia, constipation, diarrhea, elevated liver function test results, nausea, pseudomembranous colitis, vomiting
GU: Elevated BUN and serum creatinine levels, hematuria, renal failure, vaginitis
RESP: Apnea, dyspnea
SKIN: Diaper rash from candidiasis (children), pruritus, rash
Other: Anaphylaxis; injection site inflammation, pain, or phlebitis

Nursing Considerations
- Obtain body fluid and tissue specimens, as ordered, for culture and sensitivity testing. Expect to review test results, if possible, before giving first dose of meropenem.
- If you'll be administering drug by I.V. bolus, add 10 ml of sterile water for injection to 500-mg/20-ml vial, or 20 ml of diluent to 1-g/30-ml vial of drug. Shake to dissolve. Use within 2 hours if stored at 15° to 25° C (59° to 77° F) or within 12 hours if refrigerated. Further dilute this solution with appropriate diluent if you'll be administering drug by I.V. infusion.

- Prepare infusion bottles (available as 500 mg and 1 g) using 100 ml of D_5W, NS, or 0.45NS. Use solution prepared with D_5W within 1 hour if stored at 15° to 25° C (59° to 77° F) or within 8 hours if refrigerated. Use solution prepared with NS within 2 hours if stored at 15° to 25° C (59° to 77°) or within 18 hours if refrigerated. Be aware that drug's stability varies, depending on the drug form used, type and amount of diluent, and storage method. Consult manufacturer's insert for specific guidelines.
- **WARNING** Be aware that fatal hypersensitivity reactions have occurred with meropenem. Determine whether patient has had previous reactions to antibiotics or other allergens.
- Be prepared to administer emergency treatment for anaphylaxis, including epinephrine, corticosteroids, and oxygen.
- Take seizure precautions, according to facility policy, for patients with bacterial meningitis or CNS or renal disorders because they're at increased risk for seizures with meropenem.
- Observe for signs of secondary infection, such as oral candidiasis or pseudomembranous colitis, caused by overgrowth of nonsusceptible fungi or bacteria.
- Before reconstituting meropenem, store it at 20° to 25° C (68° to 77° F).

PATIENT TEACHING
- Advise patient to report diarrhea, difficulty breathing, injection site pain, mouth soreness, or vaginal irritation.

metaraminol bitartrate

Aramine

Class and Category

Chemical: Sympathomimetic amine
Therapeutic: Vasopressor
Pregnancy category: C

Indications and Dosages

▶ *To treat hypotension secondary to spinal anesthesia or as adjunct to treat hypotension caused by hemorrhage, adverse drug reactions, surgical complications, or shock resulting from brain damage secondary to trauma or tumor*

I.V. INFUSION
Adults. 15 to 100 mg (base) mixed in 500 ml of NS or D_5W; dosage individualized to maintain desired blood pressure.

▶ *To treat severe shock*
I.V. INJECTION
Adults. 500 mcg (0.5 mg) to 5 mg (base), followed by I.V. infusion individualized to maintain desired blood pressure.

Route	Onset	Peak	Duration
I.V.	1 to 2 min	Unknown	20 to 60 min

Mechanism of Action
Thought to directly stimulate alpha-adrenergic receptors and inhibit activity of the intracellular enzyme adenyl cyclase, which then inhibits production of cAMP. Inhibition of cAMP causes arterial and venous constriction and increases peripheral vascular resistance and systolic blood pressure. Metaraminol also directly stimulates beta-adrenergic receptors in the myocardium and increases adenyl cyclase activity, producing positive inotropic and chronotropic effects.

Incompatibilities
Don't mix metaraminol with barbiturates, penicillins, phenytoin, sodium salts, or other drugs that have poor solubility in acidic solutions.

Contraindications
Hypersensitivity to metaraminol or its components, including sulfites; use with cyclopropane or halothane anesthesia unless clinically warranted

Interactions
DRUGS
alpha blockers, other drugs with alpha-blocking effects: Possibly decreased peripheral vasoconstrictive and hypertensive effects of metaraminol
beta blockers (ophthalmic): Decreased effects of metaraminol; increased risk of bronchospasm, wheezing, decreased pulmonary function, and respiratory failure
beta blockers (systemic): Increased risk of bronchospasm, decreased effects of both drugs
digoxin: Increased risk of arrhythmias
diuretics and other antihypertensives: Possibly reduced effectiveness of these drugs
doxapram: Possibly increased vasopressor effects of both drugs
ergot alkaloids: Increased vasopressor effects

guanadrel, guanethidine, mecamylamine, methyldopa: Possibly decreased effects of these drugs and increased risk of adverse effects
hydrocarbon inhalation anesthetics: Increased risk of atrial and ventricular arrhythmias
MAO inhibitors: Intensified and extended cardiac stimulation and vasopressor effects; possibly severe hypertension
maprotiline, tricyclic antidepressants: Increased vasopressor response; increased risk of prolonged QTc interval, arrhythmias, hypertension, and hyperpyrexia
methylphenidate: Possibly increased vasopressor effect of metaraminol
nitrates: Possibly reduced antianginal effects of nitrates, decreased vasopressor effect
other sympathomimetics (such as dopamine): Possibly increased cardiac effects and adverse reactions
oxytocin: Possibly severe hypertension
thyroid hormones: Increased effects of both drugs, increased risk of coronary insufficiency in patients with coronary artery disease

Adverse Reactions
CNS: Anxiety, dizziness, headache, nervousness, seizures, weakness
CV: Angina, arrhythmias (including bradycardia, tachycardia, and ventricular arrhythmias), hypertension, hypotension, palpitations, peripheral vasoconstriction
GI: Nausea, vomiting
RESP: Dyspnea
SKIN: Extravasation with tissue necrosis and sloughing
Other: Injection site abscess

Nursing Considerations
- Before starting metaraminol therapy, expect to administer blood, plasma volume expanders, I.V. fluids, and electrolyte replacement therapy, as ordered, to correct conditions that caused hypotension, such as hemorrhage or hypovolemia.
- Discard vial if you observe discoloration or precipitates.
- To prepare an I.V. infusion, add 15 to 100 mg of metaraminol to 500 ml of appropriate solution, such as NS or D_5W. (You may use a smaller or larger amount of solution, depending on patient's fluid needs.) Use within 24 hours.
- Expect to use large veins for I.V. administration, such as antecubital fossa or a vein in the thigh. Administer infusion using an infusion pump to provide a controlled rate.

- Monitor blood pressure, cardiac rate and rhythm, central venous pressure, and urine output during administration. Be aware that vasoconstrictive effects of prolonged metaraminol administration may prevent volume expansion and prolong shock state. If this occurs, expect to administer blood and plasma volume expanders, as ordered.
- Allow at least 10 minutes to pass between dosage adjustments to let dose achieve maximum effect. Adjust infusion rate to patient response, as ordered.
- **WARNING** Assess for allergic reactions—including anaphylaxis and, possibly, life-threatening asthmatic episodes— because drug contains sodium bisulfite.
- Expect to discontinue metaraminol infusion gradually. Continue to monitor patient's blood pressure after infusion has stopped; elevated blood pressure may persist from drug's cumulative effects. Expect to restart metaraminol, as prescribed, if hypotension recurs.
- Be aware that patients with a history of cardiovascular disease (including hypertension) or hyperthyroidism and chronically ill patients are at increased risk for drug's adverse cardiovascular effects. Monitor patients with acute MI for worsening of condition because metaraminol can intensify or prolong myocardial ischemia.
- Monitor patients with cirrhosis for arrhythmias and diuresis. Expect to administer electrolytes, as prescribed, if diuresis occurs.
- Assess patients with angle-closure glaucoma for signs of an exacerbation, such as eye pain or blurred vision.
- Assess circulation in patients with a history of occlusive vascular disease, such as atherosclerosis, diabetic endarteritis, and Raynaud's disease, because metaraminol may cause decreased circulation and increase the risk of necrosis or gangrene. Inspect I.V. site periodically for signs of extravasation.
- **WARNING** Be aware that headache, euphoria, arrhythmias, severe hypertension, and MI are some of the symptoms of metaraminol overdose. Contact prescriber immediately if patient experiences such symptoms, and expect to provide supportive treatment.
- Monitor patients with a history of malaria for signs of a metaraminol-induced relapse, such as fever, chills, or muscle aches.
- Store drug at 15° to 30° C (59° to 86° F); protect from freezing and light.

- Advise patient to immediately report any discomfort at metaraminol infusion site, such as pain, swelling, or redness.
- Instruct patient to report adverse reactions, including chest pain, difficulty breathing, dizziness, irregular heartbeat, headache, and weakness.

methicillin sodium
Staphcillin

Class and Category
Chemical: Penicillinase-resistant penicillin
Therapeutic: Antibiotic
Pregnancy category: B

Indications and Dosages
▶ *To treat general infections, such as sepsis, sinusitis, and skin and soft-tissue infections, caused by susceptible organisms (including penicillinase-producing and non-penicillinase-producing strains of* Staphylococcus epidermidis, Staphylococcus saprophyticus, *and* Streptococcus pneumoniae*)*

I.V. INFUSION
Adults and children who weigh 40 kg (88 lb) or more. 1 g q 6 hr. *Maximum:* 24 g/day.
Children who weigh less than 40 kg. 25 mg/kg q 6 hr.
DOSAGE ADJUSTMENT For adults and children with cystic fibrosis, dosage decreased to 50 mg/kg q 6 hr.
▶ *To treat bacterial meningitis*

I.V. INFUSION
Neonates who weigh 2 kg (4.4 lb) or more. 50 mg/kg q 8 hr for first wk after birth and then 50 mg/kg q 6 hr.
Neonates who weigh less than 2 kg. 25 to 50 mg/kg q 12 hr for first wk after birth and then 50 mg/kg q 8 hr.

Mechanism of Action
Kills bacterial cells by inhibiting bacterial cell wall synthesis. In susceptible bacteria, the rigid, cross-linked cell wall is assembled in several steps. In the final stage of cross-linking, methicillin binds with and inactivates penicillin-binding proteins (enzymes responsible for linking cell wall strands), resulting in bacterial cell lysis and death. *Staphylococcus aureus* has developed resistance to methicillin by altering its penicillin-binding proteins.

Incompatibilities

Don't mix methicillin in same syringe or I.V. solution with other drugs. Don't mix methicillin with dextrose solutions because their low acidity may damage drug. Administer methicillin at least 1 hour before or after aminoglycosides and at different sites to prevent mutual inactivation.

Contraindications

Hypersensitivity to methicillin sodium, other penicillins, or their components

Interactions

DRUGS

aminoglycosides: Substantial aminoglycoside inactivation
chloramphenicol, erythromycins, sulfonamides, tetracyclines: Possibly decreased therapeutic effects of methicillin
methotrexate: Increased risk of methotrexate toxicity
probenecid: Possibly decreased renal clearance, increased blood level, and increased risk of toxicity of methicillin

Adverse Reactions

CNS: Aggressiveness, agitation, anxiety, confusion, depression, headache, seizures
EENT: Oral candidiasis
GI: Abdominal pain, diarrhea, hepatotoxicity, nausea, pseudomembranous colitis, vomiting
GU: Interstitial nephritis, vaginitis
HEME: Leukopenia, neutropenia, thrombocytopenia
SKIN: Exfoliative dermatitis, pruritus, rash, urticaria
Other: Anaphylaxis; infusion site redness, swelling, and tenderness; serum sickness–like reaction

Nursing Considerations

- **WARNING** Be aware that methicillin is not a first-line treatment for the indications listed previously because of the prevalence of methicillin-resistant *Staphylococcus aureus.*
- Before giving first dose, obtain appropriate body fluid or tissue specimens for culture and sensitivity tests, as ordered, and review test results if available.
- Add 1.5 ml, 5.7 ml, or 8.6 ml of sterile water for injection or 0.9% sodium chloride injection to 1-g, 4-g, or 6-g vial, respectively, to yield a concentration of 500 mg/ml. Dilute further with 25 ml of NS for each 500 mg (1 ml) of drug. Use concentrations of 2 to 20 mg/ml within 8 hours if stored at room temperature.

- Observe infusion site closely during administration for redness, swelling, and tenderness.
- Monitor fluid intake and output and renal function test results during methicillin therapy.
- Observe for signs of superinfection, such as diarrhea, vaginal itching, and white patches or sores in mouth or on tongue. Notify prescriber if they occur.
- Closely monitor renal function test results, including serum creatinine level; about one-third of patients experience interstitial nephritis after 10 days of methicillin therapy.
- Monitor liver function test results, and observe for signs of hepatotoxicity, such as fever and nausea. Notify prescriber if such signs occur.
- When calculating sodium intake for patients on a sodium-restricted diet, keep in mind that each gram of methicillin contains approximately 2.24 mEq of sodium.
- Store drug at 15° to 30° C (59° to 86° F).

PATIENT TEACHING
- Unless contraindicated, instruct patient to drink extra fluids during methicillin therapy.
- Advise patient to report diarrhea, infusion site pain, mouth sores, or rash.

methocarbamol

Carbacot, Robaxin, Skelex

Class and Category

Chemical: Carbamate derivative of guaifenesin
Therapeutic: Skeletal muscle relaxant
Pregnancy category: C

Indications and Dosages

▶ *To relieve discomfort caused by acute, painful musculoskeletal conditions*

I.V. INJECTION (100 MG/ML)

Adults and adolescents. Up to 3,000 mg/day administered q 8 hr for 3 consecutive days. Regimen repeated as prescribed after patient is drug-free for 48 hr.

▶ *To provide supportive therapy for tetanus*

I.V. INFUSION OR INJECTION (100 MG/ML)

Adults and adolescents. 1,000 to 3,000 mg by infusion or 1,000 to 2,000 mg by direct injection q 6 hr. *Maximum:* 3 g/day.
Children. 15 mg/kg q 6 hr.

Route	Onset	Peak	Duration
I.V.	Immediate	Almost immediate	Unknown

Mechanism of Action
May depress the CNS, which leads to sedation and reduced skeletal muscle spasms. Methocarbamol also alters the perception of pain.

Contraindications
Hypersensitivity to methocarbamol or its components, renal disease

Interactions
DRUGS
CNS depressants: Increased CNS depression
ACTIVITIES
alcohol use: Increased CNS depression

Adverse Reactions
CNS: Dizziness, drowsiness, fever, headache, light-headedness, seizures, syncope, vertigo, weakness
CV: Bradycardia, hypotension, thrombophlebitis
EENT: Blurred vision, conjunctivitis, diplopia, metallic taste, nasal congestion, nystagmus
GI: Nausea
GU: Black, brown, or green urine
SKIN: Flushing, pruritus, rash, urticaria
Other: Anaphylaxis, injection site sloughing

Nursing Considerations
• To prepare solution for I.V. infusion, add 10 ml of methocarbamol to no more than 250 ml of D_5W or NS. Infuse directly through I.V. infusion line at no more than 300 mg (3 ml)/minute to avoid hypotension and seizures.
• Keep patient recumbent during I.V. administration and for at least 15 minutes afterward. Then have him rise slowly.
• Monitor I.V. site regularly for signs of phlebitis.
• Keep epinephrine, antihistamines, and corticosteroids available in case patient experiences anaphylactic reaction to parenterally administered drug.
• Monitor renal function test results, as ordered, for signs of impaired renal function, especially if patient has received methocarbamol for 3 days or longer.

- Monitor patients with a history of epilepsy because they may be at increased risk for seizures during methocarbamol therapy.
- Store drug at 15° to 30° C (59° to 86° F); don't freeze.

PATIENT TEACHING
- Inform patient that urine may turn green, black, or brown during methocarbamol therapy but that this will resolve when drug is discontinued.
- Advise patient to avoid potentially hazardous activities until drug's CNS effects are known.
- Instruct patient to avoid alcohol and other CNS depressants during methocarbamol therapy.

methotrexate sodium
Folex, Folex PFS, Mexate, Mexate-AQ

Class and Category
Chemical: Folic acid analogue
Therapeutic: Antipsoriatic
Pregnancy category: X

Indications and Dosages
▶ *To treat severe psoriasis that is unresponsive to other therapy*
I.V. INJECTION
Adults. 10 mg/wk. *Maximum:* 25 mg/wk.
▶ *To treat acute lymphocytic leukemia*
I.V. INFUSION OR INJECTION
Adults. *Induction:* 3.3 mg (base)/m² q day in combination with prednisone or other drugs. *Maintenance:* 2.5 mg/kg q 14 days.
▶ *To treat osteosarcoma*
I.V. INFUSION
Adults. 12 g/m² over 4 hr on weeks 4, 5, 6, 7, 11, 12, 15, 16, 29, 30, 44, and 45 after surgery, in combination with other drugs. Dosage may be increased to 15 g/m² to reach peak blood methotrexate concentration of 1×10^{-3} M/L.

Route	Onset	Peak	Duration
I.V.*	3 to 6 wk	Unknown	Unknown

*For severe psoriasis.

Mechanism of Action

May exert its immunosuppressive effects by inhibiting the replication and function of T lymphocytes and, possibly, B lymphocytes, which are involved in immune and inflammatory processes. Methotrexate also slows the growth of rapidly proliferating cells, such as epithelial skin cells associated with psoriasis. This action may result from the drug's ability to inhibit dihydrofolate reductase, the enzyme that reduces folic acid to tetrahydrofolic acid. Inhibition of tetrahydrofolic acid interferes with DNA synthesis and cell reproduction in rapidly proliferating cells.

Contraindications

Breast-feeding, hypersensitivity to methotrexate or its components, pregnancy

Interactions

DRUGS

blood-dyscrasia–causing drugs (such as cephalosporins and sulfasalazine): Increased risk of leukopenia and thrombocytopenia

bone marrow depressants: Possibly increased bone marrow depression

folic acid: Possibly decreased effectiveness of methotrexate

hepatotoxic drugs: Increased risk of hepatotoxicity

NSAIDs, penicillins, probenecid, salicylates: Increased risk of methotrexate toxicity

oral anticoagulants: Increased risk of bleeding

phenytoin: Increased risk of methotrexate toxicity

probenecid: Possibly decreased methotrexate excretion and increased blood methotrexate level

sulfonamides: Increased risk of hepatotoxicity

theophylline: Possibly increased blood theophylline level

vaccines, killed virus: Possibly decreased antibody response to vaccine

vaccines, live virus: Possibly decreased antibody response to vaccine, increased adverse effects of vaccine, and severe infection

ACTIVITIES

alcohol use: Increased risk of hepatotoxicity

Adverse Reactions

CNS: Cerebral thrombosis, chemical arachnoiditis, chills, demyelination, drowsiness, fatigue, fever, headache, increased CSF pressure, leukoencephalopathy

CV: Chest pain, deep vein thrombosis, hypotension, pericardial effusion, pericarditis, thromboembolism

EENT: Blurred vision, conjunctivitis, gingivitis, glossitis, pharyngitis, stomatitis, tinnitus
GI: Anorexia, diarrhea, enteritis, GI bleeding or ulceration, hepatotoxicity, intestinal perforation, nausea, pancreatitis, vomiting
GU: Azotemia, cystitis, hematuria, nephropathy, renal failure, tubular necrosis
HEME: Anemia, leukopenia, thrombocytopenia
MS: Arthralgia, myalgia
RESP: Dry cough, dyspnea, pneumonitis, pulmonary fibrosis, pulmonary infiltrates
SKIN: Acne, alopecia, boils, cutaneous vasculitis, ecchymosis, erythema, pallor, photosensitivity, pruritus, psoriatic lesions, rash, Stevens-Johnson syndrome, sunburn reactivation, urticaria
Other: Hyperuricemia; increased risk of infection, such as bacterial infection or septicemia

Nursing Considerations

- Follow facility policy for proper handling of methotrexate and disposal of used equipment because handling parenteral form poses a risk of carcinogenicity, mutagenicity, and teratogenicity. Avoid skin contact.
- Dilute preservative-free preparations immediately before use, and discard unused portions.
- Monitor results of CBC, chest X-ray, liver and renal function tests, and urinalysis before and during treatment.
- Examine patient's mouth for stomatitis before administering each dose of methotrexate.
- **WARNING** Make sure that leucovorin is available before administering high doses of methotrexate (for example, when drug is used to treat osteosarcoma). Administer leucovorin rescue as an antidote, as ordered, after methotrexate administration.
- Be aware that adverse reactions can vary when methotrexate is administered in combination therapy. Review information for all drugs administered as part of a specific regimen, including drug interactions and adverse effects.
- Expect methotrexate therapy to be interrupted if diarrhea, ulcerative stomatitis, or pulmonary symptoms occur because of the risk of progressive adverse effects. Be alert for a dry, unproductive cough, which may signal impending pulmonary toxicity.
- **WARNING** Be aware that patients who are receiving high doses or have renal impairment are at high risk for methotrexate toxicity. Renal impairment can severely alter drug

elimination by causing formation of crystals that obstruct urine flow. Alkalinize patient's urine with sodium bicarbonate tablets, as ordered, to prevent drug precipitation.

- Unless contraindicated, increase patient's fluid intake to 2 to 3 L/day to reduce the risk of adverse GU reactions. Administer allopurinol, as ordered, for uric acid nephropathy.
- Assess for signs of bleeding and infection.
- Follow standard precautions when caring for patient because drug can cause immunosuppression.
- If patient develops thrombocytopenia, implement protective precautions according to facility policy.
- Be aware that patients who are receiving concurrent or consecutive radiation therapy are at risk for additive bone marrow depression.
- If patient becomes dehydrated from vomiting, notify prescriber and expect to withhold drug until patient recovers.
- Once patient achieves an adequate antipsoriatic response to drug, expect dosage to be decreased gradually to lowest dosage and longest rest period that maintains clinical response. Also expect prescriber to return patient to conventional therapy for psoriasis, including topical drugs.
- Be aware that patients receiving long-term methotrexate therapy for severe psoriasis may develop drug resistance.
- Before diluting drug, store it at 15° to 30° C (59° to 86° F) and protect from light.

PATIENT TEACHING
- Instruct patient to avoid alcohol during methotrexate therapy.
- Advise patient to have dental work completed before beginning methotrexate therapy, if possible, or to defer such work until blood counts return to normal because methotrexate can delay healing and cause gingival bleeding. Teach patient proper oral hygiene, and advise him to use a soft-bristled toothbrush to reduce the risk of mouth sores.
- Instruct patient to use sunblock when he's outdoors.
- Advise patient to report bruising, chills, cough, fever, dark or bloody urine, mouth sores, shortness of breath, sore throat, and yellow skin or eyes.
- Urge patient and persons who live in same household to avoid immunizations unless approved by prescriber. Also instruct patient to avoid people who have received immunizations or to wear a mask if he must be around them.

- Instruct patient who develops bone marrow depression to avoid people with infections as well as contact sports and other activities that increase his risk of bleeding or injury.
- Advise patient to avoid salicylate-containing products and NSAIDs to prevent methotrexate toxicity.
- Urge women of childbearing age to use contraception during methotrexate therapy.

methyldopate hydrochloride
Aldomet

Class and Category
Chemical: 3,4-dihydroxyphenylalanine (DOPA) analogue
Therapeutic: Antihypertensive
Pregnancy category: C

Indications and Dosages
▶ *To manage hypertension, to treat hypertensive crisis*
I.V. INFUSION
Adults. 250 to 500 mg diluted in D_5W and infused over 30 to 60 min q 6 hr. *Maximum:* 1,000 mg q 6 hr.
Children. 20 to 40 mg/kg infused over 30 to 60 min q 6 hr. *Maximum:* 65 mg/kg or 3,000 mg/day.

Route	Onset	Peak	Duration
I.V.	Unknown	4 to 6 hr	10 to 16 hr

Mechanism of Action
Is decarboxylated in the body to produce alpha-methylnorepinephrine, a metabolite that stimulates central inhibitory alpha-adrenergic receptors. This action may reduce blood pressure by decreasing sympathetic stimulation of the heart and peripheral vascular system.

Incompatibilities
Don't administer methyldopate through same I.V. line as barbiturates or sulfonamides.

Contraindications
Active hepatic disease; hypersensitivity to methyldopa, methyldopate, or their components; impaired hepatic function from previous methyldopa or methyldopate therapy; use within 14 days of MAO inhibitor therapy

Interactions

DRUGS

antihypertensives: Increased hypotension

appetite suppressants, NSAIDs, tricyclic antidepressants: Possibly decreased therapeutic effects of methyldopa

central anesthetics: Possibly need for reduced anesthetic dosage

CNS depressants: Possibly increased CNS depression

haloperidol: Increased risk of adverse CNS effects

levodopa: Possibly decreased therapeutic effects of levodopa and increased risk of adverse CNS effects

lithium: Increased risk of lithium toxicity

MAO inhibitors: Possibly hallucinations, headaches, hyperexcitability, and severe hypertension

oral anticoagulants: Possibly increased therapeutic effects of anticoagulants

sympathomimetics: Possibly decreased therapeutic effects of methyldopa and increased vasopressor effects of sympathomimetics

ACTIVITIES

alcohol use: Possibly increased CNS depression

Adverse Reactions

CNS: Decreased concentration, depression, dizziness, drowsiness, fever, headache, involuntary motor activity, memory loss (transient), nightmares, paresthesia, parkinsonism, sedation, vertigo, weakness

CV: Angina, bradycardia, edema, heart failure, myocarditis, orthostatic hypotension

EENT: Black or sore tongue, dry mouth, nasal congestion

ENDO: Gynecomastia

GI: Constipation, diarrhea, flatulence, hepatic necrosis, hepatitis, nausea, pancreatitis, vomiting

GU: Decreased libido, impotence

HEME: Agranulocytosis, hemolytic anemia, leukopenia, positive Coombs' test, positive tests for ANA and rheumatoid factor, thrombocytopenia

SKIN: Eczema, rash, urticaria

Other: Weight gain

Nursing Considerations

• Expect to monitor CBC and differential results before and periodically during methyldopa therapy.

• Add methyldopate to 100 ml of D_5W, and administer over 30 to 60 minutes.

• Monitor blood pressure regularly during therapy.

- Monitor results of Coombs' test; a positive result after several months of treatment indicates that patient has hemolytic anemia. Expect prescriber to discontinue drug.
- Assess for weight gain and edema. If they occur, administer a diuretic, as prescribed.
- Notify prescriber if patient experiences abnormal liver function test results, signs of heart failure (dyspnea, edema, hypertension), jaundice, fever, or involuntary jerky movements.
- Be aware that hypertension may return within 48 hours after drug is discontinued. Expect prescriber to convert patient to oral methyldopa, typically at same dosage as parenteral form. Maximum adult oral dosage is 3,000 mg/day.
- Store drug at 15° to 30° C (59° to 86° F); don't freeze.

PATIENT TEACHING

- Instruct patient to avoid potentially hazardous activities until methyldopate's CNS effects are known.
- Advise patient to change position slowly to minimize effects of orthostatic hypotension.
- Direct patient to report bruising, chest pain, fever, involuntary jerky movements, prolonged dizziness, rash, or yellow eyes or skin.

methylprednisolone sodium succinate

A-methaPred, Solu-Medrol

Class and Category

Chemical: Synthetic glucocorticoid
Therapeutic: Anti-inflammatory, immunosuppressant
Pregnancy category: Not rated

Indications and Dosages

▶ *To treat ulcerative colitis*

I.V. INFUSION

Adults. 40 to 120 mg 3 to 7 times/wk for 2 or more wk. Later doses based on patient's condition and response.

Children. 0.14 to 0.84 mg/kg/day in divided doses q 12 to 24 hr.

▶ *To treat a wide range of immune and inflammatory disorders, including allergic rhinitis, asthma, Crohn's disease, and systemic lupus erythematosus*

I.V. INFUSION

Adults. *Initial:* 10 to 40 mg infused over several min. Later doses based on patient's condition and response.

Children. 0.14 to 0.84 mg/kg q 12 to 24 hr.

▶ *To treat acute exacerbations of multiple sclerosis*
I.V. INJECTION
Adults. 160 mg q.d. for 1 wk, followed by 64 mg q.o.d. for 1 mo.

Route	Onset	Peak	Duration
I.V.	Rapid	30 min	Unknown

Mechanism of Action
Binds to intracellular glucocorticoid receptors and suppresses inflammatory and immune responses by:
- inhibiting the accumulation of neutrophils and monocytes at inflammation sites
- stabilizing lysosomal membranes
- suppressing the antigen response of macrophages and helper T cells
- inhibiting the synthesis of inflammatory response mediators, such as cytokines, interleukins, and prostaglandins.

Incompatibilities
Don't mix methylprednisolone with any drug without first consulting pharmacist.

Contraindications
Fungal infection, hypersensitivity to methylprednisolone or its components

Interactions
DRUGS
acetaminophen: Increased risk of hepatotoxicity
amphotericin B, carbonic anhydrase inhibitors: Possibly severe hypokalemia
anabolic steroids, androgens: Increased risk of edema and worsening of acne
anticholinergics: Possibly increased intraocular pressure
asparaginase: Increased risk of hyperglycemia and toxicity
aspirin, NSAIDs: Increased risk of adverse GI effects and bleeding
cyclosporine: Increased risk of seizures
digoxin: Possibly hypokalemia-induced arrhythmias and digitalis toxicity
ephedrine, phenobarbital, phenytoin, rifampin: Decreased blood methylprednisolone level
estrogens, oral contraceptives: Possibly increased therapeutic and toxic effects of methylprednisolone

isoniazid: Possibly decreased therapeutic effects of isoniazid
mexiletine: Possibly decreased blood mexiletine level
neuromuscular blockers: Possibly increased neuromuscular blockade, causing respiratory depression or apnea
oral anticoagulants, thrombolytics: Increased risk of GI ulceration and hemorrhage, possibly decreased therapeutic effects of these drugs
potassium-depleting drugs (such as thiazide diuretics): Possibly severe hypokalemia
potassium supplements: Possibly decreased effects of these supplements
somatrem, somatropin: Possibly decreased therapeutic effects of these drugs
streptozocin: Increased risk of hyperglycemia
troleandomycin: Increased blood methylprednisolone level
vaccines: Decreased antibody response and increased risk of neurologic complications
ACTIVITIES
alcohol use: Increased risk of adverse GI effects and bleeding

Adverse Reactions

CNS: Ataxia, behavioral changes, depression, dizziness, euphoria, fatigue, headache, increased ICP with papilledema, insomnia, malaise, mood changes, paresthesia, restlessness, seizures, steroid psychosis, syncope, vertigo
CV: Arrhythmias (from hypokalemia), edema, fat embolism, heart failure, hypertension, hypotension, thromboembolism, thrombophlebitis
EENT: Exophthalmos, glaucoma, increased intraocular pressure, nystagmus, posterior subcapsular cataracts
ENDO: Adrenal insufficiency, cushingoid symptoms (moon face, buffalo hump, central obesity, supraclavicular fat pad enlargement), diabetes mellitus, growth suppression in children, hyperglycemia, negative nitrogen balance from protein catabolism
GI: Abdominal distention, hiccups, increased appetite, melena, nausea, pancreatitis, peptic ulcer, ulcerative esophagitis, vomiting
GU: Amenorrhea, glycosuria, menstrual irregularities, perineal burning or tingling
HEME: Easy bruising, leukocytosis
MS: Arthralgia; aseptic necrosis of femoral and humeral heads; compression fractures; muscle atrophy, twitching, or weakness; myalgia; osteoporosis; spontaneous fractures; steroid myopathy; tendon rupture

SKIN: Acne; altered skin pigmentation; diaphoresis; erythema; hirsutism; necrotizing vasculitis; petechiae; purpura; rash; scarring; sterile abscess; striae; subcutaneous fat atrophy; thin, fragile skin; urticaria

Other: Anaphylaxis, hypocalcemia, hypokalemia, hypokalemic alkalosis, impaired wound healing, masking of infection, metabolic alkalosis, suppressed skin test reaction, weight gain

Nursing Considerations

- **WARNING** Don't administer methylprednisolone preparations that contain benzyl alcohol to neonates or premature infants because this preservative has been linked to a fatal toxic syndrome characterized by CNS, respiratory, circulatory, and renal impairment and metabolic acidosis.
- Don't administer acetate injectable form by I.V. route; this form is used for intra-articular, intralesional, I.M., and soft-tissue injections.
- After reconstituting drug according to manufacturer's directions, use it within 48 hours.
- Discard parenteral products if you observe discoloration or particles.
- Arrange for low-sodium diet with added potassium, as prescribed.
- Protect patient from falling, especially elderly patient at risk for fractures from osteoporosis.
- Closely monitor patient for signs of infection because drug may mask them.
- Assess for possible depression or psychotic episodes during therapy.
- Monitor blood glucose level; dosage of insulin or oral antidiabetic drug may need to be adjusted for diabetic patient.
- **WARNING** To avoid possibly fatal acute adrenocortical insufficiency, expect to taper long-term therapy when it must be discontinued.
- Store drug at a controlled room temperature of 20° to 25° C (68° to 77° F), and protect from light.

PATIENT TEACHING

- Urge patient receiving methylprednisolone to immediately report dark or tarry stools; signs of impending adrenocortical insufficiency, such as anorexia, dizziness, fainting, fatigue, fever, joint pain, muscle weakness, or nausea; and sudden weight gain or swelling.

- Inform patient with diabetes that his blood glucose level will be checked frequently during therapy because methylprednisolone may affect glucose level.
- Advise patient to notify prescriber if he develops another illness or requires surgery during therapy or if his condition recurs or worsens after dosage is reduced or therapy is discontinued.
- Instruct patient not to obtain vaccinations unless approved by prescriber.
- Urge patient to take vitamin D, calcium supplements, or both if recommended by prescriber.
- Instruct patient on long-term therapy to follow a low-sodium, high-potassium, high-protein diet, if prescribed, to help minimize weight gain. Advise him to inform prescriber if he's on a special diet.
- Inform patient that insomnia and restlessness usually resolve after 1 to 3 weeks of therapy.
- Caution patient to avoid people with contagious diseases, such as chicken pox or measles.
- Discuss the need for regular exercise or physical therapy to maintain muscle mass.
- Urge patient to avoid alcoholic beverages during therapy because alcohol increases the risk of GI bleeding.
- Encourage patient to keep regularly scheduled follow-up medical appointments, even after therapy stops.
- Instruct patient to undergo periodic ophthalmic examinations.
- Advise patient to carry medical identification that documents his need for long-term corticosteroid therapy.

metoclopramide hydrochloride
Reglan

Class and Category
Chemical: Benzamide
Therapeutic: Antiemetic, upper GI stimulant
Pregnancy category: B

Indications and Dosages
▶ *To treat diabetic gastroparesis*
I.V. INJECTION
Adults and adolescents. 10 mg t.i.d. or q.i.d. for severe symptoms; dosage adjusted as needed.

▶ *To prevent chemotherapy-induced vomiting*
I.V. INFUSION
Adults and adolescents. 3 mg/kg before chemotherapy and then 0.5 mg/kg/hr for 8 hr.
I.V. INJECTION
Adults and adolescents. 1 to 2 mg/kg 30 min before chemotherapy and then repeated q 2 to 3 hr, as needed.
Children. 1 mg/kg as a single dose, repeated in 1 hr. *Maximum:* 2 mg/kg.
DOSAGE ADJUSTMENT Usual dose reduced by 50% if creatinine clearance is less than 40 ml/min/1.73 m^2.

Route	Onset	Peak	Duration
I.V.	1 to 3 min	Unknown	1 to 2 hr

Mechanism of Action
May enhance gastric motility by antagonizing the inhibitory neurotransmitter effect of dopamine on GI smooth muscle. This results in gastric contraction, promoting gastric emptying and increased peristalsis. Metoclopramide also blocks dopaminergic receptors in the chemoreceptor trigger zone, thereby preventing nausea and vomiting.

Incompatibilities
Don't administer metoclopramide through same I.V. line as calcium gluconate, cephalothin sodium, chloramphenicol sodium, cisplatin, erythromycin lactobionate, furosemide, methotrexate, penicillin G potassium, or sodium bicarbonate.

Contraindications
Concurrent use of butyrophenones, phenothiazines, or other drugs that may cause extrapyramidal reactions; GI hemorrhage, mechanical obstruction, or perforation; hypersensitivity to metoclopramide or its components; pheochromocytoma; seizure disorders

Interactions
DRUGS
anticholinergics, opioid analgesics: Possibly decreased therapeutic effects of metoclopramide
apomorphine: Possibly decreased antiemetic effect of apomorphine, possibly increased CNS depression

bromocriptine, pergolide: Possibly decreased therapeutic effects of these drugs
cimetidine: Possibly decreased absorption and therapeutic effects of cimetidine
CNS depressants: Possibly increased CNS depression
cyclosporine: Increased blood cyclosporine level
digoxin: Decreased gastric absorption of digoxin
levodopa: Possibly decreased levodopa effectiveness
MAO inhibitors: Increased risk of severe hypertension in patients with essential hypertension
mexiletine: Possibly faster mexiletine absorption
succinylcholine: Possibly prolonged therapeutic action of succinylcholine
ACTIVITIES
alcohol use: Increased risk of excessive sedation

Adverse Reactions

CNS: Agitation, anxiety, depression, dizziness, drowsiness, extrapyramidal reactions (motor restlessness, parkinsonism, tardive dyskinesia), fatigue, headache, insomnia, irritability, lassitude, panic reaction, restlessness
CV: Hypertension, hypotension, tachycardia
EENT: Dry mouth
ENDO: Galactorrhea, gynecomastia
GI: Constipation, diarrhea, nausea
GU: Menstrual irregularities
HEME: Agranulocytosis
SKIN: Rash
Other: Restless leg syndrome

Nursing Considerations

- Before administering metoclopramide, assess for signs of intestinal obstruction, such as abnormal bowel sounds, diarrhea, nausea, and vomiting. Notify prescriber if you detect such signs.
- Be aware that you don't need to dilute doses of 10 mg or less, unless ordered. Give these doses slowly, over 1 to 2 minutes. Dilute doses larger than 10 mg in 50 ml of NS, 0.45NS, D_5W, Ringer's injection, or LR, and infuse over at least 15 minutes.
- Use diluted solutions within 24 hours if protected from light. Discard unused portions in vial or ampule because drug doesn't contain preservatives.
- Avoid too-rapid I.V. administration because it may cause intense anxiety, restlessness, and then drowsiness.

- **WARNING** Notify prescriber if patient displays signs of toxicity, such as disorientation, drowsiness, and extrapyramidal reactions.
- Monitor blood pressure, especially in patients with a history of hypertension, because metoclopramide may aggravate this condition.
- Be aware that patients with Parkinson's disease are also at risk for an exacerbation from metoclopramide therapy.
- Monitor patient for signs of depression, even if he has no prior history.
- Assess patients with a history of asthma for increasing shortness of breath, wheezing, or difficulty breathing because drug may increase their risk of bronchospasm.
- Store drug at 15° to 30° C (59° to 86° F), and protect from light.

PATIENT TEACHING
- Advise patient to avoid activities that require alertness for about 2 hours after each dose of metoclopramide.
- Urge patient to avoid alcohol and CNS depressants while receiving metoclopramide because they may increase CNS depression.
- Advise patient to avoid potentially hazardous activities until drug's CNS effects are known.
- Instruct patient to immediately report involuntary movements of the face, eyes, tongue, or hands.

metoprolol tartrate
Apo-Metoprolol (Type L), Betaloc (CAN), Lopresor (CAN), Lopressor, Novometoprol (CAN), Nu-Metop (CAN)

Class and Category
Chemical: Beta$_1$-adrenergic antagonist
Therapeutic: Antianginal, MI prophylaxis and treatment
Pregnancy category: C

Indications and Dosages
▶ *To treat acute MI or evolving acute MI*
I.V. INJECTION, TABLETS
Adults. *Initial:* 5 mg by I.V. bolus q 2 min for 3 doses, followed by 50 mg P.O. for patients who tolerate total I.V. dose (or 25 to 50 mg P.O. for patients who can't tolerate total I.V. dose) q 6 hr for 48 hr, starting 15 min after final I.V. dose; after 48 hr, 100 mg b.i.d., followed by maintenance dosage. *Maintenance:* 100 mg P.O. b.i.d. for at least 3 mo.

Route	Onset	Peak	Duration
I.V.	Unknown	20 min	Unknown
P.O.	60 min	1 to 2 hr	Unknown

Mechanism of Action

Inhibits stimulation of beta$_1$-receptor sites, located primarily in the heart, resulting in decreased cardiac excitability, cardiac output, and myocardial oxygen demand. These effects help relieve angina.

Contraindications

Acute heart failure, bradycardia below 45 beats/minute, cardiogenic shock, hypersensitivity to metoprolol or its components, second- or third-degree AV block

Interactions

DRUGS

aluminum salts, barbiturates, calcium salts, cholestyramine, colestipol, NSAIDs, rifampin, salicylates, sulfinpyrazone: Decreased therapeutic effects of metoprolol

amiodarone, digitalis glycosides, diltiazem, verapamil: Increased risk of complete AV block

calcium channel blockers: Increased risk of heart failure, increased therapeutic effects of both drugs

cimetidine: Increased blood metoprolol level

clonidine, diazoxide, guanabenz: Increased risk of hypotension

estrogens: Possibly decreased antihypertensive effect of metoprolol

general anesthetics: Increased risk of hypotension and heart failure

insulin, oral antidiabetic drugs: Decreased blood glucose control, possible masking of signs and symptoms of hypoglycemia

lidocaine: Increased risk of lidocaine toxicity

MAO inhibitors: Increased risk of hypertension

neuromuscular blockers: Possibly enhanced and prolonged neuromuscular blockade

other antihypertensives: Additive hypotensive effect

phenothiazines: Possibly increased blood levels of both drugs

propafenone: Increased blood level and half-life of metoprolol

sympathomimetics, xanthines: Possibly decreased therapeutic effects of these drugs or metoprolol

FOODS

all foods: Increased bioavailability of metoprolol

Adverse Reactions

CNS: Anxiety, confusion, depression, dizziness, drowsiness, fatigue, hallucinations, headache, insomnia, weakness
CV: Arrhythmias (including AV block and bradycardia), chest pain, heart failure, orthostatic hypotension
EENT: Nasal congestion
GI: Constipation, diarrhea, nausea, vomiting
GU: Impotence
HEME: Leukopenia, thrombocytopenia
MS: Back pain, myalgia
RESP: Bronchospasm, dyspnea
SKIN: Rash

Nursing Considerations

- If patient with acute MI delays treatment or can't tolerate initial metoprolol dosage, start with maintenance dosage, as prescribed and tolerated.
- **WARNING** If patient receives more than 400 mg/day, monitor for bronchospasm and dyspnea because metoprolol competitively blocks beta₂-adrenergic receptors in bronchial and vascular smooth muscles. Patients with bronchospastic disease are at highest risk.
- Expect elderly patients to be either more or less sensitive to drug's effects.
- **WARNING** When substituting metoprolol for clonidine, expect to gradually reduce clonidine dosage and increase metoprolol dosage over several days, as prescribed. Giving these drugs together causes additive hypotensive effects.
- Be aware that patients who take metoprolol may be at risk for AV block. If AV block results from depressed AV node conduction, prepare to administer appropriate drug, as prescribed, or assist with temporary pacemaker insertion.
- Be aware that patients with left ventricular dysfunction are at increased risk for heart failure from metoprolol therapy.
- Expect drug's negative inotropic effect to further depress cardiac output in patients with chronic heart failure. (Lower dosages may be beneficial for some patients with chronic heart failure.)
- Check for signs of poor glucose control in patients with diabetes mellitus because metoprolol may interfere with therapeutic effects of insulin and oral antidiabetic drugs. Drug also may mask signs of hypoglycemia, such as palpitations, tachycardia, and tremor, but doesn't mask diaphoresis and hypertension.

- Monitor patients with myasthenia gravis for increased muscle weakness and diplopia because beta blockers may worsen these symptoms.
- Assess patients with psoriasis for an exacerbation during metoprolol therapy. Notify prescriber if this occurs.
- **WARNING** Expect to taper metoprolol dosage when drug is discontinued; abrupt discontinuation can cause myocardial ischemia, MI, ventricular arrhythmias, or severe hypertension, especially in patients with cardiac disease. It also may precipitate thyroid storm in patients with hyperthyroidism or thyrotoxicosis.
- Store drug at 15° to 30° C (59° to 86° F); protect from freezing and light.

PATIENT TEACHING
- Instruct patient receiving metoprolol to immediately report dizziness or drowsiness.
- Inform diabetic patient that his blood glucose level will be checked frequently during metoprolol therapy.
- Advise patient to avoid potentially hazardous activities until drug's CNS effects are known.
- Instruct patient to take metoprolol tablets with food at the same time each day.
- Caution patient not to stop taking oral metoprolol abruptly.
- Teach patient how to measure his radial pulse. Advise him to notify prescriber if pulse rate falls below 60 beats/minute or is significantly lower than usual.

metronidazole
Flagyl (CAN), Flagyl I.V. RTU, Metro I.V.
metronidazole hydrochloride
Flagyl I.V.

Class and Category
Chemical: Nitroimidazole derivative
Therapeutic: Antibiotic
Pregnancy category: B

Indications and Dosages
▶ *To treat systemic anaerobic infections caused by* Bacteroides fragilis, Clostridium difficile, Clostridium perfringens, Eubacterium, Fusobacterium, Peptococcus, Peptostreptococcus, *and* Veillonella *species*

I.V. INFUSION
Adults and adolescents. *Initial:* 15 mg/kg and then 7.5 mg/kg up to 1,000 mg q 6 hr for 7 days or longer. *Maximum:* 4,000 mg/day.
Children. 7.5 mg/kg q 6 hr or 10 mg/kg q 8 hr.
▶ *To prevent perioperative bowel infection*
I.V. INFUSION
Adults and adolescents. 15 mg/kg 1 hr before surgery and then 7.5 mg/kg 6 and 12 hr after initial dose.

Mechanism of Action
After undergoing intracellular chemical reduction during anaerobic metabolism, damages DNA's helical structure and breaks its strands. These actions inhibit bacterial nucleic acid synthesis and cause cell death.

Incompatibilities
Don't administer metronidazole with aluminum needles or hubs or through same I.V. line as other drugs.

Contraindications
Breast-feeding, hypersensitivity to metronidazole or its components, trichomoniasis during first trimester of pregnancy

Interactions
DRUGS
cimetidine: Possibly delayed elimination and increased blood level of metronidazole
disulfiram: Possibly combined toxicity, resulting in confusion and psychotic reactions
neurotoxic drugs: Increased risk of neurotoxicity
oral anticoagulants: Possibly increased anticoagulant effect
phenobarbital: Increased metabolism and decreased blood level and half-life of metronidazole
phenytoin: Decreased phenytoin clearance
ACTIVITIES
alcohol use: Possibly disulfiram-like effects

Adverse Reactions
CNS: Ataxia, dizziness, encephalopathy, fever, headache, light-headedness, peripheral neuropathy, seizures (high doses)
EENT: Dry mouth, metallic taste

GI: Abdominal cramps or pain, anorexia, diarrhea, nausea, pancreatitis, vomiting
GU: Darkened urine, vaginal candidiasis, dysuria, urinary frequency
HEME: Leukopenia
SKIN: Erythema, pruritus, rash, urticaria
Other: Infusion site edema, pain, or tenderness

Nursing Considerations

- To prepare metronidazole hydrochloride for I.V. infusion, add 4.4 ml of sterile water for injection, 0.9% sodium chloride injection, or bacteriostatic water for injection to each 500-mg vial to yield a concentration of 100 mg/ml. Use within 96 hours if stored at room temperature and protected from light.
- Further dilute with 100 ml of NS, D$_5$W, or LR. Neutralize solution with 5 mEq of sodium bicarbonate for each 500 mg. To prevent precipitation, don't exceed final concentration of 8 mg/ml of neutralized metronidazole hydrochloride. Relieve pressure from gas buildup in container, as needed. Use within 24 hours if stored at room temperature; don't refrigerate because a precipitate may form.
- Be aware that prefilled plastic containers that require no further dilution or buffering (neutralization) are available. Avoid using I.V. lines with series connections to prevent air embolism.
- Administer metronidazole by slow infusion over 1 hour; don't give by direct I.V. injection.
- Discontinue primary I.V. infusion during metronidazole infusion.
- **WARNING** If patient experiences adverse CNS reactions, such as seizures or peripheral neuropathy, notify prescriber and stop drug immediately.
- Monitor patients with impaired hepatic function for signs of metronidazole toxicity because drug is metabolized in the liver. If toxicity occurs, expect prescriber to reduce dosage.
- Be aware that candidiasis symptoms may be more pronounced during metronidazole therapy. Monitor for such signs as white patches in mouth or vaginal discharge or irritation.
- Monitor CBC and culture and sensitivity test results if therapy lasts longer than 10 days or if second course of treatment is needed.
- Store drug at room temperature, and protect from light.

PATIENT TEACHING
- Advise patient to avoid potentially hazardous activities until metronidazole's CNS effects are known.

- Instruct female patient to notify prescriber if she is or intends to get pregnant or if she's breast-feeding.
- Caution patient to avoid alcohol during therapy and for at least 1 day afterward.
- Inform patient that his urine may be darker during metronidazole therapy.
- Suggest ice chips or sugarless hard candy or gum to relieve dry mouth; encourage patient to see dentist if dryness lasts longer than 2 weeks.

mezlocillin sodium
Mezlin

Class and Category
Chemical: Acyclaminopenicillin
Therapeutic: Antibiotic
Pregnancy category: B

Indications and Dosages
▶ *To treat moderate to severe infections, including bacteremia, bone and joint infections, gynecologic infections (such as endometritis, pelvic cellulitis, and pelvic inflammatory disease), intra-abdominal infections (such as cholangitis, cholecystitis, hepatic abscess, intra-abdominal abscess, and peritonitis), lower respiratory tract infections (such as pneumonia and lung abscess), meningitis, septicemia caused by susceptible bacteria, or skin and soft-tissue infections (such as cellulitis and diabetic foot ulcer); to manage febrile neutropenia*
I.V. INFUSION
Adults and adolescents. 3 g q 4 hr or 4 g q 6 hr.
▶ *To treat life-threatening infections of the types listed above*
I.V. INFUSION
Adults and adolescents. Up to 350 mg/kg/day. *Maximum:* 24,000 mg/day.
Children and infants. 50 mg/kg q 4 hr.
Neonates over age 7 days who weigh 2,000 g (4 lb, 6 oz) or less. 75 mg/kg q 8 hr.
Neonates age 7 days or less who weigh 2,000 g or less. 75 mg/kg q 12 hr.
Neonates age 7 days or less who weigh more than 2,000 g. 75 mg/kg q 6 hr.
▶ *To treat uncomplicated UTIs*
I.V. INFUSION
Adults. 1.5 to 2 g q 6 hr.

▶ *To treat complicated UTIs*
I.V. INFUSION
Adults. 3 g q 6 hr.
DOSAGE ADJUSTMENT Dosing interval extended to q 6 to 8 hr, if needed, for patients with creatinine clearance of 10 to 30 ml/min/1.73 m². Dosing interval extended and dosage reduced to 1.5 to 2 g for patients with creatinine clearance of less than 10 ml/min/1.73 m².

▶ *To treat uncomplicated gonorrhea caused by susceptible strains of* Neisseria gonorrhoeae
I.V. INFUSION
Adults. 1 to 2 g as a single dose given with 1 g of probenecid P.O. (or probenecid given up to 30 min before mezlocillin).

▶ *To prevent infection from potentially contaminated surgical procedures*
I.V. INFUSION
Adults. 4 g 30 min before surgery and then 4 g q 6 hr for 2 more doses.

▶ *To prevent infection in cesarean section*
I.V. INFUSION
Adults. 4 g as soon as umbilical cord is clamped; then 4 g q 4 hr for 2 more doses, starting 4 hr after initial dose.

Mechanism of Action

Inhibits bacterial cell wall synthesis. In susceptible bacteria, the rigid, cross-linked cell wall is assembled in several steps. Mezlocillin exerts its effects in the final stage of the cross-linking process by binding with and inactivating penicillin-binding proteins (enzymes responsible for linking cell wall strands). This action causes bacterial cell lysis and death.

Incompatibilities

Administer mezlocillin at separate sites and at least 1 hour before or after aminoglycosides. Don't mix mezlocillin in same I.V. bag, bottle, or tubing as other drugs.

Contraindications

Hypersensitivity to mezlocillin, other penicillins, or their components

Interactions

DRUGS
aminoglycosides: Substantial aminoglycoside inactivation
chloramphenicol, erythromycins, sulfonamides, tetracyclines: Possibly decreased therapeutic effects of mezlocillin

methotrexate: Increased risk of methotrexate toxicity
probenecid: Increased blood level and prolonged half-life of
mezlocillin

Adverse Reactions

CNS: Depression, headache, seizures
EENT: Oral candidiasis
GI: Abdominal pain, diarrhea, pseudomembranous colitis, nausea,
vomiting
GU: Vaginitis
HEME: Leukopenia, neutropenia
SKIN: Exfoliative dermatitis, pruritus, rash, urticaria
Other: Anaphylaxis; hypokalemia; injection site pain, redness,
and swelling; serum sickness–like reaction

Nursing Considerations

- **WARNING** Before administering first dose of mezlocillin,
  make sure patient has had no previous hypersensitivity reactions to penicillins.
- Expect mezlocillin therapy to continue for at least 2 days after
  signs and symptoms have resolved—typically 7 to 10 days, depending on severity of infection. Complicated infections may
  need longer treatment. Group A beta-hemolytic streptococcal
  infections usually are treated for at least 10 days to reduce the
  risk of rheumatic fever or glomerulonephritis.
- Reconstitute each gram of mezlocillin with 10 ml of sterile water for injection, D_5W, or sodium chloride for injection and
  shake vigorously. Don't exceed a concentration of 100 mg/ml
  (10%). Be aware that stability of reconstituted solution varies,
  depending on type of diluent used, concentration, and storage
  temperature. Consult manufacturer's insert for specific storage
  guidelines. If a precipitate forms during refrigeration, warm solution to 37° C (98.6° F) using a water bath for 20 minutes.
  Shake well. Inject slowly, directly into I.V. tubing, over 3 to
  5 minutes.
- For intermittent infusion, further dilute to desired volume (50
  to 100 ml) with an appropriate I.V. solution and administer
  over 30 minutes. Discontinue other infusions during mezlocillin
  administration.
- Be aware that mezlocillin powder and reconstituted solution
  may darken slightly but that potency isn't affected.
- Periodically monitor serum potassium level of patients receiving
  long-term therapy, as appropriate.

• When calculating sodium intake for patients on a sodium-restricted diet, keep in mind that each gram of mezlocillin contains approximately 1.9 mEq of sodium.
• During long-term therapy, monitor for signs and symptoms of superinfection, such as oral candidiasis and vaginitis.
• Before reconstituting drug, store it at less than 30° (86° F).

PATIENT TEACHING
• Instruct patient receiving mezlocillin to immediately report increased bruising or other bleeding tendencies.
• Advise patient to report diarrhea and to check with prescriber before taking an antidiarrheal because it may mask symptoms of pseudomembranous colitis.

midazolam hydrochloride
Versed

Class, Category, and Schedule
Chemical: Benzodiazepine
Therapeutic: Sedative-hypnotic
Pregnancy category: D
Controlled substance: Schedule IV

Indications and Dosages
▶ *To induce preoperative sedation or amnesia, to control preoperative anxiety*
I.V. INJECTION
Adults age 60 and older. 1.5 mg over 2 min immediately before procedure. After 2-min waiting period, dosage adjusted to desired level in 25% increments, as ordered. *Maximum:* 1 mg in 2 min.
Adults under age 60 and adolescents. Up to 2.5 mg over 2 min immediately before procedure. After 2-min waiting period, dosage adjusted to desired level in 25% increments, as ordered. *Maximum:* 5 mg.
Children ages 6 to 12. *Initial:* 0.025 to 0.05 mg/kg, up to 0.4 mg/kg, if needed. *Maximum:* 10 mg.
Children ages 6 months to 5 years. *Initial:* 0.05 to 0.1 mg/kg, up to 0.6 mg/kg, if needed. *Maximum:* 6 mg.
▶ *To relieve agitation and anxiety in mechanically ventilated patients*
I.V. INFUSION
Adults. *Initial:* 0.01 to 0.05 mg/kg infused over several min, repeated at 10- to 15-min intervals until adequate sedation occurs.

Maintenance: 0.02 to 0.1 mg/kg/hr initially, adjusted to desired level in 25% to 50% increments, as ordered. After achieving desired level of sedation, infusion rate decreased by 10% to 25% every few hr, as ordered, until minimum effective infusion rate is determined.

Children. *Initial:* 50 to 200 mcg/kg over 2 to 3 min followed by 1 to 2 mcg/kg/min by continuous infusion. *Maintenance:* 0.4 to 6 mcg/kg/min.

Infants age 32 weeks or older. 1 mcg/kg/min by continuous infusion.

Infants under age 32 weeks. 0.5 mcg/kg/min by continuous infusion.

Route	Onset	Peak	Duration
I.V.*	1.5 to 5 min	Rapid	2 to 6 hr

Mechanism of Action

May exert its sedating effect by increasing the activity of gamma-aminobutyric acid, a major inhibitory neurotransmitter in the brain. As a result, midazolam produces a calming effect, relaxes skeletal muscles, and—at high doses—induces sleep.

Contraindications

Acute angle-closure glaucoma; alcohol intoxication; coma; hypersensitivity to midazolam, other benzodiazepines, or their components; shock

Interactions

DRUGS

antihypertensives: Increased risk of hypotension

cimetidine, diltiazem, erythromycin, fluconazole, indinavir, itraconazole, ketoconazole, ranitidine, ritonavir, roxithromycin, saquinavir, verapamil: Prolonged sedation caused by reduced midazolam metabolism

CNS depressants: Possibly increased CNS and respiratory depression and hypotension

rifampin: Decreased blood midazolam level

FOODS

grapefruit, grapefruit juice: Possibly increased blood midazolam level and risk of toxicity

---

* For sedation.

ACTIVITIES
alcohol use: Possibly increased CNS and respiratory depression and hypotension

Adverse Reactions

CNS: Agitation, delirium, or dreaming during emergence from anesthesia; anxiety; ataxia; chills; combativeness; confusion; dizziness; drowsiness; euphoria; excessive sedation; headache; insomnia; lethargy; nervousness; nightmares; paresthesia; prolonged emergence from anesthesia; restlessness; retrograde amnesia; sleep disturbance; slurred speech; weakness; yawning

CV: Cardiac arrest, hypotension, nodal rhythm, PVCs, tachycardia, vasovagal episodes

EENT: Blurred vision, diplopia, or other vision changes; increased salivation; laryngospasm; miosis; nystagmus; toothache

GI: Hiccups, nausea, retching, vomiting

RESP: Airway obstruction, bradypnea, bronchospasm, coughing, decreased tidal volume, dyspnea, hyperventilation, respiratory arrest, shallow breathing, tachypnea, wheezing

SKIN: Pruritus, rash, urticaria

Other: Infusion site burning, edema, induration, pain, redness, and tenderness

Nursing Considerations

- **WARNING** Be aware that I.V. midazolam is given only in hospitals or ambulatory care settings that allow continuous monitoring of respiratory and cardiac function. Keep resuscitative drugs and equipment readily available.
- As needed, combine midazolam injection with D_5W, NS, or LR. Solutions mixed with D_5W or NS remain stable for 24 hours; solutions mixed with LR remain stable for 4 hours.
- As needed, mix injection in same syringe with atropine sulfate, meperidine hydrochloride, morphine sulfate, or scopolamine hydrobromide. The resulting solution remains stable for 30 minutes.
- Expect child's dosage to be based on ideal body weight. This is especially important for an obese child.
- **WARNING** Be aware that midazolam contains the preservative benzyl alcohol, which may cause a fatal toxic syndrome in neonates and premature infants, characterized by CNS, respiratory, circulatory, and renal impairment and metabolic acidosis. Because the 5-mg/ml and 1-mg/ml vials contain the same amount of benzyl alcohol, using the 5-mg/ml vial to

prepare neonatal doses may decrease the amount of benzyl alcohol the patient receives.

- Be aware that neonates have a higher risk of respiratory depression than other pediatric or adult patients.
- Assess LOC frequently because the range between sedation and unconsciousness or disorientation is narrower with midazolam than with other benzodiazepines.
- Be aware that recovery time is usually 2 hours but may take up to 6 hours.
- Store drug at 15° to 30° C (59° to 86° F); don't freeze.

PATIENT TEACHING

- Inform patient that he may not remember procedure because midazolam produces amnesia.
- Advise patient to avoid potentially hazardous activities until drug's adverse CNS effects, such as dizziness and drowsiness, have worn off.
- Instruct patient to avoid alcohol and other CNS depressants for 24 hours after receiving drug, unless directed otherwise by prescriber.

milrinone lactate
Primacor

Class and Category
Chemical: Bipyridine derivative
Therapeutic: Inotropic agent, vasodilator
Pregnancy category: C

Indications and Dosages
▶ *To provide short-term treatment of acute heart failure*
I.V. INFUSION
Adults. *Loading:* 50 mcg/kg over 10 min (at least 0.375 mcg/kg/min). *Usual:* 0.375 to 0.75 mcg/kg/min. *Maximum:* 1.13 mg/kg/day.
DOSAGE ADJUSTMENT Dosage adjusted according to cardiac output, pulmonary artery wedge pressure (PAWP), and clinical response. For patients with renal impairment, dosage reduced as follows: for creatinine clearance of 30 to 39 ml/min/1.73 m^2, 0.33 mcg/kg/min; for creatinine clearance of 20 to 29 ml/min/1.73 m^2, 0.28 mcg/kg/min; for creatinine clearance of 10 to 19 ml/min/1.73 m^2, 0.23 mcg/kg/min; and for creatinine clearance of 5 to 9 ml/min/1.73 m^2, 0.20 mcg/kg/min.

Route	Onset	Peak	Duration
I.V.	5 to 15 min	Unknown	3 to 6 hr

Mechanism of Action

An inotropic drug, milrinone increases the force of myocardial contraction—and cardiac output—by blocking the enzyme phosphodiesterase, which is normally activated by hormones binding to cell membrane receptors. As shown top right, phosphodiesterase normally degrades intracellular cAMP, which restricts calcium movement into myocardial cells. By inhibiting phosphodiesterase, as shown bottom right, milrinone slows the rate of cAMP degradation, increasing the intracellular cAMP level and the amount of calcium that enters myocardial cells. In blood vessels, increased cAMP causes smooth-muscle relaxation, which improves cardiac output by reducing preload and afterload.

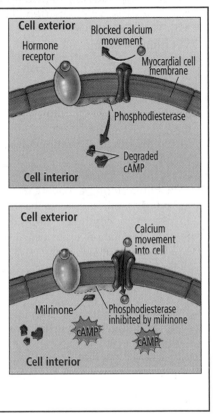

Incompatibilities

Don't administer milrinone through same I.V. line as furosemide because a precipitate will form. Don't add other drugs to premixed milrinone flexible containers.

Contraindications

Hypersensitivity to milrinone or its components

Interactions

DRUGS

antihypertensives: Possibly hypotension

Adverse Reactions

CNS: Headache, tremor
CV: Angina, hypotension, supraventricular arrhythmias, ventricular ectopic activity, ventricular fibrillation, ventricular tachycardia
HEME: Thrombocytopenia
RESP: Bronchospasm
Other: Hypokalemia

Nursing Considerations

• Make sure ECG equipment is available for continuous monitoring during milrinone therapy.
• Check platelet count before and periodically during infusion, as ordered. Expect to discontinue drug if platelet count falls below 150,000/mm^3.
• Discard drug if it contains particles or is discolored.
• When administering a loading dose, directly infuse undiluted drug into I.V. line with a compatible infusing solution. When administering a continuous infusion, dilute drug with 0.45NS, NS, or D$_5$W. Dilution isn't needed when using premixed milrinone flexible containers.
• Administer loading dose using a controlled-rate infusion device. Administer continuous infusion using a calibrated electronic infusion device.
• Monitor cardiac output, PAWP, blood pressure, heart rate, weight, and fluid status during therapy to determine drug effectiveness.
• Monitor renal function test results and serum electrolyte levels. Notify prescriber of abnormalities.
• If severe hypotension develops, notify prescriber immediately and expect to discontinue drug.
• Anticipate that patient also will receive digoxin before starting milrinone because milrinone can increase the ventricular response rate.
• Before using drug, store vials and cartridges at 15° to 30° C (59° to 86° F) and flexible containers at 25° C (77° F). Don't freeze or expose to excessive heat.

PATIENT TEACHING
• Reassure patient that you'll be present and that he'll be monitored constantly during milrinone therapy.

minocycline hydrochloride
Minocin

Class and Category
Chemical: Tetracycline
Therapeutic: Antibiotic, antiprotozoal
Pregnancy category: D

Indications and Dosages
▶ *To treat bartonellosis, brucellosis, chancroid, granuloma inguinale, inclusion conjunctivitis, lymphogranuloma venereum, nongonococcal urethritis, plague, psittacosis, Q fever, relapsing fever, respiratory tract infections (including pneumonia), rickettsial pox, Rocky Mountain spotted fever, tularemia, typhus, and UTIs caused by gram-negative organisms (including* Bartonella bacilliformis, Brucella *species,* Haemophilus ducreyi, Haemophilus influenzae, Vibrio cholerae, *and* Yersinia pestis*), susceptible gram-positive organisms (including certain strains of* Streptococcus pneumoniae*), and other organisms (including* Actinomyces *species,* Bacillus anthracis, Borrelia recurrentis, Chlamydia *species,* Mycoplasma pneumoniae, *and* Rickettsiae*); as adjunct to treat intestinal amebiasis and as alternative to treat listeriosis caused by* Listeria monocytogenes, *syphilis caused by* Treponema pallidum, *and yaws caused by* Treponema pertenue *for nonpregnant patients allergic to penicillin*

I.V. INJECTION

Adults and adolescents. *Initial:* 200 mg. *Maintenance:* 100 mg q 12 hr. *Maximum:* 400 mg q.d.

Children over age 8. *Initial:* 4 mg/kg. *Maintenance:* 2 mg/kg q 12 hr.

Route	Onset	Peak	Duration
I.V.	Unknown	Unknown	6 to 12 hr

Mechanism of Action
Inhibits bacterial protein synthesis by competitively binding to the 30S ribosomal subunit of the mRNA-ribosome complex of certain organisms.

Incompatibilities
Don't mix minocycline in same syringe with a solution that contains calcium because a precipitate will form.

Contraindications

Hypersensitivity to minocycline, other tetracyclines, or their components

Interactions

DRUGS

digoxin: Possibly increased blood digoxin level and digitalis toxicity

insulin: Possibly decreased need for insulin

lithium: Possibly increased or decreased blood lithium level

methoxyflurane: Increased risk of nephrotoxicity

oral anticoagulants: Possibly potentiated anticoagulant effects

oral contraceptives containing estrogen: Decreased contraceptive effectiveness, increased risk of breakthrough bleeding

penicillin: Interference with bactericidal action of penicillin

vitamin A: Possibly benign intracranial hypertension

Adverse Reactions

CNS: Dizziness, fever, headache, light-headedness, unsteadiness, vertigo

CV: Pericarditis

EENT: Blurred vision, darkened or discolored tongue, glossitis, papilledema, tooth discoloration (children), vision changes

GI: Abdominal cramps or pain, anorexia, diarrhea, dysphagia, enterocolitis, esophageal irritation and ulceration, hepatitis, hepatotoxicity, indigestion, nausea, pancreatitis, vomiting

GU: Genital candidiasis, nephrotoxicity

HEME: Eosinophilia, hemolytic anemia, neutropenia, thrombocytopenia, thrombocytopenic purpura

MS: Arthralgia, myopathy (transient)

RESP: Pulmonary infiltrates (with eosinophilia)

SKIN: Erythema multiforme, exfoliative dermatitis, brown pigmentation of skin and mucous membranes, erythematous and maculopapular rash, jaundice, onycholysis, photosensitivity, pruritus, purpura (anaphylactoid), Stevens-Johnson syndrome, urticaria

Other: Anaphylaxis, angioedema, serum sickness–like reaction, systemic lupus erythematosus exacerbation

Nursing Considerations

- **WARNING** Notify prescriber if patient is breast-feeding because minocycline appears in breast milk and may have toxic effects on infant.
- Avoid giving minocycline to children younger than age 8 because drug may cause permanent discoloration and enamel hypoplasia of developing teeth and may slow skeletal growth rate.

- Monitor results of renal and liver function tests before and periodically during long-term therapy. Expect to adjust dosage for patients with hepatic disease to prevent drug accumulation.
- Reconstitute each 100-mg vial with 5 to 10 ml of sterile water for injection. Further dilute in 500 to 1,000 ml of NS, D_5W, D_5NS, LR, or Ringer's solution. Administer final dilution immediately, but avoid rapid administration.
- Store reconstituted drug at room temperature, and use within 24 hours.
- Assess patient for signs of superinfection; if they appear, notify prescriber and expect to discontinue minocycline and start appropriate therapy, as ordered.
- Monitor PT in patients who also take an anticoagulant during minocycline therapy.
- Before reconstituting drug, store it at 15° to 30° C (59° to 86° F) and protect from light.

PATIENT TEACHING
- Instruct patient receiving minocycline to immediately report blurred vision, dizziness, headache, known or suspected pregnancy, and unsteadiness.
- Advise patient to avoid prolonged exposure to sun or sunlamps during therapy.
- Counsel female patient to avoid becoming pregnant during minocycline therapy because drug may permanently discolor teeth and slow skeletal growth rate of fetus. If she uses an oral contraceptive, encourage her to use an additional contraceptive method during minocycline therapy

mitoxantrone
Novantrone

Class and Category
Chemical: Anthracenedione
Therapeutic: Antineoplastic
Pregnancy category: D

Indications and Dosages
▶ *To reduce neurologic disability and frequency of relapses in patients with secondary (chronic) progressive, progressive relapsing, or worsening relapsing-remitting multiple sclerosis (MS) whose neurologic status is significantly abnormal between relapses*

I.V. INFUSION

Adults. 12 mg/m^2 given over 5 to 15 min q 3 mo. *Maximum:* Cumulative dose of 140 mg/m^2.

▶ *As adjunct to treat pain related to advanced hormone-refractory prostate cancer*

I.V. INFUSION

Adults. 12 to 14 mg/m^2 given over 5 to 15 min q 21 days.

▶ *As adjunct to treat acute nonlymphocytic leukemia (ANLL)*

I.V. INFUSION

Adults. *Initial:* 12 mg/m^2 given over at least 3 min on days 1 to 3, along with 100 mg/m^2 of cytarabine as a continuous 24-hour infusion on days 1 to 7. If patient's antileukemic response is inadequate or incomplete, a second induction course given at same dosage. *Maintenance:* 6 wk after induction, 12 mg/m^2 given over at least 3 min on days 1 and 2, along with 100 mg/m^2 of cytarabine as a continuous 24-hour infusion on days 1 to 5. A second maintenance course given 4 wk after first course, if needed and tolerated.

Mechanism of Action

By binding to hydrogen, intercalates into DNA, causing breakage of cross-links and strands. Mitoxantrone also interferes with RNA synthesis and is a potent inhibitor of topoisomerase II, an enzyme responsible for uncoiling and repairing damaged DNA. It produces a cytocidal effect on both proliferating and nonproliferating cells and does not appear to be cell-cycle–phase specific. Mitoxantrone's role in multiple sclerosis is unknown, but the drug is known to inhibit proliferation of B cells, T cells, and macrophages and to impair antigen function.

Incompatibilities

Don't mix mitoxantrone in same infusion as heparin (because a precipitate may form) or with any other drugs.

Contraindications

Hypersensitivity to mitoxantrone or its components

Interactions

DRUGS

allopurinol, colchicine, probenecid, sulfinpyrazone: Possible interference with antihyperuricemic action of these drugs

blood-dyscrasia–causing drugs (such as cephalosporins and sulfasalazine): Increased risk of leukopenia and thrombocytopenia
bone marrow depressants (such as carboplatin and lomustine): Possibly additive bone marrow depression
daunorubicin, doxorubicin: Increased risk of cardiotoxicity
vaccines, killed virus: Decreased antibody response to vaccine
vaccines, live virus: Possibly decreased antibody response to vaccine, increased adverse effects of vaccine, and severe infection

Adverse Reactions
CNS: Headache, seizures
CV: Arrhythmias (including bradycardia), chest pain, decreased left ventricular ejection fraction, ECG changes, heart failure
EENT: Blue cornea, conjunctivitis, mucositis, stomatitis
GI: Abdominal pain, diarrhea, GI bleeding, nausea, vomiting
GU: Blue-green urine, renal failure
HEME: Leukopenia, thrombocytopenia
RESP: Cough, dyspnea
SKIN: Alopecia, extravasation, jaundice
Other: Allergic reaction, hyperuricemia, infection, infusion site pain or redness

Nursing Considerations
• Expect patient to undergo an echocardiogram, ECG studies, and radionuclide angiography before beginning mitoxantrone therapy and periodically thereafter to evaluate cardiac status. Also expect to obtain hematocrit, hemoglobin level, and CBC with platelet count before and during therapy.
• Be aware that drug should not be given to a patient with MS whose neutrophil count is less than 1,500 cells/mm^3.
• Obtain liver function test results, as ordered, before beginning each course of mitoxantrone. Be aware that drug should not be given to a patient with MS whose hepatic function is abnormal.
• Expect to obtain a pregnancy test before each course of mitoxantrone for female patients with MS who are of childbearing age. Notify prescriber of test results.
• Follow facility policy for handling antineoplastic drugs. Manufacturer recommends the use of goggles, gloves, and protective gowns during drug preparation and administration.
• Before infusing drug, dilute it in at least 50 ml of NS or D$_5$W.
• **WARNING** Be aware that drug should not be administered intrathecally because paralysis may occur.

- If mitoxantrone solution comes in contact with your skin or mucosa, wash it off thoroughly with warm water. If drug comes in contact with your eye, irrigate eye thoroughly with water or NS.
- Discard unused portion of diluted solution because it contains no preservatives. After stopper of vial has been penetrated, undiluted drug may be stored for up to 7 days at room temperature or 14 days in refrigerator. Avoid freezing drug.
- If extravasation occurs, stop infusion immediately and notify prescriber. Then resume the infusion in another vein. Although mitoxantrone is a nonvesicant, observe the extravasation site for signs of necrosis or phlebitis.
- Monitor patients with herpes zoster and those who currently have, or have recently been exposed to, chicken pox for signs and symptoms of severe, generalized disease.
- Monitor blood uric acid levels for signs of hyperuricemia in patients with a history of gout or renal calculi. Expect to give allopurinol, as prescribed, to patients with leukemia or lymphoma who have elevated blood uric acid levels to prevent uric acid nephropathy.
- Monitor patients with heart disease for signs and symptoms of cardiotoxicity, such as arrhythmias and chest pain. The risk of cardiotoxicity increases for cancer patients who reach a cumulative dose of 140 mg/m^2 and for MS patients who reach a cumulative dose of 100 mg/m^2.
- **WARNING If patient develops severe or life-threatening hematologic or nonhematologic toxicity during the first induction course, expect to withhold second induction course until toxicity resolves.**
- If patient develops thrombocytopenia, implement protective precautions according to facility policy.
- Assess for signs of infection, such as fever, if patient develops leukopenia. Expect to obtain appropriate specimens for culture and sensitivity testing.

PATIENT TEACHING

- Advise patient to have dental work completed before treatment begins, if possible, or to defer such procedures until blood counts return to normal because mitoxantrone may delay healing and cause gingival bleeding. Instruct patient in proper oral hygiene, and advise him to use a soft-bristled toothbrush.
- Encourage patient to drink plenty of fluids to increase urine output and help excrete uric acid.

- Advise patient to immediately report GI upset but to continue taking drug unless otherwise directed.
- Stress the importance of complying with the dosage regimen and of keeping follow-up medical appointments and appointments for laboratory tests.
- Inform patient that urine may turn blue-green and the whites of his eyes may turn blue during therapy and for 24 hours afterward. Stress that these effects are temporary and harmless.
- Explain the possibility of hair loss; reassure patient that hair should regrow after completion of therapy.
- Caution patient to avoid receiving immunizations unless approved by prescriber, and urge him to avoid people who have recently received vaccines or to wear a protective mask over his nose and mouth when he's around them.
- Instruct patient with bone marrow depression to avoid people with infections. Advise him to contact prescriber if he experiences fever, chills, cough, hoarseness, lower back or side pain, or painful or difficult urination because these may be signs and symptoms of an infection.
- Advise patient to contact prescriber immediately if he notices unusual bleeding or bruising, black or tarry stools, blood in urine or stools, or red pinpoint spots on skin.
- Instruct patient to avoid touching his eyes or inside of his nose unless he washes his hands immediately beforehand.
- Stress the importance of avoiding accidental cuts from sharp objects, such as razors or fingernail clippers, because excessive bleeding or infection may occur.
- Urge patient to avoid contact sports and other activities that increase his risk of bruising or injury.

morphine sulfate

Astramorph PF, Duramorph, Epimorph (CAN), Morphine Extra-Forte (CAN), Morphine Forte (CAN), Morphine H.P. (CAN)

Class, Category, and Schedule
Chemical: Phenanthrene derivative
Therapeutic: Opioid analgesic
Pregnancy category: C
Controlled substance: Schedule II

Indications and Dosages

▶ *To relieve acute or chronic moderate to severe pain; as adjunct to treat pulmonary edema caused by left-sided heart failure; to supplement general, local, or regional anesthesia*

I.V. INFUSION

Adults. *Initial:* 15 mg (or more), followed by 0.8 to 10 mg/hr; increased as needed for effectiveness. *Maintenance:* 0.8 to 80 mg/hr.

Children. 0.01 to 0.04 mg/kg/hr postoperatively, 0.025 to 2.6 mg/kg/hr for severe chronic cancer pain, or 0.03 to 0.15 mg/kg/hr for sickle cell crisis.

Neonates. *Initial:* 0.010 mg/kg/hr (10 mcg/kg/hr) postoperatively. *Maintenance:* 0.015 to 0.02 mg/kg/hr (15 to 20 mcg/kg/hr).

I.V. INJECTION

Adults. 2.5 to 15 mg injected slowly.

Children. 0.5 to 0.1 mg/kg administered slowly.

EPIDURAL INFUSION (PRESERVATIVE-FREE)

Adults. *Initial:* 2 to 4 mg/24 hr, increased by 1 to 2 mg/24 hr, as directed, to achieve sufficient pain relief.

EPIDURAL INJECTION (PRESERVATIVE-FREE)

Adults. *Initial:* 5 mg into lumbar region. If pain isn't relieved after 1 hr, 1- to 2-mg doses given at appropriate intervals to relieve pain. *Maximum:* 10 mg/24 hr.

INTRATHECAL INJECTION (PRESERVATIVE-FREE)

Adults. 0.2 to 1 mg as a single dose.

▶ *To relieve MI pain*

I.V. INJECTION

Adults. 1 to 4 mg by slow I.V. injection. Repeated up to q 5 min, if needed. *Maximum:* 2 to 15 mg.

Route	Onset	Peak	Duration
I.V.	Unknown	20 min	4 to 5 hr
Epidural, intrathecal	15 to 60 min	Unknown	Up to 24 hr

Mechanism of Action

Binds with and activates opioid receptors (primarily mu receptors) in the brain and spinal cord to produce analgesia and euphoria.

Contraindications

For all drug forms: Asthma, hypersensitivity to morphine or its components, labor (with premature delivery), prematurity (in infants), respiratory depression, upper airway obstruction

For I.V. injection: Acute alcoholism, alcohol withdrawal syndrome, arrhythmias, brain tumor, heart failure caused by chronic lung disease, seizure disorders

For epidural or intrathecal injection: Anticoagulant therapy, bleeding tendency, injection site infection, parenteral corticosteroid treatment (or other treatment or condition that prohibits drug administration by intrathecal or epidural route) within 2 weeks

Interactions
DRUGS

amitriptyline, clomipramine, nortriptyline: Increased CNS and respiratory depression

anticholinergics: Possibly severe constipation leading to ileus, urine retention

antidiarrheals (such as loperamide and paregoric): CNS depression, possibly severe constipation

antihistamines, chloral hydrate, glutethimide, MAO inhibitors, methocarbamol: Increased CNS and respiratory depressant effects of morphine

antihypertensives, other hypotension-producing drugs: Increased hypotension, risk of orthostatic hypotension

buprenorphine: Decreased therapeutic effects of morphine, increased respiratory depression, possibly withdrawal symptoms

cimetidine: Increased analgesic and CNS and respiratory depressant effects of morphine

CNS depressants (antiemetics, general anesthetics, hypnotics, phenothiazines, sedatives, tranquilizers): Possibly coma, hypotension, respiratory depression, severe sedation

diuretics: Decreased diuretic efficacy

hydroxyzine: Increased analgesic, CNS depressant, and hypotensive effects of morphine

metoclopramide: Possibly antagonized metoclopramide effect on GI motility

mixed agonist-antagonist analgesics: Possibly withdrawal symptoms

naloxone: Antagonized analgesic and CNS and respiratory depressant effects of morphine, possibly withdrawal symptoms

naltrexone: Possibly induction or worsening of withdrawal symptoms if morphine given within 7 to 10 days before naltrexone

neuromuscular blockers: Increased or prolonged respiratory depression

other opioid analgesics (such as alfentanil and sufentanil): Increased CNS and respiratory depression, increased hypotension

zidovudine: Decreased zidovudine clearance

ACTIVITIES

alcohol use: Increased CNS and respiratory depression, increased hypotension

Adverse Reactions

CNS: Amnesia, anxiety, coma, confusion, decreased concentration, delirium, delusions, depression, dizziness, drowsiness, euphoria, fever, hallucinations, headache, insomnia, lethargy, lightheadedness, malaise, psychosis, restlessness, sedation, seizures, syncope, tremor

CV: Bradycardia, cardiac arrest, hypotension, orthostatic hypotension, palpitations, shock, tachycardia

EENT: Blurred vision, diplopia, dry mouth, laryngeal edema or laryngospasm (allergic), miosis, nystagmus, rhinitis

GI: Abdominal cramps or pain, anorexia, biliary tract spasm, constipation, diarrhea, dysphagia, elevated liver function test results, gastroesophageal reflux, hiccups, ileus and toxic megacolon (in patients with inflammatory bowel disease), indigestion, nausea, vomiting

GU: Decreased ejaculate potency, decreased libido, difficult ejaculation, impotence, prolonged labor, urinary hesitancy, urine retention

HEME: Anemia, leukopenia, thrombocytopenia

MS: Arthralgia

RESP: Apnea, asthma exacerbation, atelectasis, bronchospasm, depressed cough reflex, hypoventilation, pulmonary edema, respiratory arrest and depression, wheezing

SKIN: Diaphoresis, flushing, pallor, pruritus

Other: Allergic reaction; facial edema; injection site edema, pain, rash, or redness; physical and psychological dependence; withdrawal symptoms

Nursing Considerations

- Before giving morphine, make sure an opioid antagonist and equipment for administering oxygen and controlling respiration are available.
- Before therapy begins, assess patient's current drug use, including all prescription and OTC drugs.
- Discard injection solution if it's discolored or darker than pale yellow or if it contains precipitates that don't disappear with shaking.

- **WARNING** Avoid using highly concentrated morphine solutions (such as 10 to 25 mg/ml) for single-dose I.V. administration. These solutions are intended for use in continuous, controlled microinfusion devices.
- Instruct patient to lie down during morphine administration to minimize dizziness, light-headedness, nausea, and vomiting.
- For direct I.V. injection, dilute appropriate dose with 4 to 5 ml of sterile water for injection. Inject 2.5 to 15 mg directly into tubing of free-flowing I.V. solution over 4 to 5 minutes. Rapid I.V. injection may increase adverse reactions.
- For continuous I.V. infusion, dilute drug in D_5W and administer with infusion-control device. Adjust dose and rate based on patient response, as prescribed.
- For intrathecal injection, expect prescriber to give no more than 2 ml of 0.5-mg/ml solution or 1 ml of 1-mg/ml solution. Intrathecal dosage should be about one-tenth of epidural dosage.
- **WARNING** Monitor respiratory and cardiovascular status carefully and frequently during morphine therapy. Be alert for respiratory depression and hypotension. Patients having an acute asthma attack, those with chronic respiratory disease, and elderly, debilitated, or very ill patients are at increased risk for respiratory depression; patients with a history of hypothyroidism are at increased risk for respiratory and prolonged CNS depression.
- Monitor for excessive or persistent sedation; dosage may need to be adjusted.
- Be aware that morphine may cause physical and psychological dependence, especially in patients with a history of drug abuse, emotional instability, or suicidal ideation. Monitor closely for drug tolerance and withdrawal symptoms, such as body aches, diaphoresis, diarrhea, fever, piloerection, rhinorrhea, sneezing, and yawning.
- If patient develops a tolerance to morphine, expect prescriber to increase dosage.
- Be aware that morphine may have a prolonged duration and cumulative effect in patients with impaired hepatic or renal function. It also may prolong labor by reducing the strength, duration, and frequency of uterine contractions.
- Be aware that opioid analgesics may induce or exacerbate arrhythmias or seizures in patients with a history of these conditions and may mask symptoms of acute abdominal disorders.

- Be aware that morphine may mask or worsen gallbladder pain.
- Assess urine output; decreasing output may signal urine retention. Patients with prostatic hypertrophy, obstructive urethral stricture, or recent UTI are at increased risk.
- Monitor for signs of drug-induced CNS depression or increased CSF pressure, such as altered LOC, restlessness, or irritability, in patients with a head injury, intracranial lesions, or other conditions that cause these effects. Patients who are taking, or have recently taken, drugs that depress the CNS are also more susceptible to these effects. Take appropriate safety precautions.
- When discontinuing morphine in patients receiving more than 30 mg/day, expect prescriber to reduce daily dose by about 50% for 2 days and then by 25% every 2 days thereafter until total dose reaches initial amount recommended for patients who haven't previously received opioids (15 to 30 mg/day). This regimen minimizes the risk of withdrawal symptoms.
- Store morphine sulfate at 15° to 30° C (59° to 86° F).

PATIENT TEACHING

- Advise patient receiving morphine to report adverse reactions, such as constipation, severe nausea, and shortness of breath.
- Encourage patient to change position slowly to minimize effects of orthostatic hypotension.
- Instruct patient to report worsening or breakthrough pain.
- Instruct patient to administer morphine exactly as prescribed and not to change dosage without consulting prescriber.
- Urge patient to avoid alcohol and other CNS depressants during morphine therapy.
- Caution ambulatory patient to take extra precautions because of the risk of drowsiness.
- Advise patient to avoid potentially hazardous activities during morphine therapy.
- Inform patient that morphine may be habit-forming. Urge him to report anxiety, decreased appetite, excessive tearing, irritability, muscle aches or twitching, rapid heart rate, or yawning, which may be signs and symptoms of withdrawal.
- Advise female patient to report if she becomes pregnant. Regular morphine use during pregnancy may cause physical dependence in fetus and withdrawal symptoms in neonate.

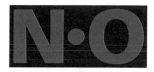

nafcillin sodium

Nafcil, Nallpen, Unipen

Class and Category

Chemical: Penicillin
Therapeutic: Antibiotic
Pregnancy category: B

Indications and Dosages

▶ *To treat infections caused by penicillinase-producing* Staphylococcus aurcus

I.V. INFUSION

Adults and adolescents. 500 to 1,500 mg q 4 hr. *Maximum:* 20,000 mg/day.

Children from birth to age 12. 10 to 20 mg/kg q 4 hr, or 20 to 40 mg/kg q 8 hr.

▶ *To treat bone and joint infections, endocarditis, meningitis, and pericarditis caused by susceptible organisms*

I.V. INFUSION

Adults and adolescents. 1,500 to 2,000 mg q 4 to 6 hr. *Maximum:* 20,000 mg/day.

Children from birth to age 12. 10 to 20 mg/kg q 4 hr or 20 to 40 mg/kg q 8 hr. For meningitis in neonates weighing up to 2 kg (4.4 lb), 25 to 50 mg/kg q 12 hr for first week after birth and then 50 mg/kg q 8 hr. For neonates weighing 2 kg or more, 50 mg/kg q 8 hr during first week after birth and then 50 mg/kg q 6 hr.

Mechanism of Action

Binds to certain penicillin-binding proteins inside bacterial cell walls, thereby inhibiting the third and final stage of bacterial cell wall synthesis. The result is cell lysis. Nafcillin's action is bolstered by its chemical composition; its unique side chain resists destruction by beta-lactamases.

Incompatibilities

Don't mix nafcillin in same I.V. bag as aminoglycosides; these drugs are chemically incompatible.

Contraindications
Hypersensitivity to nafcillin, other penicillins, or their components

Interactions
DRUGS
aminoglycosides: Substantial mutual inactivation
chloramphenicol, erythromycins, sulfonamides, tetracyclines: Possibly decreased therapeutic effects of nafcillin
hepatotoxic drugs: Increased risk of hepatotoxicity
methotrexate: Increased risk of methotrexate toxicity
probenecid: Increased blood nafcillin level

Adverse Reactions
CNS: Depression, headache, seizures
EENT: Oral candidiasis
GI: Abdominal pain, diarrhea, nausea, pseudomembranous colitis, vomiting
GU: Interstitial nephritis, vaginitis
HEME: Leukopenia, neutropenia
SKIN: Exfoliative dermatitis, pruritus, rash, urticaria
Other: Anaphylaxis; hypokalemia; infusion site pain, redness, and swelling; serum sickness–like reaction

Nursing Considerations
- Obtain body fluid or tissue specimens for culture and sensitivity testing, as prescribed, and obtain test results, if possible, before giving nafcillin.
- **WARNING** Before starting nafcillin therapy, make sure patient has had no previous hypersensitivity reactions to penicillins.
- Dilute with appropriate diluent to a concentration of 2 to 40 mg/ml. Infuse over 30 to 60 minutes.
- Give nafcillin at least 1 hour before or after aminoglycosides, especially if patient has renal disease.
- When giving drug to patient at risk for hypertension or fluid overload, be aware that each gram of nafcillin contains 2.5 mEq of sodium.
- **WARNING** Don't administer nafcillin preparations that contain benzyl alcohol to neonates or premature infants because this preservative has been linked to a fatal toxic syndrome characterized by CNS, respiratory, circulatory, and renal impairment and metabolic acidosis.

- Monitor for signs of superinfection, such as oral candidiasis and pseudomembranous colitis, especially in elderly, immunocompromised, or debilitated patients who receive large doses of nafcillin.
- Store drug at 15° to 30° C (59° to 86° F).

PATIENT TEACHING

- Advise patient to report chills, fever, or rash. If she develops diarrhea, tell her to check with prescriber before taking an antidiarrheal to avoid masking of pseudomembranous colitis.

nalbuphine hydrochloride
Nubain

Class and Category
Chemical: Phenanthrene derivative
Therapeutic: Anesthesia adjunct, opioid analgesic
Pregnancy category: Not rated

Indications and Dosages
▶ *To relieve moderate to severe pain*
I.V. INJECTION
Adults who weigh 70 kg (154 lb). 10 mg q 3 to 6 hr, p.r.n. Dosage adjusted for patients who weigh more or less.
▶ *As adjunct to anesthesia*
I.V. INJECTION
Adults. 0.3 to 3 mg/kg over 10 to 15 min, followed by 0.25 to 0.5 mg/kg, as needed.
DOSAGE ADJUSTMENT For patients who have repeatedly received an opioid agonist, initial dose possibly reduced to 25% of usual dosage. For patients who haven't developed a tolerance to drug's effects, maximum usually is 20 mg/dose or 160 mg/day.

Route	Onset	Peak	Duration
I.V.	2 to 3 min	30 min	3 to 4 hr

Mechanism of Action
Binds with and stimulates mu and kappa opioid receptors in the spinal cord and higher levels in the CNS. In this way, nalbuphine alters the perception of, and emotional response to, pain.

Incompatibilities

Don't administer nalbuphine with diazepam or pentobarbital. Use a separate I.V. line or flush line well before and after administration.

Contraindications

Hypersensitivity to nalbuphine or its components

Interactions

DRUGS

alfentanil, CNS depressants, fentanyl, sufentanil: Increased risk of hypotension and CNS and respiratory depression

anticholinergics: Increased risk of severe constipation and urine retention

antidiarrheals (such as difenoxin and atropine, loperamide, and paregoric): Increased risk of severe constipation and increased CNS depression

antihypertensives: Increased risk of hypotension

buprenorphine: Possibly decreased therapeutic effects of nalbuphine and increased risk of respiratory depression

hydroxyzine: Increased risk of CNS depression and hypotension

MAO inhibitors: Risk of possibly fatal increased CNS excitation or depression

metoclopramide: Possibly antagonized effects of metoclopramide

naloxone, naltrexone: Decreased pharmacologic effects of nalbuphine

neuromuscular blockers: Increased risk of prolonged CNS and respiratory depression

ACTIVITIES

alcohol use: Increased risk of coma, hypotension, profound sedation, and respiratory depression

Adverse Reactions

CNS: Confusion, depression, dizziness, euphoria, fatigue, hallucinations, headache, nervousness, restlessness, syncope, tiredness, weakness

CV: Hypertension, hypotension, tachycardia

EENT: Blurred vision, diplopia, dry mouth

GI: Abdominal cramps, anorexia, constipation, nausea, vomiting

GU: Decreased urine output, ureteral spasm

RESP: Dyspnea, respiratory depression, wheezing

SKIN: Diaphoresis, flushing, pruritus, rash, sensation of warmth, urticaria

Other: Injection site burning, pain, redness, swelling, and warmth

Nursing Considerations

- Instruct patient to lie down during nalbuphine administration to minimize dizziness, light-headedness, nausea, and vomiting. Avoid rapid administration, which can cause serious adverse reactions, including anaphylaxis, hypotension, and severe respiratory depression.
- For direct I.V. injection through an I.V. line with a compatible infusing solution, give drug slowly—no more than 10 mg over 3 to 5 minutes. Inject into free-flowing NS, D_5W, or LR solution.
- Keep resuscitation equipment and naloxone readily available to reverse nalbuphine's effects, if needed.
- Monitor for signs of respiratory depression, such as apnea and decreased respiratory rate, especially in patients with impaired respiration from such conditions as asthma, infection, uremia, and respiratory obstruction and in patients taking other drugs that can cause respiratory depression.
- Assess patients with impaired renal or hepatic function for signs of increased malabsorption because drug is metabolized in the liver and excreted by the kidneys.
- Monitor for signs of drug-induced CNS depression or increased CSF pressure, such as altered LOC, restlessness, and irritability, in patients with a head injury, intracranial lesions, or other conditions that cause these effects. Patients who are taking, or have recently taken, drugs that depress the CNS are also more susceptible to these effects. Take appropriate safety precautions.
- Be aware that nalbuphine may induce or exacerbate arrhythmias or seizures in patients with a history of these conditions and may mask symptoms of acute abdominal disorders.
- Be aware that patients with a history of drug abuse (including acute alcoholism), emotional instability, or suicidal ideation or attempts are at increased risk for opioid abuse; however, the risk of drug dependence is lower with nalbuphine than with other opioid analgesics.
- Be aware that nalbuphine may mask or worsen gallbladder pain.
- **WARNING** Monitor opioid-dependent patients for withdrawal symptoms, such as abdominal cramps, anorexia, anxiety, backache, bone or joint pain, confusion, depression, diaphoresis, dysphoria, erythema, fear, fever, irritability, labile blood pressure and pulse, lacrimation, muscle spasms, myalgia, mydriasis, nasal congestion, nausea, opioid craving, piloerection, restlessness, rhinorrhea, sensation of crawling skin, sleep disturbances, tremor, uneasiness, vomiting, and yawning.

- **WARNING** Be aware that drug may obscure neurologic assessment findings in patients with cerebral aneurysm, head injury, or increased ICP.
- During prolonged use, expect to give a stool softener to minimize constipation.
- Store drug at 15° to 30° C (59° to 86° F); protect from freezing and light.

PATIENT TEACHING
- Advise patient to avoid potentially hazardous activities until nalbuphine's CNS effects are known.
- Counsel patient against making important decisions while receiving drug because it may cloud her judgment.

nalmefene hydrochloride
Revex

Class and Category
Chemical: 6-Methylene analogue of naltrexone
Therapeutic: Opioid antagonist
Pregnancy category: B

Indications and Dosages
▶ *To treat known or suspected opioid overdose*
I.V. INJECTION
Adults. 500 mcg/70 kg (154 lb) of body weight, followed by second dose of 1,000 mcg/70 kg in 2 to 5 min, as indicated. *Maximum:* 1,500 mcg/70 kg.
▶ *To treat postoperative opioid-induced respiratory depression*
I.V. INJECTION
Adults. *Initial:* 0.25 mcg/kg q 2 to 5 min until desired degree of reversal is achieved. *Maximum:* 1 mcg/kg.
DOSAGE ADJUSTMENT Initial and subsequent doses possibly reduced to 0.1 mcg/kg for patients at increased risk for CV complications.

Route	Onset	Peak	Duration
I.V.	2 to 5 min	Unknown	30 to 60 min*

Contraindications
Hypersensitivity to nalmefene or its components

---

* For partial reversal of opioid effects; up to several hr for full reversal.

Mechanism of Action

Antagonizes mu, kappa, and sigma opioid receptors in the CNS, thus reversing the analgesia, hypotension, respiratory depression, and sedation caused by most opioids. Mu receptors are responsible for analgesia, euphoria, miosis, and respiratory depression. Kappa receptors are responsible for analgesia and sedation. Sigma receptors control dysphoria and other delusional states.

Interactions

DRUGS

opioid analgesics (including alfentanil, fentanyl, and sufentanil): Reversal of these drugs' analgesic and adverse effects, possibly withdrawal symptoms in opioid-dependent patients

Adverse Reactions

CNS: Agitation, chills, confusion, depression, dizziness, fever, hallucinations, headache, nervousness, somnolence, tremor
CV: Arrhythmias, hypertension, hypotension, tachycardia, vasodilation
EENT: Dry mouth, pharyngitis
GI: Diarrhea, nausea, vomiting
GU: Urine retention
SKIN: Pruritus
Other: Withdrawal symptoms

Nursing Considerations

- **WARNING** Read the label carefully before administering nalmefene because drug comes in concentrations of 100 mcg/ml and 1 mg/ml.
- Monitor patients with hepatic or renal dysfunction for signs of increased nalmefene effects because drug is metabolized by liver and excreted by kidneys.
- Monitor heart rate, respiratory rate, and blood pressure to detect CV complications. Patients who have received a cardiotoxic drug and those with cardiac disease are at increased risk.
- Continue to monitor patient after nalmefene administration because symptoms of opioid toxicity may return if opioid's duration of action is longer than that of nalmefene.
- **WARNING** Monitor for withdrawal symptoms, especially in opioid-dependent patients. Symptoms include abdominal cramps, anorexia, anxiety, backache, bone or joint pain, con-

fusion, depression, diaphoresis, dysphoria, erythema, fear, fever, irritability, labile blood pressure and pulse, lacrimation, muscle spasms, myalgia, mydriasis, nasal congestion, nausea, opioid craving, piloerection, restlessness, rhinorrhea, sensation of crawling skin, sleep disturbances, tremor, uneasiness, vomiting, and yawning.

• Be prepared to provide mechanical or assisted ventilation if reversal of opioid-induced respiratory depression is incomplete.

• Store drug at 15° to 30° C (59° to 86° F).

PATIENT TEACHING

• Inform patient or family members that nalmefene is administered to reverse opioid-induced adverse reactions.

• Urge opioid-dependent patient to seek drug rehabilitation.

naloxone hydrochloride
Narcan

Class and Category
Chemical: Thebaine derivative
Therapeutic: Opioid antagonist
Pregnancy category: B

Indications and Dosages
▶ *To treat known or suspected opioid overdose*
I.V. INJECTION
Adults, children age 5 and older, and children under age 5 who weigh more than 20 kg (44 lb). 0.4 to 2 mg repeated q 2 to 3 min, p.r.n. If no response after 10 mg, patient may not have narcotic-induced respiratory depression.
Infants and children under age 5 who weigh less than 20 kg. 0.01 mg/kg as a single dose; if no improvement, another 0.1 mg/kg, as prescribed. Alternatively, 0.1 mg/kg repeated q 2 to 3 min, as needed.
I.V. INJECTION
Neonates. 0.01 mg/kg repeated q 2 to 3 min, as prescribed, until desired response occurs. Alternatively, initial dose of 0.1 mg/kg.
▶ *To treat postoperative opioid-induced respiratory depression*
I.V. INJECTION
Adults and adolescents. *Initial:* 0.1 to 0.2 mg q 2 to 3 min until desired response occurs. Additional doses given q 1 to 2 hr, if needed, based on patient response.

Children. *Initial:* 0.005 to 0.01 mg q 2 to 3 min until desired response occurs. Additional doses given q 1 to 2 hr, if needed, based on patient response.

▶ *To reverse opioid-induced asphyxia*

I.V. INJECTION

Neonates. *Initial:* 0.01 mg/kg q 2 to 3 min until desired response occurs. Additional doses given q 1 to 2 hr, if needed, based on patient response.

▶ *As adjunct to treat hypotension caused by septic shock*

I.V. INFUSION OR INJECTION

Adults. 0.03 to 0.2 mg/kg over 5 min, followed by continuous infusion of 0.03 to 0.3 mg/kg/hr for 1 to 24 hr, as needed, based on patient response.

Route	Onset	Peak	Duration
I.V.	1 to 2 min	5 to 15 min	45 min or longer

Mechanism of Action

Briefly and competitively antagonizes mu, kappa, and sigma opioid receptors in the CNS, thus reversing the analgesia, hypotension, respiratory depression, and sedation caused by most opioids. Mu receptors are responsible for analgesia, euphoria, miosis, and respiratory depression. Kappa receptors are responsible for analgesia and sedation. Sigma receptors control dysphoria and other delusional states.

Incompatibilities

Don't mix naloxone with any other solution unless you verify that drugs are compatible; drug is incompatible with alkaline, bisulfite, and metabisulfite solutions.

Contraindications

Hypersensitivity to naloxone or its components

Interactions

DRUGS

butorphanol, nalbuphine, pentazocine: Reversal of these drugs' analgesic and adverse effects

opioid analgesics: Reversal of these drugs' analgesic and adverse effects, possibly withdrawal symptoms in opioid-dependent patients

Adverse Reactions

CNS: Excitement, irritability, nervousness, restlessness, seizures, tremor, violent behavior

CV: Hypertension (severe), hypotension, ventricular fibrillation, ventricular tachycardia
GI: Nausea, vomiting
RESP: Pulmonary edema
SKIN: Diaphoresis
Other: Withdrawal symptoms

Nursing Considerations

• Keep resuscitation equipment readily available during naloxone administration.
• If needed, dilute naloxone with sterile water before administering I.V. injection. To prepare a continuous infusion, add 2 mg of naloxone to 500 ml of NS or D_5W to yield a concentration of 4 mcg/ml. Use within 24 hours.
• Give repeat doses as prescribed, depending on patient's response. Continue to monitor patient after naloxone administration because symptoms of opioid toxicity may return if opioid's duration of action is longer than that of naloxone.
• Be aware that rapid reversal of opioid effects can cause diaphoresis, nausea, and vomiting.
• **WARNING** Monitor for withdrawal symptoms, especially in opioid-dependent patients. Symptoms may include abdominal cramps, anorexia, anxiety, backache, bone or joint pain, confusion, depression, diaphoresis, dysphoria, erythema, fear, fever, irritability, labile blood pressure and pulse, lacrimation, muscle spasms, myalgia, mydriasis, nasal congestion, nausea, opioid craving, piloerection, restlessness, rhinorrhea, sensation of crawling skin, sleep disturbances, tremor, uneasiness, vomiting, and yawning.
• Monitor cardiac and respiratory status of patients with a history of CV or pulmonary disease for signs of exacerbation.
• Expect patient with hepatic or renal dysfunction to have increased circulating blood naloxone level.
• Store naloxone at 15° to 30° C (59° to 86° F); protect from freezing and light.

PATIENT TEACHING
• Inform patient or family that naloxone is administered to reverse opioid-induced adverse reactions.
• Urge opioid-dependent patient to seek drug rehabilitation.

neostigmine methylsulfate
Prostigmin

Class and Category
Chemical: Quaternary ammonium compound
Therapeutic: Anticholinesterase, curare antidote
Pregnancy category: C

Indications and Dosages
▶ *To reverse nondepolarizing neuromuscular blockade*
I.V. INJECTION
Adults. 0.5 to 2 mg by slow push, repeated as needed up to
5 mg; 0.6 to 1.2 mg of atropine or 0.2 to 0.6 mg of glycopyrrolate
is given with or a few minutes before neostigmine, as ordered.
Children. 0.04 mg/kg by slow push; 0.02 mg/kg of atropine is
given I.M. or S.C. with each dose or with alternate doses.

Route	Onset	Peak	Duration
I.V.	4 to 8 min	30 min	2 to 4 hr

Mechanism of Action
Inhibits the action of cholinesterase, an enzyme that destroys acetylcholine at
myoneuronal junctions, thereby increasing acetylcholine accumulation at
myoneuronal junctions and facilitating nerve impulse transmission across the
junctions. This action reverses the effects of nondepolarizing neuromuscular
blockers.

Contraindications
Hypersensitivity to neostigmine, other anticholinesterases, bro-
mides, or their components; mechanical obstruction of intestinal
or urinary tract; peritonitis

Interactions
DRUGS
*aminoglycosides, anesthetics, capreomycin, colistimethate, colistin, lido-
caine, lincomycins, polymyxin B, quinine:* Increased risk of neuromuscular blockade
anticholinergics: Possibly masked signs of cholinergic crisis

guanadrel, guanethidine, mecamylamine, trimethaphan: Possibly antagonized effects of neostigmine, possibly decreased antihypertensive effects

neuromuscular blockers: Possibly prolonged action of depolarizing—and antagonized action of nondepolarizing—neuromuscular blockers

procainamide, quinidine: Possibly antagonized effects of neostigmine

quinine: Decreased neostigmine effectiveness

Adverse Reactions

CNS: Dizziness, drowsiness, headache, seizures, syncope, weakness

CV: Arrhythmias (AV block, bradycardia, nodal rhythm, tachycardia), cardiac arrest, ECG changes, hypotension

EENT: Increased salivation, lacrimation, miosis, vision changes

GI: Abdominal cramps, diarrhea, flatulence, increased peristalsis, nausea, vomiting

GU: Urinary frequency

MS: Arthralgia, dysarthria, muscle spasms

RESP: Bronchospasm, dyspnea, increased bronchial secretions, respiratory arrest or depression

SKIN: Flushing, diaphoresis, rash, urticaria

Nursing Considerations

- If also giving atropine, be sure to administer it with or before neostigmine, as prescribed.
- Make sure patient is well ventilated and airway remains patent until normal respiration is assured.
- **WARNING** Monitor for signs of neostigmine overdose, which can cause life-threatening cholinergic crisis (increased muscle weakness, including respiratory muscles). Expect to stop neostigmine and atropine, as ordered.
- Be aware that patients with postoperative atelectasis, pneumonia, UTI, or asthma may experience an exacerbation of their condition if given neostigmine.
- Store drug at 15° to 30° C (59° to 86° F); protect from freezing and light.

PATIENT TEACHING

- Instruct patient to report muscle weakness, excessive salivation, dizziness, urinary frequency, or other adverse reactions after receiving neostigmine.

nesiritide

Natrecor

Class and Category

Chemical: Human B-type natriuretic peptide
Therapeutic: Arterial and venous smooth-muscle cell relaxant
Pregnancy category: C

Indications and Dosages

▶ *To reduce dyspnea at rest or with minimal activity in patients with acute decompensated heart failure*

I.V. INJECTION OR INFUSION

Adults. 2-μg/kg bolus, followed by a continuous infusion of 0.01 μg/kg/min for up to 48 hr.

Route	Onset	Peak	Duration
I.V.	In 15 min	1 hr	3 hr

Mechanism of Action

Binds to the guanylate cyclase receptor of vascular smooth-muscle and endothelial cells. This action increases intracellular levels of cGMP, which leads to arterial and venous smooth-muscle cell relaxation. Ultimately, nesiritide reduces pulmonary artery wedge pressure and systemic arterial pressure in patients with heart failure, thereby decreasing the heart's workload and subsequently relieving dyspnea.

Incompatibilities

Don't infuse nesiritide through the same I.V. line as bumetanide, enalaprilat, ethacrynate sodium, furosemide, heparin, hydralazine, or insulin because these drugs are chemically and physically incompatible with nesiritide. Don't infuse drugs that contain the preservative sodium metabisulfite through the same I.V. line as nesiritide because they're incompatible.

Contraindications

Hypersensitivity to nesiritide or its components, patients with a systolic blood pressure less than 90 mm Hg, primary therapy for cardiogenic shock

Interactions

DRUGS

ACE inhibitors: Increased risk of symptomatic hypotension

Adverse Reactions

CNS: Anxiety, dizziness, headache, insomnia
CV: Angina, bradycardia, hypotension, PVCs, ventricular tachycardia
GI: Abdominal pain, nausea, vomiting
GU: Elevated serum creatinine level
MS: Back pain

Nursing Considerations

• **WARNING** Be aware that nesiritide is not recommended for patients for whom vasodilating drugs are inappropriate, such as those with significant valvular stenosis, restrictive or obstructive cardiomyopathy, constrictive pericarditis, pericardial tamponade, or other conditions in which cardiac output is dependent upon venous return, or for patients suspected of having low cardiac filling pressures.

• Reconstitute 1.5-mg vial by adding 5 ml of diluent removed from a 250-ml plastic I.V. bag containing preservative-free D_5W, NS, $D_5/0.45NS$, or $D_5/0.2NS$.

• Don't shake vial. To ensure complete reconstitution, rock vial gently so that all surfaces, including the stopper, come in contact with diluent. Inspect drug for particles and discoloration; if present, discard drug.

• Withdraw entire contents of reconstituted solution and add it to the same 250-ml plastic I.V. bag used to withdraw the diluent to yield a solution with a concentration of approximately 6 µg/ml. Invert I.V. bag several times to ensure that solution is completely mixed.

• After preparing infusion bag, withdraw bolus volume from infusion bag and administer it over approximately 60 seconds. Immediately after administering bolus, infuse drug at a flow rate of 0.1 ml/kg/hour, which will deliver a dose of 0.01 µg/kg/minute.

• Prime I.V. tubing with 25 ml of solution before connecting to I.V. line and before administering bolus dose or starting infusion.

• Flush I.V. line between administration of nesiritide and incompatible drugs.

• Because nesiritide binds to heparin and could bind to heparin lining of a heparin-coated catheter, don't administer drug through a central heparin-coated catheter.

• Store reconstituted vials at room temperature (20° to 25° C [68° to 77° F]) or refrigerate (2° to 8° C [36° to 46° F]) for up to 24 hours.

- Because nesiritide contains no antimicrobial preservatives, discard reconstituted solution after 24 hours.
- Monitor blood pressure and heart rate and rhythm frequently during drug therapy. If hypotension occurs, notify prescriber and expect dosage to be reduced or drug to be discontinued. Implement measures to support blood pressure, as prescribed.
- Assess breath sounds and respiratory rate, rhythm, depth, and quality frequently during nesiritide therapy.
- Monitor serum creatinine level during therapy and notify prescriber of abnormal results.
- Store unopened drug at controlled room temperature or refrigerate. Keep in carton until time of use.

PATIENT TEACHING
- Instruct patient to report dizziness during nesiritide therapy because this may indicate hypotension.
- Reassure patient that her blood pressure, heart rate, and breathing will be monitored frequently.

netilmicin sulfate
Netromycin

Class and Category
Chemical: Aminoglycoside
Therapeutic: Antibiotic
Pregnancy category: D

Indications and Dosages
▶ *To treat serious systemic infections, such as intra-abdominal infections, lower respiratory tract infections, septicemia, and skin and soft-tissue infections, caused by* Enterobacter aerogenes, Escherichia coli, Klebsiella pneumoniae, Proteus mirabilis, Pseudomonas aeruginosa, Serratia *species, and* Staphylococcus aureus

I.V. INFUSION
Adults and children age 12 and older. 1.3 to 2.2 mg/kg q 8 hr or 2 to 3.25 mg/kg q 12 hr for 7 to 14 days. *Maximum:* 7.5 mg/kg/day.
Children ages 6 weeks to 12 years. 1.8 to 2.7 mg/kg q 8 hr or 2.7 to 4 mg/kg q 12 hr for 7 to 14 days.
Infants up to age 6 weeks. 2 to 3.25 mg/kg q 12 hr for 7 to 14 days.

▶ *To treat complicated UTIs caused by* Citrobacter *species,* Enterobacter *species,* E. coli, K. pneumoniae, P. mirabilis, P. aeruginosa, Serratia *species, and* Staphylococcus *species*
I.V. INFUSION
Adults and adolescents. 1.5 to 2 mg/kg q 12 hr for 7 to 14 days. *Maximum:* 7.5 mg/kg/day.

Mechanism of Action

Is transported into bacterial cells, where it competes with messenger RNA to bind with a specific receptor protein on the 30S ribosomal subunit of DNA. This action causes abnormal, nonfunctioning proteins to form. A lack of functional proteins causes bacterial cell death.

Incompatibilities
Don't mix netilmicin with beta-lactam antibiotics (penicillins and cephalosporins) because substantial mutual inactivation may result. If these drugs are prescribed concurrently, administer them at separate sites.

Contraindications
Hypersensitivity to netilmicin, other aminoglycosides, or their components

Interactions
DRUGS
capreomycin, other aminoglycosides: Increased risk of nephrotoxicity, neuromuscular blockade, and ototoxicity
cephalosporins, nephrotoxic drugs: Increased risk of nephrotoxicity
loop diuretics, ototoxic drugs: Increased risk of ototoxicity
methoxyflurane, polymyxins (parenteral): Increased risk of nephrotoxicity and neuromuscular blockade
neuromuscular blockers: Increased neuromuscular blockade

Adverse Reactions
CNS: Disorientation, dizziness, encephalopathy, headache, myasthenia gravis–like syndrome, neuromuscular blockade (acute muscle paralysis and apnea), paresthesia, peripheral neuropathy, seizures, vertigo, weakness
CV: Hypotension, palpitations
EENT: Blurred vision, hearing loss, nystagmus, tinnitus
GI: Diarrhea, elevated liver function tests results, nausea, vomiting

GU: Elevated BUN and serum creatinine levels, nephrotoxicity, oliguria, proteinuria
HEME: Anemia, eosinophilia, leukopenia, prolonged PT, thrombocytopenia, thrombocytosis
MS: Muscle twitching
RESP: Apnea
SKIN: Allergic dermatitis, erythema, pruritus, rash
Other: Angioedema; hyperkalemia; injection site hematoma, induration, and pain

Nursing Considerations

- To prepare netilmicin for I.V. use, dilute each dose in 50 to 200 ml of suitable diluent, such as NS, D$_5$W, or LR solution, and administer slowly over 30 to 60 minutes. When giving drug to children, adjust amount of diluent proportionately, as required. Prepared solution typically may be stored for up to 72 hours at room temperature; however, storage times vary, depending on type of diluent used, type of container, concentration, and storage method. Consult manufacturer's insert for specific stability and storage information.
- Ensure adequate hydration during therapy to maintain adequate renal function.
- Monitor blood netilmicin level; optimum peak level is 6 to 10 mcg/ml and trough level is 0.5 to 2 mcg/ml.
- Check BUN and serum creatinine levels, urine specific gravity, and creatinine clearance during netilmicin therapy, as ordered.
- Anticipate higher risk of nephrotoxicity in infants, elderly patients, those with impaired renal function or dehydration, and those receiving high-dose or prolonged netilmicin therapy.
- Decrease dosage or discontinue drug, as ordered, if signs of drug-induced ototoxicity or vestibular toxicity occur, to reduce the risk of permanent damage. Patients with cranial nerve VIII impairment are at increased risk for both types of toxicity.
- Be aware that infants with botulism and patients with myasthenia gravis or Parkinson's disease may experience increased muscle weakness.
- Store drug at 15° to 30° C (59° to 86° F); don't freeze.

PATIENT TEACHING
- Encourage patient to drink plenty of fluids during netilmicin therapy.

- Instruct patient to immediately report dizziness, hearing loss, muscle twitching, nausea, numbness and tingling, ringing or buzzing in ears, seizures, significant changes in amount of urine or frequency of urination, and vomiting.
- Urge patient to keep follow-up appointments—for example, for audiometric and renal function tests—to monitor progress.

niacin
(nicotinic acid, vitamin B₃)
niacinamide
(nicotinamide, vitamin B₃)

Class and Category
Chemical: B complex vitamin
Therapeutic: Nutritional supplement
Pregnancy category: C (for doses above the RDA)

Indications and Dosages
▶ *To prevent niacin deficiency based on U.S. and Canadian recommended daily allowances (RDAs)*
I.V. INFUSION
Adults and children. Dosage individualized based on severity of deficiency, as prescribed, and given as part of total parenteral nutrition solution.
▶ *To treat niacin deficiency*
I.V. INJECTION
Adults and children age 11 and older. 25 to 100 mg at least b.i.d.
Children. Up to 300 mg q.d.

Mechanism of Action
Acts as a dietary supplement for vitamin B₃. After conversion to niacinamide, niacin becomes a compound of two coenzymes, which are needed for tissue respiration; glycogenolysis; and metabolism of lipids, amino acids, proteins, and purines.

Contraindications
Active peptic ulcer disease; arterial bleeding; hepatic impairment (significant or unexplained); hypersensitivity to niacin, niacinamide, or their components

Interactions
DRUGS
HMG-CoA reductase inhibitors: Increased risk of rhabdomyolysis and acute renal failure

Adverse Reactions
CNS: Dizziness, headache (niacin), syncope
CV: Arrhythmias, peripheral vasodilation (niacin)
EENT: Dry eyes
ENDO: Hyperglycemia
GI: Diarrhea, epigastric pain, nausea, vomiting
GU: Hyperuricemia
MS: Myalgia
SKIN: Dry skin, flushing (niacin), pruritus, sensation of warmth (niacin)
Other: Anaphylaxis

Nursing Considerations
- Follow manufacturer's directions for preparing niacinamide for I.V. injection or infusion. To prepare niacin, dilute injection solution to a concentration of 2 mg/ml for direct I.V. injection. Administer either preparation at a rate not exceeding 2 mg/minute.
- For intermittent or continuous infusion, dilute appropriate dose of niacin in 500 ml of NS or other compatible solution and administer at a rate not exceeding 2 mg/minute.
- Monitor patient for "niacin flush," a reaction caused by dilation of peripheral cutaneous blood vessels, which increases blood flow and causes redness, mainly in the face, neck, and chest. Expect patient to develop tolerance to this effect after 2 weeks of therapy. If flushing persists, notify prescriber, who may order aspirin to be taken before each niacin dose to control this effect.
- Expect to monitor liver function tests every 6 months during therapy or as clinically indicated. Expect niacin to be discontinued if serum transaminase levels rise to 3 times the upper limit of normal or if patient exhibits clinical symptoms of hepatic dysfunction.
- Monitor patients with peptic ulcer disease for possible exacerbation of symptoms because nicotinic acid can stimulate histamine release, leading to increased gastric acid production.
- Monitor patients with, or predisposed to, gout for exacerbation of symptoms because drug can cause hyperuricemia when given in high doses.

- Monitor patients with diabetes mellitus for altered glucose control because high doses of niacin may cause hyperglycemia.
- Monitor CBC, especially in patients with thrombocytopenia or coagulopathy and those who are on anticoagulant therapy, because niacin may cause slight decrease in platelet count or increased prothrombin time.
- Be aware that additional dosage considerations, adverse reactions, and nursing considerations apply to patients who are taking *oral* niacin or niacinamide. Oral niacin may be prescribed to treat hyperlipidemia.

PATIENT TEACHING

- Instruct patient to avoid activities requiring mental alertness, such as driving or operating machinery, until full CNS effects of niacin are known because vasodilatory response to drug may be dramatic at start of treatment.
- Inform patient that she may experience skin flushing, mainly in the face, neck, and chest, but that she may develop a tolerance to this effect after 2 weeks of therapy. Advise her to notify prescriber of persistent or intolerable flushing because prescriber may adjust drug dosage or recommend that patient take aspirin before each niacin dose to control flushing.

nicardipine hydrochloride

Cardene, Cardene I.V., Cardene SR

Class and Category

Chemical: Dihydropyridine derivative
Therapeutic: Antianginal, antihypertensive
Pregnancy category: C

Indications and Dosages

▶ *To manage angina pectoris and Prinzmetal's angina, to manage hypertension*

I.V. INFUSION

Adults. 0.5 to 2.2 mg/hr by continuous infusion.

CAPSULES

Adults and adolescents. 20 to 40 mg t.i.d., increased q 3 days, as prescribed.

E.R. CAPSULES

Adults. 30 mg b.i.d.

▶ *To control acute hypertension*
I.V. INFUSION
Adults. *Initial:* 5 mg/hr by continuous infusion; increased by 2.5 mg/hr q 5 to 15 min, as prescribed. *Maximum:* 15 mg/hr.

Route	Onset	Peak	Duration
I.V.	Immediate	Unknown	Unknown
P.O.	20 min	1 to 2 hr	Unknown
P.O. (E.R.)	20 min	1 to 2 hr	12 hr

Mechanism of Action

May slow extracellular calcium movement into myocardial and vascular smooth-muscle cells by deforming calcium channels in cell membranes, inhibiting ion-controlled gating mechanisms, and interfering with calcium release from the sarcoplasmic reticulum. By decreasing the intracellular calcium level, nicardipine inhibits smooth-muscle–cell contraction and dilates coronary and systemic arteries. As with other calcium channel blockers, these actions lead to decreased myocardial oxygen requirements and reduced peripheral resistance, blood pressure, and afterload.

Incompatibilities

Don't mix nicardipine with, or administer through same I.V. line as, sodium bicarbonate or LR solution.

Contraindications

Advanced aortic stenosis, hypersensitivity to any calcium channel blocker, second- or third-degree AV block in patient without artificial pacemaker

Interactions

DRUGS
anesthetics (hydrocarbon inhalation): Possibly hypotension
beta blockers, other antihypertensives, prazosin: Increased risk of hypotension
calcium supplements: Possibly impaired action of nicardipine
cimetidine: Increased nicardipine bioavailability
digoxin: Transiently increased blood digoxin level, increased risk of digitalis toxicity
disopyramide, flecainide: Increased risk of bradycardia, conduction defects, and heart failure
estrogens: Possibly increased fluid retention and decreased therapeutic effects of nicardipine

lithium: Increased risk of neurotoxicity
NSAIDs, sympathomimetics: Possibly decreased therapeutic effects of nicardipine
procainamide, quinidine: Possibly prolonged QT interval
FOODS
grapefruit, grapefruit juice: Possibly increased bioavailability of nicardipine
high-fat meals: Decreased blood nicardipine level
ACTIVITIES
alcohol use: Increased hypotensive effect

Adverse Reactions

CNS: Anxiety, asthenia, ataxia, confusion, dizziness, drowsiness, headache, nervousness, paresthesia, psychiatric disturbance, syncope, tremor, weakness
CV: Bradycardia, chest pain, heart failure, hypotension, orthostatic hypotension, palpitations, peripheral edema, tachycardia
EENT: Altered taste, blurred vision, dry mouth, epistaxis, gingival hyperplasia, pharyngitis, rhinitis, tinnitus
ENDO: Gynecomastia, hyperglycemia
GI: Anorexia, constipation, diarrhea, elevated liver function test results, indigestion, nausea, thirst, vomiting
GU: Dysuria, nocturia, polyuria, sexual dysfunction, urinary frequency
HEME: Anemia, leukopenia, thrombocytopenia
MS: Joint stiffness, muscle spasms
RESP: Bronchitis, cough, upper respiratory tract infection
SKIN: Dermatitis, diaphoresis, erythema multiforme, flushing, photosensitivity, pruritus, rash, Stevens-Johnson syndrome, urticaria
Other: Hypokalemia, weight gain

Nursing Considerations

- Check blood pressure and pulse rate before nicardipine therapy begins, during dosage changes, and periodically throughout therapy. During prolonged therapy, periodically assess ECG tracings for arrhythmias and other changes.
- Dilute each 25-mg ampule of nicardipine with 240 ml of a compatible solution to yield 0.1 mg/ml. Mixture is stable at room temperature for 24 hours when prepared with D_5W, D_5NS, D_5/0.45NS, 0.45NS, or NS.
- Administer continuous infusion by I.V. pump or controller, and adjust according to patient's blood pressure, as prescribed.
- Change peripheral I.V. site every 12 hours, if feasible.

- Give first dose of oral nicardipine 1 hour before stopping I.V. infusion, as prescribed.
- Monitor fluid intake and output and daily weight for signs of fluid retention, which may precipitate heart failure. Also assess for signs of heart failure, such as crackles, dyspnea, jugular vein distention, peripheral edema, and weight gain.
- Monitor liver and renal function test results periodically during long-term therapy. Patients with impaired hepatic or renal function may require dosage adjustment. Expect elevated liver function test results to return to normal after drug is discontinued.
- Monitor serum potassium level during prolonged therapy. Hypokalemia increases the risk of arrhythmias.
- Because of drug's negative inotropic effect on some patients, closely monitor patients who take a beta blocker or have heart failure or significant left ventricular dysfunction.
- **WARNING** Expect to taper dosage gradually before discontinuing drug to prevent angina or dangerously high blood pressure.
- Store drug at 20° to 25° C (68° to 77° F); protect from light and elevated temperatures.

PATIENT TEACHING
- Advise patient to change position slowly during nicardipine therapy to minimize effects of orthostatic hypotension.
- Urge patient to avoid potentially hazardous activities until drug's CNS effects are known.
- Advise patient to immediately report chest pain that is not relieved by rest or nitroglycerin, constipation, irregular heartbeat, nausea, pronounced dizziness, severe or persistent headache, and swelling of hands or feet.
- Urge patient to take oral nicardipine as prescribed, even if she feels well.
- Instruct patient to swallow E.R. capsules whole, not to chew, crush, cut, or open them.
- Advise patient not to take drug within 1 hour of eating a high-fat meal or grapefruit product. Urge her not to alter the amount of grapefruit products in her diet without consulting prescriber.
- **WARNING** Caution patient against stopping nicardipine abruptly because angina or dangerously high blood pressure could result.
- Teach patient how to take her pulse, and urge her to notify prescriber immediately if it falls below 50 beats/minute.

- Teach patient how to measure her blood pressure, and advise her to do so weekly if nicardipine was prescribed for hypertension. Suggest that she keep a log of blood pressure readings to take to follow-up appointments with her doctor.
- Encourage patient to comply with suggested lifestyle changes, such as alcohol moderation, low-sodium or low-fat diet, regular exercise, smoking cessation, stress management, and weight loss.
- Inform patient that saunas, hot tubs, and prolonged hot showers may cause dizziness or fainting.
- Instruct patient to avoid prolonged sun exposure and to use sunscreen when going outdoors.

nitroglycerin
(glyceryl trinitrate)
Nitro-Bid I.V., Nitroject, Tridil

Class and Category
Chemical: Nitrate
Therapeutic: Antianginal, antihypertensive, vasodilator
Pregnancy category: C

Indications and Dosages
▶ *To prevent or treat angina, to manage hypertension or heart failure*
I.V. INFUSION
Adults. 5 mcg/min, increased by 5 mcg/min q 3 to 5 min to 20 mcg/min, as prescribed, and then increased by 10 to 20 mcg/min q 3 to 5 min until desired effect occurs.

Route	Onset	Peak	Duration
I.V.	1 to 2 min	Unknown	3 to 5 min

Incompatibilities
Don't administer nitroglycerin through I.V. bags or tubing made of polyvinyl chloride. Don't mix drug with other solutions.

Contraindications
Angle-closure glaucoma, cerebral hemorrhage, constrictive pericarditis, head trauma, hypersensitivity to nitrates, hypotension, hypovolemia, inadequate cerebral circulation, increased ICP, orthostatic hypotension, pericardial tamponade, severe anemia

Mechanism of Action

Nitroglycerin may interact with nitrate receptors in vascular smooth-muscle–cell membranes. This interaction reduces nitroglycerin to nitric oxide, which activates the enzyme guanylate cyclase, increasing intracellular formation of cGMP, as shown.

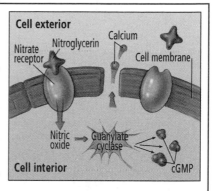

The increased cGMP level may relax vascular smooth muscle by forcing calcium out of muscle cells, causing vasodilation. Venous dilation decreases venous return to the heart, reducing left ventricular end-diastolic pressure and pulmonary artery wedge pressure. Arterial dilation decreases systemic vascular resistance, systolic arterial pressure, and mean arterial pressure. As a result, nitroglycerin reduces preload and afterload, decreasing myocardial workload and oxygen demand. Nitroglycerin also dilates coronary arteries, increasing blood flow to ischemic myocardial tissue.

Interactions

DRUGS

acetylcholine, norepinephrine: Possibly decreased therapeutic effects of these drugs
heparin: Possibly decreased anticoagulant effect of heparin
opioid analgesics, other antihypertensives, vasodilators: Possibly increased orthostatic hypotension
sildenafil: Possibly potentiated hypotensive effect of nitroglycerin
sympathomimetics: Possibly decreased antianginal effect of nitroglycerin and increased risk of hypotension

ACTIVITIES

alcohol use: Possibly increased orthostatic hypotension

Adverse Reactions

CNS: Agitation, anxiety, dizziness, headache, insomnia, restlessness, syncope, weakness
CV: Arrhythmias (including tachycardia), edema, hypotension, orthostatic hypotension, palpitations
EENT: Blurred vision, dry mouth
GI: Abdominal pain, diarrhea, indigestion, nausea, vomiting
GU: Dysuria, impotence, urinary frequency
HEME: Methemoglobinemia

MS: Arthralgia
RESP: Bronchitis, pneumonia
SKIN: Flushing of face and neck, rash

Nursing Considerations

- Dilute I.V. nitroglycerin in D_5W or NS, and avoid mixing with other infusions. Add drug to a glass bottle, not a container made of polyvinyl chloride (PVC). Don't use a filter because plastic absorbs drug. Administer with infusion pump.
- Check label carefully to verify concentration available for dilution. Also check manufacturer's insert for specific dilution, dosage, and administration recommendations, which can vary among products. Use diluted solution within 24 hours.
- Be aware that PVC tubing absorbs a portion of nitroglycerin from prepared solution.
- **WARNING Before infusion, test infusion pump for proper flow and interruption of flow when pump is turned off. Non-PVC infusion pumps may not infuse solution accurately or may not stop infusion completely when turned off.**
- Store premixed containers in the dark; don't freeze them.
- Check vital signs before every dosage adjustment and frequently during therapy.
- Frequently monitor heart and breath sounds, LOC, fluid intake and output, and pulmonary artery wedge pressure, if possible.
- **WARNING Assess for signs of overdose, such as confusion, diaphoresis, dyspnea, flushing, headache, hypotension, nausea, palpitations, tachycardia, vertigo, vision changes, and vomiting. Treat as prescribed by discontinuing nitroglycerin infusion, if possible; elevating the legs above heart level; and administering an alpha-adrenergic agonist, such as phenylephrine, as prescribed, to treat severe hypotension.**
- Store drug at 15° to 30° C (59° to 86° F); protect from freezing and light.

PATIENT TEACHING
- Teach patient to recognize signs and symptoms of angina pectoris, including chest fullness, pain, and pressure, which may be accompanied by sweating and nausea. Pain may radiate down left arm or into neck or jaw. Inform female patients and those with diabetes mellitus or hypertension that they may experience only fatigue and shortness of breath.
- Inform patient that nitroglycerin commonly causes headache, which typically resolves after a few days of continuous therapy. Suggest that she take acetaminophen as needed.

- Advise patient to immediately report blurred vision, dizziness, and severe headache.
- Instruct patient to change position slowly to minimize effects of orthostatic hypotension.
- Advise patient to avoid potentially hazardous activities until drug's CNS effects are known.
- Urge patient to avoid alcohol during therapy.

nitroprusside sodium

Nipride, Nitropress

Class and Category

Chemical: Cyanonitrosylferrate
Therapeutic: Antihypertensive, vasodilator
Pregnancy category: C

Indications and Dosages

▶ *To treat hypertensive crisis and manage severe heart failure*

I.V. INFUSION

Adults and children. *Initial:* 0.25 to 0.3 mcg/kg/min, increased gradually q few minutes until blood pressure reaches desired level. *Maintenance:* 3 mcg/kg/min (range, 0.25 to 10 mcg/kg/min). *Maximum:* 10 mcg/kg/min for 10 min.

Route	Onset	Peak	Duration
I.V.	1 to 2 min	Immediate	1 to 10 min

Mechanism of Action

May interact with nitrate receptors in vascular smooth-muscle–cell membranes. This interaction reduces nitroprusside to nitric oxide, which activates the enzyme guanylate cyclase, increasing intracellular formation of cGMP. The increased cGMP level may relax vascular smooth muscle by forcing calcium out of muscle cells. Smooth-muscle relaxation causes arteries and veins to dilate, which reduces peripheral vascular resistance and blood pressure.

Incompatibilities

Don't mix nitroprusside with any other drug.

Contraindications

Acute heart failure with decreased peripheral vascular resistance, congenital optic atrophy, decreased cerebral perfusion, hypersensitivity to nitroprusside or its components, hypertension from aortic coarctation or AV shunting, tobacco-induced amblyopia

Interactions
DRUGS

dobutamine: Increased cardiac output, decreased pulmonary artery wedge pressure

ganglionic blockers, general anesthetics, hypotension-producing drugs: Increased hypotensive effect

sympathomimetics: Decreased antihypertensive effect of nitroprusside

Adverse Reactions
CNS: Anxiety, dizziness, headache, increased ICP, nervousness, restlessness

CV: Hypotension, tachycardia

ENDO: Hypothyroidism

GI: Abdominal pain, ileus, nausea, vomiting

HEME: Methemoglobinemia

MS: Muscle twitching

SKIN: Diaphoresis, flushing, rash

Other: Infusion site phlebitis

Nursing Considerations
- Obtain baseline vital signs before administering nitroprusside.
- **WARNING** Don't infuse drug undiluted. Reconstitute with 2 ml of D_5W, and add solution to 250 to 500 ml of D_5W to produce 200 mcg/ml or 100 mcg/ml, respectively.
- Be aware that solution is stable at room temperature for 24 hours when protected from light. Don't use reconstituted solution if it contains particles or is blue, green, red, or darker than faint brown.
- Use an infusion pump. Place opaque covering over infusion container because drug is metabolized by light. I.V. tubing doesn't need to be covered.
- Keep patient supine when starting drug or titrating dose up or down.
- Monitor blood pressure continuously with intra-arterial pressure monitor. Record blood pressure every 5 minutes at start of infusion and every 15 minutes thereafter.
- If patient has severe heart failure, expect to administer an inotropic drug, such as dopamine or dobutamine, as prescribed.
- Monitor level of serum thiocyanate (which forms during nitroprusside metabolism) at least every 72 hours; levels exceeding 100 mcg/ml are associated with toxicity.

- **WARNING** Monitor patients receiving prolonged or high-dose nitroprusside therapy for signs of thiocyanate toxicity (ataxia, blurred vision, delirium, dizziness, dyspnea, headache, hyperreflexia, loss of consciousness, nausea, tinnitus, vomiting). Toxicity can cause arrhythmias, metabolic acidosis, severe hypotension, and death.
- **WARNING** Assess for signs of cyanide toxicity (absence of reflexes, coma, distant heart sounds, hypotension, metabolic acidosis, mydriasis, pink skin, shallow respirations, and weak pulse). If you detect such signs, discontinue nitroprusside, as ordered, and give 4 to 6 mg/kg of sodium nitrite over 2 to 4 minutes to convert hemoglobin to methemoglobin. Follow with 150 to 200 mg/kg of sodium thiosulfate. Repeat this regimen at one-half the original doses after 2 hours, as ordered.
- Monitor infusion site for redness, swelling, and pain.
- Store drug at 15° to 30° C (59° to 86° F), and protect from light.

PATIENT TEACHING
- Advise patient to change position slowly during nitroprusside therapy to minimize dizziness from sudden, severe hypotension.
- Instruct patient to report adverse reactions, such as rash, dizziness, headache, and abdominal pain.

norepinephrine bitartrate
(levarterenol bitartrate)
Levophed

Class and Category
Chemical: Catecholamine
Therapeutic: Cardiac stimulant, vasopressor
Pregnancy category: C

Indications and Dosages
▶ *To treat acute hypotension, cardiogenic shock, and septic shock*
I.V. INFUSION
Adults. *Initial:* 0.5 to 1 mcg/min; increased, as ordered, until systolic blood pressure reaches desired level. *Maintenance:* 2 to 12 mcg/min.
Children. 0.1 mcg/kg/min. *Maximum:* 1 mcg/kg/min.
▶ *To treat refractory shock*
I.V. INFUSION
Adults. Up to 30 mcg/min.

Route	Onset	Peak	Duration
I.V.	Rapid	Unknown	1 to 2 min

Mechanism of Action

At high doses (more than 4 mcg/min), directly stimulates alpha-adrenergic receptors and inhibits activity of the intracellular enzyme adenyl cyclase, which then inhibits cAMP production. Inhibition of cAMP causes arterial and venous constriction and increases peripheral vascular resistance and systolic blood pressure. At low doses (less than 2 mcg/min), norepinephrine directly stimulates beta-adrenergic receptors in the myocardium and increases adenyl cyclase activity, producing positive inotropic and chronotropic effects.

Incompatibilities

Don't mix norepinephrine with iron salts, alkalies, or oxidizing solutions. Don't mix norepinephrine with NS alone.

Contraindications

Concurrent use of hydrocarbon inhalation anesthetics, hypersensitivity to norepinephrine or its components, hypovolemia, mesenteric or peripheral vascular thrombosis

Interactions

DRUGS

alpha blockers: Decreased vasopressor effects of norepinephrine
beta blockers: Decreased cardiac-stimulating effect of norepinephrine, possibly decreased therapeutic effects of both drugs
digoxin: Increased risk of arrhythmias, possibly potentiated inotropic effect
doxapram: Possibly increased vasopressor effects of both drugs
ergonovine, ergotamine, methylergonovine, methysergide, oxytocin: Possibly increased vasoconstriction
general anesthetics: Increased risk of arrhythmias
guanadrel, guanethidine: Increased vasopressor response to norepinephrine, possibly severe hypertension
MAO inhibitors: Possibly life-threatening adverse effects, including arrhythmias, hyperpyrexia, severe headache, severe hypertension, and vomiting
maprotiline, tricyclic antidepressants: Possibly potentiated cardiovascular and pressor effects of norepinephrine, including arrhythmias, severe hypertension, and hyperpyrexia

methylphenidate: Possibly potentiated vasopressor effect of norepinephrine

nitrates: Possibly decreased therapeutic effects of both drugs

phenoxybenzamine: Possibly arrhythmias or hypotension

sympathomimetics: Increased risk of adverse cardiovascular effects

thyroid hormones: Increased risk of coronary insufficiency

Adverse Reactions

CNS: Anxiety, dizziness, headache, insomnia, nervousness, tremor, weakness

CV: Angina, bradycardia, ECG changes, edema, hypertension, hypotension, palpitations, peripheral vascular insufficiency (including gangrene), PVCs, sinus tachycardia

GI: Nausea, vomiting

GU: Decreased renal perfusion

RESP: Apnea, dyspnea

SKIN: Pallor

Other: Infusion site sloughing and tissue necrosis, metabolic acidosis

Nursing Considerations

- Dilute norepinephrine concentrate for infusion in D_5W or D_5NS before administering. Concentrations typically range from 16 to 32 mcg/ml. Discard any unused portion of prepared solution.
- Make sure solution contains no particles and isn't discolored before administering.
- Administer drug with infusion pump or other flow-control device.
- Check blood pressure every 2 to 3 minutes, preferably by direct intra-arterial monitoring, until stabilized and then every 5 minutes.
- **WARNING** Because extravasation can cause severe tissue damage and necrosis, expect prescriber to give multiple S.C. injections of phentolamine (5 to 10 mg diluted in 10 to 15 ml of NS) around extravasated infusion site.
- If blanching occurs along vein, change infusion site and notify prescriber immediately.
- Monitor ECG tracing continuously during drug administration.
- Store drug in light-resistant container at 15° to 30° C (59° to 86° F); don't freeze.

PATIENT TEACHING

- Urge patient receiving norepinephrine to immediately report burning, leaking, or tingling around I.V. site.

octreotide acetate

Sandostatin

Class and Category

Chemical: Cyclic octapeptide, somatostatin analogue
Therapeutic: Antidiarrheal, hormone suppressant
Pregnancy category: B

Indications and Dosages

▶ *To treat symptoms of acromegaly, to suppress the release of growth hormone from pituitary tumors*

I.V. INFUSION, I.V. OR S.C. INJECTION

Adults. *Initial:* 50 mcg t.i.d. *Usual:* 100 mcg t.i.d. *Maximum:* 1,500 mcg/day.

I.M. INJECTION

Adults currently receiving S.C. injections. 20 mg q 4 wk for 3 mo, then adjusted as prescribed in response to serum growth hormone level. *Maximum:* 40 mg q 4 wk.

Route	Onset	Peak	Duration
S.C.	Unknown	Unknown	Up to 12 hr

Mechanism of Action

Controls many types of secretory diarrhea by inhibiting secretion of serotonin and pituitary and GI hormones (including insulin, glucagon, growth hormone, thyrotropin, and possibly thyroid-stimulating hormone) as well as vasoactive intestinal peptides and pancreatic polypeptides (including gastrin, secretin, and motilin). Inhibition of serotonin and peptides increases intestinal absorption of water and electrolytes, decreases pancreatic and gastric acid secretions, and increases intestinal transit time by slowing gastric motility.

By inhibiting hormones involved in vasodilation, octreotide increases splanchnic arterial resistance and decreases GI blood flow, hepatic vein wedge pressure, hepatic blood flow, portal vein pressure, and intravariceal pressure, thus raising seated and standing blood pressures. By inhibiting serotonin secretion, the drug decreases symptoms of acromegaly, including diarrhea, flushing, wheezing, and urinary excretion of 5-hydroxyindoleacetic acid.

Incompatibilities

Don't mix octreotide in same syringe with fat emulsions or total parenteral nutrition solutions.

Contraindications

Hypersensitivity to octreotide or its components

Interactions

DRUGS

beta blockers, calcium channel blockers: Additive cardiovascular effects of these drugs

cisapride: Decreased effectiveness of both drugs

cyclosporine: Decreased blood cyclosporine level

diuretics: Increased risk of fluid and electrolyte imbalances

insulin, oral antidiabetic drugs: Increased risk of hypoglycemia

vitamin B₁₂: Decreased blood levels of vitamin B_{12}

Adverse Reactions

CNS: Dizziness, drowsiness, fatigue, headache

CV: Arrhythmias (including conduction abnormalities), edema, hypotension, orthostatic hypotension

EENT: Vision changes

ENDO: Hyperglycemia, hypoglycemia

GI: Abdominal pain, acute cholecystitis, ascending cholangitis, biliary obstruction, cholelithiasis, cholestatic hepatitis, constipation, flatulence, nausea, pancreatitis, vomiting

GU: Increased urine output

Other: Dehydration, electrolyte imbalances, injection site irritation

Nursing Considerations

- Administer octreotide by rapid I.V. injection only in an emergency, as prescribed.
- To prepare drug for I.V. administration, dilute octreotide acetate injection in 50 to 200 ml of D₅W or NS and use within 24 hours. Discard solution if it contains particles or is discolored. Administer by I.V. infusion over 15 to 30 minutes or by I.V. injection over 3 minutes.
- Don't administer depot injection (long-acting suspension form) by S.C. or I.V. route; administer only by I.M. route and only to patients who respond to and tolerate S.C. drug, as prescribed.
- To prepare depot injection, let powder and diluent warm to room temperature and then reconstitute according to manufacturer's instructions. Gently inject 2 ml of supplied diluent down side of vial without disturbing depot powder. Let diluent saturate powder. After 2 to 5 minutes, check sides and bottom of

vial without inverting it. Once powder is completely saturated, swirl—don't shake—vial for 30 to 60 seconds to form suspension. Use immediately after reconstituting.
- To minimize pain, use smallest injection volume to deliver desired dose and rotate injection sites.
- Avoid using deltoid site for I.M. injection because injection site reactions and pain may result. Intragluteal injection is recommended.
- **WARNING To avoid worsening of symptoms, expect to continue S.C. injections when switching to I.M. injections, as prescribed.**
- Be aware that octreotide increases the risk of acute cholecystitis, ascending cholangitis, biliary obstruction, cholestatic hepatitis, and pancreatitis.
- Monitor vital signs, bowels sounds, and stool consistency. Assess for abdominal pain and signs of gallbladder disease.
- Monitor serum liver enzyme levels, as appropriate.
- Monitor for signs of electrolyte imbalance and dehydration.
- Closely monitor diabetic patient for altered glucose control.
- Expect to give additional doses of S.C. octreotide temporarily, as prescribed, for periodic flare-ups of symptoms.
- Before diluting octreotide, store it at 2° to 8° C (36° to 46° F), and protect from light. Drug may be kept at room temperature for up to 14 days.

PATIENT TEACHING
- Advise patient to change position slowly during octreotide therapy to minimize effects of orthostatic hypotension.
- Instruct patient to report adverse reactions, especially abdominal pain, which may indicate pancreatitis.
- Inform diabetic patient that his blood glucose level will be monitored frequently.

ofloxacin

Floxin

Class and Category

Chemical: Fluoroquinolone
Therapeutic: Antibiotic
Pregnancy category: C

Indications and Dosages

▶ *To treat acute, uncomplicated cystitis caused by* Escherichia coli *or* Klebsiella pneumoniae

I.V. INFUSION

Adults. 200 mg q 12 hr for 3 days.

▶ *To treat uncomplicated cystitis caused by* Citrobacter diversus, Enterobacter aerogenes, Proteus mirabilis, *or* Pseudomonas aeruginosa

I.V. INFUSION

Adults. 200 mg q 12 hr for 7 days.

▶ *To treat complicated UTIs caused by* C. diversus, E. coli, K. pneumoniae, P. mirabilis, *or* P. aeruginosa

I.V. INFUSION

Adults. 200 mg q 12 hr for 10 days.

▶ *To treat uncomplicated gonorrhea*

I.V. INFUSION

Adults and adolescents. 400 mg as a single dose.

▶ *To treat urethritis or cervicitis caused by* Chlamydia trachomatis *or* Neisseria gonorrhoeae

I.V. INFUSION

Adults and adolescents. 300 mg b.i.d. for 7 days as an alternative to doxycycline or azithromycin.

▶ *To treat pelvic inflammatory disease caused by susceptible organisms*

I.V. INFUSION

Adults and adolescents. 400 mg q 12 hr with metronidazole I.V.; after 24 hr, switched to oral therapy, as prescribed. Complete course of therapy lasts 14 days.

TABLETS

Adults and adolescents. 400 mg b.i.d. with metronidazole P.O. for 10 to 14 days.

▶ *To treat prostatitis caused by* E. coli

I.V. INFUSION

Adults. 300 mg q 12 hr for 6 wk.

▶ *To treat lower respiratory tract infections caused by* Haemophilus influenzae *or* Streptococcus pneumoniae *and skin and soft-tissue infections caused by* Staphylococcus aureus *or* Streptococcus pyogenes

I.V. INFUSION

Adults. 400 mg q 12 hr for 10 days.

DOSAGE ADJUSTMENT For patients with creatinine clearance of 20 to 50 ml/min/1.73 m^2, dosing frequency possibly reduced to q 24 hr; with creatinine clearance of less than 20 ml/

min/1.73 m², dosing frequency possibly reduced to q 24 hr and dosage possibly reduced by 50%.

Mechanism of Action

Normally, the enzyme DNA gyrase is responsible for unwinding and supercoiling of bacterial DNA before it replicates, as shown top right. Ofloxacin inhibits synthesis of this enzyme, as shown bottom right, by counteracting the excessive supercoiling of DNA during replication and transcription. In this way, ofloxacin causes the death of of both rapidly growing and slow-growing bacterial cells.

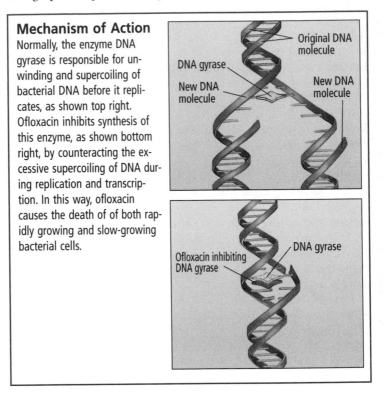

Incompatibilities

Don't mix ofloxacin with other I.V. drugs or additives.

Contraindications

Hypersensitivity to ofloxacin, other fluoroquinolones, or their components

Interactions

DRUGS

aluminum-, calcium-, or magnesium-containing antacids; didanosine; ferrous sulfate; multivitamins; sevelamer; sucralfate; zinc: Decreased absorption of oral ofloxacin

probenecid: Decreased ofloxacin excretion, increased risk of toxicity

procainamide: Decreased renal clearance of procainamide

warfarin: Possibly increased anticoagulant activity and risk of bleeding

Adverse Reactions

CNS: Dizziness, drowsiness, headache, insomnia
GI: Abdominal cramps or pain, diarrhea, nausea, pseudomembranous colitis, vomiting
GU: Vaginal candidiasis
MS: Tendinitis; tendon inflammation, pain, or rupture
SKIN: Blisters, diaphoresis, erythema, erythema multiforme, exfoliative dermatitis, photosensitivity, pruritus, rash, Stevens-Johnson syndrome, toxic epidermal necrolysis, urticaria
Other: Infusion site phlebitis

Nursing Considerations

- When preparing ofloxacin for I.V. infusion, dilute it in NS or D$_5$W to at least 4 mg/ml. Use within 72 hours if stored below 24° C (75° F) or within 14 days if refrigerated. Prepared solution may also be frozen for up to 6 months. Thaw at room temperature or in refrigerator; don't use microwave or warm water to thaw. Discard solution if it contains particles or is discolored; also discard any unused portion. Infuse over 60 minutes to minimize the risk of hypotension.
- Stop drug and notify prescriber immediately if patient has severe (toxic) photosensitivity reaction or tendon pain.
- Maintain adequate hydration to prevent highly concentrated urine and crystalluria.
- Expect an increased risk of drug toxicity in patients with severe hepatic disease, including cirrhosis.
- Be aware that ofloxacin may stimulate the CNS and aggravate seizure disorders.
- If patient develops diarrhea, consider the possibility of pseudomembranous colitis, a complication of long-term use.
- Be alert for signs and symptoms of secondary fungal infection.
- Before diluting drug, store it at 30° C (86° F); protect from freezing and light.

PATIENT TEACHING

- Advise patient to immediately report burning skin, hives, itching, rapid heart rate, rash, and tendon pain during ofloxacin therapy.
- Urge patient to seek medical attention immediately if he develops trouble breathing or swallowing, which may signal an allergic reaction.
- Encourage patient to take oral doses with a full glass of water.

- Instruct patient not to take antacids, didanosine, multivitamins, sucralfate, or iron or zinc preparations within 2 hours of oral ofloxacin to prevent decreased or delayed drug absorption.
- Caution patient to avoid excessive exposure to sun and other forms of ultraviolet light to prevent skin reactions, such as blistering or burning.

ondansetron hydrochloride
Zofran

Class and Category
Chemical: Carbazole
Therapeutic: Antiemetic
Pregnancy category: B

Indications and Dosages
▶ *To prevent chemotherapy-induced nausea and vomiting*
I.V. INFUSION
Adults. 32 mg infused over 15 min, starting 30 min before chemotherapy; or 8 mg infused over 15 min, starting 30 min before chemotherapy, followed by continuous infusion of 1 mg/hr for 24 hr.
Children ages 4 to 18. 3 to 5 mg/m^2 infused over 15 min immediately before chemotherapy, followed by 4 mg P.O. q 8 hr for 5 days or less.
I.V. INFUSION (3-DOSE REGIMEN)
Adults and children ages 4 to 18. 150 mcg/kg infused over 15 min, starting 30 min before chemotherapy; then 150 mcg/kg 4 and 8 hr after first dose.
▶ *To prevent postoperative nausea and vomiting*
I.V. INFUSION
Adults and children age 12 and older. 4 mg as a single dose just before anesthesia induction or if nausea or vomiting develops shortly after surgery.
Children ages 2 to 12 who weigh more than 40 kg (88 lb). 4 mg as a single dose just before anesthesia induction or if nausea or vomiting develops shortly after surgery.
Children ages 2 to 12 who weigh 40 kg or less. 0.1 mg/kg as a single dose just before anesthesia induction or if nausea or vomiting develops shortly after surgery.
DOSAGE ADJUSTMENT For patients with hepatic impairment, maximum dosage limited to 8 mg/day.

Mechanism of Action
Blocks serotonin receptors centrally in the chemoreceptor trigger zone and peripherally at vagal nerve terminals in the intestine. This action reduces nausea and vomiting by preventing serotonin release in the small intestine (the probable cause of chemotherapy-induced nausea and vomiting) and by blocking signals to the CNS. Ondansetron may also bind to other serotonin receptors and to mu opioid receptors.

Incompatibilities
Don't administer ondansetron through same I.V. line as acyclovir, allopurinol, aminophylline, amphotericin B, ampicillin, ampicillin and sulbactam, amsacrine, cefepime, cefoperazone, furosemide, ganciclovir, lorazepam, methylprednisolone, mezlocillin, piperacillin, or sargramostim. Alkaline solutions and highly concentrated solutions of fluorouracil are also physically incompatible with ondansetron.

Contraindications
Hypersensitivity to ondansetron or its components

Interactions
DRUGS
cisplatin, cyclophosphamide: Possibly altered blood levels of these drugs
hepatic enzyme inducers and inhibitors (such as phenytoin and oral estrogen–containing contraceptives): Possibly altered half-life of ondansetron
ACTIVITIES
alcohol use: Increased stimulant and sedative effects, including mood changes and physical sensations

Adverse Reactions
CNS: Akathisia, ataxia, dizziness, fever, headache, restlessness, seizures, weakness
CV: Chest pain, hypotension, pulmonary embolism, tachycardia
EENT: Accommodation disturbances, altered taste, blurred vision, dry mouth
GI: Abdominal pain, anorexia, constipation, diarrhea, elevated liver function test results, flatulence, indigestion, intestinal obstruction, thirst
SKIN: Flushing, hyperpigmentation, maculopapular rash, pruritus
Other: Injection site burning, pain, and redness

Nursing Considerations
- Be aware that patients with a history of hypersensitivity to dolasetron or granisetron may also be hypersensitive to ondansetron.
- Dilute up to 4 mg of odansetron in 50 ml of D₅W or NS. Administer prepared solution within 48 hours if stored at room temperature under normal room lighting. Shake vial to dissolve precipitate, which may form where stopper and vial meet.
- **WARNING** Be aware that ondansetron may mask symptoms of adynamic ileus or gastric distention after abdominal surgery.
- Before diluting drug, store it at 2° to 30° C (36° to 86° F); protect from freezing and light.

PATIENT TEACHING
- Advise patient to immediately report signs of hypersensitivity reaction, such as rash, flushing, or trouble breathing, during ondansetron therapy.
- Review with patient possible adverse reactions, such as headache or abdominal pain, and instruct him to report any that occur. Also advise him to report persistent nausea.
- Advise parents of a child who is taking ondansetron oral solution after I.V. administration to use calibrated container or oral syringe to measure dose.

orphenadrine citrate
Aniflex, Banflex, Flexoject, Miolin, Mio-Rel, Myotrol, Norflex, Orfro, Orphenate

Class and Category
Chemical: Tertiary amine
Therapeutic: Skeletal muscle relaxant
Pregnancy category: C

Indications and Dosages
▶ *To relieve muscle spasms in painful musculoskeletal conditions*
I.V. INJECTION
Adults and adolescents. 60 mg q 12 hr, p.r.n.

Route	Onset	Peak	Duration
I.V.	Immediate	Unknown	4 to 6 hr

Mechanism of Action

May reduce muscle spasms by acting on the cerebral motor centers or the medulla. Postganglionic anticholinergic effects and some antihistaminic and local anesthetic action contribute to skeletal muscle relaxation.

Contraindications

Angle-closure glaucoma; hypersensitivity to orphenadrine or its components; myasthenia gravis; obstruction of bladder neck, duodenum, or pylorus; prostatic hypertrophy; stenosing peptic ulcers

Interactions

DRUGS

amantadine, amitriptyline, amoxapine, antimuscarinics, atropine, bupropion, carbinoxamine, chlorpromazine, clemastine, clomipramine, clozapine, cyclobenzaprine, diphenhydramine, disopyramide, doxepin, imipramine, maprotiline, mesoridazine, methdilazine, nortriptyline, phenothiazines, procainamide, promazine, promethazine, protriptyline, thioridazine, triflupromazine, trimeprazine, trimipramine: Possibly additive anticholinergic effects

CNS depressants: Increased CNS depression

haloperidol: Increased schizophrenic symptoms, possibly tardive dyskinesia

propoxyphene: Increased risk of anxiety, confusion, and tremor

ACTIVITIES

alcohol use: Increased CNS depression

Adverse Reactions

CNS: Agitation, confusion, dizziness, drowsiness, light-headedness, syncope, tremor

CV: Palpitations, tachycardia

EENT: Blurred vision, dry eyes and mouth, increased contact lens awareness

GI: Abdominal distention, constipation, nausea, vomiting

GU: Urine retention

Nursing Considerations

- Be aware that orphenadrine shouldn't be given to patients with tachycardia or cardiac insufficiency.
- Administer drug over 5 minutes with patient in supine position. Have patient remain in this position for 5 to 10 minutes to minimize adverse reactions. Then assist him to sitting position.
- Be aware that drug can aggravate myasthenia gravis and cause tachycardia.

- Anticipate that drug's anticholinergic effects may cause blurred vision, dry eyes, and increased contact lens awareness.
- Be aware that elderly patients may be at increased risk for adverse CNS effects, such as confusion and syncope.
- Monitor blood count and liver and renal function test results periodically for patients receiving long-term orphenadrine therapy.
- Before using drug, store it at 15° to 30° C (59° to 86° F); protect from freezing and light.

PATIENT TEACHING

- Advise patient to avoid potentially hazardous activities until orphenadrine's CNS effects are known.
- Inform patient that dry mouth can be relieved by ice chips, sugarless candy or gum, and increased intake of fluid.
- Suggest that patient use artificial tears during therapy (especially if he wears contact lenses) to reduce discomfort from dry eyes.
- Instruct patient to avoid alcohol and other CNS depressants during orphenadrine therapy.

oxacillin sodium

Bactocill, Prostaphlin

Class and Category

Chemical: Penicillin
Therapeutic class: Antibiotic
Pregnancy category: B

Indications and Dosages

▶ *To treat mild to moderate infections caused by penicillinase-producing strains of* Staphylococcus *or other susceptible organisms*

I.V. INFUSION

Adults and children who weigh 40 kg (88 lb) or more. 250 to 500 mg q 4 to 6 hr.

Infants and children who weigh less than 40 kg. 50 mg/kg/day in divided doses q 4 to 6 hr.

Neonates over age 7 days who weigh 2,000 g or more. 25 to 50 mg/kg q 6 hr.

Neonates over age 7 days who weigh less than 2,000 g. 25 to 50 mg/kg q 8 hr.

Neonates age 7 days and younger who weigh more than 2,000 g. 25 to 50 mg/kg q 8 hr.

Neonates age 7 days and younger who weigh 2,000 g or less. 25 to 50 mg/kg q 12 hr.
▶ *To treat severe infections caused by penicillinase-producing strains of* Staphylococcus *or other susceptible organisms*
I.V. INFUSION
Adults and children who weigh 40 kg or more. 1,000 mg q 4 to 6 hr.
Infants and children who weigh less than 40 kg. 100 to 200 mg/kg/day in divided doses q 4 to 6 hr.
Neonates over age 7 days who weigh 2,000 g or more. 25 to 50 mg/kg q 6 hr.
Neonates over age 7 days who weigh less than 2,000 g. 25 to 50 mg/kg q 8 hr.
Neonates age 7 days and younger who weigh more than 2,000 g. 25 to 50 mg/kg q 8 hr.
Neonates age 7 days and younger who weigh 2,000 g or less. 25 to 50 mg/kg q 12 hr.
▶ *To treat endocarditis caused by methicillin-susceptible* Staphylococcus aureus *in patients without a prosthetic valve*
I.V. INFUSION
Adults. 2 g q 4 hr for 4 to 6 wk.
▶ *To treat endocarditis caused by methicillin-susceptible* S. aureus *in patients with a prosthetic valve*
I.V. INFUSION
Adults. 2 g q 4 hr for at least 6 wk.

Mechanism of Action
Inhibits bacterial cell wall synthesis. In susceptible bacteria, the rigid, cross linked cell wall is assembled in several steps. Oxacillin exerts its effects in the final stage of the cross-linking process by binding with and inactivating penicillin-binding proteins (enzymes responsible for linking the cell wall strands). This action causes bacterial cell lysis and death.

Incompatibilities
Don't give oxacillin at same time or in same admixture as aminoglycosides because they are chemically and physically incompatible.

Contraindications
Hypersensitivity to oxacillin, penicillins, or their components

Interactions

DRUGS

aminoglycosides: Inactivation of both drugs
chloramphenicol, erythromycins, sulfonamides, tetracyclines: Decreased therapeutic effects of oxacillin
oral contraceptives: Decreased contraceptive efficacy
probenecid: Increased blood oxacillin level

Adverse Reactions

CNS: Anxiety, depression, fatigue, hallucinations, headache, seizures
EENT: Oral candidiasis
GI: Diarrhea, hepatotoxicity, nausea, pseudomembranous colitis, vomiting
GU: Interstitial nephritis, vaginal candidiasis
HEME: Agranulocytosis, anemia, granulocytopenia, neutropenia
SKIN: Exfoliative dermatitis, pruritus, rash, urticaria
Other: Anaphylaxis

Nursing Considerations

- Obtain body fluid or tissue specimens for culture and sensitivity testing, as prescribed, and obtain test results, if possible, before giving oxacillin.
- Before starting oxacillin therapy, make sure that patient has had no prior hypersensitivity reactions to penicillins.
- Administer oxacillin at least 1 hour before other antibiotics.
- Before reconstituting drug, loosen powder by tapping bottle several times. Reconstitute only with NS or D_5W. Be aware that oxacillin is available in several concentrations. Consult manufacturer's insert for specific dilution guidelines. Use diluted solutions with a concentration of up to 40 mg/ml within 72 hours if stored at room temperature or within 7 days if refrigerated. Shake vial until solution is clear.
- Before reconstituting drug, store it at 15° to 30° C (59° to 86° F).

PATIENT TEACHING

- Instruct patient receiving oxacillin to immediately report a rash, shortness of breath, or fever.
- Advise patient to report diarrhea and to consult prescriber before taking an antidiarrheal to avoid masking signs of pseudomembranous colitis.
- Advise female patient who uses an oral contraceptive to use an additional contraceptive method during oxacillin therapy.

oxymorphone hydrochloride
Numorphan

Class, Category, and Schedule
Chemical: Phenanthrene derivative
Therapeutic: Opioid analgesic
Pregnancy category: Not rated
Controlled substance: Schedule II

Indications and Dosages
▶ *To relieve moderate to severe pain, to relieve anxiety in patients with dyspnea from pulmonary edema due to acute left ventricular dysfunction*
I.V. INJECTION
Adults. *Initial:* 0.5 mg, repeated q 3 to 6 hr, p.r.n.

Route	Onset	Peak	Duration
I.V.	5 to 10 min	15 to 30 min	3 to 4 hr

Mechanism of Action
Alters the perception of, and emotional response to, pain at the spinal cord and higher levels of the CNS by blocking the release of inhibitory neurotransmitters, such as gamma-aminobutyric acid and acetylcholine.

Contraindications
Acute or severe asthma; hypersensitivity to oxymorphone, other morphine analogues, or their components; ileus; pulmonary edema from a chemical respiratory irritant; severe respiratory depression; upper airway obstruction

Interactions
DRUGS
anticholinergics: Possibly urine retention and severe constipation
antidiarrheals, antiperistaltics: Increased risk of severe constipation, CNS depression
antihypertensives, diuretics, hypotension-producing drugs: Increased hypotensive effects
buprenorphine: Reduced oxymorphone effectiveness if buprenorphine is given first, possibly withdrawal symptoms in oxymorphone-dependent patients
CNS depressants: Additive CNS depressant effects, increased risk of habituation
hydroxyzine, other opioid analgesics: Increased analgesia, CNS depression, and hypotensive effects

MAO inhibitors: Increased risk of unpredictable, severe, sometimes fatal adverse reactions

metoclopramide: Antagonized effects of metoclopramide on GI motility

naloxone: Antagonized analgesic, CNS, and respiratory depressant effects of oxymorphone

naltrexone: Withdrawal symptoms in oxymorphone-dependent patients

neuromuscular blockers: Additive respiratory depression

ACTIVITIES

alcohol use: Additive CNS depressant effects, increased risk of habituation

Adverse Reactions

CNS: Confusion, delusions, depersonalization, dizziness, drowsiness, euphoria, headache, light-headedness, nervousness, nightmares, restlessness, seizures, tiredness, tremor, weakness

CV: Bradycardia, hypertension, hypotension, palpitations, tachycardia

EENT: Blurred vision, diplopia, dry mouth, laryngeal edema, laryngospasm, tinnitus

GI: Abdominal cramps or pain, constipation, hepatotoxicity, nausea, vomiting

GU: Decreased urine output, dysuria, urinary frequency

MS: Muscle rigidity (with large doses), uncontrolled muscle movements

RESP: Atelectasis, bradypnea, bronchospasm, dyspnea, irregular breathing, respiratory depression, wheezing

SKIN: Diaphoresis, erythema, flushing of face, pruritus, rash, urticaria

Other: Anaphylaxis, facial edema, injection site burning, pain, redness, and swelling

Nursing Considerations

- Instruct patient to lie down during oxymorphone administration and for a period afterward to minimize dizziness, light-headedness, nausea, and vomiting.
- **WARNING** Avoid rapid administration of oxymorphone, which may cause serious adverse effects, including anaphylaxis, severe respiratory depression, hypotension, peripheral circulatory collapse, and cardiac arrest.
- Monitor vital signs during oxymorphone therapy to detect respiratory depression and hypotension. Elderly, severely ill, or de-

bilitated patients and patients with chronic respiratory disease are at increased risk for drug's respiratory depressant effects.
- Monitor urinary and bowel elimination status. Decreasing urine output may signal urine retention. Constipation may become so severe that it causes ileus.
- Offer fluids to relieve dry mouth.
- Monitor for signs of drug-induced CNS depression or increased CSF pressure, such as altered LOC and restlessness, in patients with a head injury, intracranial lesions, or other conditions that could cause these effects. Patients who are taking, or have recently taken, drugs that depress the CNS are also more susceptible to these effects. Take appropriate safety precautions.
- Be aware that oxymorphone may induce or exacerbate arrhythmias or seizures in patients with a history of these conditions and may mask symptoms of acute abdominal conditions.
- Be aware that patients with a history of drug abuse (including acute alcoholism), emotional instability, or suicidal ideation or attempts are at increased risk for opioid abuse.
- Monitor patients with a history of common bile duct disorders for signs of increased biliary pressure, such as pain in upper midline area that may radiate to back and right shoulder.
- Monitor for worsening condition in patients with diarrhea caused by poisoning or pseudomembranous colitis. Patients who have recently had GI tract surgery are also at risk for adverse effects because of oxymorphone's effect on GI motility.
- Be aware that patients with hypothyroidism are at increased risk for respiratory depression and prolonged CNS depression.
- Store drug at 15° to 30° C (59° to 86° F); protect from freezing and light.

PATIENT TEACHING
- Instruct patient to immediately report a rash, facial swelling, or difficulty breathing during oxymorphone therapy.
- Advise patient to rise slowly from a sitting or lying position.
- Stress importance of receiving drug before pain becomes severe.
- Suggest increased fluid and fiber intake to prevent constipation.
- Caution patient to avoid potentially hazardous activities until drug's CNS effects are known.
- Urge patient not to drink alcohol or use CNS depressants during therapy without first consulting prescriber.
- Advise female patient to stop drug and notify prescriber if she becomes, or suspects she might be, pregnant.

paclitaxel

Taxol

Class and Category

Chemical: Diterpenoid taxane
Therapeutic: Antimicrotubule antineoplastic
Pregnancy category: D

Indications and Dosages

▶ *To treat ovarian cancer*

I.V. INFUSION

Previously untreated adults. 135 mg/m^2 infused over 24 hr, followed by 75 mg/m^2 of cisplatin; repeated q 21 days. Alternatively, 175 mg/m^2 over 3 hr, followed by 75 mg/m^2 of cisplatin; repeated q 21 days.

Previously treated adults. 135 mg/m^2 or 175 mg/m^2 over 3 hr q 21 days.

▶ *To treat metastatic breast cancer, as a single agent or in combination with other drugs, as first-line treatment; to treat metastatic breast cancer if initial chemotherapy regimen fails or if relapse occurs within 6 months of adjuvant chemotherapy that included an anthracycline antineoplastic*

I.V. INFUSION

Adults. 175 mg/m^2 over 3 hr q 21 days.

▶ *To treat node-positive breast cancer sequentially with doxorubicin-containing combination therapy*

I.V. INFUSION

Adults. 175 mg/m^2 over 3 hr q 21 days for 4 courses, administered sequentially with doxorubicin-containing combination chemotherapy

▶ *To treat non–small-cell lung cancer*

I.V. INFUSION

Adults. 135 mg/m^2 over 24 hr, followed by 75 mg/m^2 of cisplatin.

▶ *To treat AIDS-related Kaposi's sarcoma*

I.V. INFUSION

Adults. 135 mg/m^2 over 3 hr q 21 days. Alternatively, 100 mg/m^2 over 3 hr q 14 days.

DOSAGE ADJUSTMENT Subsequent dosage reduced by 20% if peripheral neuropathy occurs or if patient's neutrophil count falls below 500/mm^3 for 1 week or longer during paclitaxel therapy.

Mechanism of Action

Stabilizes microtubules, which normally contribute to cell structure and movement, and promotes microtubule assembly. In this way, paclitaxel inhibits the normal reorganization of the microtubule network, which is active during interphase and mitotic cellular functions. Paclitaxel also causes abnormal groups of microtubules to form throughout the cell cycle and multiple asters of microtubules to form during mitosis, when cell division normally occurs.

Incompatibilities

Don't let paclitaxel come in contact with plasticized polyvinyl chloride (PVC) equipment or devices, such as infusion bags or sets, to avoid exposing patient to plasticizer DEHP, which can be leached from these materials.

Contraindications

Hypersensitivity to paclitaxel or its components; hypersensitivity to other drugs formulated in polyoxyethylated castor oil, such as cyclosporine or teniposide; patients with solid tumors whose baseline neutrophil count is less than 1,500/mm^3; patients with AIDS-related Kaposi's sarcoma whose baseline neutrophil count is less than 1,000/mm^3

Interactions

DRUGS

blood-dyscrasia–causing drugs (such as cephalosporins and sulfasalazine): Increased risk of leukopenia and thrombocytopenia
bone marrow depressants (such as carboplatin and lomustine): Possibly additive bone marrow depression
vaccines, killed virus: Possibly decreased antibody response to vaccine
vaccines, live virus: Possibly decreased antibody response to vaccine, increased adverse effects of vaccine, and severe infection

Adverse Reactions

CNS: Motor dysfunction, paresthesia, peripheral neuropathy, seizures
CV: Arrhythmias (including bradycardia and ventricular tachycardia), AV block, chest pain, ECG changes, hypotension, MI
EENT: Mucositis

GI: Anorexia, diarrhea, elevated liver function test results, esophageal necrosis and ulceration, nausea, vomiting
GU: Nephrotoxicity
HEME: Anemia, leukopenia, neutropenia, thrombocytopenia
MS: Arthralgia, myalgia
RESP: Dyspnea
SKIN: Alopecia, extravasation with phlebitis or cellulitis, rash, urticaria
Other: Anaphylaxis, angioedema, hypersensitivity reaction, infection

Nursing Considerations

- Follow facility protocols for preparation and handling of antineoplastic drugs and for appropriate disposal of used equipment.
- Monitor CBC, including hematocrit, platelet count, and WBC with differential, before and frequently during paclitaxel therapy, as ordered.
- **WARNING Don't administer paclitaxel to patients with AIDS-related Kaposi's sarcoma whose neutrophil count is below 1,000/mm³. For all other indications, don't administer paclitaxel if neutrophil count falls below 1,500/mm³.**
- If paclitaxel solution comes in contact with your skin or mucosa, wash it off thoroughly with warm water. If drug comes in contact with your eye, irrigate it thoroughly with water or NS.
- Dilute and store drug in glass or polypropylene bottles or in plastic bags made of polypropylene or polyolefin, and administer it through polyethylene-line administration sets to avoid exposing patient to plasticizer DEHP, which can be leached from PVC supplies.
- Dilute paclitaxel with NS, D₅W, D₅NS, or D₅LR to a final concentration of 0.3 to 1.2 mg/ml. Use solution within 27 hours if stored at controlled room temperature and in ambient lighting.
- Use an in-line filter no greater than 0.22 micron when administering paclitaxel. Be aware that filter may need to be changed periodically if clogging occurs during infusion.
- To prevent a hypersensitivity reaction, expect to premedicate patient, as ordered, with 20 mg P.O. of dexamethasone (10 mg P.O for treatment of AIDS-associated Kaposi's sarcoma) about 12 and 6 hours before paclitaxel administration; 50 mg of diphenhydramine I.V. 30 to 60 minutes before paclitaxel admin-

istration; and 300 mg of cimetidine or 50 mg of ranitidine 30 to 60 minutes before paclitaxel administration.

- Observe patient continuously for first 30 minutes of each paclitaxel infusion and frequently thereafter. If anaphylaxis occurs, administer epinephrine, antihistamines, corticosteroids, or oxygen, as prescribed.

- Monitor vital signs during paclitaxel therapy, especially during the first hour of administration, assessing for signs of bradycardia or hypotension. Patients with a history of angina, cardiac conduction abnormalities, MI within past 6 months, or heart failure may be at increased risk for adverse cardiac effects.

- Maintain continuous cardiac monitoring, as prescribed, of patients with a history of cardiac conduction abnormalities.

- Be aware that adverse reactions can vary when paclitaxel is administered in combination therapy. Review information for all drugs administered as part of a specific regimen, including drug interactions and adverse effects.

- If extravasation occurs, stop the infusion immediately and notify prescriber. Then resume the infusion in another vein.

- Monitor patients who have, or have recently been exposed to, chicken pox and those who have herpes zoster for signs and symptoms of severe generalized disease.

- Be aware that patients who have previously received cytotoxic therapy and those who are receiving concurrent or consecutive radiation therapy are at risk for additive bone marrow depression.

- If patient develops thrombocytopenia, implement protective precautions according to facility policy.

- Assess for signs of infection, such as fever, if patient develops leukopenia. Expect to obtain appropriate specimens for culture and sensitivity testing.

- Before diluting paclitaxel, store it at controlled room temperature of 20° to 25° C (68° to 77° F). Protect from light.

PATIENT TEACHING

- Advise patient to have dental work completed before beginning paclitaxel treatment, if possible, or to defer such work until blood counts return to normal because drug can delay healing and cause gingival bleeding. Teach patient proper oral hygiene, and advise her to use a soft-bristled toothbrush.

- Advise patient to immediately report burning at injection site or other signs of extravasation.
- Also instruct patient to immediately report unusual bleeding or bruising, black or tarry stools, blood in urine or stools, or red pinpoint spots on skin.
- Stress the importance of avoiding accidental cuts from sharp objects, such as razor blades and fingernail clippers, because excessive bleeding or infection may occur.
- Caution patient to avoid contact sports and other activities that put her at risk for bruising or injury.
- Suggest that patient with mucositis eat bland, soft foods served cold or at room temperature to decrease irritation.
- Instruct patient who develops bone marrow depression to avoid people with infections. Advise her to report fever, chills, cough, hoarseness, lower back or side pain, and painful or difficult urination because these signs and symptoms may signal an infection.
- Instruct patient to wash her hands immediately before touching her eyes or inside of her nose.
- Caution patient to avoid receiving immunizations unless approved by prescriber. Instruct her to avoid people who have recently received vaccines or to wear a protective mask that covers her nose and mouth when in their presence.
- Stress the importance of complying with the dosage regimen and of keeping follow-up medical appointments and appointments for laboratory tests.
- Inform patient that her hair should grow back after paclitaxel therapy has been completed.
- Advise patient to use contraception because of the risk of fetal harm from paclitaxel therapy. Instruct her to notify prescriber immediately if she becomes pregnant.

pamidronate disodium
Aredia

Class and Category
Chemical: Bisphosphonate
Therapeutic: Antihypercalcemic, bone resorption inhibitor
Pregnancy category: C

Indications and Dosages

▶ *To treat cancer-induced hypercalcemia that is inadequately managed by oral hydration alone*

I.V. INFUSION

Adults. 60 to 90 mg over 2 to 24 hr as a single dose when corrected serum calcium level is 12 to 13.5 mg/dl; 90 mg over 2 to 24 hr when corrected serum calcium level is greater than 13.5 mg/dl. May be repeated as prescribed after 7 days if hypercalcemia recurs.

DOSAGE ADJUSTMENT For patients with renal failure, dosage limited to 30 mg over 4 to 24 hr, as prescribed. For patients with cardiac or renal failure, drug is given in a smaller volume of fluid or at a slower rate, as prescribed.

▶ *To treat moderate to severe Paget's disease of bone*

I.V. INFUSION

Adults. 30 mg/day over 4 hr on 3 consecutive days for a total dose of 90 mg. Repeated as needed and tolerated.

▶ *To treat osteolytic bone metastasis associated with breast cancer*

I.V. INFUSION

Adults. 90 mg over 2 hr q 3 to 4 wk.

▶ *To treat osteolytic bone metastasis associated with multiple myeloma*

I.V. INFUSION

Adults. 90 mg over 4 hr q mo.

Mechanism of Action

Inhibits bone resorption, possibly by impairing attachment of osteoclast precursors to mineralized bone matrix, thus reducing the rate of bone turnover in Paget's disease and osteolytic metastasis. Pamidronate also reduces the flow of calcium from resorbing bone into the blood.

Incompatibilities

Don't mix pamidronate with calcium-containing infusion solutions, such as LR. Also avoid mixing pamidronate with, or administering it through same I.V. line as, other drugs.

Contraindications

Hypersensitivity to pamidronate, other bisphosphonates, or their components

Interactions

DRUGS

calcium-containing preparations, vitamin D preparations (such as calcife-diol and calcitriol): Antagonized pamidronate effects when used to treat hypercalcemia

Adverse Reactions

CNS: Confusion, fever, psychosis

GI: Abdominal cramps, anorexia, GI bleeding, indigestion, nausea, vomiting

GU: Azotemia

HEME: Leukopenia, lymphopenia

MS: Bone pain, muscle spasms or stiffness

Other: Hypocalcemia, hypokalemia, hypomagnesemia, hypophosphatemia, injection site pain and swelling

Nursing Considerations

- Reconstitute each 30- or 90-mg vial of pamidronate with 10 ml of sterile water for injection to yield a concentration of 30 mg/10 ml or 90 mg/10 ml. Allow all particles to dissolve. Use within 24 hours if stored at 2° to 8° C (36° to 46° F).
- To treat cancer-induced hypercalcemia, dilute prescribed dose in 1,000 ml of 0.45NS, NS, or D₅W. Use within 24 hours if stored at room temperature.
- To treat Paget's disease, dilute 30-mg dose of pamidronate in 500 ml of 0.45NS, NS, or D₅W. To treat osteolytic bone metastasis from breast cancer, dilute 90-mg dose in 250 ml of 0.45NS, NS, or D₅W. To treat osteolytic bone metastasis of multiple myeloma, dilute 90-mg dose in 500 ml of 0.45NS, NS, or D₅W.
- Be alert for fever during first 3 days of pamidronate therapy, especially in patients receiving high doses. If patient develops fever, obtain CBC with differential, as ordered.
- Monitor CBC with differential, hematocrit, and hemoglobin as well as serum creatinine and electrolyte levels (including calcium, phosphate, and magnesium) during pamidronate therapy, as ordered.
- Assess patient with anemia, leukopenia, or thrombocytopenia for worsening condition during first 2 weeks of therapy.
- Before reconstituting pamidronate, store it at less than 30° C (86° F).

PATIENT TEACHING

- Advise patient to report such adverse reactions as muscle spasms, fever, chills, sore throat, and unusual bleeding or bruising during pamidronate therapy.

- Stress the importance of complying with the prescribed administration schedule.
- Advise patient to avoid calcium and vitamin D supplements during therapy.

pantoprazole sodium

Pantoloc (CAN), Protonix, Protonix I.V.

Class and Category

Chemical: Substituted benzimidazole
Therapeutic: Antiulcer agent, gastric acid proton pump inhibitor
Pregnancy category: B

Indications and Dosages

▶ *To treat gastroesophageal reflux disease (GERD)*
I.V. INFUSION
Adults. 40 mg q.d. infused over 15 min for 7 to 10 days, followed by oral doses.
DELAYED-RELEASE TABLETS
Adults. 40 mg q.d for up to 8 wk. Dosage repeated for another 4 to 8 wk if healing isn't achieved.
▶ *To maintain healing of erosive esophagitis and reduce relapse of daytime and nighttime symptoms in patients with GERD*
DELAYED-RELEASE TABLETS
Adults. 40 mg q.d. for up to 12 mo.

Route	Onset	Peak	Duration
I.V.	1 day	Unknown	1 wk
P.O.	1 day	1 wk	1 wk

Mechanism of Action

Interferes with gastric acid secretion by inhibiting the hydrogen-potassium–adenosine triphosphatase (H^+, K^+–ATPase) enzyme system, or proton pump, in gastric parietal cells. Normally, the proton pump uses energy from the hydrolysis of ATPase to drive H^+ and chloride (Cl^-) out of parietal cells and into the stomach lumen in exchange for potassium (K^+), which leaves the stomach lumen and enters parietal cells. After this exchange, H^+ and Cl^- combine in the stomach to form hydrochloric acid (HCl). Pantoprazole irreversibly inhibits the final step in gastric acid production by blocking the exchange of intracellular H^+ and extracellular K^+, thus preventing H^+ from entering the stomach and additional HCl from forming.

Contraindications

Hypersensitivity to pantoprazole, other substituted benzimidazoles (omeprazole, lansoprazole, rabeprazole sodium), or their components

Interactions

DRUGS

ampicillin, cyanocobalamin, digoxin, iron salts, ketoconazole: Possibly impaired absorption of these drugs

Adverse Reactions

CNS: Headache, malaise
GI: Diarrhea

Nursing Considerations

- Reconstitute pantoprazole with 10 ml of NS. Use within 2 hours if stored at room temperature. Dilute with 100 ml of D_5W, NS, or LR to a final concentration of 0.4 mg/ml. Use within 12 hours if stored at room temperature.
- Use in-line filter provided by manufacturer to remove any precipitate. If administering drug at a Y-site, place in-line filter below the Y-site closest to patient.
- Flush I.V. line with D_5W, NS, or LR before and after administering pantoprazole.
- Be aware that pantoprazole is used cautiously in patients with severe hepatic dysfunction because of potential for drug accumulation. Monitor such patients for increased adverse effects.
- Don't administer pantoprazole, as prescribed, within 4 weeks of testing for *Helicobacter pylori* because antibiotics, proton pump inhibitors, and bismuth preparations suppress *H. pylori* and may lead to false-negative results.
- Before reconstituting pantoprazole, store it at 2° to 8° C (36° to 46° F); protect from freezing and light.

PATIENT TEACHING

- Instruct patient to swallow pantoprazole tablets whole and not to chew or crush them.
- Advise patient to expect relief of symptoms within 2 weeks of beginning therapy.

paricalcitol

Zemplar

Class and Category

Chemical: Sterol derivative, vitamin D analogue
Therapeutic: Antihyperparathyroid agent
Pregnancy category: Not rated

Indications and Dosages

▶ *To prevent or treat secondary hyperparathyroidism in patients with chronic renal failure*

I.V. INJECTION

Adults. *Initial:* 0.04 to 0.1 mcg/kg (2.8 to 7 mcg) no more than q.o.d. at any time during dialysis. *Maintenance:* If initial dose fails to produce a satisfactory response, 2 to 4 mcg given q 2 to 4 wk. Dosage adjusted according to individual needs. *Maximum:* 0.24 mcg/kg or up to 16.8 mcg.

DOSAGE ADJUSTMENT Dosage immediately reduced or therapy discontinued if serum calcium level is elevated or if serum calcium-phosphorus product is greater than 75. Dosage resumed at a lower dose when these levels return to normal.

Route	Onset	Peak	Duration
I.V.	Unknown	Unknown	15 hr

Mechanism of Action

Reduces serum parathyroid hormone (PTH) level by an unknown mechanism. In chronic renal failure, decreased renal synthesis of vitamin D leads to chronic hypocalcemia. In an attempt to stimulate vitamin D synthesis and normalize serum calcium levels, the parathyroid glands secrete excessive amounts of PTH; however, increased PTH levels can't result in normal serum calcium levels because of renal failure.

Contraindications

Evidence of vitamin D toxicity, hypercalcemia, hypersensitivity to paricalcitol or its components

Interactions

None known.

Adverse Reactions

CNS: Chills, fever, light-headedness, malaise
CV: Palpitations

EENT: Dry mouth
GI: GI bleeding, nausea, vomiting
RESP: Pneumonia
Other: Generalized edema, influenza, sepsis

Nursing Considerations

• Before administering paricalcitol, inspect drug for particulate matter and discoloration; if present, discard drug.
• Administer drug as an I.V. bolus and discard unused portion.
• Monitor serum calcium and phosphorus levels, as ordered, twice weekly during initiation of therapy and then monthly to guide dosage adjustments.
• **WARNING** Be aware that paricalcitol use may lead to vitamin D toxicity associated with hypercalcemia. Assess patient for early signs and symptoms, including arthralgia, constipation, dry mouth, headache, metallic taste, myalgia, nausea, somnolence, vomiting, and weakness. Also assess for late signs, including albuminuria, anorexia, arrhythmias, azotemia, conjunctivitis (calcific), decreased libido, elevated BUN and serum ALT and AST levels, generalized vascular calcification, hypercholesterolemia, hypertension, hyperthermia, irritability, mild acidosis, nephrocalcinosis, nocturia, pancreatitis, photophobia, polydipsia, polyuria, pruritus, rhinorrhea, and weight loss.
• If vitamin D toxicity occurs, notify prescriber immediately and expect to decrease dosage or discontinue drug. Place patient on bed rest and administer fluids, a low-calcium diet, and a laxative, as prescribed. If patient develops a hypercalcemic crisis and dehydration, infuse NS and a loop diuretic, such as furosemide or ethacrynic acid, to increase renal calcium excretion, as prescribed.
• Expect to monitor serum parathyroid hormone level every 3 months.
• If patient also takes digoxin, monitor for signs and symptoms of digitalis toxicity, which is potentiated by hypercalcemia.
• Store drug at 25° C (77° F).

PATIENT TEACHING
• Advise patient to follow a diet high in calcium and low in phosphorus during paricalcitol therapy.
• Inform patient that she may require phosphate binders to control serum phosphorus levels.

- Teach patient the early signs of hypercalcemia and vitamin D toxicity. Advise her to contact prescriber immediately if she develops any signs or symptoms.
- Advise patient to avoid activities that require alertness until drug's full CNS effects are known.
- If patient takes digoxin, teach her the signs and symptoms of digitalis toxicity. Urge her to contact prescriber immediately if she suspects toxicity.

penicillin G potassium
Megacillin (CAN), Pentids, Pfizerpen
penicillin G sodium

Class and Category
Chemical: Penicillin
Therapeutic: Antibiotic
Pregnancy category: B

Indications and Dosages
▶ *To treat systemic infections caused by gram-positive organisms,*
including Bacillus anthracis, Corynebacterium diphtheriae,
enterococci, Listeria monocytogenes, Staphylococcus aureus, *and*
Staphylococcus epidermidis; *gram-negative organisms, including*
Neisseria gonorrhoeae, Neisseria meningitidis, Pasteurella
multocida, *and* Streptobacillus moniliformis *(rat-bite fever); and*
gram-positive anaerobes, including Actinomyces israelii *(actinomy-*
cosis), Clostridium perfringens, Clostridium tetani, Pasteurella
multocida, Peptococcus *species,* Peptostreptococcus *species, and*
spirochetes, especially Treponema carateum *(pinta),* Treponema
pallidum, *and* Treponema pertenue *(yaws)*
I.V. INFUSION
Adults and adolescents. 1 to 5 million U q 4 to 6 hr. *Maximum:*
80 million U/day.
Children. 8,333 to 16,667 U/kg q 4 hr or 12,500 to 25,000 U/kg
q 6 hr.
Premature and full-term neonates. 30,000 U/kg q 12 hr.
▶ *To treat bacterial meningitis*
I.V. INFUSION
Adults. 50,000 U/kg q 4 hr or 24 million U/day in divided doses
q 2 to 4 hr.

Mechanism of Action

Inhibits final stage of bacterial cell wall synthesis by competitively binding to penicillin-binding proteins inside the cell wall. Penicillin-binding proteins are responsible for various steps in bacterial cell wall synthesis. By binding to these proteins, penicillin leads to cell wall lysis.

Contraindications

Hypersensitivity to penicillin or its components

Incompatibilities

Don't mix any penicillin in the same syringe or container with aminoglycosides to prevent mutual inactivation. Don't mix penicillin G potassium with oxidizing or reducing agents, such as alcohol or glycol, to prevent inactivation of penicillin. Don't mix penicillin G sodium with acids, alkalies, or oxidizing agents or with carbohydrate solutions with an alkaline pH.

Interactions

DRUGS

ACE inhibitors, potassium-containing drugs, potassium-sparing diuretics: Increased risk of hyperkalemia (with penicillin G potassium)
aminoglycosides: Possibly mutual inactivation of both drugs, risk of decreased blood aminoglycoside level when drugs are administered by different routes
chloramphenicol, erythromycin, sulfonamides, tetracycline, thrombolytics: Possibly interference with penicillin's bactericidal effect
methotrexate: Decreased methotrexate clearance, increased risk of toxicity
probenecid: Increased blood penicillin level

Adverse Reactions

CNS: Confusion, dizziness, dysphasia, hallucinations, headache, lethargy, sciatic nerve irritation, seizures
CV: Labile blood pressure, palpitations
EENT: Black "hairy" tongue, oral candidiasis, stomatitis, taste perversion
GI: Abdominal pain, diarrhea, elevated liver function test results (transient), indigestion, nausea, pseudomembranous colitis
GU: Interstitial nephritis (acute), vaginal candidiasis
MS: Muscle twitching
SKIN: Rash
Other: Electrolyte imbalances; injection site necrosis, pain, or redness

Nursing Considerations
- Obtain body tissue and fluid specimens for culture and sensitivity tests, as ordered, before giving first dose of penicillin G. Expect to begin drug therapy before test results are known.
- Before starting drug therapy, make sure patient has had no previous hypersensitivity reactions to penicillin.
- **WARNING** Check label closely to make sure you're administering only penicillin G potassium or penicillin G sodium. Be aware that penicillin G procaine should not be administered by I.V. route. I.V. injection may be fatal, and intra-arterial injection may cause extensive tissue and organ necrosis.
- Reconstitute vials of penicillin for injection with sterile water for injection, D_5W, or sodium chloride for injection. Use reconstituted drug within 7 days if refrigerated or within 24 hours if stored at room temperature.
- Administer penicillin at least 1 hour before other antibiotics.
- Assess for signs of secondary infection, such as profuse diarrhea.
- Monitor serum sodium level and assess for early signs of heart failure in patients receiving high doses of penicillin G sodium.
- Store drug at 15° to 30° C (59° to 86° F).

PATIENT TEACHING
- Instruct patient to immediately report adverse reactions, including fever, hives, and difficulty breathing, during penicillin therapy.
- Advise patient to report diarrhea and to consult prescriber before taking an antidiarrheal because it may mask signs of pseudomembranous colitis.

pentamidine isethionate
Pentacarinat (CAN), Pentam 300

Class and Category
Chemical: Diamidine derivative
Therapeutic: Antiprotozoal
Pregnancy category: C

Indications and Dosages
▶ *To treat* Pneumocystis carinii *pneumonia*
I.V. INFUSION
Adults and children. 4 mg/kg q.d. infused over 1 to 2 hr for 14 to 21 days.
DOSAGE ADJUSTMENT Dosage possibly reduced or I.V. infusion time or dosing interval extended for patients with renal failure.

Mechanism of Action
May bind to DNA and inhibit DNA replication in *Pneumocystis carinii*. Pentamidine also may inhibit dihydrofolate reductase, an enzyme needed to convert dihydrofolic acid to tetrahydrofolic acid in this organism. This action inhibits the formation of coenzymes that are essential to the growth and replication of *P. carinii*.

Incompatibilities
Don't mix pentamidine with other drugs or with saline solutions because precipitation may occur.

Contraindications
History of anaphylactic reaction to pentamidine or its components, hypersensitivity to pentamidine or its components

Interactions
DRUGS
blood-dyscrasia–causing drugs, bone marrow depressants: Increased risk of adverse hematologic effects
didanosine: Increased risk of pancreatitis
erythromycin: Increased risk of torsades de pointes
foscarnet: Increased risk of severe but reversible hypocalcemia, hypomagnesemia, and nephrotoxicity
nephrotoxic drugs: Increased risk of nephrotoxicity

Adverse Reactions
CNS: Chills, confusion, dizziness, fatigue, fever, hallucinations, headache
CV: Arrhythmias, edema, hypotension, prolonged QT interval, torsades de pointes, ventricular tachycardia
EENT: Bitter or metallic taste
ENDO: Diabetes mellitus, hyperglycemia, hypoglycemia
GI: Abdominal pain, anorexia, diarrhea, elevated liver function test results, nausea, vomiting, pancreatitis
GU: Elevated serum creatinine level
HEME: Anemia, leukopenia, thrombocytopenia, unusual bleeding or bruising
MS: Myalgia
SKIN: Night sweats, rash
Other: Hyperchloremic acidosis, hyperkalemia, hypocalcemia, hypomagnesemia, infusion site phlebitis

Nursing Considerations

- To prepare initial dilution, add 3 to 5 ml of sterile water for injection or D₅W to 300-mg vial of pentamidine. Use drug prepared with D₅W within 24 hours of reconstitution, and protect from light until ready to use. Further dilute in 50 to 250 ml of D₅W, and infuse over 1 to 2 hours.
- Keep patient supine during infusion, and monitor blood pressure frequently during and after administration. Keep emergency resuscitation equipment readily available.
- Assess for hypoglycemia and arrhythmias. Although uncommon, these adverse reactions can be severe.
- Monitor CBC; platelet count; liver function test results; BUN, serum creatinine and calcium, and blood glucose levels; and ECG tracing throughout therapy, as ordered.
- Monitor blood glucose level because pentamidine use can induce insulin release from pancreas, causing severe hypoglycemia that can last from 1 day to several weeks.
- Be aware that hyperglycemia and diabetes mellitus can occur up to several months after discontinuation of parenteral therapy.
- Before reconstituting pentamidine, store it at 2° to 8° C (36° to 46° F) and protect from light.

PATIENT TEACHING

- Advise patient to avoid potentially hazardous activities until pentamidine's CNS effects are known.
- Instruct patient to report unusual bleeding or bruising and to take precautions to avoid bleeding, such as using a soft-bristled toothbrush and an electric shaver.
- Caution patient about possible hypoglycemic effects of pentamidine therapy.
- Advise patient to undergo follow-up testing for diabetes mellitus, which can occur up to several months after pentamidine therapy is completed.

pentazocine lactate
Talwin

Class, Category, and Schedule
Chemical: Synthetic opioid
Therapeutic: Analgesic
Pregnancy category: C
Controlled substance: Schedule IV

Indications and Dosages

▶ *To relieve moderate to severe pain*
I.V. INJECTION
Adults. *Initial:* 30 mg q 3 to 4 hr, p.r.n. *Maximum:* 30 mg/single dose or 360 mg/24 hr.
▶ *To relieve obstetric pain*
I.V. INJECTION
Adults. 20 mg when contractions become regular; repeated 2 or 3 times q 2 to 3 hr, as prescribed.

Route	Onset	Peak	Duration
I.V.	2 to 3 min	15 to 30 min	2 to 3 hr

Mechanism of Action

Binds with opioid receptors, primarily kappa and sigma receptors, at many CNS sites to alter the perception of, and emotional response to, pain.

Incompatibilities

Don't mix pentazocine in same syringe with a soluble barbiturate because precipitation will occur.

Contraindications

Hypersensitivity to pentazocine or its components

Interactions

DRUGS
anticholinergics: Increased risk of urine retention and severe constipation
antidiarrheals, antiperistaltics: Increased risk of severe constipation and CNS depression
antihypertensives, diuretics, other hypotension-producing drugs: Additive hypotensive effects
buprenorphine: Decreased pentazocine effectiveness, increased respiratory depression
CNS depressants: Increased CNS depression, increased risk of habituation
hydroxyzine, other opioid analgesics: Increased analgesia, CNS depression, and hypotensive effects
MAO inhibitors: Increased risk of unpredictable, severe, and sometimes fatal adverse reactions

metoclopramide: Antagonized metoclopramide effects on GI motility
naloxone: Antagonized analgesic, CNS, and respiratory depressant effects of pentazocine
naltrexone: Withdrawal symptoms in patients who are physically dependent on pentazocine
neuromuscular blockers: Increased respiratory depression
ACTIVITIES
alcohol use: Additive CNS depression and increased risk of habituation

Adverse Reactions

CNS: Dizziness, drowsiness, euphoria, fatigue, headache, light-headedness, nervousness, nightmares, restlessness, weakness
CV: Hypotension, tachycardia
EENT: Blurred vision, diplopia, dry mouth, laryngeal edema, laryngospasm
GI: Constipation, hepatotoxicity, nausea, vomiting
GU: Decreased urine output, dysuria, urinary frequency
MS: Muscle rigidity (with large doses)
RESP: Atelectasis, bronchospasm, dyspnea, hypoventilation, wheezing
SKIN: Diaphoresis, facial flushing, pruritus, rash, urticaria
Other: Facial edema; injection site burning, pain, redness, or swelling; physical and psychological dependence

Nursing Considerations

- Instruct patient to lie down during pentazocine administration and for a period afterward to lessen drug's adverse effects, including dizziness, light-headedness, nausea, and vomiting.
- **WARNING** Avoid rapid administration of pentazocine, which may cause serious adverse effects, including anaphylaxis, severe respiratory depression, hypotension, peripheral circulatory collapse, and cardiac arrest.
- Monitor vital signs during pentazocine therapy to detect respiratory depression and hypotension. Patients with chronic respiratory disease and elderly, severely ill, or debilitated patients are at increased risk for drug's respiratory depressant effects.
- Assess patients with impaired hepatic or renal function for signs of increased effects of pentazocine or increased adverse reactions because drug is metabolized in the liver and excreted by the kidneys.

- Assess urine output; decreased output may indicate urine retention. Patients with a history of prostatic hypertrophy or obstruction, urethral stricture, or recent urinary tract surgery are at increased risk for urine retention.
- Monitor for signs of drug-induced CNS depression or increased CSF pressure, such as altered LOC, restlessness, and irritability, in patients with a head injury, intracranial lesions, or other conditions that could cause these effects. Be aware that pentazocine may mask neurologic signs and symptoms. Patients who are taking, or have recently taken, drugs that depress the CNS are also more susceptible to these effects. Take appropriate safety precautions.
- Be aware that pentazocine can increase cardiac workload; it also may induce or exacerbate arrhythmias or seizures in patients with a history of these conditions and may mask symptoms of acute abdominal conditions.
- Be aware that patients with a history of drug abuse (including acute alcoholism), emotional instability, or suicidal ideation or attempts are at increased risk for opioid abuse. Monitor patients with a history of physical dependence on opioid agonists because pentazocine use may lead to withdrawal symptoms.
- Monitor patients with a history of common bile duct disorders for signs of increased biliary pressure, such as pain in upper midline area that may radiate to back and right shoulder.
- Monitor for worsening condition in patients with diarrhea caused by poisoning or pseudomembranous colitis. Patients who have recently had GI tract surgery are also at risk for adverse effects because of pentazocine's effect on GI motility.
- Be aware that patients with hypothyroidism are at increased risk for respiratory depression and prolonged CNS depression.
- Expect to taper dosage gradually, as prescribed, to reduce the risk of withdrawal symptoms.
- Store drug at 15° to 30° C (59° to 86° F); don't freeze.

PATIENT TEACHING

- Advise patient to report signs of an allergic reaction to pentazocine, such as a rash or itching.
- Inform patient about drug's possible adverse CNS effects, such as dizziness and drowsiness. Advise her to avoid potentially hazardous activities until CNS effects are known.
- Caution patient that prolonged use of pentazocine may result in drug dependence.
- Urge patient not to use alcohol or OTC drugs without consulting prescriber.

pentobarbital sodium
Nembutal

Class, Category, and Schedule
Chemical: Barbiturate
Therapeutic: Anticonvulsant, sedative-hypnotic
Pregnancy category: D
Controlled substance: Schedule II

Indications and Dosages
▶ *To provide short-term treatment of insomnia*
I.V. INJECTION
Adults. *Initial:* 100 mg, with additional small doses at 1-min intervals, as prescribed. *Maximum:* 500 mg.

▶ *To provide emergency treatment of seizures associated with eclampsia, meningitis, status epilepticus, tetanus, or toxic reactions to local anesthetics or strychnine*
I.V. INJECTION
Adults. 100 mg, with additional small doses at 1-min intervals, as prescribed. *Maximum:* 500 mg.
Children. 50 mg, with additional small doses at 1-min intervals, as prescribed, until desired effect occurs.
DOSAGE ADJUSTMENT Dosage possibly reduced for elderly or debilitated patients and those with hepatic dysfunction.

Route	Onset	Peak	Duration
I.V.	In 1 min	Unknown	15 min

Mechanism of Action
Inhibits ascending conduction of impulses in the reticular formation, which controls CNS arousal to produce drowsiness, hypnosis, and sedation. Pentobarbital also decreases the spread of seizure activity in the cortex, thalamus, and limbic system. It promotes an increased threshold for electrical stimulation in the motor cortex, which may contribute to its anticonvulsant properties.

Contraindications
Hepatic disease; history of addiction to hypnotics or sedatives; hypersensitivity to pentobarbital, other barbiturates, or their components; nephritis; porphyria; severe respiratory disease with airway obstruction or dyspnea

Interactions
DRUGS

acetaminophen: Possibly decreased effects of acetaminophen (with long-term pentobarbital use)

carbamazepine, chloramphenicol, corticosteroids, cyclosporine, dacarbazine, digoxin, disopyramide, doxycycline, griseofulvin, metronidazole, oral contraceptives, phenylbutazone, quinidine, theophyllines, vitamin D: Decreased effectiveness of these drugs

CNS depressants: Increased CNS depression and risk of habituation

divalproex sodium, valproic acid: Increased risk of CNS toxicity and neurotoxicity

guanadrel, guanethidine: Possibly increased risk of orthostatic hypotension

halogenated hydrocarbon anesthetics: Increased risk of hepatotoxicity (with long-term pentobarbital use)

haloperidol: Possibly decreased blood haloperidol level, possibly altered seizure pattern or frequency

hydantoins: Possibly interference with hydantoin metabolism

leucovorin: Possibly decreased anticonvulsant effect of pentobarbital

maprotiline: Possibly enhanced CNS depression and decreased therapeutic effects of pentobarbital

mexiletine: Possibly decreased blood mexiletine level

oral anticoagulants: Possibly decreased therapeutic effects of these drugs, possibly increased risk of bleeding when pentobarbital is discontinued

tricyclic antidepressants: Possibly decreased therapeutic effects of these drugs

ACTIVITIES

alcohol use: Increased CNS depression

Adverse Reactions
CNS: Agitation, anxiety, ataxia, confusion, delusions, depression, dizziness, drowsiness, fever, hallucinations, headache, insomnia, irritability, nervousness, nightmares, paradoxical stimulation, seizures, syncope, tremor

CV: Orthostatic hypotension

EENT: Vision changes

GI: Anorexia, constipation, hepatic dysfunction, nausea, vomiting

HEME: Agranulocytosis

MS: Arthralgia, bone pain, muscle twitching or weakness

RESP: Respiratory depression

SKIN: Exfoliative dermatitis, rash, Stevens-Johnson syndrome

Other: Physical and psychological dependence, weight loss

Nursing Considerations

- Inject pentobarbital at 50 mg or less/minute to prevent adverse respiratory and circulatory reactions.
- Be aware that pentobarbital shouldn't be given during third trimester of pregnancy because repeated use can cause dependence in neonate. It also shouldn't be given to breast-feeding women because it may cause CNS depression in infants.
- Closely monitor blood pressure, pulse, and respirations during administration. Keep emergency equipment and drugs nearby in case respiratory depression or adverse hemodynamic effects occur. Be aware that patients with cardiovascular disease are at increased risk for adverse circulatory reactions, particularly if drug is administered too fast, and that those with pulmonary diseases associated with obstruction or dyspnea are at increased risk for ventilatory depression. Anticipate the risk of hypotension, even when giving drug at recommended rate.
- Monitor for hypersensitivity reactions, such as bronchospasm, difficulty breathing, facial edema, and urticaria, especially in patients with a history of asthma, angioedema, or urticaria.
- Anticipate that pentobarbital's CNS effects may exacerbate major depression, suicidal tendencies, or other mental disorders.
- Be aware that pentobarbital may cause paradoxical stimulation (excitement, euphoria, restlessness) in patients with acute pain, children, and elderly or debilitated patients. Elderly or debilitated patients are also more likely to experience such adverse CNS reactions as confusion and depression; monitor these patients closely and take safety precautions.
- Assess hyperthyroid patients for exacerbated symptoms resulting from pentobarbital use, such as increased nervousness and palpitations.
- Be aware that barbiturate-induced respiratory depression may cause complications in patients with severe anemia.
- Be aware that drug may trigger signs and symptoms in patients with acute intermittent porphyria.
- If patient shows premonitory signs of hepatic coma, withhold drug and notify prescriber immediately.
- Monitor I.V. site closely and be careful to avoid extravasation. Drug is highly alkaline and may cause local tissue damage and necrosis.
- Store drug at 2° to 15° (36° to 59° F) in a tightly closed container.

PATIENT TEACHING
- Inform patient that pentobarbital is habit-forming.
- Advise patient to avoid potentially hazardous activities until pentobarbital's CNS effects are known.
- Urge patient to avoid alcohol and other CNS depressants because they may increase drug's adverse CNS effects.

perphenazine

Apo-Perphenazine (CAN), PMS Perphenazine (CAN), Trilafon, Trilafon Concentrate

Class and Category

Chemical: Piperazine phenothiazine
Therapeutic: Antiemetic
Pregnancy category: Not rated

Indications and Dosages

▶ *To treat severe nausea and vomiting*

I.V. INFUSION OR INJECTION

Adults and adolescents. 1 mg q 1 to 2 min, up to total of 5 mg.
DOSAGE ADJUSTMENT Initial dose possibly reduced and gradually increased for elderly, emaciated, or debilitated patients. Lower end of adult dosage range possibly needed for adolescents.

Mechanism of Action

Prevents nausea and vomiting by inhibiting or blocking dopamine receptors in the medullary chemoreceptor trigger zone and peripherally by blocking the vagus nerve in the GI tract.

Contraindications

Blood dyscrasias; bone marrow depression; cerebral arteriosclerosis; coma; concurrent use of CNS depressants (large doses); coronary artery disease; hepatic impairment; hypersensitivity to perphenazine, other phenothiazines, or their components; myeloproliferative disorders; severe CNS depression; severe hypertension or hypotension; subcortical brain damage

Interactions

DRUGS

amantadine, anticholinergics, antidyskinetics, antihistamines: Increased adverse anticholinergic effects

amphetamines: Decreased therapeutic effects of both drugs
anticonvulsants: Decreased seizure threshold, inhibited metabolism and toxicity of anticonvulsant
antithyroid drugs: Increased risk of agranulocytosis
apomorphine: Additive CNS depression, decreased emetic response to apomorphine if perphenazine is given first
appetite suppressants (except phenmetrazine): Antagonized anorectic effect of appetite suppressants
beta blockers: Increased blood levels of both drugs and risk of arrhythmias, hypotension, irreversible retinopathy, and tardive dyskinesia
bromocriptine: Possibly interference with bromocriptine's effects
CNS depressants: Increased CNS and respiratory depression, increased hypotensive effects
dopamine: Antagonized peripheral vasoconstriction with high doses of dopamine
ephedrine: Decreased vasopressor response to ephedrine
epinephrine: Blocked alpha-adrenergic effects of epinephrine, possibly causing severe hypotension and tachycardia
hepatotoxic drugs: Increased risk of hepatotoxicity
hypotension-causing drugs: Increased risk of severe orthostatic hypotension
levodopa: Inhibited antidyskinetic effects of levodopa
lithium: Possibly neurotoxicity (disorientation, extrapyramidal symptoms, unconsciousness)
maprotiline, tricyclic antidepressants: Prolonged and intensified sedative and anticholinergic effects of these drugs or perphenazine
metrizamide: Decreased seizure threshold
opioid analgesics: Increased CNS and respiratory depression, increased risk of orthostatic hypotension and severe constipation
ototoxic drugs (especially antibiotics): Possibly masking of some symptoms of ototoxicity, such as dizziness, tinnitus, and vertigo
probucol, other drugs that prolong QT interval: Prolonged QT interval, which may increase risk of ventricular tachycardia
thiazide diuretics: Possibly hyponatremia and water intoxication
ACTIVITIES
alcohol use: Increased CNS and respiratory depression, hypotensive effects, and risk of heatstroke

Adverse Reactions

CNS: Behavioral changes, cerebral edema, dizziness, drowsiness, extrapyramidal reactions (such as akathisia, dystonia, pseudoparkinsonism), fever, headache, neuroleptic malignant syndrome, seizures, syncope, tardive dyskinesia (persistent)

CV: Bradycardia, cardiac arrest, hypertension, hypotension, orthostatic hypotension, tachycardia
EENT: Blurred vision, dry mouth, glaucoma, laryngeal edema, miosis, mydriasis, nasal congestion, ocular changes (corneal opacification, retinopathy)
ENDO: Decreased libido, galactorrhea, gynecomastia, syndrome of inappropriate ADH secretion
GI: Anorexia, constipation, diarrhea, fecal impaction, nausea, vomiting
GU: Bladder paralysis, ejaculation failure, menstrual irregularities, polyuria, urinary frequency, urinary incontinence, urine retention
HEME: Agranulocytosis, eosinophilia, hemolytic anemia, leukopenia, pancytopenia, thrombocytopenic purpura
RESP: Asthma
SKIN: Diaphoresis, eczema, erythema, exfoliative dermatitis, hyperpigmentation, jaundice, pallor, photosensitivity, pruritus, urticaria
Other: Anaphylaxis, angioedema

Nursing Considerations

- Wear gloves when working with perphenazine because the parenteral solution may cause contact dermatitis.
- Dilute drug to 0.5 mg/ml with sodium chloride for injection. Protect solution from light. Slight yellowing is acceptable, but discard solution if it is markedly discolored or contains precipitate.
- Be aware that some perphenazine solutions contain sulfites. Patients with a history of sulfite sensitivity may be at increased risk for a hypersensitivity reaction.
- Obtain blood samples for CBC and liver and renal function tests, as ordered, to detect adverse reactions.
- Monitor temperature frequently, and notify prescriber if it rises; a significant increase suggests drug intolerance.
- Monitor blood pressure of patient who takes large doses of perphenazine, especially if surgery is indicated, because of the increased risk of hypotension.
- **WARNING** Be alert for possible suppressed cough reflex, which increases patient's risk of aspirating vomitus.
- Monitor patients (especially children) with chronic respiratory disorders (such as severe asthma or emphysema) or acute respiratory tract infections for exacerbations of these conditions caused by perphenazine's CNS depressant effects. Be aware that patients with cardiovascular or renal disease are at increased risk for developing hypotension, heart failure, and arrhythmias.

- **WARNING** If patient develops neuroleptic malignant syndrome (hyperpyrexia, muscle rigidity, altered mental status, autonomic instability), notify prescriber immediately and expect to discontinue drug and begin intensive medical treatment. Monitor carefully for recurrence if patient resumes perphenazine therapy.
- Be aware that patients with impaired hepatic function are at risk for decreased perphenazine metabolism or further hepatic dysfunction. Monitor patients with a history of hepatic encephalopathy from cirrhosis for increased sensitivity to drug's CNS effects.
- Because of perphenazine's anticholinergic effects, monitor patients with a history of, or predisposition to, glaucoma for signs and symptoms of this disorder, such as eye pain, vision changes, or nausea and vomiting from increased intraocular pressure.
- Be aware that drug should be used cautiously in those who are exposed to organophosphorus insecticides.
- Monitor patients who have been exposed to extreme heat for heatstroke due to drug-induced suppression of temperature regulation. Symptoms include tachycardia, fever, and confusion.
- Be aware that children and elderly patients are at increased risk for developing hypotension amd extrapyramidal reactions, especially if they're acutely ill or debilitated.
- Store drug at 15° to 30° C (59 to 86° F); protect from freezing and light.

PATIENT TEACHING
- Stress the importance of reporting persistent or severe adverse reactions resulting from perphenazine therapy.
- Urge patient to avoid alcohol and other CNS depressants during perphenazine therapy and to avoid potentially hazardous activities until drug's CNS effects are known.
- Advise patient to avoid excessive sun exposure and to protect skin when outdoors.
- Advise patient, especially if elderly, to rise slowly from a supine or seated position to avoid dizziness, light-headedness, and fainting.
- Inform patient that drug may reduce body's response to heat and cold; advise her to avoid temperature extremes, as in very cold or hot showers.
- Suggest sugarless chewing gum, hard candy, and fluids to relieve dry mouth.
- Urge patient to report sudden sore throat or other signs of infection.

phenobarbital sodium
Luminal

Class, Category, and Schedule
Chemical: Barbiturate
Therapeutic: Anticonvulsant, sedative-hypnotic
Pregnancy category: D
Controlled substance: Schedule IV

Indications and Dosages
▶ *To treat seizures*
I.V. INJECTION
Adults. 100 to 320 mg, repeated as needed and as prescribed. *Maximum:* 600 mg/day.
Children. *Initial:* 10 to 20 mg/kg as a single dose. *Maintenance:* 1 to 6 mg/kg/day.
▶ *To treat status epilepticus*
I.V. INFUSION OR INJECTION
Adults. 10 to 20 mg/kg given slowly and repeated as needed and as prescribed.
Children. 15 to 20 mg/kg over 10 to 15 min.
▶ *To provide short-term treatment of insomnia*
I.V. INJECTION
Adults. 100 to 325 mg h.s.
▶ *To provide daytime sedation*
I.V. INJECTION
Adults. 30 to 120 mg/day in divided doses b.i.d. or t.i.d.
▶ *To provide preoperative sedation*
I.V. INJECTION
Children. 1 to 3 mg/kg 60 to 90 min before surgery.
DOSAGE ADJUSTMENT Dosage possibly reduced for elderly or debilitated patients to minimize confusion, depression, and excitement.

Route	Onset	Peak	Duration
I.V.	5 min	30 min	4 to 6 hr

Mechanism of Action
Inhibits ascending conduction of impulses in the reticular formation, which controls CNS arousal to produce drowsiness, hypnosis, and sedation. Phenobarbital also decreases the spread of seizure activity in the cortex, thalamus, and limbic system. It promotes an increased threshold for electrical stimulation in the motor cortex, which may contribute to its anticonvulsant properties.

Contraindications

Hepatic disease; history of addiction to hypnotics or sedatives; hypersensitivity to phenobarbital, other barbiturates, or their components; nephritis; porphyria; severe respiratory disease with airway obstruction or dyspnea

Interactions

DRUGS

acetaminophen: Decreased acetaminophen effectiveness with long-term phenobarbital therapy

anticonvulsants (hydantoin): Unpredictable effects on metabolism of anticonvulsant

anticonvulsants (succinimide, including carbamazepine): Decreased blood levels and elimination half-lives of these drugs

calcium channel blockers: Possibly excessive hypotension

carbonic anhydrase inhibitors: Enhanced osteopenia induced by phenobarbital

chloramphenicol, corticosteroids, cyclosporine, dacarbazine, digoxin, metronidazole, quinidine: Decreased effectiveness of these drugs from enhanced metabolism

CNS depressants: Additive CNS depression

cyclophosphamide: Possibly reduced half-life and increased leukopenic activity of cyclophosphamide

disopyramide: Possibly ineffectiveness of disopyramide

doxycycline, fenoprofen: Shortened half-life of these drugs

griseofulvin: Possibly decreased absorption and effectiveness of griseofulvin

guanadrel, guanethidine: Possibly increased orthostatic hypotension

halogenated hydrocarbon anesthetics: Possibly hepatotoxicity

haloperidol: Decreased seizure threshold, decreased blood haloperidol level

ketamine (high doses): Increased risk of hypotension and respiratory depression

leucovorin: Interference with phenobarbital's anticonvulsant effect

levothyroxine, oral contraceptives, phenylbutazone, tricyclic antidepressants: Decreased effectiveness of these drugs

loxapine, phenothiazines, thioxanthenes: Decreased seizure threshold

MAO inhibitors: Prolonged phenobarbital effects, possibly altered pattern of seizure activity

maprotiline: Increased CNS depression, decreased seizure threshold at high doses, decreased phenobarbital effectiveness

methoxyflurane: Possibly hepatotoxicity and nephrotoxicity

methylphenidate: Increased risk of phenobarbital toxicity

mexiletine: Decreased blood mexiletine level

oral anticoagulants: Decreased anticoagulant activity, increased risk of bleeding when phenobarbital is discontinued

pituitary hormones (posterior): Increased risk of arrhythmias and coronary insufficiency

primidone: Altered pattern of seizures, increased CNS effects of both drugs

valproate, valproic acid: Decreased phenobarbital metabolism, increased risk of barbiturate toxicity

vitamin D: Decreased phenobarbital effectiveness

xanthines: Increased xanthine metabolism, antagonized hypnotic effect of phenobarbital

ACTIVITIES

alcohol use: Additive CNS depression

Adverse Reactions

CNS: Anxiety, depression, dizziness, drowsiness, headache, irritability, lethargy, mood changes, paradoxical stimulation, sedation, vertigo

CV: Hypotension, sinus bradycardia

EENT: Miosis, ptosis

GI: Constipation, diarrhea, nausea, vomiting

GU: Decreased libido, impotence, sexual dysfunction

MS: Arthralgia, bone tenderness

RESP: Bronchospasm, respiratory depression

SKIN: Dermatitis, photosensitivity, rash, urticaria

Other: Injection site phlebitis, physical and psychological dependence

Nursing Considerations

- Be aware that phenobarbital shouldn't be given during third trimester of pregnancy because repeated use can cause dependence in neonate. It also shouldn't be given to breast-feeding women because it may cause CNS depression in infants.
- Because drug can cause respiratory depression, assess respiratory rate and depth before use, especially in patient with bronchopneumonia, pulmonary disease, respiratory tract infection, or status asthmaticus.
- Be aware that phenobarbital is available as a solution and as a powder that can be reconstituted. Reconstitute sterile powder with the recommended amount of sterile water for injection. Don't use reconstituted solution if it fails to clear within 5 minutes. Use within 30 minutes. Further dilute prescribed dose with NS or D$_5$W, and infuse over 30 to 60 minutes.

- Don't administer I.V. injection more rapidly than 60 mg/minute to prevent respiratory depression.
- Monitor blood pressure, respiratory rate, and heart rate and rhythm during administration. Anticipate an increased risk of hypotension, even when giving drug at recommended rate. Keep resuscitation equipment readily available. Patients with cardiovascular disease are at increased risk for adverse circulatory reactions, particularly if drug is administered too rapidly. Patients with pulmonary diseases associated with obstruction or dyspnea are at increased risk for ventilatory depression.
- Monitor for hypersensitivity reactions, such as bronchospasm, difficulty breathing, facial edema, and urticaria, especially in patients with a history of asthma, angioedema, or urticaria.
- Be aware that I.V. phenobarbital may not reach peak effects for up to 30 minutes. Expect to wait for drug to take effect before a second dose is ordered.
- Be aware that drug may cause physical and psychological dependence.
- Anticipate that phenobarbital's CNS effects may exacerbate major depression, suicidal tendencies, or other mental disorders.
- Take safety precautions for elderly patients, as appropriate, because they're more likely to experience confusion, depression, and excitement as adverse CNS reactions.
- Be aware that phenobarbital may cause paradoxical stimulation (excitement, euphoria, restlessness) in patients with acute pain, children, and elderly or debilitated patients. Elderly or debilitated patients are also more likely to experience such adverse CNS reactions as confusion and depression; monitor these patients closely and take safety precautions.
- Be aware that drug may trigger signs and symptoms in patients with acute intermittent porphyria.
- Assess hyperthyroid patients for exacerbated symptoms resulting from phenobarbital use, such as increased nervousness and palpitations.
- Be aware that barbiturate-induced respiratory depression may cause complications in patients with severe anemia.
- Store drug at 15° to 30° C (59° to 86° F); don't freeze.

PATIENT TEACHING
- Caution patient about possible drowsiness and reduced alertness. Advise her to avoid potentially hazardous activities until phenobarbital's CNS effects are known.
- Urge patient to avoid alcohol during therapy.

- Inform parents that their child may react to drug with paradoxical excitement. Tell them to notify prescriber if this occurs.
- Instruct female patient to report suspected, known, or intended pregnancy. Advise against breast-feeding during therapy.

phentolamine mesylate

Regitine, Rogitine (CAN)

Class and Category

Chemical: Imidazoline
Therapeutic: Antihypertensive, diagnostic aid, vasodilator
Pregnancy category: Not rated

Indications and Dosages

▶ *To diagnose pheochromocytoma*

I.V. INJECTION

Adults. 2.5 mg as a single dose. After negative result, repeat test with 5-mg dose, as prescribed.

Children. 1 mg as a single dose. After negative result, repeat test with 0.1-mg/kg dose, as prescribed.

▶ *To manage hypertension before or during pheochromocytomectomy*

I.V. INJECTION

Adults. 5 mg 1 to 2 hr before surgery, repeated as needed and as prescribed. During surgery, 5 mg, as ordered.

Children. 1 mg 1 to 2 hr before surgery, repeated as needed and as prescribed. During surgery, 1 mg, as ordered.

▶ *To prevent dermal necrosis or sloughing after extravasation of I.V. norepinephrine*

I.V. INJECTION

Adults, children, and infants. 10 mg/L of I.V. fluid that contains norepinephrine at rate determined by patient response.

Mechanism of Action

Blocks the actions of circulating epinephrine and norepinephrine by antagonizing alpha$_1$ and alpha$_2$ receptors. Phentolamine causes peripheral vasodilation through direct relaxation of vascular smooth muscle and alpha blockade. Positive inotropic and chronotropic effects increase cardiac output. A positive inotropic effect primarily raises blood pressure, but in larger doses, phentolamine causes peripheral vasodilation and can reduce blood pressure.

In patients with pheochromocytoma, phentolamine causes systolic and diastolic blood pressures to fall dramatically. In those without pheochromocytoma, it causes blood pressure to fall or rise slightly or remain the same.

Contraindications
Angina, hypersensitivity to phentolamine or its components, MI

Interactions
DRUGS
antihypertensives: Additive hypotensive effect
dopamine: Antagonized vasopressor activity of dopamine
epinephrine, methoxamine, norepinephrine, phenylephrine: Inhibited alpha-adrenergic effects of these drugs
metaraminol: Possibly decreased vasopressor effect of metaraminol
ACTIVITIES
alcohol use: Additive vasodilation, increased risk of hypotension and tachycardia

Adverse Reactions
CNS: Dizziness
CV: Angina; arrhythmias, including tachycardia; hypotension
EENT: Nasal congestion
GI: Diarrhea, nausea, vomiting
GU: Ejaculation disorders, priapism
MS: Muscle weakness
SKIN: Flushing

Nursing Considerations
- Reconstitute each 5-mg vial of phentolamine with 1 ml of sterile water for injection.
- Use reconstituted solution immediately; don't store unused portion.
- Dilute 5 to 10 mg of reconstituted solution in 500 ml of D_5W.
- Inspect drug for particles and discoloration before administering.
- When using drug to diagnose pheochromocytoma, withhold all nonessential drugs, as ordered, for at least 24 hours (preferably 48 to 72 hours) before test.
- Before giving I.V. test dose for pheochromocytoma, place patient in supine position and determine baseline blood pressure by taking readings every 10 minutes for at least 30 minutes.
- Expect patient with pheochromocytoma to have excessive hypotension after receiving drug.
- Take safety precautions according to facility policy if patient experiences dizziness.
- Store drug at 15° to 30° C (59° to 86° F).
PATIENT TEACHING
- Instruct patient to move slowly after phentolamine administration to minimize dizziness and avoid falls.

phenylephrine hydrochloride
Neo-Synephrine

Class and Category
Chemical: Sympathomimetic amine
Therapeutic: Antiarrhythmic, vasoconstrictor, vasopressor
Pregnancy category: C

Indications and Dosages
▶ *To manage mild to moderate hypotension*
I.V. INJECTION
Adults. *Initial:* 0.1 to 0.5 mg. *Usual:* 0.2 mg, repeated no more often than q 10 to 15 min, as prescribed.
▶ *To treat severe hypotension or shock*
I.V. INFUSION
Adults. *Initial:* 100 to 180 mcg/min (0.1 to 0.18 mg/min) until blood pressure is stable. *Maintenance:* 40 to 60 mcg/min (0.04 to 0.06 mg/min). Infusion concentration and flow rate, adjusted as prescribed, based on patient response.
▶ *To treat hypotension during spinal anesthesia*
I.V. INJECTION
Adults. *Initial:* 0.2 mg, increased by no more than 0.2 mg, as prescribed. *Maximum:* 0.5 mg/dose.
Children. 0.5 to 1 mg for each 11.3 kg (25 lb).
▶ *To treat paroxysmal supraventricular tachycardia*
I.V. INJECTION
Adults. *Initial:* Up to 0.5 mg by rapid injection; later doses increased to 0.1 to 0.2 mg above preceding dose, as prescribed. *Maximum:* 1 mg/dose.

Route	Onset	Peak	Duration
I.V.	Immediately	Unknown	15 to 20 min

Mechanism of Action
Directly stimulates alpha-adrenergic receptors and inhibits activity of the intracellular enzyme adenyl cyclase, which then inhibits production of cAMP. The inhibition of cAMP causes arterial and venous constriction and increases peripheral vascular resistance and systolic blood pressure. With greater-than-therapeutic doses, phenylephrine directly stimulates beta-adrenergic receptors in the myocardium, which increases the activity of adenyl cyclase and produces positive inotropic and chronotropic effects.

Contraindications

Hypersensitivity to bisulfites, phenylephrine, or their components; severe coronary artery disease or hypertension; use within 14 days of MAO inhibitor therapy; ventricular tachycardia

Interactions

DRUGS

alpha blockers, haloperidol, loxapine, phenothiazines, thioxanthenes: Possibly decreased vasoconstrictor effect of phenylephrine

antihypertensives, diuretics: Possibly decreased antihypertensive effects

atropine, methylphenidate: Possibly enhanced vasopressor effect of phenylephrine

beta blockers: Decreased therapeutic effects of both drugs

bretylium: Possibly potentiated vasopressor effect and arrhythmias

doxapram: Increased vasopressor effect of both drugs

ergot alkaloids: Possibly cerebral blood vessel rupture, increased vasopressor effect, peripheral vascular ischemia, and gangrene (with ergotamine)

guanadrel, guanethidine: Increased vasopressor effect of phenylephrine, increased risk of severe hypertension and arrhythmias

hydrocarbon inhalation anesthetics: Increased risk of serious arrhythmias

MAO inhibitors: Increased and prolonged cardiac stimulation, increased vasopressor effect, increased risk of severe cardiovascular and cerebrovascular effects, hyperpyrexia, vomiting

maprotiline, tricyclic antidepressants: Increased risk of severe cardiovascular effects (including arrhythmias, hyperpyrexia, severe hypertension); possibly increased or decreased sensitivity to phenylephrine

mecamylamine, methyldopa: Decreased hypotensive effects of these drugs, increased vasopressor effect of phenylephrine

nitrates: Possibly decreased vasopressor effect of phenylephrine and decreased antianginal effect of nitrates

other sympathomimetics (such as dopamine and isoproterenol): Possibly increased cardiovascular effects or adverse reactions

oxytocin: Possibly severe, persistent hypertension

phenoxybenzamine: Decreased vasoconstrictor effect of phenylephrine, possibly hypotension and tachycardia

thyroid hormones: Increased cardiovascular effects of both drugs

Adverse Reactions

CNS: Dizziness, headache, insomnia, nervousness, paresthesia, restlessness, tremor, weakness

CV: Angina, bradycardia, hypertension, hypotension, palpitations, peripheral vasoconstriction that may lead to necrosis or gangrene, tachycardia, ventricular arrhythmias
GI: Nausea, vomiting
RESP: Dyspnea
SKIN: Extravasation with tissue necrosis and sloughing, pallor
Other: Allergic reaction

Nursing Considerations

- Be aware that phenylephrine may not be prescribed for patients with occlusive vascular disease, such as atherosclerosis, Buerger's disease, diabetic endarteritis, or Raynaud's disease, because of the risk of decreased peripheral circulation.
- For I.V. use, dilute with D_5W or sodium chloride for injection and prepare as prescribed—usually 10 mg/500 ml. Administer infusions using an infusion pump to ensure appropriate administration rate.
- Assess for signs and symptoms of angina, arrhythmias, and hypertension because phenylephrine may increase myocardial oxygen demand and the risk of proarrhythmias and blood pressure changes.
- **WARNING** Monitor patient with thyroid disease for increased sensitivity to catecholamines and, possibly, thyrotoxicity or cardiotoxicity.
- **WARNING** Be aware that extravasation may cause tissue necrosis, gangrene, and other reactions around injection site. If extravasation occurs, expect to use phentolamine to antagonize vasoconstriction and minimize sloughing and tissue necrosis.
- Store drug at 15° to 30° C (59° to 86° F); protect from freezing and light.

PATIENT TEACHING

- Advise patient to avoid potentially hazardous activities until phenylephrine's CNS effects are known.

phenytoin sodium
Dilantin

Class and Category
Chemical: Hydantoin derivative
Therapeutic: Anticonvulsant
Pregnancy category: C

Indications and Dosages

▶ *To treat status epilepticus*
I.V. INJECTION

Adults and adolescents. *Initial:* 15 to 20 mg/kg by slow push in 50 ml of sodium chloride for injection at a rate not to exceed 50 mg/min. *Maintenance:* Beginning within 12 to 24 hr of initial dose, 100 mg q 6 to 8 hr or 5 mg/kg/day P.O. in divided doses b.i.d. to q.i.d.

Children. 15 to 20 mg/kg at no more than 1 mg/kg/min. *Maximum:* 50 mg/min.

DOSAGE ADJUSTMENT For elderly or very ill patients and those with cardiovascular or hepatic disease, dosage reduced to 25 mg/min, as prescribed, or possibly to as low as 5 to 10 mg/min to reduce the risk of adverse reactions.

▶ *To prevent or treat seizures during neurosurgery*
I.V. INJECTION

Adults. 100 to 200 mg q 4 hr at a rate not to exceed 50 mg/min during or immediately after neurosurgery.

Mechanism of Action

Limits the spread of seizure activity and the start of new seizures by regulating voltage-dependent sodium and calcium channels in neurons, inhibiting calcium movement across neuronal membranes, and enhancing sodium-potassium–adenosine triphosphatase activity in neurons and glial cells. These actions all help stabilize the neurons.

Incompatibilities

Don't mix phenytoin in same syringe with any other drugs or with any I.V. solutions other than sodium chloride for injection because a precipitate will form.

Contraindications

Adams-Stokes syndrome, hypersensitivity to phenytoin or its components, SA block, second- or third-degree heart block, sinus bradycardia

Interactions

DRUGS

acetaminophen: Possibly hepatoxicity, decreased acetaminophen effects

activated charcoal, antacids, calcium salts, enteral feedings, sucralfate: Decreased absorption of oral phenytoin *allopurinol, benzodiazepines, chloramphenicol, cimetidine, disulfiram, fluconazole, isoniazid, itraconazole, methylphenidate, metronidazole, miconazole, omeprazole, phenacemide, ranitidine, sulfonamides, trazodone, trimethoprim:* Decreased metabolism and increased effects of phenytoin

amiodarone, ticlopidine: Possibly increased blood phenytoin level

antifungals (azole): Increased blood phenytoin level, decreased blood antifungal level

antineoplastics, nitrofurantoin, pyridoxine: Decreased phenytoin effects

barbiturates: Variable effects on blood phenytoin level

bupropion, clozapine, loxapine, MAO inhibitors, maprotiline, molindone, phenothiazines, pimozide, thioxanthenes, tricyclic antidepressants: Decreased seizure threshold, decreased anticonvulsant effect of phenytoin

calcium channel blockers: Increased metabolism and decreased effects of these drugs, possibly increased blood phenytoin level

carbamazepine: Decreased blood level and effects of carbamazepine, possibly phenytoin toxicity

carbonic anhydrase inhibitors: Increased risk of osteopenia from phenytoin

chlordiazepoxide, diazepam: Possibly increased blood phenytoin level, decreased effects of these drugs

clonazepam: Possibly decreased blood level and effects of clonazepam, possibly phenytoin toxicity

corticosteroids, cyclosporine, dicumarol, digoxin, disopyramide, doxycycline, estrogens, furosemide, lamotrigine, levodopa, methadone, metyrapone, mexiletine, oral contraceptives, quinidine, sirolimus, tacrolimus, theophylline: Increased metabolism and decreased effects of these drugs

dopamine: Increased risk of severe hypotension and bradycardia

fluoxetine: Increased blood phenytoin level and risk of phenytoin toxicity

folic acid, leucovorin: Decreased blood phenytoin level, increased risk of seizures

haloperidol: Decreased effects of haloperidol, decreased anticonvulsant effect of phenytoin

halothane anesthetics: Increased risk of hepatotoxicity and phenytoin toxicity

ifosfamide: Decreased phenytoin effects, possibly increased toxicity

influenza virus vaccine: Possibly decreased phenytoin effects

insulin, oral antidiabetic drugs: Possibly hyperglycemia, increased blood phenytoin level (with tolbutamide)

levonorgestrel, mebendazole, streptozocin, sulfonylureas: Decreased effects of these drugs

lidocaine, propranolol (possibly other beta blockers): Increased cardiac depressant effects, possibly decreased blood level and increased adverse effects of phenytoin

lithium: Increased risk of lithium toxicity, increased risk of neurologic symptoms with normal blood lithium level

meperidine: Increased metabolism and decreased effects of meperidine, possibly meperidine toxicity

methadone: Possibly increased metabolism of methadone and withdrawal symptoms

neuromuscular blockers: Shorter duration of action and decreased effects of neuromuscular blockers

oral anticoagulants: Decreased metabolism and increased effects of phenytoin; early increase in anticoagulant effect followed by decrease

paroxetine: Decreased bioavailability of both drugs

phenylbutazone, salicylates: Increased phenytoin effects, possibly phenytoin toxicity

primidone: Increased primidone effects, possibly primidone toxicity

rifampin: Increased hepatic metabolism of phenytoin

valproic acid: Possibly decreased phenytoin metabolism, resulting in increased phenytoin effects; possibly decreased blood valproic acid level

vitamin D: Possibly decreased vitamin D effects, resulting in rickets or osteomalacia (with long-term use of phenytoin)

ACTIVITIES

alcohol use: Additive CNS depression, increased phenytoin clearance

Adverse Reactions

CNS: Ataxia, confusion, depression, dizziness, drowsiness, excitement, fever, headache, involuntary motor activity, lethargy, nervousness, peripheral neuropathy, restlessness, slurred speech, tremor, weakness

CV: Cardiac arrest, hypotension, vasculitis

EENT: Amblyopia, conjunctivitis, diplopia, earache, epistaxis, eye pain, gingival hyperplasia, hearing loss, loss of taste, nystagmus, pharyngitis, photophobia, rhinitis, sinusitis, taste perversion, tinnitus

ENDO: Gynecomastia, hyperglycemia

GI: Abdominal pain, anorexia, constipation, diarrhea, epigastric pain, hepatic dysfunction, hepatic necrosis, hepatitis, nausea, vomiting

GU: Glycosuria, priapism, renal failure

HEME: Acute intermittent porphyria (exacerbation), agranulocytosis, anemia, eosinophilia, leukopenia, pancytopenia, thrombocytopenia

MS: Arthralgia, arthropathy, bone fractures, muscle twitching, osteomalacia, polymyositis

RESP: Apnea, asthma, bronchitis, cough, dyspnea, hypoxia, increased sputum production, pneumonia, pneumothorax, pulmonary fibrosis

SKIN: Exfoliative dermatitis, jaundice, maculopapular or morbilliform rash, purpuric dermatitis, Stevens-Johnson syndrome, toxic epidermal necrolysis, unusual hair growth, urticaria

Other: Facial feature enlargement, injection site pain, lupuslike symptoms, lymphadenopathy, polyarteritis, weight gain or loss

Nursing Considerations

- Be aware that preferred administration routes for phenytoin are I.V. injection and oral. Phenytoin has a variable absorption rate when administered by I.M. route.
- Inspect I.V. form for particles and discoloration before administering.
- Administer I.V. injection through a large vein, using a large-gauge needle or an I.V. catheter.
- **WARNING** Avoid rapid I.V. injection because it may cause cardiac arrest, CNS depression, or severe hypotension. Administer at a rate not to exceed 50 mg/minute.
- To decrease vein irritation, follow I.V. injection with flush of sodium chloride for injection through same I.V. catheter.
- Continuously monitor ECG tracings and blood pressure when administering I.V. phenytoin.
- Frequently assess I.V. site for signs of extravasation because drug can cause tissue necrosis.
- Administer oral phenytoin at least 2 hours before or after antacids and calcium salts.
- If patient has difficulty swallowing, open prompt (rapid-release) capsules and mix contents with food or fluid.
- Shake oral suspension before measuring dose, and use a calibrated measuring device.
- To minimize GI distress, give phenytoin with or just after meals.
- If patient has an NG tube in place, minimize drug absorption by polyvinyl chloride tubing by diluting suspension threefold with sodium chloride for injection, D_5W, or sterile water. After administering drug, flush tube with at least 20 ml of diluent.

- Expect continuous enteral feedings to disrupt phenytoin absorption and, possibly, reduce blood phenytoin level. Discontinue tube feedings 1 to 2 hours before and after phenytoin administration, as prescribed. Anticipate increasing phenytoin dosage, as prescribed, to compensate for reduced bioavailability during continuous tube feedings.
- Monitor blood phenytoin level. Therapeutic level ranges from 10 to 20 mg/L.
- **WARNING Monitor hematologic status during therapy because phenytoin can cause blood dyscrasias. Patients with a history of agranulocytosis, leukopenia, or pancytopenia may have an increased risk of infection because phenytoin can cause myelosuppression.**
- Anticipate that drug may worsen intermittent porphyria.
- Frequently monitor blood glucose level of patient with diabetes mellitus because drug can stimulate glucagon and impair insulin secretion, either of which can raise blood glucose level.
- Monitor blood thyroid hormone levels of patients receiving thyroid replacement therapy, as appropriate, because phenytoin may decrease circulating thyroid hormone levels and increase thyroid-stimulating hormone level.
- Be aware that long-term phenytoin therapy may increase patient's requirements for folic acid or vitamin D supplements. However, keep in mind that a diet high in folic acid may decrease seizure control.
- Store drug at 15° to 30° C (59° to 86° F); don't freeze.

PATIENT TEACHING

- Caution patient to avoid potentially hazardous activities until phenytoin's CNS effects are known.
- Explain to patient with diabetes mellitus that she may be at increased risk for hyperglycemia and may need an increased dosage of antidiabetic drug during phenytoin therapy. Inform her that her blood glucose level will be monitored frequently.
- Instruct patient to crush or thoroughly chew phenytoin chewable tablets or to shake oral solution well before swallowing.
- Advise patient to take drug exactly as prescribed and not to change brands or dosage or stop taking drug unless instructed by prescriber.
- Instruct patient to avoid taking antacids or calcium products within 2 hours of oral phenytoin.
- Urge patient to avoid alcohol during phenytoin therapy.

- Stress the importance of good oral hygiene, and encourage patient to inform her dentist that she's taking phenytoin.
- Encourage patient to carry medical identification indicating her diagnosis and drug therapy.

physostigmine salicylate
Antilirium

Class and Category
Chemical: Salicylic acid derivative
Therapeutic: Anticholinergic antidote, cholinesterase inhibitor
Pregnancy category: Not rated

Indications and Dosages
▶ *To counteract toxic anticholinergic effects (anticholinergic syndrome)*
I.V. INJECTION
Adults and adolescents. 0.5 to 2 mg at no more than 1 mg/min; then 1 to 4 mg, repeated q 20 to 30 min as needed and as prescribed.
Children. 0.02 mg/kg at a rate not to exceed 0.5 mg/min, repeated q 5 to 10 min as needed and as prescribed. *Maximum:* 2 mg/dose.

Route	Onset	Peak	Duration
I.V.	3 to 8 min	5 min	30 to 60 min

Mechanism of Action
Inhibits the destruction of acetylcholine by acetylcholinesterase. This action increases the concentration of acetylcholine at cholinergic transmission sites and prolongs and exaggerates the effects of acetylcholine that are blocked by toxic doses of anticholinergics.

Contraindications
Asthma; cardiovascular disease; diabetes mellitus; gangrene; GI or GU obstruction; hypersensitivity to physostigmine, sulfites, or their components

Interactions
DRUGS
choline esters: Enhanced effects of carbachol and bethanechol with concurrent use of physostigmine, enhanced effects of acetylcholine and methacholine with prior use of physostigmine
succinylcholine: Prolonged neuromuscular paralysis

Adverse Reactions

CNS: CNS stimulation, fatigue, hallucinations, restlessness, seizures (with too-rapid administration), weakness
CV: Bradycardia (with too-rapid administration), irregular heartbeat, palpitations
EENT: Increased salivation, lacrimation, miosis
GI: Abdominal pain, diarrhea, nausea, vomiting
GU: Urinary urgency
MS: Muscle twitching
RESP: Bronchospasm, chest tightness, dyspnea (with too-rapid administration), increased bronchial secretions, wheezing
SKIN: Diaphoresis

Nursing Considerations

- Avoid rapid administration of physostigmine because it may lead to bradycardia, respiratory distress, or seizures.
- Frequently monitor pulse and respiratory rates, blood pressure, and neurologic status during therapy.
- Monitor ECG tracing during drug administration. Patients with a history of bradycardia may be at increased risk for drug-induced bradycardia.
- Closely monitor patients with asthma for an asthma attack; drug may precipitate an attack by causing bronchoconstriction.
- Monitor for drug-induced seizures due to drug's CNS-stimulating effects in patients with a history of seizures.
- Assess patients with Parkinson's disease for increased tremors, akinesia, or rigidity.
- **WARNING** Be alert for signs of a life-threatening cholinergic crisis, which may indicate a physostigmine overdose: confusion, diaphoresis, hypotension, miosis, muscle weakness, nausea, paralysis (including respiratory paralysis), salivation, seizures, sinus bradycardia, and vomiting. If you detect such signs, prepare to give atropine (the antidote) and use resuscitation equipment. Keep in mind that atropine counteracts only muscarinic cholinergic effects; paralytic effects may continue.
- Store drug at 15° to 30° C (59° to 86° F); protect from freezing and light.

PATIENT TEACHING

- Reassure patient that her vital signs will be monitored frequently during physostigmine administration to help prevent or detect adverse reactions.
- Instruct patient to notify prescriber immediately about signs of cholinergic crisis.

piperacillin sodium
Pipracil

Class and Category
Chemical: Piperazine derivative of ampicillin, acylureidopenicillin
Therapeutic: Antibiotic
Pregnancy category: B

Indications and Dosages
▶ *To treat moderate to severe bacterial infections, including bone and joint infections, gynecologic infections, intra-abdominal infections, lower respiratory tract infections, septicemia, and skin and soft-tissue infections, caused by susceptible strains of* Acinetobacter *species, anaerobic cocci,* Bacteroides *species,* Enterobacter *species,* Escherichia coli, Haemophilus influenzae, Klebsiella *species,* Proteus *species,* Pseudomonas aeruginosa, *and* Serratia *species*
I.V. INFUSION
Adults and adolescents. 12 to 18 g/day or 200 to 300 mg/kg/day in divided doses q 4 to 6 hr. *Maximum:* 24 g/day.
▶ *To treat bacterial meningitis*
I.V. INFUSION
Adults and adolescents. 4 g q 4 hr or 75 mg/kg q 6 hr. *Maximum:* 24 g/day.
▶ *To treat uncomplicated UTIs and community-acquired pneumonia caused by susceptible organisms, including* E. coli, Klebsiella *species, and* Serratia *species*
I.V. INFUSION
Adults. 6 to 8 g/day or 100 to 125 mg/kg/day in divided doses q 6 to 12 hr.
▶ *To treat complicated UTIs caused by susceptible organisms, including* Acinetobacter *species,* Klebsiella *species, and* Serratia *species*
I.V. INFUSION
Adults. 8 to 16 g/day or 125 to 200 mg/kg/day in divided doses q 6 to 8 hr.
▶ *To provide surgical prophylaxis in intra-abdominal procedures, including GI and biliary surgery*
I.V. INFUSION
Adults. 2 g 20 to 30 min before anesthesia, 2 g during surgery, and 2 g q 6 hr for 24 hr after surgery.
▶ *To provide surgical prophylaxis in abdominal hysterectomy*
I.V. INFUSION
Adults. 2 g 20 to 30 min before anesthesia, 2 g just after surgery, and 2 g 6 hr later.

▶ *To provide surgical prophylaxis in vaginal hysterectomy*
I.V. INFUSION
Adults. 2 g 20 to 30 min before anesthesia, then 2 g 6 and 12 hr after initial dose.
▶ *To provide surgical prophylaxis in cesarean section*
I.V. INFUSION
Adults. 2 g after cord is clamped, then 2 g 4 and 8 hr after initial dose.

Mechanism of Action

Binds to specific penicillin-binding proteins and inhibits the third and final stage of bacterial cell wall synthesis by interfering with an autolysin inhibitor. Uninhibited autolytic enzymes destroy the cell wall and result in cell lysis.

Incompatibilities

Don't mix piperacillin sodium in same container with aminoglycosides because of chemical incompatibility (depending on concentrations, diluents, pH, and temperature). Don't mix with solutions that contain only sodium bicarbonate because of chemical instability.

Contraindications

Hypersensitivity to cephalosporins, penicillins, or their components

Interactions

DRUGS
aminoglycosides: Additive or synergistic effects against some bacteria, possibly mutual inactivation
anti-inflammatory drugs (including aspirin and NSAIDs), heparin, oral anticoagulants, platelet aggregation inhibitors, sulfinpyrazone, thrombolytics: Increased risk of bleeding
hepatotoxic drugs (including labetalol and rifampin): Increased risk of hepatotoxicity
methotrexate: Increased blood methotrexate level and risk of toxicity
probenecid: Increased blood piperacillin level and risk of toxicity

Adverse Reactions

CNS: CVA, dizziness, fever, hallucinations, headache, lethargy, seizures
CV: Cardiac arrest, hypotension, palpitations, tachycardia, vasodilation, vasovagal reactions
EENT: Oral candidiasis, pharyngitis

GI: Diarrhea, epigastric distress, intestinal necrosis, nausea, pseudomembranous colitis, vomiting
GU: Hematuria, impotence, nephritis, neurogenic bladder, priapism, proteinuria, renal failure, vaginal candidiasis
HEME: Eosinophilia, leukopenia, neutropenia, thrombocytopenia
MS: Arthralgia
RESP: Dyspnea, pulmonary embolism, pulmonary hypertension
SKIN: Exfoliative dermatitis, mottling, rash
Other: Anaphylaxis; facial edema; hypokalemia; hyponatremia; injection site pain, phlebitis, and skin ulcer; superinfection

Nursing Considerations

- Obtain blood, sputum, or other specimens for culture and sensitivity testing, as ordered, before giving piperacillin. Expect to begin piperacillin therapy before results are available.
- Before initiating piperacillin therapy, make sure patient has had no previous hypersensitivity reactions to penicillins or cephalosporins.
- Be aware that sunlight may darken powder for dilution but won't alter drug potency.
- Reconstitute each gram of piperacillin with at least 5 ml of a compatible solution, such as sterile water for injection, sodium chloride for injection, D_5W, D_5NS, or bacteriostatic water that contains parabens or benzyl alcohol. Shake solution vigorously after adding diluent to help drug dissolve, and inspect for particles and discoloration before administering.
- If needed, further dilute with a compatible solution, such as NS, D_5W, D_5NS, LR, or dextran 6% in NS. If solution is diluted with LR, administer it within 2 hours.
- For intermittent infusion, infuse appropriate dose over 20 to 30 minutes.
- Assess for bleeding or excessive bruising because drug can decrease platelet aggregation.
- Monitor serum potassium level to detect hypokalemia, which may result from urinary potassium loss.
- Monitor for diarrhea during or shortly after drug therapy; diarrhea may signal pseudomembranous colitis.
- Administer aminoglycosides 1 hour before or after piperacillin, using separate site, I.V. bag, and tubing.
- When calculating sodium intake for patients on a sodium-restricted diet, keep in mind that each gram of piperacillin sodium contains 1.98 mEq of sodium.
- Store drug at 15° to 30° C (59° to 86° F).

PATIENT TEACHING
- Advise patient receiving piperacillin to report signs of superinfection, such as severe diarrhea or white patches on tongue or in mouth. Instruct her to check with prescriber before taking an antidiarrheal because it may mask signs of pseudomembranous colitis.
- Advise patient to consult prescriber before using OTC drugs during piperacillin therapy because of the risk of interactions.
- Inform patient that increased bruising may occur if she takes anti-inflammatory drugs, such as aspirin and NSAIDs, during piperacillin therapy.

piperacillin sodium and tazobactam sodium

Tazocin (CAN), Zosyn

Class and Category

Chemical: Piperazine derivative of ampicillin, acylureidopenicillin (piperacillin); penicillinate sulfone (tazobactam)
Therapeutic: Antibiotic
Pregnancy category: B

Indications and Dosages

▶ *To treat moderate to severe gram-negative or anaerobic infections, such as appendicitis, community-acquired pneumonia, diabetic foot ulcers, intra-abdominal infections, pelvic inflammatory disease, peritonitis, postpartum endometritis, and uncomplicated or complicated skin or soft-tissue infections caused by susceptible organisms, such as* Bactcroides *species (including many strains of* Bacteroides fragilis*),* Clostridium *species,* Enterobacter *species,* Enterococcus faecalis, Escherichia coli, Haemophilus influenzae, Klebsiella pneumoniae, Morganella morganii, Neisseria gonorrhoeae, Proteus mirabilis, Proteus vulgaris, Pseudomonas aeruginosa, and* Serratia *species*

I.V. INFUSION

Adults and adolescents. 3.375 g q 6 hr. *Maximum:* 4.5 g q 6 to 8 hr.

▶ *To treat nosocomial pneumonia caused by susceptible organisms*

I.V. INFUSION

Adults and adolescents. 3.375 g q 4 hr in addition to aminoglycoside therapy for 7 to 14 days.

DOSAGE ADJUSTMENT Dosage possibly decreased to 2.25 g q 6 hr for patients with creatinine clearance of 20 to 40 ml/min/1.73 m² and to 2.25 g q 8 hr for those with creatinine clearance of less than 20 ml/min/1.73 m².

Mechanism of Action

Piperacillin binds to specific penicillin-binding proteins and inhibits the third and final stage of bacterial cell wall synthesis by interfering with an autolysin inhibitor. Uninhibited autolytic enzymes destroy the cell wall, resulting in cell lysis.

Tazobactam doesn't change piperacillin's action, but it protects piperacillin against Richmond and Sykes types II, III, IV, and V beta-lactamases; staphylococcal beta-lactamases; and extended-spectrum beta-lactamases.

Incompatibilities

Don't mix piperacillin and tazobactam in same container with aminoglycosides because these drugs are chemically incompatible (depending on concentrations, diluents, pH, and temperature). Also avoid mixing with LR.

Contraindications

Hypersensitivity to beta-lactamase inhibitors, cephalosporins, penicillins, piperacillin, tazobactam, or their components

Interactions

DRUGS

aminoglycosides: Additive or synergistic effects against some bacteria, possibly mutual inactivation
anti-inflammatory drugs (including aspirin and NSAIDs), heparin, oral anticoagulants, platelet aggregation inhibitors, sulfinpyrazone, thrombolytics: Increased risk of bleeding
hepatotoxic drugs (including labetalol and rifampin): Increased risk of hepatotoxicity
methotrexate: Increased blood methotrexate level and risk of toxicity
probenecid: Increased blood piperacillin level and risk of toxicity

Adverse Reactions

CNS: Chills, CVA, dizziness, fever, hallucinations, headache, lethargy, seizures
CV: Cardiac arrest, hypotension, palpitations, tachycardia, vasodilation, vasovagal reactions
EENT: Epistaxis, oral candidiasis, pharyngitis

GI: Diarrhea, elevated liver function test results, epigastric distress, intestinal necrosis, nausea, pseudomembranous colitis, vomiting
GU: Hematuria, impotence, nephritis, neurogenic bladder, priapism, proteinuria, renal failure, vaginal candidiasis
HEME: Eosinophilia, leukopenia, neutropenia, thrombocytopenia
MS: Arthralgia, prolonged muscle relaxation
RESP: Dyspnea, pulmonary embolism, pulmonary hypertension
SKIN: Erythema multiforme, exfoliative dermatitis, mottling, rash, Stevens-Johnson syndrome
Other: Anaphylaxis, facial edema, hypokalemia, hyponatremia

Nursing Considerations

- Obtain blood, sputum, or other specimens for culture and sensitivity testing, as ordered, before giving piperacillin and tazobactam. Expect to begin therapy before results are available.
- Before initiating piperacillin and tazobactam therapy, make sure patient has had no previous hypersensitivity reactions to this drug or its components or to other penicillins, beta-lactamase inhibitors, or cephalosporins.
- Be aware that sunlight may darken powder for dilution but won't alter drug potency.
- Reconstitute each gram with 5 ml of a compatible solution, such as sterile water for injection, sodium chloride for injection, D_5W, or bacteriostatic water or saline solution that contains parabens or benzyl alcohol. Shake well after adding diluent to help drug dissolve, and inspect for particles and discoloration before administering. Use within 24 hours if stored at room temperature or 7 days if refrigerated.
- If needed, further dilute to desired final volume (50 to 150 ml except as noted) with appropriate solution, such as NS, sterile water for injection (no more than 50 ml), D_5W, or dextran 6% in NS.
- Administer over at least 30 minutes.
- **WARNING** Monitor closely for signs of anaphylaxis, which may be life-threatening. Patients at increased risk include those with a history of multiple allergies, asthma, hay fever, or urticaria and those with a hypersensitivity to penicillins or cephalosporins. If patient develops an anaphylactic reaction, discontinue drug, notify prescriber at once, and provide appropriate treatment as ordered. Anaphylaxis requires immediate treatment with epinephrine as well as airway management and corticosteroid therapy as needed.
- Assess for bleeding or excessive bruising because drug can de-

crease platelet aggregation. Monitor PT and partial thromboplastin time as ordered.

• Monitor serum potassium level to detect hypokalemia, which may result from urinary potassium loss.

• Monitor for diarrhea during or shortly after drug therapy; diarrhea may signal pseudomembranous colitis.

• Administer aminoglycosides 1 hour before or after piperacillin and tazobactam, using separate site, I.V. bag, and tubing.

• When calculating sodium intake for patients on a sodium-restricted diet, keep in mind that each gram of piperacillin and tazobactam contains between 2.35 and 2.85 mEq of sodium (amount varies, depending on type of preparation being used).

• Follow manufacturer's instructions on how to store drug before reconstitution. Instructions vary, depending on type of preparation being used. Powder form may be stored at 15° to 30° C (59° to 86° F); frozen form supplied in plastic containers should be stored at less than –20° C (–4° F).

PATIENT TEACHING

• Advise patient receiving piperacillin and tazobactam to report signs of superinfection, such as severe diarrhea or white patches on tongue or in mouth. Instruct her to check with prescriber before taking an antidiarrheal because it may mask signs of pseudomembranous colitis.

• Advise patient to consult prescriber before using OTC drugs during treatment with piperacillin and tazobactam because of the risk of interactions.

• Inform patient that she may bruise easily if she takes anti-inflammatory drugs, such as aspirin and NSAIDs, during piperacillin and tazobactam therapy.

polymyxin B sulfate

Aerosporin

Class and Category

Chemical: *Bacillus polymyxa* derivative
Therapeutic: Antibiotic
Pregnancy category: Not rated

Indications and Dosages

▶ *To treat infections that are resistant to less toxic drugs, such as bacteremia, septicemia, and UTIs caused by susceptible organisms, including* Enterobacter aerogenes, Escherichia coli, Haemophilus influenzae, *and* Klebsiella pneumoniae

I.V. INFUSION
Adults and children age 2 and older. 15,000 to 25,000 U/kg/day in divided doses q 12 hr or as a continuous infusion. *Maximum:* 2 million U/day.
Infants and children under age 2. Up to 40,000 U/kg/day in divided doses q 12 hr or as a continuous infusion.
DOSAGE ADJUSTMENT Dosage reduced by 50% for patients with creatinine clearance of 5 to 20 ml/min/1.73 m^2 and by 85% for patients with creatinine clearance of less than 5 ml/min/1.73 m^2.

▶ *To treat meningitis caused by susceptible strains of* Pseudomonas aeruginosa *or* H. influenzae
INTRATHECAL INJECTION
Adults and children age 2 and older. 50,000 U q.d. for 3 to 4 days, then 50,000 U q.o.d. for at least 2 wk after CSF cultures are negative and glucose content is normal.
Infants and children under age 2. 20,000 U q.d. for 3 to 4 days, then 25,000 U q.o.d. for at least 2 wk after CSF cultures are negative and glucose content is normal.

Mechanism of Action
Binds to cell membrane phospholipids in gram-negative bacteria, increasing the permeability of the cell membrane. Polymyxin B also acts as a cationic detergent, altering the osmotic barrier of the membrane and causing essential intracellular metabolites to leak out. Both actions lead to cell death.

Incompatibilities
Don't mix polymyxin B sulfate with amphotericin B, calcium salts, chloramphenicol, chlorothiazide, heparin sodium, magnesium salts, nitrofurantoin, penicillins, prednisolone, or tetracyclines because these drugs are incompatible.

Contraindications
Hypersensitivity to polymyxin B or its components

Interactions
DRUGS
general anesthetics, neuromuscular blockers, skeletal muscle relaxants: Increased or prolonged skeletal muscle relaxation, possibly respiratory paralysis

nephrotoxic and neurotoxic drugs (such as aminoglycosides, amphotericin B, colistin, sodium citrate, streptomycin, tobramycin, and vancomycin): Increased risk of nephrotoxicity and neurotoxicity

Adverse Reactions

CNS: Ataxia, confusion, dizziness, drowsiness, fever, giddiness, headache, increased leukocyte and protein levels in CSF, neurotoxicity, paresthesia (circumoral or peripheral), slurred speech
CV: Thrombophlebitis
EENT: Blurred vision, nystagmus
GU: Albuminuria, azotemia, cylindruria, decreased urine output, hematuria, nephrotoxicity
HEME: Eosinophilia
RESP: Respiratory muscle paralysis
SKIN: Rash, urticaria
Other: Anaphylaxis, drug-induced fever, facial flushing, injection site pain, stiff neck (with intrathecal injection), superinfection

Nursing Considerations

- Be aware that patients receiving polymyxin B sulfate are hospitalized to allow appropriate supervision.
- Obtain blood, urine, or other specimens for culture and sensitivity tests, as ordered, before giving drug. Expect to begin polymyxin B therapy before results are known. Keep in mind that baseline renal function tests should have been performed before administration. Check these test results, if available, and notify prescriber of abnormalities.
- For I.V. infusion, dissolve polymyxin B in 300 to 500 ml of D$_5$W and infuse over 60 to 90 minutes.
- For intrathecal administration, add 10 ml of sodium chloride for injection to vial of polymyxin B.
- Inspect for particles and discoloration before giving drug.
- Monitor renal function, including BUN and serum creatinine levels, during therapy, especially in patients with a history of renal insufficiency.
- **WARNING** Be aware that declining urine output and rising BUN level suggest nephrotoxicity, which also is characterized by albuminuria, azotemia, cylindruria, excessive excretion of electrolytes, hematuria, leukocyturia, and rising blood drug level. Notify prescriber immediately if you detect any of these signs.
- **WARNING** Notify prescriber immediately if patient experiences blurred vision, circumoral or peripheral paresthesia,

confusion, dizziness, drowsiness, facial flushing, giddiness, myasthenia, nystagmus, or slurred speech. These may be signs of neurotoxicity, a serious adverse reaction that may lead to respiratory arrest or paralysis if untreated.

- Assess for signs of superinfection, such as mouth sores, severe diarrhea, and white patches on tongue or in mouth, especially in debilitated or elderly patients.
- Monitor fluid intake and output, and provide adequate fluids to reduce the risk of nephrotoxicity.

PATIENT TEACHING

- Encourage patient to maintain adequate fluid intake during polymyxin B therapy.
- Instruct patient to immediately report diarrhea, mouth sores, or vaginitis, which may be early signs of superinfection.

potassium acetate
(contains 2 or 4 mEq of elemental potassium per 1 ml of injection)
potassium chloride
(contains 0.1, 0.2, 0.3, 0.4, 1.5, 2, 3, or 10 mEq of elemental potassium per 1 ml of injection)

Class and Category
Chemical: Electrolyte cation
Therapeutic: Electrolyte replacement
Pregnancy category: C

Indications and Dosages
▶ *To prevent or treat hypokalemia in patients who can't ingest sufficient dietary potassium or who are losing potassium because of certain conditions (such as hepatic cirrhosis and prolonged vomiting) or drugs (such as potassium-wasting diuretics and certain antibiotics)*

I.V. INFUSION

Adults and adolescents with serum potassium level above 2.5 mEq/L. Up to 10 mEq/hr. *Maximum:* 200 mEq/day.

Adults and adolescents with serum potassium level below 2 mEq/L, ECG changes, or paralysis. Up to 20 mEq/hr. *Maximum:* 400 mEq/day.

Children. 3 mEq/kg/day.

DOSAGE ADJUSTMENT Dosage adjusted as prescribed based on patient's ECG patterns and serum potassium level.

Mechanism of Action

Acts as the major cation in intracellular fluid, activating many enzymatic reactions that are essential for physiologic processes, including nerve impulse transmission and cardiac and skeletal muscle contraction. Potassium also helps maintain electroneutrality in cells by controlling the exchange of intracellular and extracellular ions. It also helps maintain normal renal function and acid-base balance.

Incompatibilities

Don't mix potassium chloride for injection in same syringe with amino acid solutions, lipid solutions, or mannitol because these drugs may precipitate from solution. Administration with blood or blood products can cause lysis of infused RBCs.

Contraindications

Acute dehydration, Addison's disease (untreated), concurrent use of potassium-sparing diuretics, crush syndrome, heat cramps, hyperkalemia, hypersensitivity to potassium salts or their components, renal impairment with azotemia or oliguria, severe hemolytic anemia

Interactions

DRUGS

ACE inhibitors, beta blockers, blood products, cyclosporine, heparin, NSAIDs, potassium-containing drugs, potassium-sparing diuretics: Increased risk of hyperkalemia

amphotericin B, corticosteroids (glucocorticoids or mineralocorticoids), gentamicin, penicillins, polymyxin B: Possibly hypokalemia

calcium salts (parenteral): Possibly arrhythmias

digoxin: Increased risk of digitalis toxicity

insulin, laxatives, sodium bicarbonate: Decreased serum potassium level

sodium polystyrene sulfonate: Possibly decreased serum potassium level and fluid retention

thiazide diuretics: Possibly hyperkalemia when diuretic is discontinued

FOODS

low-salt milk, salt substitutes: Increased risk of hyperkalemia

Adverse Reactions

CNS: Confusion, paralysis, paresthesia, weakness

CV: Arrhythmias, ECG changes

RESP: Dyspnea
SKIN: Rash
Other: Hyperkalemia, injection site pain and redness

Nursing Considerations

- **WARNING** Be aware that direct injection of a potassium concentrate may be immediately fatal. Dilute potassium concentrate for injection with an adequate volume of solution before I.V. use. Maximum concentration suggested is 40 mEq/L, although stronger concentrations (up to 80 mEq/L) may be used for severe hypokalemia. Inappropriate solutions or improper technique may cause extravasation, fever, hyperkalemia, hypervolemia, I.V. site infection, phlebitis, venospasm, and venous thrombosis.
- **WARNING** Be aware that only potassium chloride strengths of 0.1, 0.2, 0.3, and 0.4 mEq may be administered by a calibrated infusion device without further dilution. Carefully inspect labels on vials and ampules before use to verify concentrations.
- Monitor serum potassium level before and regularly during administration of I.V. potassium.
- Infuse potassium slowly to avoid phlebitis and decrease the risk of adverse cardiac reactions. Keep in mind that different forms of potassium salts contain different amounts of elemental potassium per gram and that not all forms are dosage equivalent.
- Regularly assess for signs of hypokalemia, such as arrhythmias, fatigue, and weakness, and for signs of hyperkalemia, such as arrhythmias, confusion, dyspnea, and paresthesia.
- Because adequate renal function is needed for potassium supplementation, monitor serum creatinine level and urine output during administration. Notify prescriber if you detect signs of decreased renal function.
- Store drug at 15° to 30° C (59° to 86° F); don't freeze.

PATIENT TEACHING

- Inform patient that potassium is a normal part of a regular diet and that most meats, seafoods, fruits, and vegetables contain sufficient potassium to meet the recommended daily intake. Also advise her not to exceed the recommended daily amount of potassium.
- Teach patient how to take her radial pulse, and advise her to report significant changes in heart rate or rhythm.
- Inform patient that her serum potassium level will be checked periodically during therapy.

potassium phosphates
sodium phosphates

Class and Category
Chemical: Anion, soluble salts
Therapeutic: Electrolyte replenisher
Pregnancy category: C

Indications and Dosages
▶ *To prevent or treat hypophosphatemia*
I.V. INFUSION (POTASSIUM PHOSPHATES)
Adults and adolescents. 10 mmol (310 mg)/day.
Children. 1.5 to 2 mmol (46.5 to 62 mg)/day.
I.V. INFUSION (SODIUM PHOSPHATES)
Adults and adolescents. 10 to 15 mmol (310 to 465 mg)/day.
Children. 1.5 to 2 mmol (46.5 to 62 mg)/day.

Mechanism of Action
Reverses symptoms of hypophosphatemia by replenishing the body's supply of phosphate.

Incompatibilities
Don't add potassium or sodium phosphates to calcium- or magnesium-containing solutions because a precipitate may form.

Contraindications
Hyperkalemia (potassium formulations only), hypernatremia (sodium formulations only), hyperphosphatemia, magnesium ammonium phosphate urolithiasis accompanied by infection, severe renal insufficiency, UTIs caused by urea-splitting organisms

Interactions
DRUGS
ACE inhibitors, cyclosporine, heparin (long-term use), NSAIDs, potassium-containing drugs, potassium-sparing diuretics: Increased risk of hyperkalemia (potassium formulations only)
anabolic steroids, androgens, corticosteroids, estrogens: Increased risk of edema (sodium formulations only)
calcium-containing drugs: Increased risk of calcium deposition in soft tissues
phosphate-containing drugs, vitamin D: Increased risk of hyperphosphatemia

salicylates: Increased blood salicylate level
zinc supplements: Reduced zinc absorption
FOODS
low-salt milk, salt substitutes: Increased risk of hyperkalemia

Adverse Reactions

CNS: Anxiety, confusion, dizziness, fatigue, headache, paresthesia, seizures, tremor, weakness
CV: Arrhythmias, edema of legs, tachycardia
GI: Thirst
GU: Decreased urine output
MS: Muscle cramps or weakness
RESP: Dyspnea
Other: Hyperkalemia, hypernatremia, hyperphosphatemia, hypocalcemia, weight gain

Nursing Considerations

• Avoid mixing potassium or sodium phosphates with solutions containing calcium or magnesium to prevent the formation of precipitates. Dilute phosphates, as prescribed, before administration.

• Monitor serum phosphorus level, as appropriate, of patients with a condition that may be associated with an elevated phosphorus level, such as chronic renal disease, hypoparathyroidism, and rhabdomyolysis; phosphates may further increase serum phosphorus level.

• Monitor serum calcium level, as appropriate, of patients with a condition that may be associated with a low calcium level, such as acute pancreatitis, chronic renal disease, hypoparathyroidism, osteomalacia, rhabdomyolysis, and rickets; phosphates may further decrease serum calcium level.

• Monitor serum potassium level, as appropriate, of patients who receive potassium phosphates and have a condition that may be associated with an elevated potassium level, such as acute dehydration, adrenal insufficiency, extensive tissue breakdown (as in severe burns), myotonia congenita, pancreatitis, rhabdomyolysis, and severe renal insufficiency; they may be at increased risk for hyperkalemia.

• Monitor serum sodium level of patients who receive sodium phosphates and have a condition that may be exacerbated by sodium excess, such as heart failure, hypernatremia, hypertension, peripheral or pulmonary edema, preeclampsia, renal impairment, and severe hepatic disease.

- Monitor ECG tracing frequently during I.V. infusion of sodium phosphates to detect arrhythmias.
- Store drug at 15° to 30° C (59° to 86° F); don't freeze.

PATIENT TEACHING
- Urge patient receiving potassium or sodium phosphates to immediately report muscle weakness or cramps, unexplained weight gain, or shortness of breath.
- Encourage increased intake of fluids (8 oz/hour, if not contraindicated) to prevent kidney stones.

pralidoxime chloride
(2-PAM chloride, 2-pyridine aldoxime methochloride)
Protopam Chloride

Class and Category
Chemical: Quaternary ammonium oxime
Therapeutic: Anticholinesterase antidote
Pregnancy category: C

Indications and Dosages
▶ *As adjunct to reverse organophosphate pesticide toxicity*
I.V. INFUSION, I.M. OR S.C. INJECTION
Adults. *Initial:* 1 to 2 g in 100 ml of NS infused over 15 to 30 min, given concurrently with atropine 2 to 6 mg q 5 to 60 min until muscarinic signs and symptoms disappear; may be repeated in 1 hr and then q 3 to 8 hr if muscle weakness persists. If I.V. route isn't feasible, administer I.M. or S.C.
Children. *Initial:* 20 mg/kg in 100 ml of NS infused over 15 to 30 min, given concurrently with atropine (dosage individualized); may be repeated in 1 hr and then q 3 to 8 hr if muscle weakness persists. If I.V. route isn't feasible, administer I.M. or S.C.
▶ *To treat anticholinesterase overdose secondary to myasthenic drugs (including ambenonium, neostigmine, and pyridostigmine)*
I.V. INJECTION
Adults. *Initial:* 1 to 2 g, followed by 250 mg q 5 min.
▶ *To treat exposure to nerve agents*
I.V. INJECTION
Adults. *Initial:* 1 atropine-containing autoinjector followed by 1 pralidoxime-containing autoinjector as soon as atropine's effects are evident; both injections repeated q 15 min for 2 additional doses if nerve agent symptoms persist.

DOSAGE ADJUSTMENT Dosage reduced for patients with renal insufficiency.

Mechanism of Action

Reverses muscle paralysis by removing the phosphoryl group from inhibited cholinesterase molecules at the neuromuscular junction of skeletal and respiratory muscles. Reactivation of cholinesterase restores the body's ability to metabolize acetylcholine, which is inhibited by the effects of organophosphate pesticides, anticholinesterase overdose, or nerve agent poisoning.

Contraindications

Hypersensitivity to pralidoxime chloride or its components

Interactions

DRUGS

aminophylline, morphine, phenothiazines, reserpine, succinylcholine, theophylline: Increased symptoms of organophosphate poisoning
barbiturates: Potentiated barbiturate effects

Adverse Reactions

CNS: Dizziness, drowsiness, headache
CV: Increased systolic and diastolic blood pressure, tachycardia
EENT: Accommodation disturbances, blurred vision, diplopia
GI: Nausea, vomiting
MS: Muscle weakness
RESP: Hyperventilation
Other: Injection site pain

Nursing Considerations

- Be aware that pralidoxime must be administered within 36 hours of toxicity to be effective.
- Use drug with extreme caution in patients with myasthenia gravis who are being treated for organophosphate poisoning because pralidoxime may precipitate myasthenic crisis.
- Reconstitute drug according to manufacturer's guidelines and administration route.
- For intermittent infusion, further dilute with NS to a volume of 100 ml and infuse over 15 to 30 minutes.
- Avoid too-rapid administration, which may cause hypertension, laryngospasm, muscle spasms, neuromuscular blockade, and tachycardia. Also be sure to avoid intradermal injection.
- Closely monitor neuromuscular status during therapy.

- Monitor BUN and serum creatinine levels, as appropriate, in patients with renal insufficiency because drug is excreted in urine.
- When pralidoxime is administered with atropine, expect signs of atropinization, such as dry mouth and nose, flushing, mydriasis, and tachycardia, to occur earlier than when atropine is given alone.
- Store drug at room temperature.

PATIENT TEACHING
- Inform patient receiving I.M. pralidoxime that she'll experience pain at the injection site for 40 to 60 minutes afterward.
- Reassure patient that she'll be closely monitored throughout therapy.

procainamide hydrochloride
Pronestyl

Class and Category
Chemical: Ethyl benzamide monohydrochloride
Therapeutic: Antiarrhythmic
Pregnancy category: C

Indications and Dosages
▶ *To treat life-threatening ventricular arrhythmias, to treat ventricular extrasystoles and arrhythmias associated with anesthesia and surgery*
I.V. INFUSION OR INJECTION
Adults. *Initial:* 100 mg diluted in D_5W and administered at a rate not to exceed 50 mg/min. Dosage repeated q 5 min until arrhythmia is controlled or maximum total dose of 1 g is reached. Alternatively, 10 to 15 mg/kg I.V. bolus administered at a rate of 25 to 50 mg/min. *Maintenance:* 1 to 4 mg/min by continuous infusion.
DOSAGE ADJUSTMENT For elderly patients or patients with cardiac or hepatic insufficiency, dosage possibly reduced or dosing intervals increased. For patients with creatinine clearance less than 50 ml/min/1.73 m^2, initial dosage reduced to 1 to 2 mg/min.

Route	Onset	Peak	Duration
I.V.	Unknown	Immediate	Unknown

Contraindications
Complete heart block, hypersensitivity to procainamide or its components, systemic lupus erythematosus, torsades de pointes

Mechanism of Action

Prolongs the recovery period after myocardial repolarization by inhibiting sodium influx through myocardial cell membranes. This action prolongs the refractory period, causing myocardial automaticity, excitability, and conduction velocity to decline.

Interactions

DRUGS

antiarrhythmics: Additive cardiac effects

anticholinergics, antidyskinetics, antihistamines: Possibly intensified atropine-like adverse effects, increased risk of ileus

antihypertensives: Additive hypotensive effects

antimyasthenics: Possibly antagonized effect of antimyasthenic on skeletal muscle

bethanechol: Possibly antagonized cholinergic effect of bethanechol

bone marrow depressants: Possibly increased leukopenic or thrombocytopenic effects

bretylium: Possibly decreased inotropic effect of bretylium and enhanced hypotension

neuromuscular blockers: Possibly increased or prolonged neuromuscular blockade

pimozide: Possibly prolonged QT interval, leading to life-threatening arrhythmias

Adverse Reactions

CNS: Chills, disorientation, dizziness, light-headedness

CV: Heart block (second degree), hypotension, pericarditis, prolonged QT interval, tachycardia

EENT: Bitter taste

GI: Abdominal distress, anorexia, diarrhea, nausea, vomiting

HEME: Agranulocytosis, neutropenia, thrombocytopenia

MS: Arthralgia, myalgia

RESP: Pleural effusion

SKIN: Pruritus, rash

Other: Drug-induced fever, lupuslike symptoms

Nursing Considerations

• Place patient in a supine position before administering procainamide to minimize hypotensive effects. Monitor blood pressure frequently and ECG tracings continuously during administration and for 30 minutes afterward.

- Inspect parenteral solution for particles and discoloration before administering; discard if particles are present or solution is darker than light amber.
- Dilute procainamide with D_5W according to manufacturer's instructions.
- For I.V. infusion, dilute 200 to 1,000 mg of procainamide with 50 to 500 ml of D_5W, respectively, to yield a concentration of 2 or 4 mg/ml.
- Administer I.V. infusion with an infusion pump or other controlled-delivery device.
- Don't administer more than 500 mg in 30 minutes by I.V. infusion or 50 mg/minute by I.V. injection because heart block or cardiac arrest may occur.
- Anticipate that patient has reached maximum clinical response when ventricular tachycardia resolves, hypotension develops, or QRS complex is 50% wider than it was originally.
- If patient is switching to oral form, expect to administer first oral dose 3 or 4 hours after last I.V. dose.
- Before diluting procainamide, store it at 15° to 30° C (59° to 86° F).

PATIENT TEACHING
- Advise patient receiving procainamide to immediately report bruising, chills, diarrhea, fever, or rash.
- Urge patient to obtain needed dental work before therapy starts or after blood count returns to normal, if possible, because drug can cause myelosuppression and increase the risk of bleeding and infection. Stress the need for good oral hygiene during therapy, and urge patient to consult prescriber before scheduling dental procedures.

prochlorperazine edisylate
Compazine

Class and Category
Chemical: Phenothiazine, piperazine
Therapeutic: Antianxiety agent, antiemetic
Pregnancy category: Not rated

Indications and Dosages
▶ *To control nausea and vomiting related to surgery*
I.V. INFUSION OR INJECTION
Adults and adolescents. 5 to 10 mg at a rate not to exceed 5 mg/ml 15 to 30 min before anesthesia or during or after sur-

gery, as needed. Dosage repeated once, if necessary. *Maximum:* 10 mg/dose, 40 mg/day.

▶ *To control severe nausea and vomiting*

I.V. INFUSION OR INJECTION

Adults and adolescents. 2.5 to 10 mg at a rate not to exceed 5 mg/min. *Maximum:* 40 mg/day.

▶ *To provide short-term treatment of anxiety*

I.V. INFUSION OR INJECTION

Adults and adolescents. 2.5 to 10 mg at a rate not to exceed 5 mg/min. *Maximum:* 40 mg/day.

DOSAGE ADJUSTMENT Initial dose usually reduced and subsequent dosage increased more gradually for elderly, emaciated, and debilitated patients.

Route	Onset	Peak	Duration
I.V.	Unknown	Up to 6 mo	Unknown

Mechanism of Action

Alleviates nausea and vomiting by centrally blocking dopamine receptors in the medullary chemoreceptor trigger zone and by peripherally blocking the vagus nerve in the GI tract. In addition, prochlorperazine's anticholinergic effects and alpha-adrenergic blockade reduce anxiety by decreasing arousal and filtering internal stimuli to the reticular activating system.

Incompatibilities

Don't mix prochlorperazine in same syringe with other drugs. A precipitate may form when prochlorperazine edisylate is mixed in same syringe with morphine sulfate.

Contraindications

Age younger than 2 years, blood dyscrasias, bone marrow depression, cerebral arteriosclerosis, coma, coronary artery disease, hepatic dysfunction, hypersensitivity to phenothiazines, myeloproliferative disorders, pediatric surgery, severe CNS depression, severe hypertension or hypotension, subcortical brain damage, use of large quantities of CNS depressants, weight less than 9 kg (20 lb)

Interactions

DRUGS

amantadine, anticholinergics, antidyskinetics, antihistamines: Possibly intensified anticholinergic adverse effects, increased risk of prochlorperazine-induced hyperpyretic effect *amphetamines:* Decreased stimulant effect of amphetamines, decreased antipsychotic effect of prochlorperazine

anticonvulsants: Lowered seizure threshold

antithyroid drugs: Increased risk of agranulocytosis

apomorphine: Possibly decreased emetic response to apomorphine, additive CNS depression

appetite suppressants: Possibly antagonized anorectic effect of appetite suppressants (except for phenmetrazine)

astemizole, cisapride, disopyramide, erythromycin, pimozide, probucol, procainamide: Additive QT interval prolongation, increased risk of ventricular tachycardia

beta blockers: Increased risk of additive hypotensive effects, irreversible retinopathy, arrhythmias, and tardive dyskinesia

bromocriptine: Decreased effectiveness of bromocriptine

CNS depressants: Additive CNS depression

dopamine: Possibly antagonized peripheral vasoconstriction (with high doses of dopamine)

ephedrine, epinephrine: Decreased vasopressor effects of these drugs

hepatotoxic drugs: Increased incidence of hepatotoxicity

hypotension-producing drugs: Possibly severe hypotension with syncope

levodopa: Inhibited antidyskinetic effect of levodopa

lithium: Reduced absorption of oral prochlorperazine, increased excretion of lithium, increased extrapyramidal effects, possibly masking of early symptoms of lithium toxicity

MAO inhibitors, maprotiline, tricyclic antidepressants: Possibly prolonged and intensified anticholinergic and sedative effects, increased blood antidepressant levels, inhibited prochlorperazine metabolism, and increased risk of neuroleptic malignant syndrome

mephentermine: Possibly antagonized antipsychotic effect of prochlorperazine and vasopressor effect of mephentermine

metrizamide: Increased risk of seizures

opioid analgesics: Increased risk of CNS and respiratory depression, orthostatic hypotension, severe constipation, and urine retention

ototoxic drugs: Possibly masking of some symptoms of ototoxicity, such as dizziness, tinnitus, and vertigo

phenytoin: Possibly inhibited phenytoin metabolism and increased risk of phenytoin toxicity

thiazide diuretics: Possibly potentiated hyponatremia and water intoxication

ACTIVITIES

alcohol use: Additive CNS depression

Adverse Reactions

CNS: Akathisia, altered temperature regulation, dizziness, drowsiness, extrapyramidal reactions (such as dystonia, pseudoparkinsonism, tardive dyskinesia)
CV: Hypotension, orthostatic hypotension, tachycardia
EENT: Blurred vision, dry mouth, nasal congestion, ocular changes, pigmentary retinopathy
ENDO: Galactorrhea, gynecomastia
GI: Constipation, epigastric pain, nausea, vomiting
GU: Dysuria, ejaculation disorders, menstrual irregularities, urine retention
SKIN: Decreased sweating, photosensitivity, pruritus, rash
Other: Weight gain

Nursing Considerations

• Wear gloves when working with prochlorperazine because the parenteral solution may cause contact dermatitis.
• Be aware that I.V. form may be administered undiluted as an injection or diluted in isotonic solution as an infusion. Don't administer more than 10 mg as a single dose or exceed a rate of 5 mg/minute.
• Be aware that parenteral solution may develop a slight yellowing that won't affect potency. Don't use if discoloration is pronounced or precipitate is present.
• **WARNING** Monitor closely for numerous adverse reactions that may be serious.
• **WARNING** Monitor patients with chronic respiratory disorders (such as severe asthma or emphysema) or acute respiratory tract infections for exacerbations of these conditions caused by prochlorperazine's CNS depressant effects. Be alert for possible suppressed cough reflex, which increases patient's risk of aspirating vomitus.
• Be aware that patients with cardiovascular or renal disease are at increased risk for developing hypotension, heart failure, and arrhythmias.
• **WARNING** If patient develops neuroleptic malignant syndrome (hyperpyrexia, muscle rigidity, altered mental status, autonomic instability), notify prescriber immediately and expect to discontinue drug and begin intensive medical treatment.

- Be aware that patients with impaired hepatic function are at risk for decreased prochlorperazine metabolism or further hepatic dysfunction. Monitor patients with a history of hepatic encephalopathy from cirrhosis for increased sensitivity to drug's CNS effects.
- Because prochlorperazine may have anticholinergic effects, monitor patients with a history of, or predisposition to, glaucoma for signs and symptoms of this disorder, such as eye pain, vision changes, or nausea and vomiting from increased intraocular pressure.
- Be aware that drug should be used cautiously in those who are exposed to organophosphorus insecticides.
- Monitor patients who have been exposed to extreme heat for heatstroke due to drug-induced suppression of temperature regulation. Symptoms include tachycardia, fever, and confusion.
- Be aware that pediatric and elderly patients are at increased risk for developing hypotension and extrapyramidal reactions, especially if they're acutely ill or debilitated.
- Store drug at less than 30° C (86° F); protect from freezing and light.

PATIENT TEACHING
- Advise patient to rise slowly from a lying or sitting position during prochlorperazine therapy to minimize effects of orthostatic hypotension.
- Instruct patient to avoid potentially hazardous activities because of the risk of drowsiness and impaired judgment and coordination.
- Urge patient to report involuntary movements and restlessness.
- Advise patient to report sudden sore throat or other signs of infection.
- Inform patient that drug may reduce body's response to heat and cold; advise her to avoid temperature extremes, such as very cold or hot showers.
- Suggest sugarless chewing gum, hard candy, and fluids to relieve dry mouth.
- Urge patient to avoid alcohol and OTC drugs that may contain CNS depressants.
- Instruct patient to avoid excessive sun exposure and to wear sunscreen when outdoors.

promethazine hydrochloride

Anergan 25, Anergan 50, Antinaus 50, Histantil (CAN), Pentazine, Phenazine 25, Phenazine 50, Phencen-50, Phenergan, Phenerzine, Phenoject-50, Pro-50, Promacot, Pro-Med 50, Promet, Prorex-25, Prorex-50, Prothazine, Shogan, V-Gan-25, V-Gan-50

Class and Category

Chemical: Phenothiazine derivative
Therapeutic: Antiemetic, antihistamine, sedative-hypnotic
Pregnancy category: C

Indications and Dosages

▶ *To prevent or treat nausea and vomiting associated with certain types of anesthesia and surgery*

I.V. INJECTION

Adults and adolescents. 12.5 to 25 mg q 4 hr, p.r.n. *Maximum:* 150 mg/day.

▶ *To treat signs and symptoms of allergic response*

I.V. INJECTION

Adults and adolescents. 25 mg, repeated within 2 hr, if needed.

▶ *To provide nighttime, preoperative, or postoperative sedation*

I.V. INJECTION

Adults and adolescents. 25 to 50 mg as a single dose. Alternatively, for preoperative and postoperative sedation, 25 to 50 mg combined with appropriately reduced dosages of analgesics and anticholinergics.

DOSAGE ADJUSTMENT Dosage usually decreased for elderly patients.

▶ *To provide obstetric sedation*

I.V. INJECTION

Adults and adolescents. 50 mg for early stages of labor, followed by 1 or 2 doses of 25 to 75 mg after labor is definitely established and repeated q 4 hr during course of normal labor.

Route	Onset	Peak	Duration
I.V.	3 to 5 min	Unknown	4 to 6 hr

Mechanism of Action

Competes with histamine for H$_1$-receptor sites, thereby antagonizing many histamine effects and reducing allergy signs and symptoms. Promethazine also prevents nausea by acting centrally on the medullary chemoreceptive trigger zone and by decreasing vestibular stimulation and labyrinthine function in the inner ear. In addition, it promotes sedation and relieves anxiety by blocking receptor sites within the CNS, directly reducing stimuli to the brain.

Contraindications

Angle-closure glaucoma, benign prostatic hyperplasia, bladder neck obstruction, bone marrow depression, breast-feeding, coma, hypersensitivity to promethazine or its components, hypertensive crisis, pyloroduodenal obstruction, stenosing peptic ulcer, use of large quantities of CNS depressants

Interactions

DRUGS

amphetamines: Decreased stimulant effect of amphetamines
anticholinergics: Possibly intensified anticholinergic adverse effects
anticonvulsants: Lowered seizure threshold
appetite suppressants: Possibly antagonized anorectic effect of appetite suppressants
beta blockers: Increased risk of additive hypotensive effects, irreversible retinopathy, arrhythmias, and tardive dyskinesia
bromocriptine: Decreased effectiveness of bromocriptine
CNS depressants: Additive CNS depression
dopamine: Possibly antagonized peripheral vasoconstriction (with high doses of dopamine)
ephedrine, metaraminol, methoxamine: Decreased vasopressor response to these drugs
epinephrine: Blocked alpha-adrenergic effects of epinephrine, increased risk of hypotension
guanadrel, guanethidine: Decreased antihypertensive effects of these drugs
hepatotoxic drugs: Increased risk of hepatotoxicity
hypotension-producing drugs: Possibly severe hypotension with syncope
levodopa: Inhibited antidyskinetic effects of levodopa
MAO inhibitors: Possibly prolonged and intensified anticholinergic and CNS depressant effects of promethazine

metrizamide: Increased risk of seizures
ototoxic drugs: Possibly masking of some symptoms of ototoxicity, such as dizziness, tinnitus, and vertigo
quinidine: Additive cardiac effects
riboflavin: Increased riboflavin requirements
ACTIVITIES
alcohol use: Additive CNS depression

Adverse Reactions
CNS: Akathisia, CNS stimulation, confusion, dizziness, drowsiness, dystonia, insomnia, irritability, paradoxical stimulation, pseudoparkinsonism, restlessness, tardive dyskinesia
CV: Hypotension, tachycardia
EENT: Blurred vision; dry mouth, nose, and throat; tinnitus; vision changes
GI: Anorexia, ileus
GU: Dysuria
RESP: Tenacious bronchial secretions
SKIN: Diaphoresis, photosensitivity, rash

Nursing Considerations
- Be aware that elderly patients may be more sensitive to promethazine's effects.
- **WARNING** Avoid inadvertent intra-arterial injection of promethazine because it can cause arteriospasm; impaired circulation may lead to gangrene.
- Administer I.V. injection at a rate not to exceed 25 mg/minute; rapid I.V. administration may produce a transient fall in blood pressure.
- Monitor respiratory function because drug may suppress cough reflex and cause thickening of bronchial secretions, aggravating such conditions as asthma and COPD.
- Be aware that patients with a history of epilepsy are at increased risk for severe seizures when given I.V. promethazine.
- Assess for worsening condition in patients with jaundice.
- Assess for extrapyramidal effects, such as muscle spasms or trembling of hands, which may be confused with CNS signs of Reye's syndrome.
- Be aware that patient shouldn't undergo intradermal allergen tests within 72 hours of receiving promethazine because drug may cause significant alterations of flare response.
- Store drug at 15° to 30° C (59° to 86° F); protect from freezing and light.

PATIENT TEACHING
- Instruct patient receiving promethazine to immediately report involuntary movements and restlessness.
- Advise patient to avoid potentially hazardous activities until drug's CNS effects are known.
- Suggest that patient relieve dry mouth with frequent rinsing and use of sugarless gum or hard candy.
- Instruct patient to avoid OTC drugs unless approved by prescriber.
- Advise patient to avoid excessive sun exposure and to use sunscreen when outdoors.
- Urge patient to avoid alcohol and other CNS depressants while taking promethazine.

propofol
(disoprofol)
Diprivan

Class and Category
Chemical: 2,6-Diisopropylphenol derivative
Therapeutic: Sedative-hypnotic
Pregnancy category: B

Indications and Dosages
▶ *To provide sedation for critically ill patients in intensive care*
I.V. INFUSION
Adults. 2.8 to 130 mcg/kg/min. *Usual:* 27 mcg/kg/min.

Route	Onset	Peak	Duration
I.V.	Within 40 sec	Unknown	3 to 5 min

Mechanism of Action
Decreases cerebral blood flow, cerebral metabolic oxygen consumption, and ICP and increases cerebrovascular resistance, which may play a role in propofol's hypnotic effects.

Incompatibilities
Don't mix propofol with other drugs before administration. Don't administer propofol through same I.V. line as blood or plasma products because globular component of emulsion will aggregate.

Contraindications
Hypersensitivity to propofol or its components

Interactions
DRUGS
CNS depressants: Additive CNS depressant, respiratory depressant, and hypotensive effects; possibly decreased emetic effects of opioids
droperidol: Possibly decreased control of nausea and vomiting
ACTIVITIES
alcohol use: Additive CNS depressant, respiratory depressant, and hypotensive effects

Adverse Reactions
CV: Bradycardia, hypotension
GI: Nausea, vomiting
MS: Involuntary muscle movements (transient)
RESP: Apnea
Other: Injection site burning, pain, or stinging

Nursing Considerations
- If ordered to dilute propofol before administration, use only D₅W to yield a final concentration of 2 mg/ml or more.
- Consult prescriber about pretreating injection site with 1 ml of 1% lidocaine to minimize pain, burning, or stinging that may occur with propofol administration. Administering drug through a larger vein in the forearm or antecubital fossa may also minimize injection site discomfort.
- Shake container well before using, and administer drug promptly after opening.
- Use a drop counter, syringe pump, or volumetric pump to safely control infusion rate. Don't infuse drug through filter with a pore size of less than 5 microns because doing so could cause emulsion to break down.
- Discard all unused portions of propofol solution as well as reservoirs, I.V. tubing, and solutions immediately after or within 12 hours of administration (6 hours if propofol was transferred from original container) to prevent bacterial growth in stagnant solution. Also, protect solution from light.
- Be aware that dosage may be reduced for debilitated or hypovolemic patients and in those older than age 55. Propofol is not approved to treat sedation in children.
- Expect patient to recover from sedation within 8 minutes.

- Monitor patients with cardiac disease, peripheral vascular disease, impaired cerebral circulation, or increased ICP for signs of exacerbation because drug may aggravate these disorders.
- Store drug at 4° to 22° C (40° to 72° F); don't refrigerate. Protect from light.

PATIENT TEACHING

- Encourage patient and family to voice concerns and ask questions before propofol administration.
- Reassure patient that she'll be closely monitored throughout drug administration and that her vital functions, including breathing, will be supported as needed.

propranolol hydrochloride
Inderal

Class and Category
Chemical: Beta-adrenergic blocker
Therapeutic: Antiarrhythmic
Pregnancy category: C

Indications and Dosages
▶ *To treat supraventricular arrhythmias and ventricular tachycardia*
I.V. INJECTION
Adults. 1 to 3 mg at a rate not to exceed 1 mg/min; repeated after 2 min and again after 4 hr, if needed.
Children. 0.01 to 0.1 mg/kg at a rate not to exceed 1 mg/min; repeated q 6 to 8 hr, as needed. *Maximum:* 1 mg/dose.

Mechanism of Action
As a nonselective beta-adrenergic blocking agent, produces a decrease in the heart rate, which helps resolve tachyarrhythmias.

Contraindications
Asthma, cardiogenic shock, AV block greater than first-degree, heart failure (unless secondary to tachyarrhythmia that is responsive to propranolol), hypersensitivity to propranolol or its components, sinus bradycardia

Interactions
DRUGS
allergen immunotherapy, allergenic extracts for skin testing: Increased risk of serious systemic adverse reactions or anaphylaxis

amiodarone: Additive depressant effects on conduction, negative inotropic effects
beta blockers: Additive beta blockade effects
calcium channel blockers, clonidine, diazoxide, guanabenz, reserpine, other hypotension-producing drugs: Additive hypotensive effect and, possibly, other beta blockade effects
cimetidine: Possibly interference with propranolol clearance
estrogens: Decreased antihypertensive effect of propranolol
fentanyl, fentanyl derivatives: Possibly increased risk of initial bradycardia after induction doses of fentanyl or a derivative (with long-term propranolol use)
glucagon: Possibly blunted hyperglycemic response
hydrocarbon inhalation anesthetics: Increased risk of myocardial depression and hypotension
insulin, oral antidiabetic drugs: Possibly impaired glucose control, masking of tachycardia in response to hypoglycemia
lidocaine: Decreased lidocaine clearance, increased risk of lidocaine toxicity
MAO inhibitors: Increased risk of significant hypertension
neuromuscular blockers: Possibly potentiated and prolonged action of these drugs
NSAIDs: Possibly decreased hypotensive effects
phenothiazines: Increased blood levels of both drugs
phenytoin: Additive cardiac depressant effects (with parenteral phenytoin)
propafenone: Increased blood level and half-life of propranolol
sympathomimetics, xanthines: Possibly mutual inhibition of therapeutic effects
ACTIVITIES
nicotine chewing gum, smoking cessation, smoking deterrents: Increased therapeutic effects of propranolol

Adverse Reactions

CNS: Anxiety, depression, dizziness, drowsiness, fatigue, insomnia, lethargy, nervousness, weakness
CV: AV conduction disorders, cold extremities, heart failure, hypotension, sinus bradycardia
EENT: Nasal congestion
GI: Abdominal pain, constipation, diarrhea, nausea, vomiting
GU: Sexual dysfunction
MS: Muscle weakness
RESP: Bronchospasm, dyspnea, wheezing

Nursing Considerations

- Monitor blood pressure, apical and radial pulses, fluid intake and output, daily weight, respiration, and circulation in extremities before and during propranolol therapy.
- Administer I.V. injection at a rate not to exceed 1 mg/minute.
- Be aware that a patient undergoing surgery may receive an I.V. dose that is one-tenth of oral dose.
- **WARNING** Institute continuous ECG monitoring, as ordered. Have emergency drugs and equipment available to intervene in case hypotension or cardiac arrest occurs.
- Because drug's negative inotropic effect can depress cardiac output, monitor cardiac output in patients with heart failure, particularly those with severely compromised left ventricular dysfunction.
- Be aware that propranolol can mask tachycardia that occurs in hyperthyroidism and that abrupt withdrawal of drug in patients with hyperthyroidism or thyrotoxicosis can precipitate thyroid storm.
- Monitor diabetic patient who is receiving antidiabetic drugs because propranolol can prolong hypoglycemia or promote hyperglycemia. Propranolol also can mask signs of hypoglycemia, especially tachycardia, palpitations, and tremor, but it doesn't suppress diaphoresis or hypertensive response to hypoglycemia.
- **WARNING** Be aware that abrupt discontinuation may cause myocardial ischemia, MI, ventricular arrhythmias, or severe hypertension, particularly in patients with preexisting cardiac disease.
- Store drug at 15° to 30° C (59° to 86° F); protect from freezing and light.

PATIENT TEACHING

- Advise patient to immediately report shortness of breath during propranolol therapy.
- Inform diabetic patient that her blood glucose level will be monitored regularly and her urine tested for ketones.
- Advise patient to consult prescriber before taking OTC drugs, especially cold remedies.
- Urge patient to avoid potentially hazardous activities until drug's CNS effects are known.
- Advise smoker to notify prescriber immediately if she stops smoking because smoking cessation may decrease drug metabolism, calling for dosage adjustments.

protamine sulfate

Class and Category

Chemical: Simple low-molecular-weight protein
Therapeutic: Heparin antagonist
Pregnancy category: C

Indications and Dosages

▶ *To treat heparin toxicity or hemorrhage associated with heparin therapy*

I.V. INJECTION

Adults and children. 1 mg for each 100 U of heparin to be neutralized, or as indicated by coagulation test results. *Maximum:* 100 mg (within 2-hr period).

Route	Onset	Peak	Duration
I.V.	5 min	Unknown	2 hr

Mechanism of Action

Combines with strongly acidic heparin complex to form an inactive stable salt, thereby neutralizing the anticoagulant activity of both drugs.

Incompatibilities

Don't mix protamine sulfate in same syringe with other drugs unless they're known to be compatible. Several cephalosporins, penicillins, and other antibiotics are incompatible with protamine.

Contraindications

Allergy to fish, hypersensitivity to protamine or its components

Interactions

DRUGS

heparin: Neutralized anticoagulant effect of both drugs

Adverse Reactions

CNS: Weakness
CV: Bradycardia, hypertension, hypotension, shock
GI: Nausea, vomiting
HEME: Unusual bleeding or bruising
RESP: Dyspnea, pulmonary edema (noncardiogenic), pulmonary hypertension
SKIN: Flushing, sensation of warmth
Other: Anaphylaxis

Nursing Considerations

- Expect to administer protamine undiluted. However, dilute drug if needed (for patients other than neonates) with 5 ml of bacteriostatic water for injection containing 0.9% benzyl alcohol.
- **WARNING** When administering drug to neonates or premature infants, reconstitute with preservative-free sterile water for injection. Avoid using solutions that contain benzyl alcohol because they can cause a fatal toxic syndrome in infants, characterized by CNS, respiratory, circulatory, and renal impairment and metabolic acidosis.
- Inject drug slowly at a rate of 5 mg/minute; administer no more than 50 mg in 10 minutes or 100 mg in 2 hours.
- Discard any unused portion because protamine contains no preservatives.
- **WARNING** Be aware that rapid administration may cause severe hypotension and anaphylaxis.
- Be prepared to obtain coagulation studies (APTT, activated clotting time) 5 to 15 minutes after administering drug and to repeat studies in 2 to 8 hours to assess for heparin-rebound hypotension, shock, and bleeding.
- Monitor vital signs, hemodynamic parameters, and fluid intake and output, and assess for flushing sensation.
- Have fluids—epinephrine 1:1,000, dobutamine, or dopamine—available for allergic or hypotensive reactions.
- Be aware that vasectomized males have an increased risk of hypersensitivity reaction because of possible accumulation of antiprotamine antibodies.
- Store drug at 2° to 8° C (36° to 46° F); don't freeze.

PATIENT TEACHING

- Instruct patient receiving protamine to report adverse reactions immediately.

pyridostigmine bromide
Mestinon, Mestinon-SR (CAN), Mestinon Timespans, Regonol (CAN)

Class and Category
Chemical: Bromide dimethylcarbamate
Therapeutic: Antimyasthenic
Pregnancy category: Not rated

Indications and Dosages

▶ *To treat symptoms of myasthenia gravis*

I.V. INJECTION

Adults and adolescents. 2 mg q 2 to 3 hr.

▶ *To reverse the effects of neuromuscular blockers*

I.V. INJECTION

Adults and adolescents. 10 to 20 mg after 0.6 to 1.2 mg of I.V. atropine has been given.

DOSAGE ADJUSTMENT Dosage possibly reduced for patients with renal impairment.

Route	Onset	Peak	Duration
I.V.	2 to 5 min	Unknown	2 to 4 hr

Mechanism of Action

Improves muscle strength compromised by myasthenia gravis or neuromuscular blockade by competing with acetylcholine for its binding site on acetylcholinesterase. This action potentiates the effects of acetylcholine on skeletal muscle and the GI tract. Inhibited destruction of acetylcholine allows freer transmission of nerve impulses across the neuromuscular junction.

Contraindications

Hypersensitivity to pyridostigmine or its components, mechanical obstruction of GI or urinary tract

Interactions

DRUGS

aminoglycosides (systemic), capreomycin, hydrocarbon inhalation anesthetics, lidocaine (I.V.), lincomycins, polymyxins, quinine: Possibly antagonized effect of pyridostigmine on skeletal muscle; possibly decreased neuromuscular blocking activity of these drugs (with large doses of pyridostigmine)

anticholinergics: Possibly masking of signs of pyridostigmine overdose and reduced intestinal motility

cholinesterase inhibitors: Increased risk of additive toxicity

edrophonium: Possibly worsening of patient's condition

guanadrel, guanethidine, mecamylamine, neuromuscular blockers, procainamide: Possibly prolonged phase I blocking effect or reversal of nondepolarization blockade

local anesthetics: Inhibited neuronal transmission, increased anesthesia effects *quinidine, trimethaphan:* Possibly antagonized effects of pyridostigmine

Adverse Reactions

CV: Thrombophlebitis
EENT: Increased salivation, lacrimation, miosis
GI: Abdominal cramps, diarrhea, increased peristalsis, nausea, vomiting
GU: Urinary frequency, incontinence, or urgency
MS: Fasciculations, muscle spasms or weakness
RESP: Increased tracheobronchial secretions
SKIN: Diaphoresis, rash

Nursing Considerations

- **WARNING** Maintain a rigid dosing schedule because a missed or late dose of pyridostigmine can precipitate myasthenic crisis.
- Observe for cholinergic reactions, such as muscle weakness, during drug administration.
- Monitor BUN and serum creatinine levels, as ordered, in patients with renal disease because pyridostigmine is mainly excreted unchanged by the kidneys.
- **WARNING** Be aware that pyridostigmine overdose may obscure the diagnosis of myasthenic crisis because the primary symptom in both is muscle weakness. Respiratory muscle involvement can lead to death. Be prepared to treat cholinergic crisis by immediately stopping pyridostigmine therapy, administering atropine as prescribed, and assisting with endotracheal intubation and mechanical ventilation, if needed.
- Be aware that reversal of neuromuscular blockade usually occurs in 15 to 30 minutes. Be prepared to maintain patent airway and ventilation until normal voluntary respiration returns completely. Assess respiratory measurements and muscle tone with peripheral nerve stimulator device, as indicated.
- Store drug at 15° to 30° C (59° to 86° F); protect from freezing and light.

PATIENT TEACHING

- Instruct patient receiving pyridostigmine to report muscle weakness, difficulty breathing, diarrhea, nausea, or vomiting.
- Ask patient to record pyridostigmine dosage, times taken, and effects to help determine optimal dosage and schedule for her needs.
- Urge patient to carry medical identification describing her condition and drug regimen.

pyridoxine hydrochloride
(vitamin B₆)

Beesix, Doxine, Nestrex, Pyri, Rodex, Vitabee 6

Class and Category

Chemical: Water-soluble B complex vitamin
Therapeutic: Nutritional supplement
Pregnancy category: A

Indications and Dosages

▶ *To prevent vitamin B₆ deficiency based on U.S. and Canadian recommended daily allowances (RDAs)*

I.V. INFUSION

Adults and children. Dosage individualized as part of total parenteral nutrition.

▶ *To treat pyridoxine dependency syndrome*

I.V. INJECTION

Adults and children age 11 and older. 30 to 600 mg q.d.
Infants with seizures. *Initial:* 10 to 100 mg, then individualized based on severity of deficiency, as prescribed.

▶ *To treat drug-induced pyridoxine deficiency*

I.V. INJECTION

Adults and children age 11 and older. 50 to 200 mg/day for 3 wk, then 25 to 100 mg/day as needed.

Mechanism of Action

Replaces vitamin in pyridoxine deficiency. In erythrocytes, pyridoxine breaks down to pyridoxal and pyridoxamine, which act as coenzymes in fat, protein, and carbohydrate metabolism. Pyridoxine is used to help convert tryptophan to niacin or serotonin, to break down glycogen to glucose-1-phosphate, and to convert oxalate to glycine. It's also essential in the synthesis of both gamma-aminobutyric acid (within the CNS) and heme.

Contraindications

Hypersensitivity to pyridoxine or its components

Interactions

DRUGS

azathioprine, chlorambucil, corticosteroids, cyclophosphamide, cycloserine, cyclosporine, ethionamide, hydralazine, isoniazid, mercaptopurine, penicillamine: Possibly anemia or peripheral neuritis
estrogens, oral contraceptives: Possibly increased RDA of pyridoxine
levodopa: Reversal of levodopa's antiparkinsonian effects

Adverse Reactions

CNS: Sensory neuropathy

Nursing Considerations

- Assess patient's daily intake of pyridoxine, including any OTC sources. If patient has been ingesting high doses (2 to 6 g/day) for several months, assess for sensory neuropathy, characterized by unstable gait and numbness in feet and hands. If symptoms occur, notify prescriber and expect to discontinue drug.
- Evaluate drug's effectiveness in reversing deficiency by assessing for resolution of signs and symptoms, including xanthurenic aciduria, sideroblastic anemia, neurologic problems, seborrheic dermatitis, and cheilosis.
- Store drug at 15° to 30° C (59° to 86° F); protect from freezing and light.

PATIENT TEACHING

- Instruct patient to report unsteadiness while walking or numbness of hands or feet during pyridoxine therapy.
- Inform patient that vitamin is not a substitute for proper diet. Inform her that best sources of dietary pyridoxine include bananas, egg yolks, lima beans, meat, peanuts, and whole grain cereals.

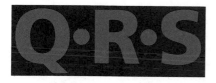

quinidine gluconate

Class and Category

Chemical: Dextrorotatory isomer of quinine
Therapeutic: Class IA antiarrhythmic
Pregnancy category: C

Indications and Dosages

▶ *To prevent or treat cardiac arrhythmias, including established atrial fibrillation, atrial flutter, paroxysmal atrial fibrillation, paroxysmal atrial tachycardia, paroxysmal AV junctional rhythm, paroxysmal ventricular tachycardia not associated with complete heart block, and premature atrial and ventricular contractions*

I.V. INFUSION

Adults. 800 mg in 40 ml of D_5W at a rate of up to 0.25 mg/kg/min.

Mechanism of Action

Depresses excitability, conduction velocity, and contractility of the myocardium and increases the effective refractory period to suppress arrhythmic activity in the atria, ventricles, and His-Purkinje system.

Contraindications

Digitalis toxicity; history of quinidine-induced thrombocytopenic purpura or torsades de pointes; hypersensitivity to quinidine, other cinchona derivatives, or their components; long QT syndrome; myasthenia gravis; pacemaker-dependent conduction disturbances

Interactions

DRUGS

antiarrhythmics, phenothiazines, rauwolfia alkaloids, and other drugs that prolong QT interval: Additive cardiac effects
anticholinergics: Possibly intensified atropine-like adverse effects
antimyasthenics: Antagonized antimyasthenic effects on skeletal muscle

barbiturates, rifampin: Possibly accelerated elimination and decreased effectiveness of quinidine

cimetidine: Increased elimination half-life, possibly leading to quinidine toxicity

digoxin: Possibly digitalis toxicity

hepatic enzyme inducers: Possibly decreased blood quinidine level

hepatic enzyme inhibitors: Possibly increased blood quinidine level

neuromuscular blockers: Possibly potentiated neuromuscular blockade

oral anticoagulants: Additive hypoprothrombinemia, increased risk of bleeding

pimozide: Risk of arrhythmias

quinine: Increased risk of quinidine toxicity

urinary alkalizers (such as antacids, carbonic anhydrase inhibitors, citrates, sodium bicarbonate, and thiazide diuretics): Increased renal tubular reabsorption of quinidine, possibly leading to quinidine toxicity

verapamil: Possibly AV block, bradycardia, pulmonary edema, significant hypotension, and ventricular tachycardia

Adverse Reactions

CNS: Anxiety, asthenia, ataxia, confusion, delirium, difficulty speaking, dizziness, drowsiness, extrapyramidal reactions, fever, headache, hypertonia, syncope, vertigo

CV: Complete heart block, orthostatic hypotension, palpitations, peripheral edema, prolonged QT interval, torsades de pointes, vasculitis, ventricular arrhythmias, widening QRS complex

EENT: Blurred vision, change in color perception, diplopia, dry mouth, hearing loss (high-frequency), pharyngitis, photophobia, rhinitis, tinnitus

GI: Abdominal pain, anorexia, constipation, diarrhea, indigestion, nausea, vomiting

HEME: Agranulocytosis, hemolytic anemia, leukopenia, neutropenia, thrombocytopenia, thrombocytopenic purpura

MS: Arthralgia, myalgia

RESP: Dyspnea

SKIN: Diaphoresis, eczema, exfoliative dermatitis, flushing, hyperpigmentation, photosensitivity, pruritus, psoriasis, purpura, rash, urticaria

Other: Angioedema, flulike symptoms, weight gain

Nursing Considerations
- For intermittent I.V. infusion, dilute quinidine in 40 ml of D_5W and administer using an infusion pump at a rate of 0.25 mg/kg/minute or less. Rapid administration may cause hypotension. Use diluted solutions within 24 hours if stored at room temperature or within 48 hours if refrigerated. Monitor ECG tracings and blood pressure throughout administration.
- Monitor therapeutic blood level of quinidine, as ordered, in all patients receiving drug.
- Monitor heart rate and rhythm closely because quinidine may cause serious adverse reactions and can be cardiotoxic, especially at dosages exceeding 2.4 g/day. Implement continuous cardiac monitoring, as ordered.
- Monitor serum electrolyte levels, especially potassium, as prescribed to identify electrolyte imbalances, which increase patient's risk of developing adverse cardiac reactions such as torsades de pointes.
- Assess for early signs and symptoms of cinchonism, including blurred vision, change in color perception, confusion, diplopia, headache, and tinnitus, which may indicate quinidine toxicity.
- Before diluting quinidine, store it at 15° to 30° C (59° to 86° F).

PATIENT TEACHING
- Urge patient receiving quinidine to immediately report blurred or double vision, change in color perception, confusion, diarrhea, fever, headache, loss of hearing, or tinnitus.

quinupristin and dalfopristin
Synercid

Class and Category
Chemical: Pristinamycin I and IIa derivative, streptogramin
Therapeutic: Antibiotic
Pregnancy category: B

Indications and Dosages
▶ *To treat serious or life-threatening infections, such as bacteremia, caused by vancomycin-resistant* Enterococcus faecium
I.V. INFUSION
Adults and adolescents age 16 and older. 7.5 mg/kg q 8 hr.
▶ *To treat complicated skin and soft-tissue infections caused by methicillin-susceptible strains of* Staphylococcus aureus *or* Streptococcus pyogenes

I.V. INFUSION
Adults and adolescents age 16 and older. 7.5 mg/kg q 12 hr
for at least 7 days.

Mechanism of Action
Inhibits bacterial protein synthesis by irreversibly blocking ribosome functioning. Quinupristin inhibits the late phase of protein synthesis by binding to the
50S ribosomal subunit. Dalfopristin inhibits the early phase of protein synthesis by binding to the 70S or 50S ribosomal subunit. This combined activity
also inhibits transfer RNA (tRNA) synthetase activity, which decreases the
amount of free tRNA within the cell. Without tRNA, the bacterial cell cannot
incorporate amino acids into peptide chains and eventually dies.

Incompatibilities
Don't mix quinupristin and dalfopristin in saline solutions, including NS, 0.45NS, 3% sodium chloride, and 5% sodium chloride, because drug is physically incompatible with these solutions.

Contraindications
Hypersensitivity to quinupristin or dalfopristin, other streptogramin antibiotics, or their components

Interactions
DRUGS
*alfentanil, alprazolam, carbamazepine, delavirdine, diazepam, diltiazem,
disopyramide, dofetilide, donepezil, erythromycin, ethinyl estradiol, felo-
dipine, fexofenadine, indinavir, lidocaine, lovastatin, methylprednisolone,
nevirapine, norethindrone, quinidine, ritonavir, saquinavir, simvastatin,
tacrolimus, triazolam, trimetrexate, verapamil, vinblastine:* Decreased
elimination of these drugs, possibly resulting in toxicity
astemizole, cisapride: Decreased elimination of these drugs, possibly
prolonged QT interval
cyclosporine, midazolam, nifedipine: Possibly increased blood levels of
these drugs
terfenadine: Decreased elimination and increased blood level of
terfenadine, possibly prolonged QT interval

Adverse Reactions
CNS: Anxiety, confusion, dizziness, fever, headache, hypertonia,
insomnia, paresthesia

CV: Chest pain, palpitations, peripheral edema, thrombophlebitis, vasodilation
EENT: Oral candidiasis, stomatitis
GI: Abdominal pain, constipation, diarrhea, elevated liver function test results, indigestion, nausea, pancreatitis, pseudomembranous colitis, vomiting
GU: Hematuria, vaginitis
MS: Arthralgia, gout, muscle spasms, myalgia, myasthenia
RESP: Dyspnea, pleural effusion
SKIN: Diaphoresis, pruritus, rash, urticaria
Other: Injection site edema, inflammation, pain, or thrombophlebitis

Nursing Considerations

- **WARNING** Reconstitute and further dilute quinupristin and dalfopristin only with dextrose in water or sterile water for injection. Don't use saline solutions because drug is physically incompatible with them.
- Reconstitute 500-mg vial (150 mg quinupristin and 350 mg dalfopristin) only with 5 ml of 5% dextrose for injection or sterile water for injection to yield a concentration of 100 mg/ml.
- Swirl gently to mix; don't shake. Let foam dissipate until solution is clear.
- Further dilute reconstituted solution within 30 minutes. Vials are for single use only. Discard any unused portion.
- Dilute prescribed dose in 250 ml of D$_5$W. Use diluted solution as soon as possible to avoid possible microbial contamination—within 5 hours if stored at room temperature or within 54 hours if refrigerated; don't freeze. Infuse drug over 1 hour through a peripheral I.V. line. If administered by central venous catheter, dilute prescribed dose in 100 ml of D$_5$W. Central venous administration may decrease incidence of infusion site reaction. Use an infusion pump or device to control rate of infusion.
- Don't flush I.V. catheter with saline or heparin flush solution because of possible incompatibility. Flush I.V. catheter only with D$_5$W before and after drug administration.
- Monitor patient for diarrhea, a possible indication of overgrowth of normal intestinal flora, such as *Clostridium difficile*. Be aware that pseudomembranous colitis may result from a toxin produced by *C. difficile*.
- If you suspect that patient has pseudomembranous colitis, notify prescriber and expect to stop drug immediately.

- If patient develops pseudomembranous colitis, be aware that drugs that inhibit peristalsis are contraindicated because of the risk of toxic megacolon.
- Assess infusion area for redness or swelling, and ask patient if he feels discomfort. If irritation occurs, expect to change infusion site, increase amount of diluent to 500 or 750 ml, or administer drug by peripherally inserted central catheter, if ordered.
- Store unopened vials of quinupristin and dalfopristin in refrigerator.

PATIENT TEACHING
- Advise patient receiving quinupristin and dalfopristin to immediately report diarrhea or abdominal pains.
- Emphasize the importance of completing the full course of quinupristin and dalfopristin therapy, as prescribed.
- Inform patient that if he requires long-term therapy, drug will be administered either in the hospital or clinic or by a home health care nurse.

ranitidine hydrochloride
Zantac

Class and Category
Chemical: Aminoalkyl-substituted puran derivative
Therapeutic: Antiulcer agent, gastric acid secretion inhibitor
Pregnancy category: B

Indications and Dosages
▶ *To provide short-term treatment of active duodenal and benign gastric ulcers*
CONTINUOUS I.V. INFUSION
Adults and adolescents. 6.25 mg/hr. *Maximum:* 400 mg/day.
INTERMITTENT I.V. INFUSION
Adults and adolescents. 50 mg diluted to total volume of 100 ml and infused over 15 to 20 min q 6 to 8 hr. *Maximum:* 400 mg/day.
Children. 2 to 4 mg/kg/day diluted to a suitable volume and infused over 15 to 20 min.
I.V. INJECTION
Adults and adolescents. 50 mg diluted to total volume of 20 ml and injected slowly, over no less than 5 min, q 6 to 8 hr. *Maximum:* 400 mg/day.

▶ *To treat acute gastroesophageal reflux disease*
INTERMITTENT I.V. INFUSION
Children. 2 to 8 mg/kg diluted to suitable volume and infused over 15 to 20 min t.i.d.

▶ *To treat hypersecretory GI conditions, such as Zollinger-Ellison syndrome, systemic mastocytosis, and multiple endocrine adenoma syndrome*
CONTINUOUS I.V. INFUSION
Adults and adolescents. *Initial:* 1 mg/kg/hr, increased by 0.5 mg/kg/hr up to 2.5 mg/kg/hr. *Maximum:* 400 mg/day.
INTERMITTENT I.V. INFUSION
Adults. 50 mg diluted to total volume of 100 ml and infused over 15 to 20 min q 6 to 8 hr. *Maximum:* 400 mg/day.
I.V. INJECTION
Adults and adolescents. 50 mg diluted to total volume of 20 ml and injected slowly, over no less than 5 min, q 6 to 8 hr. *Maximum:* 400 mg/day.
DOSAGE ADJUSTMENT For adult patients with creatinine clearance of less than 50 ml/min/1.73 m², 50 mg q 18 to 24 hr; dosage interval increased to q 12 hr as needed. Dosage reduction may also be necessary for patients with hepatic dysfunction.

Route	Onset	Peak	Duration
I.V.	Unknown	1 to 3 hr	13 hr

Mechanism of Action
Inhibits basal and nocturnal secretion of gastric acid and pepsin by competitively inhibiting the action of histamine at H_2 receptors on gastric parietal cells. This action reduces total volume of gastric juices and, thus, irritation of GI mucosa.

Contraindications
Acute porphyria, hypersensitivity to ranitidine or its components

Interactions
DRUGS
bone marrow depressants: Increased risk of neutropenia or other blood dyscrasias
diazepam, itraconazole, ketoconazole, sucralfate: Decreased absorption of these drugs

glipizide, glyburide, metoprolol, midazolam, nifedipine, phenytoin, theophylline, warfarin: Increased effects of these drugs, possibly leading to toxic reactions

Adverse Reactions
CNS: Dizziness, drowsiness, headache, insomnia
GI: Abdominal distress, constipation, diarrhea, nausea, vomiting
GU: Impotence
MS: Arthralgia, myalgia

Nursing Considerations
- Be aware that ranitidine must be diluted for I.V. administration if premixed solution is not being used. For I.V. injection, dilute to total volume of 20 ml with NS, D_5W or $D_{10}W$, LR, or 5% sodium bicarbonate. For I.V. infusion, dilute to total volume of 100 ml with any of the above solutions. Use diluted solution within 48 hours if stored at room temperature.
- Administer I.V. injection at no more than 4 ml/minute, intermittent I.V. infusion at 5 to 7 ml/minute, and continuous I.V. infusion at 6.25 mg/hour (except in patients with hypersecretory conditions, for whom initial infusion rate is 1 mg/kg/hour and then gradually increased after 4 hours, as needed, in increments of 0.5 mg/kg/hour).
- Don't introduce additives into premixed solution.
- Stop primary I.V. solution infusion during piggyback administration.
- Store undiluted ranitidine below 30° C (86° F); store premixed form at 2° to 25° C (36° to 77° F). Protect drug from freezing and light.

PATIENT TEACHING
- Instruct patient to report discomfort at ranitidine infusion site.
- Inform patient about potential adverse reactions, such as dizziness, headache, and myalgia, and advise her to report them.
- Inform patient that healing of an ulcer may require 4 to 8 weeks of therapy.

remifentanil hydrochloride
Ultiva

Class, Category, and Schedule
Chemical: Fentanyl analogue
Therapeutic: Anesthesia adjunct
Pregnancy category: C
Controlled substance: Schedule II

Indications and Dosages

▶ *As adjunct to induce general anesthesia*
INTERMITTENT I.V. INFUSION
Adults and children age 2 and older. 0.5 to 1 mcg/kg in addition to inhalation or I.V. anesthetic.

▶ *To maintain general anesthesia*
INTERMITTENT I.V. INFUSION
Adults and children age 2 and older. 0.05 to 0.2 mcg/kg, followed by 0.5 to 1 mcg/kg q 2 to 5 min, as needed.

▶ *To continue analgesic effect in immediate postoperative period*
CONTINUOUS I.V. INFUSION
Adults and children age 2 and older. *Initial:* 0.1 mcg/kg/min, adjusted in increments of 0.025 mcg/kg/min q 5 min, as prescribed, to balance level of analgesia and respiratory rate. *Maximum:* 0.2 mcg/kg/min.

▶ *To supplement local or regional anesthesia in a monitored anesthetic setting*
I.V. INFUSION
Adults and children age 2 and older. *With a benzodiazepine:* 0.05 mcg/kg/min, beginning 5 min before placement of local or regional block; after placement of block, decreased to 0.025 mcg/kg/min and then further adjusted in increments of 0.025 mcg/kg/min q 5 min, as needed. *Without a benzodiazepine:* 0.1 mcg/kg/min, beginning 5 min before placement of local or regional block; after placement of block, decreased to 0.05 mcg/kg/min and then further adjusted in increments of 0.025 mcg/kg/min q 5 min, as needed.

I.V. INJECTION
Adults and children age 2 and older. *With a benzodiazepine:* 0.5 mcg/kg administered over 30 to 60 sec as a single dose 60 to 90 sec before local anesthetic is administered. *Without a benzodiazepine:* 1 mcg/kg administered over 30 to 60 sec as a single dose 60 to 90 sec before local anesthetic is administered.

DOSAGE ADJUSTMENT For elderly patients, starting dose possibly reduced by 50%. For patients who weigh more than 30% over ideal body weight, starting dose based on ideal body weight.

Route	Onset	Peak	Duration
I.V.	1 min	1 to 2 min	5 to 10 min

Mechanism of Action

Remifentanil decreases the transmission and perception of pain by stimulating mu-opioid receptors in neurons. This action decreases the activity of adenyl cyclase in neurons, which in turn decreases cAMP production. With less cAMP available, potassium (K⁺) is forced out of neurons, and calcium (Ca⁺⁺) is prevented from entering neurons, as shown. As a result, neuron excitability declines, and fewer neurotransmitters (such as substance P) leave the neurons, leading to decreased pain transmission.

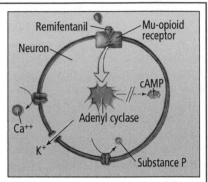

Incompatibilities

Don't administer remifentanil through same I.V. line as blood because nonspecific esterases in blood products may inactivate drug.

Contraindications

Epidural or intrathecal administration, hypersensitivity to remifentanil or other fentanyl analogues

Interactions

DRUGS

anesthetics (barbiturate, inhalation), benzodiazepines, propofol: Possibly synergistic effects, increasing risk of hypotension and respiratory depression

atropine, glycopyrrolate: Possibly reversal of remifentanil-induced bradycardia

ephedrine, epinephrine, norepinephrine: Possibly reversal of remifentanil-induced hypotension

neuromuscular blockers: Prolonged remifentanil-induced skeletal muscle rigidity

opioid antagonists: Possibly reversal of remifentanil's effects

Adverse Reactions

CNS: Headache
CV: Bradycardia, hypotension
GI: Nausea, vomiting
MS: Skeletal muscle rigidity
RESP: Apnea, dyspnea, respiratory depression

Nursing Considerations

- Be aware that remifentanil dosage for obese patients (those weighing at least 30% over ideal body weight) should be based on ideal body weight, not actual weight.
- Verify contents of vial before reconstituting drug. Add 1 ml of suitable diluent per milligram of remifentanil to yield a concentration of 1 mg/ml. Further dilute with appropriate diluent to a final concentration of 25, 50, or 250 (for 5-mg vial) mcg/ml. Use solutions prepared with D₅W, D₅NS, NS, 0.45NS, or D₅LR within 24 hours if stored at room temperature. Use solutions prepared with LR within 4 hours if stored at room temperature.
- Discard solution if you observe particles.
- Inject remifentanil into I.V. tubing at, or as close as possible to, a venous cannula.
- Use an infusion device to administer continuous infusion.
- **WARNING** Be aware that rapid administration of remifentanil may result in skeletal muscle rigidity. To decrease the risk of chest wall rigidity and glottic closure, don't administer more than 1 mcg/kg over 30 to 60 seconds by I.V. injection or more than 0.1 mcg/kg/minute by I.V. infusion.
- Monitor vital signs and oxygenation continuously during administration. Make sure that equipment and drugs needed for endotracheal intubation and resuscitation—including oxygen and an opioid antagonist—are available for immediate administration if ordered.
- Because analgesic effects dissipate rapidly when drug is discontinued, expect to start adequate postoperative analgesia, as prescribed, before stopping drug.
- **WARNING** Clear I.V. tubing after the infusion is discontinued to prevent inadvertent administration of remifentanil when another drug is infused through the same I.V. line.
- Monitor respiratory status continuously because residual effects of other anesthetics increase the risk of respiratory depression for up to 30 minutes after infusion is discontinued.
- Store drug at 2° to 25° C (36° to 77° F).

PATIENT TEACHING
- Explain expected effects of remifentanil to patient, and reassure her that she'll be monitored continuously during drug administration.

reteplase

Retavase

Class and Category

Chemical: Recombinant plasminogen activator (r-PA)
Therapeutic: Thrombolytic
Pregnancy category: C

Indications and Dosages

▶ *To improve ventricular function, prevent heart failure, and reduce mortality after acute MI*

I.V. INJECTION

Adults. 10 U over 2 min; repeated after 30 min.

Mechanism of Action

Converts plasminogen to plasmin, which works to break up fibrin clots that have formed in the coronary arteries. Elimination of the clots improves cardiac blood and oxygen flow to the area, thus improving ventricular function.

Incompatibilities

Don't add other drugs to, or administer them through same I.V. line as, reteplase injection solution.

Contraindications

Active internal bleeding, aneurysm, arteriovenous malformation, bleeding diathesis, brain tumor, history of CVA or other cerebro-vascular disease, hypersensitivity to reteplase or its components, intracranial or intraspinal surgery or trauma during previous 2 months, severe uncontrolled hypertension (systolic blood pressure of 200 mm Hg or higher, diastolic blood pressure of 110 mm Hg or higher)

Interactions

DRUGS

antifibrinolytics (including aminocaproic acid, aprotinin, and tranexamic acid): Decreased effectiveness of reteplase

antineoplastics, antithymocyte globulin, certain cephalosporins (such as cefamandole, cefoperazone, and cefotetan), heparin, oral anticoagulants, platelet aggregation inhibitors (such as abciximab, aspirin, and dipyri-damole), strontium-89 chloride, sulfinpyrazone, valproic acid: Increased risk of bleeding

Adverse Reactions

CNS: Intracranial hemorrhage

GI: GI bleeding, nausea, vomiting
HEME: Thrombocytopenia
RESP: Hemoptysis
SKIN: Bleeding from wounds, ecchymosis, hematoma, purpura
Other: Anaphylaxis, injection site bleeding

Nursing Considerations

• Expect to begin reteplase therapy, as prescribed, as soon as possible after MI symptoms begin.

• Closely monitor patient with atrial fibrillation, severe hypertension, or other cardiac disease for signs and symptoms of cerebral embolism.

• Reconstitute drug using diluent, syringe, needle, and dispensing pin provided. Withdraw 10 ml of preservative-free sterile water for injection. Remove and discard needle from syringe, and connect dispensing pin to syringe. Remove protective cap from spike end of dispensing pin, and insert spike into reteplase vial. Inject 10 ml of sterile water into the vial. With the spike still in the vial, swirl gently—don't shake—to dissolve the powder. Expect to see slight foaming. Let vial stand for several minutes. When bubbles dissipate, withdraw 10 ml of reconstituted solution into syringe (about 0.7 ml may remain in vial). Now detach syringe from dispensing pin and attach 20G needle.

• Use solution within 4 hours. Discard if it appears discolored or contains particles.

• Don't administer heparin and reteplase in same solution. Instead, flush heparin line with NS or D$_5$W before and after reteplase injection.

• Because fibrin is lysed during therapy, closely monitor all possible bleeding sites (catheter insertions, arterial and venous punctures, cutdowns, and needle punctures).

• Avoid I.M. injections, venipunctures, and nonessential handling of patient during therapy.

• If arterial puncture is necessary, use an arm vessel that can be compressed, if possible. After sample is obtained, apply pressure for at least 30 minutes, and then apply a pressure dressing. Check site frequently for bleeding.

• If bleeding occurs and can't be controlled by local pressure, notify prescriber immediately. Be prepared to stop concurrent anticoagulant therapy immediately and to discontinue second reteplase bolus, as prescribed.

- Anticipate that reperfusion arrhythmias—premature ventricular contractions, ventricular tachycardia—may follow coronary thrombolysis.
- Store drug at 2° to 25° C (36° to 77° F), and protect from light.

PATIENT TEACHING

- Advise patient to immediately report adverse reactions to reteplase, including bleeding or bruising, headache, rash, or difficulty breathing.
- Instruct patient to maintain strict bed rest while receiving reteplase to prevent or minimize bleeding.

rifampin
(rifampicin)
Rifadin, Rifadin IV, Rimactane, Rofact (CAN)

Class and Category
Chemical: Semisynthetic antibiotic derivative of rifamycin
Therapeutic: Antimycobacterial antitubercular
Pregnancy category: C

Indications and Dosages
▶ *As adjunct to treat tuberculosis caused by all strains of* Mycobacterium tuberculosis
I.V. INFUSION, CAPSULES, ORAL SUSPENSION
Adults. 10 mg/kg q.d. in combination with other antituberculars for 2 mo. *Maximum:* 600 mg/day.
Infants and children. 10 to 20 mg/kg q.d. in combination with other antituberculars for 2 mo. *Maximum:* 600 mg/day.
▶ *To eliminate meningococci from nasopharynx of asymptomatic carriers of* Neisseria meningitidis
I.V. INFUSION
Adults. 600 mg q 12 hr for 2 days (total of 4 doses).
Infants age 1 month and older and children. 10 mg/kg q 12 hr for 2 days (total of 4 doses). *Maximum:* 600 mg/day.
Infants under age 1 month. 5 mg/kg q 12 hr for 2 days (total of 4 doses). *Maximum:* 600 mg/day.
DOSAGE ADJUSTMENT For patients with hepatic impairment, maximum dosage of 8 mg/kg/day. For patients with creatinine clearance of 10 ml/min/1.73 m^2 or less, recommended dosage usually decreased by 50%.

Incompatibilities
Don't administer rifampin through same I.V. line as diltiazem.

Mechanism of Action
Inhibits bacterial and mycobacterial RNA synthesis by binding to DNA-dependent RNA polymerase, thereby blocking RNA transcription. Rifampin exhibits dose-dependent bactericidal or bacteriostatic action. It's highly effective against rapidly dividing bacilli in extracellular cavitary lesions, such as those found in the nasopharynx.

Contraindications
Concurrent use of nonnucleoside reverse transcriptase inhibitors or protease inhibitors by patients with HIV infection, hypersensitivity to rifampin or other rifamycins

Interactions
DRUGS

aminophylline, oxtriphylline, theophylline: Increased metabolism and clearance of these theophylline preparations

beta blockers, chloramphenicol, clofibrate, corticosteroids, cyclosporine, dapsone, digitalis glycosides, disopyramide, hexobarbital, itraconazole, ketoconazole, mexiletine, oral anticoagulants, oral antidiabetic drugs, phenytoin, propafenone, quinidine, tocainide, verapamil (oral): Increased metabolism, resulting in lower blood levels of these drugs

bone marrow depressants: Increased leukopenic or thrombocytopenic effects

clofazimine: Reduced absorption of rifampin, resulting in delayed peak concentration and increased half-life

diazepam: Enhanced elimination of diazepam, resulting in decreased drug effectiveness

estramustine, estrogens, oral contraceptives: Decreased estrogenic effects

hepatotoxic drugs, hydrocarbon inhalation anesthetics (except isoflurane), isoniazid: Increased risk of hepatotoxicity

methadone: Possibly impaired absorption of methadone, leading to withdrawal symptoms

nonnucleoside reverse transcriptase inhibitors, protease inhibitors (indinavir, nelfinavir, ritonavir, saquinavir): Accelerated metabolism of these drugs by patients with HIV infection, resulting in subtherapeutic levels; delayed metabolism of rifampin, increasing risk of toxicity

probenecid: Increased blood level or prolonged duration of rifampin, increasing risk of toxicity

trimethoprim: Increased elimination and shortened elimination half-life of trimethoprim

ACTIVITIES
alcohol use: Increased risk of hepatotoxicity

Adverse Reactions

CNS: Chills, dizziness, drowsiness, fatigue, headache, paresthesia
EENT: Discolored saliva, tears, and sputum; mouth or tongue soreness; periorbital edema
GI: Abdominal cramps, anorexia, diarrhea, discolored feces, elevated liver function test results, epigastric discomfort, flatulence, heartburn, hepatitis, nausea, pseudomembranous colitis, vomiting
GU: Discolored urine
MS: Arthralgia, myalgia
SKIN: Discolored skin and sweat
Other: Facial edema, flulike symptoms

Nursing Considerations

- Obtain blood samples or other specimens for culture and sensitivity testing, as ordered, before giving rifampin and throughout therapy to monitor patient's response to drug.
- Expect to monitor liver function test results before and every 2 to 4 weeks during therapy. Notify prescriber immediately of abnormalities.
- Reconstitute by adding 10 ml of sterile water for injection to 600-mg vial of rifampin. Swirl gently to dissolve. Withdraw appropriate dose, add to 500 ml of D₅W (preferred solution) or NS, and infuse over 3 hours. Alternatively, withdraw appropriate dose, add to 100 ml of D₅W (preferred solution) or NS, and infuse over 30 minutes. Use reconstituted drug promptly because rifampin may precipitate out of D₅W solution after 4 hours. Solution prepared in NS is stable for up to 24 hours at room temperature.
- Be aware that patient receiving intermittent therapy (once or twice weekly) is at increased risk for adverse reactions.
- Expect drug to cause reddish orange to reddish brown discoloration of skin and body fluids.
- Be aware that rifampin can cause myelosuppression and increase the risk of infection. Notify prescriber immediately if patient develop signs of infection such as fever.
- Store drug at less than 40° C (104° F).

PATIENT TEACHING
- Urge patient receiving rifampin to report flulike symptoms, anorexia, darkened urine, fever, joint pain or swelling, malaise, nausea, vomiting, and yellowish skin or eyes, which may indicate hepatitis.

- Instruct patient to take oral rifampin 1 hour before or 2 hours after a meal with a full glass of water. Stress the need to take drug exactly as prescribed. Explain that interruptions can lead to increased adverse reactions.
- Explain that drug may turn urine, feces, saliva, sputum, sweat, tears, and skin reddish orange to reddish brown.
- Caution patient against wearing soft contact lenses during therapy because drug may permanently stain them.
- Advise patient who takes an oral contraceptive to use an additional form of birth control during rifampin therapy.
- Advise patient to avoid alcohol during rifampin therapy.
- Instruct patient to notify prescriber if no improvement occurs within 2 to 3 weeks.

rituximab

Rituxan

Class and Category

Chemical: Chimeric murine/human monoclonal antibody
Therapeutic: Antineoplastic
Pregnancy category: C

Indications and Dosages

▶ *To treat relapsed or refractory, low-grade or follicular, CD20-positive, B-cell non-Hodgkin's lymphoma*

I.V. INFUSION

Adults. *Initial:* 375 mg/m^2 q wk for 4 or 8 wk. *Retreatment:* 375 mg/m^2 q wk for 4 wk.

Mechanism of Action

Binds to the antigen CD20, a hydrophobic transmembrane protein that mediates B-cell lysis. Found on pre-B and mature B lymphocytes and in more than 90% of B-cell non-Hodgkin's lymphomas, CD20 regulates early steps in cell cycle initiation and differentiation and may also act as a calcium ion channel.

Contraindications

History of anaphylaxis or IgE-mediated hypersensitivity to murine proteins or to rituximab or its components

Interactions
DRUGS
antihypertensives: Possibly increased risk of hypotension
cisplatin: Possibly increased risk of renal toxicity
vaccines, killed virus: Possibly inhibited response to vaccine
vaccines, live virus: Possibly inhibited response to vaccine, increased risk of adverse effects of vaccine, and severe or fatal infection

Adverse Reactions
CNS: Agitiation, anxiety, chills, fever, headache, hypoesthesia, insomnia, malaise, nervousness, paresthesia
CV: Angina, arrhythmias, hypertension, hypotension, peripheral edema
EENT: Altered taste, conjunctivitis, pharyngitis, rhinitis
ENDO: Hypoglycemia
GI: Abdominal distention or pain, anorexia, diarrhea, indigestion, nausea, vomiting
HEME: Anemia, leukopenia, neutropenia, thrombocytopenia
MS: Arthralgia, back pain
RESP: Bronchospasm, cough, dyspnea
SKIN: Flushing of face, paraneoplastic pemphigus, Stevens-Johnson syndrome, toxic epidermal necrolysis, urticaria
Other: Angioedema, infusion site pain, tumor lysis syndrome (acute renal failure, hyperkalemia, hyperuricemia, and hyperphosphatemia)

Nursing Considerations
- Be aware that prescriber may order antihypertensives to be withheld if scheduled for administration within 12 hours of rituximab infusion because rituximab may cause transient hypotension.
- Dilute rituximab with NS or D_5W to a final concentration of 1 to 4 mg/ml. Invert the bag and mix gently. Discard any unused rituximab because it contains no preservatives. Use within 24 hours if stored at 2° to 8° C (36° to 46° F).
- Administer acetaminophen and diphenhydramine before each infusion of rituximab, if ordered, to lessen severity of infusion reactions.
- Don't administer rituximab as an I.V. bolus or injection. Begin first infusion at a rate of 50 mg/hour. Increase rate in increments of 50 mg/hour every 30 minutes up to a maximum of 400 mg/hour if no hypersensitivity or infusion reactions occur. If patient experiences a mild to moderate reaction, expect to slow or discontinue infusion and administer bronchodilators,

antihistamines, corticosteroids, epinephrine, oxygen, and I.V. fluids, if ordered. If symptoms improve, be prepared to continue infusion at 50% of previous rate.

- **WARNING** Monitor patient closely for signs and symptoms of a severe infusion reaction, which is most likely to occur during the first infusion. If a severe infusion reaction occurs, discontinue infusion and notify prescriber immediately. Be alert for signs of acute respiratory distress syndrome, angioedema, cardiogenic shock, hypoxia, MI, pulmonary infiltrates, and ventricular fibrillation.

- If no infusion reaction occurs, initiate subsequent infusions at a rate of 100 mg/hour and increase in increments of 100 mg/hour every 30 minutes to a maximum of 400 mg/hour. If a reaction occurred during initial infusion, follow initial infusion guidelines for subsequent infusions.

- Expect to discontinue infusion if serious or life-threatening cardiac arrhythmias occur. Maintain continuous cardiac monitoring during and immediately after rituximab infusion for patients who develop arrhythmias during rituximab infusion and for those with preexisting cardiac conditions, such as arrhythmias or angina.

- Monitor CBC and platelet counts periodically during therapy (more often in patients who develop cytopenias). If patient develops thrombocytopenia, implement protective measures according to facility policy.

- Before diluting rituximab, store it at 2° to 8° C (36° to 46° F). Protect from direct sunlight.

PATIENT TEACHING

- Instruct patient to immediately report possible signs or symptoms of a hypersensitivity or infusion reaction, including difficulty breathing, rash, palpitations, and nausea.

- Advise patient to immediately report unusual bleeding or bruising, black or tarry stools, blood in urine or stools, or red pinpoint spots on skin.

scopolamine hydrobromide

Class and Category
Chemical: Belladonna alkaloid, tertiary amine
Therapeutic: Anesthesia adjunct, anticholinergic, antiemetic, antispasmodic, antivertigo agent
Pregnancy category: C

Indications and Dosages

▶ *To treat biliary tract disorders, enuresis, nausea and vomiting, and nocturia*

I.V. INJECTION

Adults and adolescents. 300 to 600 mcg (0.3 to 0.6 mg) as a single dose.

Children. 6 mcg (0.006 mg)/kg as a single dose.

▶ *As adjunct to anesthesia to induce sleep and calmness*

I.V. INJECTION

Adults and adolescents. 0.6 mg t.i.d. or q.i.d.

▶ *As adjunct to anesthesia to induce amnesia*

I.V. INJECTION

Adults and adolescents. 0.32 to 0.65 mg.

DOSAGE ADJUSTMENT Dosage reduction possible for elderly patients because of their increased sensitivity to scopolamine.

Route	Onset	Peak	Duration
I.V.*	10 min	50 to 80 min	2 hr

Mechanism of Action

Competitively inhibits acetylcholine at autonomic postganglionic cholinergic receptors. Because the most sensitive receptors are in the salivary, bronchial, and sweat glands, this action reduces secretions from these glands. Scopolamine also decreases nasal and oropharyngeal secretions, GI smooth-muscle tone and bladder detrusor muscle tone, and gastric secretions and GI motility. It also relaxes smooth muscles in the bronchi and bronchioles, resulting in decreased airway resistance.

In addition, scopolamine blocks neural pathways in the inner ear. This action relieves motion sickness and depresses the cerebral cortex to produce sedation and hypnotic effects.

Contraindications

Angle-closure glaucoma; hemorrhage with hemodynamic instability; hepatic dysfunction; hypersensitivity to barbiturates, scopolamine, other belladonna alkaloids, or their components; ileus; intestinal atony; myasthenia gravis; myocardial ischemia; obstructive GI disease, such as pyloric stenosis; obstructive uropathy, as

---

* For amnesia.

in prostatic hyperplasia; renal impairment; tachycardia; toxic megacolon; ulcerative colitis

Interactions
DRUGS

antimyasthenics: Possibly reduced intestinal motility

CNS depressants: Possibly potentiated effects of either drug, resulting in additive sedation

cyclopropane: Increased risk of ventricular arrhythmias

haloperidol: Decreased antipsychotic effect of haloperidol

ketoconazole: Decreased absorption of ketoconazole

lorazepam (parenteral): Possibly hallucinations, irrational behavior, and sedation

metoclopramide: Possibly antagonized effect of metoclopramide on GI motility

opioid analgesics: Increased risk of severe constipation and ileus

other anticholinergics: Possibly intensified anticholinergic effects

potassium chloride: Possibly increased severity of potassium chloride–induced GI lesions

urinary alkalizers (antacids, carbonic anhydrase inhibitors, citrates, sodium bicarbonate): Delayed excretion of scopolamine, possibly leading to increased therapeutic and adverse effects

ACTIVITIES

alcohol use: Additive CNS effects

Adverse Reactions
CNS: Dizziness, drowsiness, euphoria, insomnia, memory loss, paradoxical stimulation

CV: Palpitations, tachycardia

EENT: Blurred vision; dry eyes, mouth, nose, and throat; mydriasis

GI: Constipation, dysphagia

GU: Urinary hesitancy, urine retention

SKIN: Decreased sweating, dry skin, flushing

Other: Injection site irritation or redness

Nursing Considerations
• Dilute scopolamine with sterile water for injection.

• Assess for bladder distention and monitor urine output because drug's antimuscarinic effects on ureters and bladder can cause urine retention.

• Monitor for pain. In presence of pain, drug may act as a stimulant and produce delirium if used without morphine or meperidine.

- Monitor heart rate for transient tachycardia, which may occur with high doses of scopolamine. Expect normal rate to return within 30 minutes.
- Store scopolamine at 15° to 30° C (59° to 86° F) in a light-resistant container; don't freeze.

PATIENT TEACHING
- Advise patient to avoid potentially hazardous activities until scopolamine's CNS effects are known.
- Instruct patient to avoid alcohol while receiving scopolamine.
- Suggest lubricating drops to relieve dry eyes.

sodium bicarbonate

Class and Category
Chemical: Electrolyte
Therapeutic: Electrolyte replenisher, systemic and urinary alkalizer
Pregnancy category: C

Indications and Dosages
▶ *To provide urinary alkalization*
I.V. INFUSION
Adults and children. 2 to 5 mEq/kg over 4 to 8 hr.
▶ *To treat metabolic acidosis during cardiac arrest*
I.V. INJECTION
Adults and children. *Initial:* 1 mEq/kg, followed by 0.5 mEq/kg q 10 min while arrest continues.
▶ *To treat less urgent forms of metabolic acidosis*
I.V. INFUSION
Adults and children. 2 to 5 mEq/kg over 4 to 8 hr.
DOSAGE ADJUSTMENT Dosage reduction possible for elderly patients because of age-related renal impairment.

Mechanism of Action
Increases plasma bicarbonate level, buffers excess hydrogen ions, and raises blood pH, thereby reversing metabolic acidosis. Sodium bicarbonate also increases the excretion of free bicarbonate ions in urine, raising urine pH; increased alkalinity of urine may help to dissolve uric acid calculi.

Incompatibilities
Don't mix sodium bicarbonate in same solution or administer through same I.V. line as other drugs because a precipitate may form.

Contraindications

Hypocalcemia in which alkalosis may lead to tetany; hypochloremic alkalosis secondary to vomiting, diuretics, or nasogastric suction; preexisting metabolic or respiratory alkalosis

Interactions

DRUGS

amphetamines, quinidine: Decreased urinary excretion of these drugs, possibly resulting in toxicity

anticholinergics: Decreased anticholinergic absorption and effectiveness

chlorpropamide, lithium, salicylates, tetracyclines: Increased renal excretion of these drugs

ciprofloxacin, norfloxacin, ofloxacin: Decreased solubility of these drugs, leading to crystalluria and nephrotoxicity

citrates: Increased risk of systemic alkalosis; increased risk of calcium calculus formation and hypernatremia in patients with history of uric acid calculi

digoxin: Possibly elevated blood digoxin level

ephedrine: Increased ephedrine half-life and duration of action

mecamylamine: Decreased excretion and prolonged effect of mecamylamine

methenamine: Decreased methenamine effectiveness

mexiletine: Possibly mexiletine toxicity

potassium supplements: Decreased serum potassium level

urinary acidifiers (ammonium chloride, ascorbic acid, potassium and sodium phosphates): Counteracted effects of urinary acidifiers

Adverse Reactions

CNS: Mental or mood changes

CV: Irregular heartbeat, peripheral edema (with large doses), weak pulse

EENT: Dry mouth

GI: Abdominal cramps, thirst

MS: Muscle spasms, myalgia

SKIN: Extravasation with necrosis, tissue sloughing, or ulceration

Nursing Considerations

• Dilute sodium bicarbonate with NS, D_5W, or other standard electrolyte solution before administration.

• **WARNING** Avoid rapid I.V. infusion, which can cause severe alkalosis. However, be aware that during cardiac arrest, the risk of death from acidosis may outweigh the risks associated with rapid infusion. In addition, rapid administration in children under age 2 poses a risk of hypernatremia accompanied by decreased CSF pressure and, possibly, intracranial hemorrhage.

• Monitor urine pH, as ordered, to determine drug's effectiveness as urinary alkalizer.

• Be aware that parenteral formulations are hypertonic and that increased sodium intake can produce edema and weight gain. Patients with impaired renal function, heart failure, or other conditions that predispose them to sodium retention or edema are at increased risk.

• Assess I.V. site frequently for signs and symptoms of extravasation. If this occurs, notify prescriber immediately and remove I.V. catheter. Elevate the extremity, apply warm compresses, and expect prescriber to administer a local injection of hyaluronidase or lidocaine.

• When calculating sodium intake for patients on a sodium-restricted diet, keep in mind that sodium bicarbonate contains varying amounts of sodium, depending on concentration of solution used; check label to calculate amount of sodium that patient is receiving.

• Store drug at 15° to 30° C (59° to 86° F); don't freeze.

PATIENT TEACHING

• Advise patient receiving sodium bicarbonate to report pain, swelling, or redness at I.V. insertion site.

• Instruct patient to avoid taking OTC drugs without prescriber's approval because many drugs interact with sodium bicarbonate.

sodium ferric gluconate
(contains 62.5 mg of elemental iron per 5 ml)
Ferrlecit

Class and Category
Chemical: Iron salt, mineral
Therapeutic: Antianemic
Pregnancy category: B

Indications and Dosages
▶ *To treat iron-deficiency anemia in chronic hemodialysis patients receiving erythropoietin*
I.V. INFUSION OR INJECTION
Adults. 125 mg of elemental iron, repeated at lowest dose necessary to maintain target levels of hemoglobin and hematocrit and acceptable blood iron levels, up to a total dose of 1 g.

Mechanism of Action

Acts to replenish iron stores lost during hemodialysis because of increased blood loss or increased iron utilization from epoetin therapy. Iron is an essential component of hemoglobin, myoglobin, and several enzymes, including cytochromes, catalase, and peroxidase, and is needed for catecholamine metabolism and normal neutrophil function. Sodium ferric gluconate also normalizes RBC production by binding with hemoglobin or being stored as ferritin in reticuloendothelial cells of the liver, spleen, and bone marrow.

Incompatibilities

Don't mix sodium ferric gluconate with other drugs or with parenteral nutrition solutions for I.V. infusion.

Contraindications

Anemia other than iron deficiency type, hypersensitivity to iron salts or their components, iron overload

Interactions

DRUGS

oral iron preparations: Possibly reduced absorption of oral iron

Adverse Reactions

CNS: Asthenia, dizziness, fatigue, fever, headache, hypertonia, nervousness, paresthesia, syncope
CV: Chest pain, edema, hypertension, hypotension, tachycardia
EENT: Dry mouth
GI: Abdominal pain, diarrhea, nausea, vomiting
HEME: Hemorrhage
MS: Back pain, leg cramps
RESP: Cough, dyspnea, upper respiratory tract infection
SKIN: Pruritus
Other: Allergic or hypersensitivity reaction, generalized pain, hyperkalemia, infusion or injection site reaction

Nursing Considerations

- To reconstitute sodium ferric gluconate for I.V. infusion, dilute prescribed dose in 100 ml of NS immediately before infusion. Infuse over 1 hour. Discard any unused diluted solution.
- Inspect drug for particles and discoloration before administration; discard if present.
- Administer undiluted drug by slow I.V. injection at a rate of up to 12.5 mg/minute, not to exceed 125 mg per injection.

- Be aware that most patients require a minimum cumulative dose of 1 g of elemental iron administered over 8 sessions at sequential dialysis treatments.
- **WARNING** Assess patient for signs and symptoms of an allergic reaction, including chills, facial flushing, pruritus, and rash, and of a hypersensitivity reaction, including diaphoresis, dyspnea, nausea, severe lower back pain, vomiting, and wheezing. If patient develops either type of reaction, discontinue drug, notify prescriber immediately, and be prepared to provide emergency interventions.
- **WARNING** Assess blood pressure frequently after drug administration because hypotension may be related to rate of infusion (avoid rapid infusion) or total cumulative dose. Be prepared to provide I.V. fluids for volume expansion.
- Expect to monitor blood hemoglobin and hematocrit levels, serum ferritin level, and transferrin saturation, as ordered, before, during, and after sodium ferric gluconate therapy. Make sure that serum iron levels are tested 48 hours after last dose. Notify prescriber and expect to discontinue therapy if blood iron levels are normal or elevated, to prevent iron toxicity.
- Assess patient for possible iron overload, characterized by sedation, decreased activity, pale conjunctivae, and bleeding in GI tract and lungs.
- Store drug at 20° to 25° C (68° to 77° F), although excursions to 15° to 30° C (59° to 86° F) are permitted; don't freeze.

PATIENT TEACHING
- Caution patient not to take any oral iron preparations during sodium ferric gluconate therapy without first consulting prescriber.
- Inform patient that symptoms of iron deficiency may include decreased stamina, learning problems, shortness of breath, and fatigue.
- Stress the importance of keeping scheduled follow-up appointments and obtaining prescribed diagnostic tests to monitor treatment outcomes.

sodium thiosalicylate
Rexolate, Tusal

Class and Category
Chemical: Salicylic acid derivative
Therapeutic: Analgesic, anti-inflammatory
Pregnancy category: Not rated

Indications and Dosages

▶ *To relieve symptoms of acute gout*
I.V. INJECTION
Adults. *Initial:* 100 mg q 3 to 4 hr for 2 days, followed by 100 mg/day.

▶ *To relieve pain from musculoskeletal conditions*
I.V. INJECTION
Adults. 50 to 100 mg q.d. or q.o.d.

▶ *To relieve symptoms of osteoarthritis*
I.V. INJECTION
Adults. 100 mg 3 times/wk for several wk, followed by 100 mg once/wk, usually up to a total dose of 2.5 g. After 1 to 2 wk, another course of treatment may be given.

▶ *To treat rheumatic fever*
I.V. INJECTION
Adults. *Initial:* 100 to 150 mg q 4 to 8 hr for 3 days, followed by 100 mg b.i.d.

Mechanism of Action

Exerts peripherally Induced analgesic and anti-inflammatory effects by blocking pain impulses and inhibiting prostaglandin synthesis.

Contraindications

GI bleeding; hemophilia; hemorrhage; hypersensitivity to sodium thiosalicylate, NSAIDs, or their components; Reye's syndrome

Interactions

DRUGS

ACE inhibitors, beta blockers: Decreased antihypertensive effect of these drugs

activated charcoal: Decreased sodium thiosalicylate absorption

antacids, urinary alkalizers: Increased sodium thiosalicylate excretion, leading to reduced effectiveness and shortened half-life

carbonic anhydrase inhibitors (such as acetazolamide): Increased risk of salicylate toxicity; possibly displacement of acetazolamide from protein-binding sites, resulting in toxicity

corticosteroids: Possibly increased sodium thiosalicylate excretion

insulin, oral antidiabetic drugs: Altered glucose control (with large doses of sodium thiosalicylate)

loop diuretics: Possibly decreased effectiveness of loop diuretics in patients with renal or hepatic impairment

methotrexate: Increased risk of methotrexate toxicity

nizatidine: Increased blood sodium thiosalicylate level
probenecid, sulfinpyrazone: Decreased uricosuric effects
spironolactone: Possibly inhibited diuretic effect of spironolactone
urinary acidifiers (including ammonium chloride, ascorbic acid, and methionine): Decreased sodium thiosalicylate excretion, possibly leading to salicylate toxicity
ACTIVITIES
alcohol use: Increased risk of GI ulceration

Adverse Reactions

GI: Anorexia, diarrhea, GI bleeding, heartburn, hepatotoxicity, indigestion, nausea, thirst, vomiting
HEME: Leukopenia, platelet dysfunction, prolonged bleeding time, thrombocytopenia
RESP: Bronchospasm
SKIN: Rash, urticaria
Other: Angioedema

Nursing Considerations

- Inspect vial of sodium thiosalicylate before administration. If you detect a slight precipitate from oxidation, shake vial well. Discard if precipitate doesn't dissolve.
- Administer drug by slow injection.
- Monitor for signs of a hypersensitivity reaction, such as angioedema, bronchospasm, and rash. Patients with asthma, chronic urticaria, or nasal polyps are more prone to drug hypersensitivity.
- Expect to monitor hepatic and renal function during long-term drug therapy.
- After repeated administration or large doses, assess for signs of salicylate toxicity: CNS depression, confusion, diaphoresis, diarrhea, difficulty hearing, dizziness, headache, hyperventilation, lassitude, tinnitus, and vomiting.
- Be aware that tinnitus usually means that blood sodium thiosalicylate level has reached or exceeded upper limits for therapeutic effects.
- Store drug at 15° to 30° C (59° to 86° F).
PATIENT TEACHING
- Instruct patient to report bleeding or symptoms of salicylate toxicity immediately.

streptokinase

Kabikinase, Streptase

Class and Category

Chemical: Purified beta-hemolytic *Streptococcus* filtrate
Therapeutic: Thrombolytic
Pregnancy category: C

Indications and Dosages

▶ *To lyse coronary artery thrombi*

I.V. INFUSION

Adults. 1,500,000 IU within 60 min of event.

INTRACORONARY INFUSION

Adults. 20,000-IU bolus, followed by 2,000 IU/min for 60 min for total dose of 140,000 IU.

▶ *To lyse acute arterial thromboembolism or thrombosis, acute pulmonary embolism, or deep vein thrombosis*

I.V. INFUSION

Adults. 250,000-IU bolus over 30 min, followed by 100,000 IU/hr for 24 to 72 hr.

▶ *To clear occluded arteriovenous cannula*

I.V. INJECTION

Adults. 100,000 to 250,000 IU instilled slowly into each occluded lumen.

Route	Onset	Peak	Duration
I.V.	Immediate	20 to 120 min	4 hr

Mechanism of Action

Binds to fibrin in a thrombus and converts trapped plasminogen to plasmin. Plasmin breaks down fibrin, fibrinogen, and other clotting factors, thereby dissolving the thrombus.

Incompatibilities

Don't mix streptokinase in same syringe or administer through same I.V. line as other drugs.

Contraindications

Active internal bleeding, arteriovenous malformation or aneurysm, bleeding diathesis, CVA or intracranial or intraspinal surgery within the past 2 months, hypersensitivity to streptokinase or its components, intracranial cancer, severe uncontrolled hypertension

Interactions
DRUGS
anticoagulants, enoxaparin, heparin, NSAIDs, platelet aggregation inhibitors: Increased risk of bleeding
antifibrinolytics: Antagonized effects of both drugs
antihypertensives: Increased risk of severe hypotension, especially when streptokinase is administered rapidly to treat coronary artery occlusion
cefamandole, cefoperazone, cefotetan, plicamycin, valproic acid: Possibly hypoprothrombinemia and increased risk of severe hemorrhage
corticosteroids, ethacrynic acid, salicylates: Possibly GI ulceration or bleeding

Adverse Reactions
CNS: Chills, fever
CV: Arrhythmias, hypotension
HEME: Unusual bleeding or bruising
Other: Allergic reaction

Nursing Considerations
- Obtain hematocrit, platelet count, APTT, PT, and INR, as ordered, before, during, and after streptokinase therapy.
- Consult manufacturer's instructions for reconstituting and diluting drug for I.V. and intracoronary infusions. If drug will be used to clear occluded arteriovenous cannula, slowly reconstitute 250,000-IU vial with 2 ml of sodium chloride injection or 5% dextrose injection.
- To prevent foaming, don't shake drug during reconstitution.
- Frequently assess for bleeding at I.V. site and for blood in urine and stools. Perform neurologic assessment to detect intracranial bleeding.
- Monitor the following patients for signs and symptoms of bleeding or hemorrhage because they're at increased risk during streptokinase therapy: pregnant women and patients with acute pericarditis (risk of hemopericardium, possibly leading to cardiac tamponade); cerebrovascular disease; hemorrhagic ophthalmic conditions; history of major surgery, GI or GU bleeding, or trauma within past 10 days; hypertension; mitral stenosis with atrial fibrillation (risk of embolism); septic thrombophlebitis; severe hepatic or renal disease; or subacute bacterial endocarditis.
- Closely monitor all puncture sites, such as catheter insertion and needle puncture sites, for bleeding.

- If serious spontaneous bleeding occurs and can't be controlled by local pressure, stop streptokinase infusion immediately and notify prescriber.
- Monitor for signs of a hypersensitivity reaction, such as nausea, pruritus, rash, or wheezing. Keep equipment and drugs used to treat anaphylaxis, such as epinephrine, glucocorticoids, and antihistamines, nearby.
- Monitor heart rate and rhythm by continuous ECG, as ordered.
- Avoid giving I.M. injections and handling patient unnecessarily during streptokinase therapy. Perform venipuncture only when necessary, using a 23G or smaller needle.
- If an arterial puncture is needed after streptokinase administration, use an arm vessel that allows easy manual compression. Apply manual pressure for 30 minutes. Then apply a pressure dressing and check puncture site frequently for bleeding.
- Treat fever with acetaminophen, as prescribed, rather than aspirin to reduce the risk of bleeding.
- Store drug at 15° to 30° C (59° to 86° F).

PATIENT TEACHING

- Explain to patient that he'll be on bed rest during streptokinase therapy.
- Inform patient that minor bleeding may occur at arterial puncture or surgical sites. Reassure him that appropriate care measures will be taken if bleeding occurs.
- Advise patient to obtain medical alert identification stating that he's receiving streptokinase.
- If patient experiences chest pain within 12 months of receiving streptokinase, instruct him to inform health care providers about his streptokinase therapy because repeated administration within 12 months may be ineffective.

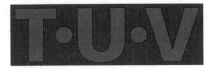

tenecteplase
TNKase

Class and Category
Chemical: Purified glycoprotein
Therapeutic: Thrombolytic
Pregnancy category: C

Indications and Dosages
▶ *To reduce mortality associated with acute MI*
I.V. INJECTION
Adults. Single bolus administered over 5 sec in individualized dosage based on patient's weight, as follows: 30 mg (6 ml) for patients who weigh less than 60 kg; 35 mg (7 ml) for patients who weigh 60 to 69 kg; 40 mg (8 ml) for patients who weigh 70 to 79 kg; 45 mg (9 ml) for patients who weigh 80 to 89 kg; 50 mg (10 ml) for patients who weigh 90 kg or more. *Maximum:* 50 mg total dose.

Mechanism of Action
Activates plasminogen, a naturally occurring substance secreted by endothelial cells in response to arterial wall injury that contributes to clot formation. Plasminogen is converted into plasmin, which breaks down the fibrin mesh that binds the clot together, resulting in dissolution of the clot.

Incompatibilities
Don't administer tenecteplase through an I.V. line containing dextrose because precipitation may occur.

Contraindications
Active internal bleeding, aneurysm, arteriovenous malformation, bleeding diathesis, brain tumor, history of CVA, hypersensitivity to tenecteplase or its components, intracranial or intraspinal surgery or trauma within past 2 months, severe uncontrolled hypertension

Interactions
DRUGS

abciximab, aspirin, clopidogrel, dipyridamole, heparin, oral anticoagulants, ticlopidine: Possibly increased risk of bleeding

Adverse Reactions

CNS: Intracranial hemorrhage
EENT: Epistaxis, gingival bleeding, pharyngeal bleeding
GI: GI and retroperitoneal bleeding
GU: Genitourinary bleeding, prolonged or heavy menstrual bleeding
HEME: Hematoma
RESP: Hemoptysis
SKIN: Bleeding at puncture sites, surgical incision sites, or venous cutdown sites

Nursing Considerations

- **WARNING** Reconstitute tenecteplase for injection immediately before use because drug contains no antibacterial preservatives. If reconstituted drug isn't used immediately, refrigerate vial at 2° to 8° C (36° to 46° F). Discard solution if not used within 8 hours.

- To reconstitute and administer drug, use supplied 10-ml syringe with dual cannula device. Withdraw 10 ml of supplied (preservative-free) sterile water for injection into syringe, and inject entire contents into vial containing tenecteplase dry powder, directing stream of diluent into powder. Gently swirl—don't shake—vial until contents are completely dissolved. If slight foaming occurs during reconstitution, allow drug to stand undisturbed for a few minutes to allow large bubbles to dissipate. Then, using supplied syringe, withdraw prescribed dose of tenecteplase from reconstituted drug in vial. Make sure that reconstituted preparation is a colorless to pale yellow transparent solution. Discard any unused portion.

- Administer drug as a single I.V. bolus over 5 seconds. Although supplied syringe is intended for use with needleless I.V. systems, be aware that it is also compatible with a conventional needle. Follow manufacturer's directions for use with each system. Flush any dextrose-containing I.V. lines with saline solution before and after administering tenecteplase.

- **WARNING** Monitor for signs and symptoms of GI bleeding, including bloody or black, tarry stools; bloody or coffee-ground vomitus; and severe stomach pain. Notify prescriber at once if patient develops any of these signs or symptoms.

- Assess tenecteplase injection site for signs and symptoms of hematoma, including deep, dark purple bruises under skin and itching, pain, redness, or swelling. Also monitor for superficial bleeding, delayed bleeding at puncture sites, and bleeding from surgical incisions.
- Assess for signs and symptoms of intracranial bleeding (such as decreased LOC), retroperitoneal bleeding (such as abdominal pain or swelling and back pain), genitourinary bleeding (such as hematuria), or respiratory tract bleeding (such as hemoptysis). Notify prescriber immediately if patient develops any of these signs or symptoms.
- If serious bleeding (not controllable by local pressure) occurs, expect to discontinue concomitant heparin or oral antiplatelet therapy immediately.
- If possible, avoid I.M. injections and nonessential handling of patient for first few hours after drug administration.
- If arterial puncture becomes necessary during first few hours after tenecteplase administration, expect to use an upper extremity that is accessible to manual compression. Apply pressure for at least 30 minutes after procedure, use a pressure dressing, and frequently monitor puncture site for signs of bleeding.
- Before reconstituting tenecteplase, store it at controlled room temperature or refrigerate it.

PATIENT TEACHING
- Instruct patient to limit physical activity during tenecteplase administration to reduce the risk of injury or bleeding.
- Advise patient to immediately report any bleeding, including from nose or gums.

theophylline in dextrose injection

Class and Category
Chemical: Xanthine derivative
Therapeutic: Bronchodilator
Pregnancy category: C

Indications and Dosages
▶ *As loading dose to treat reversible airway obstruction in patients not currently receiving theophylline*
I.V. INFUSION
Adults and children. 5 mg/kg infused over 20 to 30 min.

▶ *As partial loading dose to treat reversible airway obstruction in patients currently receiving theophylline*
I.V. INFUSION
Adults and children. Dosage individualized based on blood theophylline level, as prescribed. Loading dose based on principle that 0.5 mg/kg of theophylline will produce a 1-mcg/ml increase in blood theophylline level.
▶ *To provide maintenance treatment of reversible airway obstruction associated with asthma or COPD*
I.V. INFUSION
Adults and adolescents age 16 and older. 0.4 mg/kg/hr for nonsmokers, 0.7 mg/kg/hr for smokers.
Children ages 9 to 16. 0.7 mg/kg/hr.
Children ages 1 to 9. 0.8 mg/kg/hr.
Full-term infants up to age 1. Dosage highly individualized, as prescribed.
DOSAGE ADJUSTMENT For elderly patients and adults with cardiac decompensation, cor pulmonale, or hepatic impairment, dosage reduced to 0.2 mg/kg/hr.

Mechanism of Action

Inhibits phosphodiesterase enzymes, causing bronchodilation. Normally, these enzymes inactivate cAMP and cGMP, which are responsible for bronchial smooth-muscle relaxation. Theophylline also may cause calcium translocation, antagonize prostaglandins and adenosine receptors, stimulate catecholamines, and inhibit cGMP metabolism.

Incompatibilities

Don't mix parenteral theophylline solution with any additives. Don't infuse theophylline through same I.V. line as Hetastarch (Hespan), a colloidal plasma volume expander, which is incompatible with theophylline.

Contraindications

Hypersensitivity to theophylline or its components, peptic ulcer disease, uncontrolled seizure disorder

Interactions

DRUGS
adenosine: Decreased adenosine effectiveness
allopurinol, cimetidine, ciprofloxacin, clarithromycin, disulfiram, enoxacin, erythromycin, fluvoxamine, interferon alfa (human recombi-

nant), methotrexate, mexiletine, pentoxifylline, propafenone, propranolol, tacrine, thiabendazole, ticlopidine, troleandomycin, verapamil: Increased blood theophylline level and risk of toxicity

aminoglutethimide, carbamazepine, isoproterenol (I.V.), moricizine, oral contraceptives (containing estrogen), phenobarbital, phenytoin, rifampin: Decreased blood level and possibly effectiveness of theophylline

benzodiazepines: Possibly reversal of benzodiazepine sedation

beta blockers: Possibly decreased bronchodilator effect of theophylline

ephedrine: Increased adverse effects, including insomnia, nausea, and nervousness

halothane anesthetics: Increased risk of ventricular arrhythmias

ketamine: Lowered seizure threshold

lithium: Decreased lithium effectiveness

neuromuscular blockers: Possibly antagonized neuromuscular blockade

FOODS

caffeine: Possibly increased risk of adverse CNS effects

high-carbohydrate, low-protein diet: Possibly decreased theophylline elimination

low-carbohydrate, high-protein diet; daily intake of charbroiled beef: Possibly increased theophylline elimination

ACTIVITIES

alcohol use: Increased blood theophylline level and risk of toxicity

smoking: Increased drug clearance, decreased drug effectiveness

smoking cessation: Possibly decreased drug clearance

Adverse Reactions

CNS: Agitation, anxiety, behavioral changes, confusion, disorientation, headache, insomnia, nervousness, seizures, tremor

CV: Hypotension, tachycardia, ventricular arrhythmias

ENDO: Hyperglycemia

GI: Abdominal pain, diarrhea, heartburn, nausea, vomiting

GU: Increased urine output

Nursing Considerations

- Be aware that ideal body weight is used to calculate theophylline dosages because drug doesn't bind well in body fat.
- Discard unused portions of theophylline and dextrose solutions because they contain no preservatives.
- Infuse theophylline loading dose, bolus, or intermittent infusion at a rate not exceeding 25 mg/minute.
- Administer continuous theophylline infusion with a rate-controlled infusion device.
- Frequently assess heart rate and rhythm because theophylline can exacerbate existing arrhythmias.

- Monitor blood theophylline level, as ordered, to gauge therapeutic level and detect toxicity.
- Be especially alert for signs of toxicity in patients with acute pulmonary edema, hypothyroidism, prolonged fever, sepsis with multiple organ failure, shock, or viral pulmonary infection and those who have recently received an influenza vaccine because drug clearance is decreased in these patients. Patients with uncorrected acidemia also have an increased risk of toxicity.
- Suspect toxicity if patient experiences vomiting; be prepared to obtain blood theophylline level.
- Expect patients with cystic fibrosis or hyperthyroidism to experience increased theophylline clearance and decreased drug effectiveness. Monitor blood theophylline level, as ordered.
- Store drug at 15° to 30° C (59° to 86° F); don't freeze.

PATIENT TEACHING

- Advise patient to report if she develops a fever, makes a significant dietary change, or starts or stops smoking or taking other drugs because these factors may alter blood theophylline level.
- Urge patient to avoid excessive intake of caffeine (found in coffee, tea, cola, and chocolate), which can increase her risk of developing adverse CNS reactions, such as agitation and nervousness.

thiamine hydrochloride
(vitamin B₁)

Betaxin (CAN), Biamine

Class and Category

Chemical: Water-soluble B-complex vitamin
Therapeutic: Nutritional supplement
Pregnancy category: A (parenteral), not rated (oral)

Indications and Dosages

▶ *To provide nutritional supplementation based on U.S. and Canadian recommended daily allowances (RDAs), to prevent thiamine deficiency*

I.V. INFUSION

Adults and children. Dosage individualized and added to total parenteral nutrition solution.

▶ *To treat beriberi*

I.V. INJECTION

Adults. *Initial:* 5 to 100 mg q 8 hr, then switched to P.O. therapy as soon as possible and continued for 1 mo.

Children and infants. 10 to 25 mg/day.

ELIXIR, TABLETS
Adults. 5 to 10 mg t.i.d.
Children and infants. 10 mg/day.
▶ *To treat Wernicke's encephalopathy*
I.V. INJECTION
Adults. *Initial:* 100 mg. *Maintenance:* 50 to 100 mg q.d. until normal RDA is achieved.

Mechanism of Action

Replaces vitamin in thiamine deficiency, which can lead to beriberi or Wernicke's encephalopathy. Thiamine combines with ATP to produce thiamine pyrophosphate, a coenzyme needed for carbohydrate metabolism. Thiamine is necessary for the conversion of pyruvic acid to acetyl-CoA so that it can enter the Krebs cycle; in patients without adequate thiamine, pyruvic acid accumulates in the blood, where it's converted to lactic acid.

Incompatibilities

Don't add thiamine to alkaline or neutral solutions or mix it with oxidizing and reducing agents, including barbiturates, carbonates, citrates, and copper ions.

Contraindications

Hypersensitivity to thiamine preparations or their components

Interactions

None known.

Adverse Reactions

CNS: Restlessness, weakness
EENT: Sneezing, throat tightness
GI: Nausea, vomiting
SKIN: Diaphoresis, pruritus, sensation of warmth, urticaria

Nursing Considerations

- Be aware that symptoms of thiamine deficiency may appear as a syndrome of nonspecific symptoms that include headache, malaise, myalgia, and nausea.
- **WARNING** Severe thiamine deficiency causes beriberi, which can affect the CNS and cardiovascular system. Monitor patient for neurologic effects, such as ataxia, confabulation, impaired ability to learn, neuropathy, and retrograde amnesia, as well as cardiovascular effects, such as biventricular failure, edema, and peripheral vasodilation.

- Expect an intradermal test dose to be prescribed before I.V. administration of thiamine.
- Use thiamine immediately if mixed in solutions containing sodium bisulfite as an antioxidant or preservative because drug stability is poor in such solutions.
- Be aware that a high-carbohydrate diet and dextrose-containing I.V. solutions may increase thiamine requirements and worsen symptoms of thiamine deficiency.
- Be aware that thiamine absorption is decreased in patients with alcoholism, cirrhosis, or GI disease.
- Assess patient and laboratory test results for signs of lactic acidosis. In patients with a thiamine deficiency, pyruvic acid accumulates in the blood and is converted to lactic acid.
- Keep in mind that thiamine is a water-soluble vitamin that won't accumulate in the body.
- Store drug at 15° to 30° C (59° to 86° F); protect from freezing and light.

PATIENT TEACHING
- Inform breast-feeding patient that she and her infant must be treated with thiamine if infant has beriberi.
- Encourage patient to improve diet to prevent disease recurrence

ticarcillin disodium
Ticar

Class and Category
Chemical: Penicillin
Therapeutic: Antibiotic
Pregnancy category: B

Indications and Dosages
▶ *To treat moderate to severe infections, such as bacteremia, diabetic foot ulcers, empyema, intra-abdominal infections, lower respiratory tract infections (including pneumonia), lung abscess, peritonitis, pulmonary infections due to complications of cystic fibrosis (including bronchiectasis and pneumonia), septicemia, and skin and soft-tissue infections (including cellulitis) caused by susceptible organisms*
I.V. INFUSION
Adults and children. 200 to 300 mg/kg/day in divided doses q 4 to 6 hr. *Usual:* 3 g q 4 hr or 4 g q 6 hr.

▶ *To treat severe infections (including sepsis) caused by susceptible strains of* Pseudomonas *species,* Proteus *species, and* Escherichia coli
Neonates during first week of life who weigh less than 2 g. 75 mg/kg q 12 hr.
Neonates during first week of life who weigh more than 2 g. 75 mg/kg q 8 hr.
Neonates after first week of life who weigh less than 2 g. 75 mg/kg q 8 hr.
Neonates after first week of life who weigh more than 2 g. 100 mg/kg q 8 hr or 75 mg/kg q 6 hr.
▶ *To treat uncomplicated UTIs*
I.V. INFUSION
Adults and children who weigh 40 kg (88 lb) or more. 1 g q 6 hr.
Children over age 1 month who weigh less than 40 kg. 50 to 100 mg/kg/day in divided doses q 6 to 8 hr.
▶ *To treat complicated UTIs*
I.V. INFUSION
Adults and children. 150 to 200 mg/kg in equally divided doses q 4 to 6 hr. *Usual:* 3 g q 6 hr.
DOSAGE ADJUSTMENT Adult patients with renal impairment given a loading dose of 3 g, then dosage adjusted as follows: for creatinine clearance of 30 to 60 ml/min/1.73 m^2, 2 g q 4 hr; for creatinine clearance of 10 to 30 ml/min/1.73 m^2, 2 g q 8 hr; for creatinine clearance of less than 10 ml/min/1.73 m^2, 2 g q 12 hr; for creatinine clearance of less than 10 ml/min/1.73 m^2 *and* impaired hepatic function, 2 g q 24 hr; for patients who undergo hemodialysis, 2 g q 12 hr and 3 g after each dialysis session; for patients who undergo peritoneal dialysis, 3 g q 12 hr.

Mechanism of Action
Inhibits bacterial cell wall synthesis by binding to specific penicillin-binding proteins located inside the bacterial cell wall. Ultimately, this leads to cell wall lysis and death.

Incompatibilities
Don't administer ticarcillin through same I.V. line as amikacin, gentamicin, or tobramycin or within 1 hour of aminoglycosides.

Contraindications
Hypersensitivity to ticarcillin, other penicillins, or their components

Interactions
DRUGS
aminoglycosides: Additive or synergistic activity against some bacteria, possibly mutual inactivation
anticoagulants: Possibly interference with platelet aggregation, prolonged PT
methotrexate: Prolonged blood methotrexate level, increased risk of methotrexate toxicity
probenecid: Prolonged blood ticarcillin level

Adverse Reactions
CV: Thrombophlebitis, vasculitis
GI: Elevated liver function test results, nausea, pseudomembranous colitis, vomiting
GU: Proteinuria
HEME: Anemia, eosinophilia, hemorrhage, leukopenia, neutropenia, prolonged bleeding time, thrombocytopenia
SKIN: Erythema nodosum, exfoliative dermatitis, pruritus, rash, toxic epidermal necrolysis, urticaria
Other: Anaphylaxis, hypernatremia, hypokalemia, superinfection

Nursing Considerations
- Obtain body fluid or tissue specimens for culture and sensitivity testing, as ordered. Review test results, if possible, before giving first dose of ticarcillin.
- Before starting ticarcillin, make sure patient has had no previous hypersensitivity reactions to ticarcillin or other penicillins.
- Reconstitute each gram of ticarcillin with 4 ml of a compatible diluent, such as 5% dextrose injection or 0.9% sodium chloride injection. Further dilute reconstituted I.V. solution to 10 to 100 mg/ml with a compatible I.V. solution. To minimize vein irritation, don't exceed concentration of 100 mg/ml (concentrations of 50 mg/ml or greater are preferred). Infuse appropriate adult or children's dose over 30 to 120 minutes; infuse neonatal dose over 10 to 20 minutes.
- Assess for local injection site reaction, including thrombophlebitis, during therapy.
- **WARNING** Monitor patient's platelet count, PT, and APTT because ticarcillin may increase bleeding time and, in rare cases, may induce thrombocytopenia.
- Be aware that ticarcillin may exacerbate symptoms in patients with a history of GI disease or colitis.

- Implement seizure precautions according to facility policy for patients with renal impairment because they're at increased risk for seizures.
- Assess patient for signs of pseudomembranous colitis, such as abdominal cramps and severe watery diarrhea. Also assess for other signs of superinfection, such as oral candidiasis and rash in breast-feeding infant.
- Monitor serum electrolyte levels for hypernatremia due to drug's high sodium content and for hypokalemia due to increased urinary potassium loss.
- When calculating sodium intake for patients on a sodium-restricted diet, keep in mind that each gram of ticarcillin contains approximately 5.2 to 6.5 mEq of sodium.
- Before reconstituting drug, store it at 15° to 30° C (59° to 86° F).

PATIENT TEACHING
- Instruct patient receiving ticarcillin to immediately report adverse reactions, including rash, difficulty breathing, or fever.
- Advise patient to decrease sodium intake to reduce the risk of electrolyte imbalance.
- Advise patient to report diarrhea and to check with prescriber before taking an antidiarrheal because it may mask symptoms of pseudomembranous colitis.

ticarcillin disodium and clavulanate potassium
Timentin

Class and Category
Chemical: Penicillin
Therapeutic: Antibiotic combination
Pregnancy category: B

Indications and Dosages
▶ *To treat moderate to severe infections, such as appendicitis, bacteremia, bone and joint infections (including osteomyelitis), diabetic foot ulcers, diverticulitis, gynecologic infections (including endometritis), infectious arthritis, intra-abdominal infections, lower respiratory tract infections (including pneumonia), peritonitis, septicemia, skin and soft-tissue infections (including cellulitis), and UTIs caused by susceptible organisms; to manage febrile neutropenia*

I.V. INFUSION

Adults and children age 12 and older who weigh 60 kg (132 lb) or more. 3.1 g (3 g of ticarcillin and 100 mg of clavulanic acid) infused over 30 min q 4 to 6 hr.

Adults and children age 12 and older who weigh less than 60 kg. 200 to 300 mg/kg/day (based on ticarcillin content) in divided doses q 4 to 6 hr.

Children and infants over age 3 months. For mild to moderate infections, 200 mg/kg/day (based on ticarcillin content) in divided doses q 6 hr; for severe infections, 300 mg/kg/day (based on ticarcillin content) in divided doses q 4 to 6 hr.

DOSAGE ADJUSTMENT Adult patients with renal impairment given loading dose of 3.1 g (3 g of ticarcillin and 100 mg of clavulanic acid), then dosage adjusted as follows: for creatinine clearance of 30 to 60 ml/min/1.73 m^2, 2 g q 4 hr; for creatinine clearance of 10 to 30 ml/min/1.73 m^2, 2 g q 8 hr; for creatinine clearance of less than 10 ml/min/1.73 m^2, 2 g q 12 hr; for creatinine clearance of less than 10 ml/min/1.73 m^2 *and* impaired hepatic function, 2 g q 24 hr; for patients who undergo hemodialysis, 2 g q 12 hr and 3.1 g after each dialysis; for patients who undergo peritoneal dialysis, 3.1 g q 12 hr.

▶ *To treat pulmonary infections caused by complications of cystic fibrosis, such as bronchiectasis or pneumonia*

I.V. INFUSION

Children. 350 to 450 mg/kg/day (based on ticarcillin content) in divided doses.

Mechanism of Action

Inhibits bacterial cell wall synthesis by binding to specific penicillin-binding proteins located inside bacterial cell walls. In this way, ticarcillin ultimately leads to cell wall lysis and death. Clavulanic acid, which doesn't alter the action of ticarcillin, binds with bound and extracellular beta-lactamase, preventing beta-lactamase from inactivating ticarcillin.

Incompatibilities

Don't administer ticarcillin and clavulanate through same I.V. line as amikacin, gentamicin, or tobramycin. Don't combine with sodium bicarbonate or administer within 1 hour of aminoglycosides.

Contraindications

Hypersensitivity to ticarcillin or other penicillins, clavulanic acid, or their components

Interactions
DRUGS

aminoglycosides: Additive or synergistic activity against some bacteria, possibly mutual inactivation

anticoagulants: Possibly interference with platelet aggregation

methotrexate: Prolonged blood methotrexate level, increased risk of methotrexate toxicity

probenecid: Prolonged blood ticarcillin level

Adverse Reactions
CV: Thrombophlebitis, vasculitis

GI: Elevated liver function test results, nausea, pseudomembranous colitis, vomiting

GU: Proteinuria

HEME: Anemia, eosinophilia, hemorrhage, leukopenia, neutropenia, prolonged bleeding time, thrombocytopenia

SKIN: Erythema nodosum, exfoliative dermatitis, pruritus, rash, toxic epidermal necrolysis, urticaria

Other: Anaphylaxis, hypernatremia, hypokalemia, infusion site pain

Nursing Considerations
- Obtain body fluid or tissue specimens for culture and sensitivity testing, as ordered. Review test results, if possible, before giving first dose of ticarcillin and clavulanate.
- Before starting drug, make sure patient has had no previous hypersensitivity reactions to ticarcillin, other penicillins, or clavulanic acid.
- Keep in mind that 3.1 g of combination drug ticarcillin and clavulanate corresponds to 3 g of ticarcillin and 100 mg of clavulanic acid.
- Dilute reconstituted I.V. solution to concentration of 10 to 100 mg/ml with compatible I.V. solution. To minimize vein irritation, don't exceed concentration of 100 mg/ml. Concentrations of 50 mg/ml or greater are preferred. Infuse appropriate I.V. dose over 30 to 120 min.
- Be aware that premixed minibags are available for use in concentration of 3.1 g (3 g of ticarcillin and 100 mg of clavulanic acid) in 100 ml. Before using minibags, store them below −10° C (14° F). Allow them to thaw at room temperature. Examine contents closely before administration to make sure that ice crystals have melted. When administering minibags, don't

use I.V. lines with series connections because they may cause air embolism.

- Know that ticarcillin and clavulanate may exacerbate symptoms in patients with a history of GI disease, especially colitis.
- Assess patient for signs of pseudomembranous colitis, such as abdominal cramps and severe watery diarrhea. Also assess for other signs of superinfection, such as oral candidiasis and rash in breast-feeding infant.
- Implement seizure precautions, according to facility policy, for patients with renal impairment because they're at increased risk for seizures.
- Monitor serum electrolyte levels for hypernatremia due to drug's high sodium content and for hypokalemia due to increased urinary potassium loss.
- **WARNING** Monitor patient's platelet count, PT, and APTT because drug may increase bleeding time and, in rare cases, may induce thrombocytopenia.
- Be aware that patient receiving high doses of ticarcillin may develop pseudoproteinuria.
- When calculating sodium intake for patients on a sodium-restricted diet, keep in mind that each gram of ticarcillin contains approximately 4.75 mEq of sodium.
- Before reconstituting drug, store it at 15° to 30° C (59° to 86° F). Store premixed minibags below −10° C (14° F) before thawing.

PATIENT TEACHING
- Instruct patient receiving ticarcillin and clavulanate to immediately report adverse reactions, including fever, rash, and difficulty breathing.
- Advise patient to decrease sodium intake to reduce the risk of electrolyte imbalance.
- Advise patient to report diarrhea and to check with prescriber before taking an antidiarrheal because it may mask symptoms of pseudomembranous colitis.

tirofiban hydrochloride
Aggrastat

Class and Category
Chemical: Tyrosine derivative
Therapeutic: Platelet aggregation inhibitor
Pregnancy category: B

Indications and Dosages

▶ *To treat acute coronary syndrome*
I.V. INFUSION
Adults. 0.4 mcg/kg/min for 30 min, followed by 0.1 mcg/kg/min.
DOSAGE ADJUSTMENT For patients with creatinine clearance of less than 30 ml/min/1.73 m^2, infusion rate reduced by 50%.

Route	Onset	Peak	Duration
I.V.	Immediate	30 min	4 to 8 hr

Mechanism of Action

Binds to glycoprotein IIb/IIIa receptor sites on the surface of activated platelets. Circulating fibrinogen can bind to these receptor sites and link platelets together, forming a clot that eventually blocks a coronary artery. By binding to these receptor sites, tirofiban prevents the normal binding of fibrinogen and other factors and inhibits platelet aggregation.

Incompatibilities

Don't infuse tirofiban in same I.V. line as any drug other than heparin.

Contraindications

Acute pericarditis; arteriovenous malformation; coagulopathy; CVA within previous 30 days or history of hemorrhagic CVA; GI or GU bleeding; hemophilia; history of thrombocytopenia after tirofiban use; hypersensitivity to tirofiban or its components; intracranial aneurysm or mass, intracranial bleeding, retinal bleeding, aortic dissection, or any evidence of active abnormal bleeding within previous 30 days; major surgery or trauma within previous 6 weeks; severe uncontrolled hypertension (systolic blood pressure above 180 mm Hg, diastolic blood pressure above 110 mm Hg)

Interactions

DRUGS
antineoplastics, antithymocyte globulin, NSAIDs, oral anticoagulants, platelet aggregation inhibitors, strontium-89 chloride, thrombolytics: Increased risk of bleeding
levothyroxine, omeprazole: Increased rate of tirofiban clearance
porfimer: Decreased effectiveness of porfimer photodynamic therapy
salicylates: Increased risk of bleeding, possibly hypoprothrombinemia

Adverse Reactions

CNS: Chills, dizziness, fever, headache
CV: Edema, peripheral edema, sinus bradycardia
GI: Hematemesis, nausea, vomiting
GU: Hematuria, pelvic pain
SKIN: Diaphoresis, rash, urticaria
Other: Infusion site bleeding

Nursing Considerations

- **WARNING** Dilute 50-ml vial of tirofiban before use; *don't* dilute 500-ml container because it holds premixed solution ready for I.V. infusion. Don't use solution unless it is clear and has an intact seal.
- When administering drug from 500-ml plastic container, don't use I.V. lines with series connections because they may cause air embolism.
- Monitor platelet count, hemoglobin level, and hematocrit before and during therapy, as ordered. Expect to stop drug if platelet count is less than 90,000/mm³, or to administer a platelet transfusion, as prescribed, if platelet count falls below 50,000/mm³.
- If prescribed, administer tirofiban with heparin for 48 to 108 hours. Expect to continue infusion throughout angiography and for 12 to 24 hours after angioplasty or atherectomy.
- If bleeding can't be controlled under pressure, consult prescriber about possibly discontinuing tirofiban and heparin.
- After cardiac catheterization or percutaneous coronary angioplasty, maintain patient on bed rest and keep head of bed elevated. Ensure percutaneous site hemostasis at least 4 hours before discharge. Minimize invasive procedures to reduce the risk of bleeding.
- Store drug at 15° to 30° C (59° to 86° F), preferably at controlled temperature of 25° C (77° F); protect from freezing and light.

PATIENT TEACHING
- Advise patient to immediately report any bleeding, bruising, headache, pain, or swelling during I.V. infusion of tirofiban.

tobramycin sulfate

Nebcin, Tobi

Class and Category

Chemical: Aminoglycoside
Therapeutic: Antibiotic
Pregnancy category: D

Indications and Dosages

▶ *To treat bacteremia; bone and joint, gynecologic, intra-abdominal, lower respiratory tract, skin and soft-tissue, and urinary tract infections; endocarditis; meningitis; neonatal sepsis; pyelonephritis; and septicemia caused by susceptible strains of* Acinetobacter *species,* Aeromonas *species,* Citrobacter *species,* Enterobacter *species,* Escherichia coli, Haemophilus influenzae *(beta lactamase–negative and –positive),* Klebsiella *species,* Morganella morganii, Proteus mirabilis, Proteus vulgaris, Providencia rettgeri, Pseudomonas aeruginosa, Salmonella *species,* Serratia *species,* Shigella *species,* Staphylococcus aureus, *and* Staphylococcus epidermidis; *to treat febrile neutropenia*

I.V. INFUSION

Adults. 3 to 6 mg/kg/day in divided doses q 8 to 12 hr.

Children over age 5. 2 to 2.5 mg/kg q 8 hr.

Children under age 5. 2.5 mg/kg q 8 to 16 hr.

Neonates over age 7 days who weigh more than 2 kg (4.4 lb). 2.5 mg/kg q 8 hr.

Neonates over age 7 days who weigh 1.2 to 2 kg (2.6 to 4.4 lb). 2.5 mg/kg q 8 to 12 hr.

Neonates age 7 days and under who weigh 2 kg or more. 2.5 mg/kg q 12 hr.

Neonates age 7 days and under who weigh 1.2 to 2 kg. 2.5 mg/kg q 12 to 18 hr.

Preterm neonates who weigh 1 to 1.2 kg (2.2 to 2.6 lb). 2.5 mg/kg q 18 to 24 hr.

Preterm neonates who weigh less than 1 kg. 3.5 mg/kg q 24 hr.

▶ *To treat pulmonary infection caused by* P. aeruginosa *in patients with cystic fibrosis*

I.V. INFUSION

Adults and children. 2.5 to 3.3 mg/kg q 8 hr; dosage adjusted to achieve peak blood drug level of 8 to 12 mcg/ml and trough blood drug level of less than 2 mcg/ml.

DOSAGE ADJUSTMENT Dosage possibly reduced for patients with renal impairment.

Mechanism of Action

Inhibits bacterial protein synthesis by binding irreversibly to one of two aminoglycoside-binding sites on the 30S ribosomal subunit, resulting in bacteriostatic effects. Bactericidal effects may stem from tobramycin's ability to accumulate within cells so that the intracellular drug level exceeds the extracellular level.

Incompatibilities
Don't mix tobramycin in same solution with parenteral aminoglycosides or beta-lactam antibiotics because mutual inactivation may result.

Contraindications
Concurrent cidofovir therapy; hypersensitivity to tobramycin, aminoglycosides, sodium bisulfite, or their components

Interactions
DRUGS

acyclovir, aminoglycosides, amphotericin B, carboplatin, cisplatin, NSAIDs, vancomycin: Additive nephrotoxicity
carbenicillin, ticarcillin: Possibly inactivation of tobramycin
dimenhydrinate: Possibly masking of symptoms of ototoxicity
ethacrynic acid, furosemide: Additive ototoxicity
general anesthetics, neuromuscular blockers: Possibly exaggerated neuromuscular blockade

Adverse Reactions
CNS: Confusion, dizziness, headache, lethargy, neurotoxicity, vertigo
EENT: Hearing loss, ototoxicity, tinnitus
GI: Diarrhea, elevated liver function test results, nausea, vomiting
GU: Elevated BUN and serum creatinine levels, nephrotoxicity, oliguria, proteinuria, renal failure
HEME: Anemia, leukocytosis, leukopenia, neutropenia, thrombocytopenia
SKIN: Exfoliative dermatitis, pruritus, rash, urticaria
Other: Hypocalcemia, hypokalemia, hypomagnesemia, hyponatremia

Nursing Considerations
- Obtain body fluid and tissue specimens for culture and sensitivity testing before and during tobramycin treatment, as ordered. Review test results, if available, before therapy begins.
- After reconstituting drug with 30 ml of sterile or bacteriostatic water for injection, dilute further with NS or D$_5$W. Consult manufacturer's insert for specific instructions. Don't exceed a final concentration of 1 mg/ml when preparing diluted solutions.
- Administer each I.V. dose over 20 to 60 minutes.
- **WARNING** Don't infuse tobramycin over less than 20 minutes. Rapid infusion may result in neuromuscular blockade and greater-than-therapeutic peak blood level of drug.

- Because drug can cause bilateral and irreversible hearing loss, assess for early signs of auditory and vestibular ototoxicity, including high-frequency hearing loss and vertigo. Be aware that patients with cranial nerve VIII impairment are at increased risk.
- **WARNING** Be alert for allergic reactions, including anaphylaxis and possibly life-threatening asthmatic episodes, because some forms of drug contain sodium bisulfite.
- Monitor serum calcium, magnesium, potassium, and sodium levels to detect electrolyte imbalances.
- Discontinue tobramycin therapy 7 days before starting cidofovir therapy, as prescribed.
- Assess for signs of nephrotoxicity, such as elevated BUN and serum creatinine levels and altered urine output.
- Expect dehydration to increase the risk of nephrotoxicity. Premature infants, neonates, elderly patients, and patients with impaired renal function are also at increased risk.
- **WARNING** Monitor patient with myasthenia gravis or parkinsonism and infants with botulism for increased muscle weakness because of tobramycin's potential curare-like effect.
- When calculating sodium intake for patients on a sodium-restricted diet, keep in mind that every 50 ml of tobramycin contains 19.6 mEq of sodium.
- Store drug premixed in NS at 2° to 30° C (36° to 86° F). Store unreconstituted vials and vials containing concentrations of 10 to 80 mg/ml at 15° to 30° C (59° to 86° F); don't freeze.

PATIENT TEACHING

- Urge patient to immediately report high-frequency hearing loss and vertigo that occurs during tobramycin therapy.
- Instruct female patient to notify prescriber immediately about known or suspected pregnancy because drug poses danger to fetus.
- Stress the importance of keeping follow-up medical appointments and undergoing diagnostic tests, such as audiometric and renal function tests, if ordered.

torsemide
Demadex

Class and Category
Chemical: Anilinopyridine sulfonylurea derivative
Therapeutic: Antihypertensive, diuretic
Pregnancy category: B

Indications and Dosages

▶ *To treat edema in heart failure*
I.V. INJECTION
Adults. *Initial:* 10 to 20 mg q.d., adjusted by doubling, as prescribed, to achieve desired effect. *Maximum:* 200 mg q.d.
▶ *To treat edema in chronic renal failure*
I.V. INJECTION
Adults. *Initial:* 20 mg q.d., adjusted by doubling, as prescribed, to achieve desired effect. *Maximum:* 200 mg q.d.
▶ *To treat ascites, alone or with amiloride or spironolactone*
I.V. INJECTION
Adults. *Initial:* 5 to 10 mg q.d. *Maximum:* 40 mg q.d.

Route	Onset	Peak	Duration
I.V.	10 min	1 hr	6 to 8 hr

Mechanism of Action

Blocks active sodium and chloride reabsorption in the ascending loop of Henle by promoting rapid excretion of water, sodium, and chloride. Torsemide also increases the production of renal prostaglandins, increasing the plasma renin level and renal vasodilation. As a result, systolic and diastolic blood pressures fall, reducing preload and afterload.

Contraindications

Hypersensitivity to torsemide, sulfonamides, or their components

Interactions

DRUGS
ACE inhibitors, other antihypertensives: Additive hypotension
amiloride, spironolactone, triamterene: Possibly counteraction of torsemide-induced hypokalemia
amphotericin B: Increased risk of nephrotoxicity and severe, prolonged hypokalemia or hypomagnesemia
cisplatin: Increased risk of significant hypokalemia or hypomagnesemia, possibly permanent ototoxicity
cortisone, hydrocortisone: Increased risk of sodium retention and hypokalemia
digoxin: Increased risk of arrhythmias and digitalis toxicity due to hypokalemia or hypomagnesemia
indomethacin: Possibly decreased diuretic and antihypertensive effects of torsemide and increased risk of renal failure

lithium: Possibly lithium toxicity

metolazone, thiazide diuretics: Increased risk of severe fluid and electrolyte loss

neuromuscular blockers: Possibly increased neuromuscular blockade due to hypokalemia

probenecid: Possibly decreased diuretic effect of torsemide

quinidine and other ototoxic drugs: Increased risk of ototoxicity

salicylates: Increased risk of salicylate toxicity

ACTIVITIES

alcohol use: Additive diuresis and, possibly, dehydration

Adverse Reactions

CNS: Dizziness, drowsiness, fatigue, headache, insomnia, lethargy, nervousness, restlessness, weakness

CV: Chest pain, ECG abnormalities, edema, hypotension, tachycardia

EENT: Dry mouth, hearing loss, ototoxicity, pharyngitis, rhinitis, tinnitus

GI: Constipation, diarrhea, indigestion, nausea, thirst, vomiting

GU: Azotemia (prerenal), oliguria, urinary frequency

MS: Muscle spasms, myalgia

RESP: Cough

Other: Hypochloremia, hypokalemia, hypomagnesemia, hyponatremia, hypovolemia

Nursing Considerations

- Examine torsemide before administering it; discard if it contains particles or is discolored.
- Inject drug slowly over 2 minutes. Flush I.V. line with NS before and after administration.
- Don't exceed 200 mg in a single dose.
- Monitor serum electrolyte levels, as ordered, and fluid intake and output to detect hypovolemia.
- **WARNING** Expect drug-induced electrolyte imbalances, such as hypokalemia and hypomagnesemia, to increase the risk of toxicity and fatal arrhythmias in a patient who takes a digitalis glycoside. Hypokalemia also potentiates neuromuscular blockade effects of nondepolarizing neuromuscular blockers.
- Store drug at 15° to 30° C (59° to 86° F); don't freeze.

PATIENT TEACHING

- Advise patient to change position slowly during torsemide therapy to minimize effects of orthostatic hypotension.

• Instruct patient to immediately report drowsiness, dry mouth, hearing changes, lethargy, muscle cramps or pain, nausea, restlessness, thirst, vomiting, and weakness.
• Inform diabetic patient that her blood glucose level will be monitored frequently because torsemide may increase it.

trastuzumab
Herceptin

Class and Category
Chemical: Recombinant DNA-derived humanized monoclonal antibody
Therapeutic: Antineoplastic
Pregnancy category: B

Indications and Dosages
▶ *To treat metastatic breast cancer in patients whose tumors oxerexpress the protein human epidermal growth factor receptor 2 (HER2), either as a single agent (for those who have previously received at least one chemotherapy regimen for metastatic disease) or in combination with paclitaxel (for those who have not previously received chemotherapy for metastatic disease)*

I.V. INFUSION
Adults. *Initial:* 4 mg/kg infused over 90 min. *Maintenance:* 2 mg/kg infused over 30 min if initial dose was well tolerated.

Route	Onset	Peak	Duration
I.V.	Unknown	16 to 32 wk	Unknown

Mechanism of Action
Preferentially binds to the HER2 protein, which is associated with more aggressive forms of breast cancer. In this way, trastuzumab inhibits the proliferation of tumor cells and mediates antibody-dependent cellular toxicity in cancer cells that overexpress HER2.

Incompatibilities
Don't mix trastuzumab with dextrose solutions or any other drug.

Contraindications
None known.

Interactions
DRUGS
cyclophosphamide, doxorubicin, epirubicin: Increased risk of cardiac dysfunction
paclitaxel: Possibly increased blood level and effects of trastuzumab

Adverse Reactions
CNS: Asthenia, headache, insomnia, paresthesia
CV: Cardiomyopathy, cardiotoxicity (including heart failure), hypotension, ventricular dysfunction
EENT: Rhinitis
GI: Anorexia, diarrhea, nausea, vomiting
HEME: Anemia, leukopenia
RESP: Adult respiratory distress syndrome, bronchospasm, cough, dyspnea, hypoxia, pleural effusion, pulmonary edema (noncardiogenic), pulmonary infiltrates, pulmonary insufficiency, sinusitis, wheezing
SKIN: Rash, urticaria
Other: Allergic reaction, anaphylaxis, angioedema, infection, infusion reaction

Nursing Considerations
- Perform baseline cardiac assessment before beginning trastuzumab therapy. Expect patient to receive an echocardiogram, an ECG, or a multigated acquisition (MUGA) scan before initiation of therapy. Be aware that patients with a history of cardiac disease, including preexisting cardiac dysfunction, are at increased risk for developing cardiomyopathy. In addition, patients who have previously received a cardiotoxic drug or radiation therapy to the chest wall are at increased risk for cardiotoxicity.
- Be aware that adverse reactions can vary when trastuzumab is administered in combination therapy. Review information for all drugs administered as part of a specific regimen, including drug interactions and adverse effects.
- **WARNING** Reconstitute trastuzumab with 20 ml of the 30 ml of bacteriostatic water for injection (containing benzyl alcohol) provided by manufacturer to produce a multidose vial of 21 mg/ml. Discard the remaining 10 ml of diluent; using all of it would result in a lower-than-intended dose. Label vial with "DO NOT USE AFTER" and insert date that is 28 days after date of reconstitution. Use contents within 28 days if stored at 2° to 8° C (36° to 46° F).

- If patient is hypersensitive to benzyl alcohol, prepare initial dilution using 20 ml of sterile water for injection *without* preservative. Use immediately.
- When reconstituting drug, slowly inject the stream of diluent directly into lyophilized cake of trastuzumab. Swirl gently; don't shake. Let vial stand for about 5 minutes to allow slight foaming that may have formed to dissipate. Expect solution to be clear to slightly opalescent and colorless to pale yellow. Discard if solution contains particles.
- Dilute reconstituted trastuzumab with a 250-ml infusion bag of NS; use within 24 hours if stored at 2° to 8° C.
- Administer trastuzumab by I.V. infusion, *not* by I.V. push or bolus.
- **WARNING** Monitor patient for possibly life-threatening infusion reaction, pulmonary complications, or allergic reaction. Assess for such signs as dizziness, fever or chills, headache, nausea, rash, shortness of breath, vomiting, or weakness, particularly during administration and for at least 24 hours afterward. Be aware that infusion reaction typically occurs with the first dose but may occur with subsequent doses. Patients with preexisting pulmonary compromise from lung disease or pulmonary malignancy are at increased risk for pulmonary complications.
- Continue to assess cardiac function, including left ventricular function, in all patients during trastuzumab treatment. Prescriber may discontinue drug if patient develops a clinically significant decrease in left ventricular function. Patients who receive trastuzumab in combination with anthracyclines and cyclophosphamide are at increased risk.
- Expect to discontinue infusion if patient experiences dyspnea or clinically significant hypotension. Assess patient until signs and symptoms completely resolve. Prescriber may discontinue drug if patient develops anaphylaxis, angioedema, or acute respiratory distress syndrome.
- Before reconstituting trastuzumab, store it at 2° to 8° C.

PATIENT TEACHING

- Advise patient to immediately report signs of an infusion or allergic reaction or pulmonary complications, including difficulty breathing, rash, and facial swelling. Inform her that such reactions may occur 24 hours or longer after infusion.
- Instruct female patients not to breast-feed during trastuzumab therapy and for 6 months afterward.

- Stress the importance of complying with the dosage regimen and of keeping follow-up medical appointments and appointments for laboratory tests.

triflupromazine hydrochloride
Vesprin

Class and Category
Chemical: Phenothiazine
Therapeutic: Antiemetic, antipsychotic
Pregnancy category: Not rated

Indications and Dosages
▶ *To treat nausea and vomiting*
I.V. INJECTION
Adults. 1 mg p.r.n. *Maximum:* 3 mg/day.

Mechanism of Action
Prevents nausea and vomiting by inhibiting or blocking dopamine receptors in the medullary chemoreceptor trigger zone and, peripherally, by blocking the vagus nerve in the GI tract. Triflupromazine also blocks postsynaptic dopamine receptors, increasing dopamine turnover and decreasing dopamine neurotransmission. This action may depress the areas of the brain that control activity and aggression, including the cerebral cortex, hypothalamus, and limbic system.

Contraindications
Blood dyscrasias, bone marrow depression, cerebral arteriosclerosis, coma or severe CNS depression, concurrent use of large quantity of CNS depressants, coronary artery disease, hepatic dysfunction, hypersensitivity to phenothiazines, severe hypertension or hypotension, subcortical brain damage

Interactions
DRUGS
amantadine, anticholinergics, antidyskinetics, antihistamines: Possibly intensified adverse anticholinergic effects, increased risk of triflupromazine-induced hyperpyrexia
amphetamines: Decreased stimulant effect of amphetamines, decreased antipsychotic effect of triflupromazine
anticonvulsants: Lowered seizure threshold
antithyroid drugs: Increased risk of agranulocytosis

apomorphine: Possibly decreased emetic response to apomorphine, additive CNS depression

appetite suppressants: Decreased anorectic effect of appetite suppressants

astemizole, cisapride, disopyramide, erythromycin, pimozide, probucol, procainamide, quinidine: Prolonged QT interval, increased risk of ventricular tachycardia

beta blockers: Increased blood levels of both drugs, possibly leading to additive hypotensive effect, arrhythmias, irreversible retinopathy, and tardive dyskinesia

bromocriptine: Impaired therapeutic effects of bromocriptine

CNS depressants: Additive CNS depression

ephedrine: Decreased vasopressor response to ephedrine

epinephrine: Blocked alpha-adrenergic effects of epinephrine

extrapyramidal reaction–causing drugs (droperidol, haloperidol, metoclopramide, metyrosine, risperidone): Increased severity and frequency of extrapyramidal reactions

hepatotoxic drugs: Increased risk of hepatotoxicity

hypotension-producing drugs: Possibly severe hypotension with syncope

levodopa: Decreased antidyskinetic effect of levodopa

lithium: Possibly encephalopathy and additive extrapyramidal effects

MAO inhibitors, maprotiline, tricyclic antidepressants: Increased CNS depression, impaired triflupromazine metabolism, increased risk of neuroleptic malignant syndrome

mephentermine: Possibly antagonized antipsychotic effect of triflupromazine and vasopressor effect of mephentermine

metaraminol: Decreased vasopressor effect of metaraminol

methoxamine, phenylephrine: Decreased vasopressor effect and shortened duration of action of these drugs

metrizamide: Increased risk of seizures

opioid analgesics: Increased risk of CNS and respiratory depression, orthostatic hypotension, severe constipation, and urine retention

ototoxic drugs: Possibly masking of symptoms of ototoxicity, such as dizziness, tinnitus, and vertigo

phenytoin: Lowered seizure threshold; inhibited phenytoin metabolism, possibly leading to phenytoin toxicity

photosensitizing drugs: Possibly additive photosensitivity and intraocular photochemical damage to choroid, lens, or retina

thiazide diuretics: Possibly hyponatremia and water intoxication

ACTIVITIES

alcohol use: Increased CNS and respiratory depression, increased hypotensive effect

Adverse Reactions

CNS: Akathisia, altered temperature regulation, dizziness, drowsiness, extrapyramidal reactions (dystonia, pseudoparkinsonism, tardive dyskinesia), neuroleptic malignant syndrome

CV: Hypotension, orthostatic hypotension, tachycardia

EENT: Blurred vision, dry mouth, nasal congestion, ocular changes (deposits of fine particles in cornea and lens), pigmentary retinopathy

ENDO: Galactorrhea, gynecomastia

GI: Constipation, epigastric pain, nausea, vomiting

GU: Ejaculation disorders, menstrual irregularities, urine retention

SKIN: Decreased sweating, photosensitivity, pruritus, rash

Other: Injection site irritation and sterile abscess, weight gain

Nursing Considerations

- Be aware that I.V. triflupromazine is not recommended for use in children because of its hypotensive and severe, rapid-onset extrapyramidal effects.
- Before administering triflupromazine, observe parenteral solution, which may turn slightly yellow without altering potency. Don't use solution if discoloration is pronounced or precipitate is present.
- Don't let solution come in contact with your skin because contact dermatitis may result.
- **WARNING** Monitor patient closely for tardive dyskinesia, which may continue after treatment stops. Notify prescriber if patient exhibits such signs as uncontrolled movements of arms, body, cheeks, jaw, legs, mouth, or tongue.
- Closely monitor elderly patients and severely ill or dehydrated children because they're at increased risk for certain adverse CNS reactions. Elderly patients are also at increased risk for developing hypotension amd extrapyramidal reactions, especially if they're acutely ill or debilitated.
- Monitor patients with glaucoma for signs and symptoms of this disorder, such as eye pain, vision changes, and nausea or vomiting from increased intraocular pressure, because of drug's anticholinergic effects.
- Monitor patients with chronic respiratory disorders (such as asthma and emphysema) or acute respiratory tract infections for exacerbations due to drug's CNS depressant effects.

- Monitor patients with cardiovascular, hepatic, or renal disease because they're at increased risk for developing hypotension, heart failure, and arrhythmias.
- Be aware that triflupromazine should be used cautiously in patients who will be exposed to organophosphate insecticides.
- **WARNING** If patient develops neuroleptic malignant syndrome (hyperpyrexia, muscle rigidity, altered mental status, autonomic instability), notify prescriber immediately and expect to discontinue drug and begin intensive medical treatment.
- **WARNING** Be alert for suppressed cough reflex, which increases patient's risk of aspirating vomitus.
- Monitor patients with a history of hepatic encephalopathy due to cirrhosis for increased sensitivity to drug's CNS effects.
- Monitor patients who have been exposed to extreme heat for heatstroke due to drug-induced suppression of temperature regulation. Symptoms include tachycardia, fever, and confusion.
- Before using triflupromazine, store it at 15° to 30° C (59° to 86° F); protect from freezing and light.

PATIENT TEACHING

- Instruct patient to change position slowly during triflupromazine therapy to minimize effects of orthostatic hypotension.
- Urge patient to avoid potentially hazardous activities until drug's CNS effects are known.
- Instruct patient to immediately report difficulty swallowing or speaking and tongue protrusion.
- Caution patient to avoid alcohol during therapy.
- Urge patient to avoid exposure to the sun and extreme heat because drug may cause photosensitivity and interfere with thermoregulation. Encourage her to wear sunscreen when outdoors.

tromethamine
Tham

Class and Category
Chemical: Organic amine
Therapeutic: Alkalinizer
Pregnancy category: C

Indications and Dosages

▶ *To treat metabolic acidosis associated with cardiac arrest*

I.V. INFUSION

Adults and children. 3.6 to 10.8 g (111 to 333 ml) of 0.3 M solution.

I.V. INJECTION

Adults and children. If chest is opened, 2 to 6 g injected directly into open ventricular cavity.

▶ *To treat metabolic acidosis during cardiac bypass surgery*

I.V. INFUSION

Adults and children. 9 ml (2.7 mEq or 0.32 g) of 0.3 M solution/kg as a single dose. *Usual:* 500 ml (150 mEq or 18 g) infused over 1 hr. *Maximum:* 500 mg/kg over 1 hr.

Mechanism of Action

Combines with hydrogen ions and their associated acid anions, including lactic, pyruvic, and carbonic acid, to form salts that are excreted in urine. Tromethamine exerts additional alkalinizing effects by acting as an osmotic diuretic, promoting the excretion of alkaline urine that contains increased amounts of carbon dioxide and electrolytes.

Contraindications

Anuria, chronic respiratory acidosis, hypersensitivity to tromethamine or its components, uremia

Interactions

DRUGS

amphetamines, quinidine, other pH-dependent drugs: Altered excretion of these drugs

Adverse Reactions

CNS: Fever
CV: Vasospasm
ENDO: Hypoglycemia
GI: Hepatic necrosis (hemorrhagic)
RESP: Respiratory depression
Other: Hypervolemia; infusion site infection, phlebitis, or venous thrombosis; metabolic alkalosis

Nursing Considerations

• Evaluate blood pH, blood glucose, and serum bicarbonate and electrolyte levels, and partial pressure of arterial carbon dioxide before, during, and after tromethamine therapy, as ordered.

- Administer infusion by an indwelling catheter inserted into a large vein, such as one in the antecubital area.
- **WARNING** Be aware that exceeding the recommended dosage can cause alkalosis, respiratory depression, and reduced carbon dioxide level. Because of the risk of alkalosis, tromethamine therapy is limited to 1 day, except in life-threatening situations.
- Be aware that I.V. administration of tromethamine increases the risk of hypervolemia and subsequent pulmonary edema.
- Assess infusion site frequently for signs of infiltration, which may cause inflammation, necrosis, thrombosis, tissue sloughing, and vasospasm.
- Be aware that patients with renal failure have an increased risk of developing hyperkalemia. For such patients, be prepared to monitor ECG continuously and assess serum potassium level frequently.
- Monitor blood glucose level frequently during and after therapy because rapid administration can cause hypoglycemia for several hours.
- Protect drug from freezing and extreme heat.

PATIENT TEACHING
- Inform family members that patient's vital signs and laboratory test results will be evaluated frequently to monitor her progress.

urea
(carbamide)
Ureaphil

Class and Category
Chemical: Carbonic acid diamide salt
Therapeutic: Antiglaucoma agent, diuretic
Pregnancy category: C

Indications and Dosages
▶ *To reduce cerebral edema and ICP*
I.V. INFUSION
Adults and children age 2 and older. 500 mg to 1.5 g/kg as 30% solution in D_5W, $D_{10}W$, or 10% invert sugar solution infused over 30 min to 2 hr at 4 ml/min or as ordered, according to manufacturer's instructions. *Maximum:* 2 g/kg/day.
Children under age 2. 100 mg to 1.5 g/kg as 30% solution in D_5W, $D_{10}W$, or 10% invert sugar solution infused over 30 min to

2 hr at 4 ml/min or as ordered, according to manufacturer's instructions.

▶ *To treat malignant or secondary glaucoma*
I.V. INFUSION
Adults. 500 mg to 1.5 g/kg as 30% solution in D_5W, $D_{10}W$, or 10% invert sugar solution infused over 30 min to 2 hr at 4 ml/min or as ordered, according to manufacturer's instructions. *Maximum:* 2 g/kg/day.
DOSAGE ADJUSTMENT Dosage reduced or drug withheld for patients with renal impairment if BUN level rises to 75 mg/dl or more or if diuresis fails to occur within 2 hr after administration.

Route	Onset	Peak	Duration
I.V.	10 min	1 to 2 hr	3 to 10 hr*

Mechanism of Action
Elevates blood plasma osmolality, creating an osmotic effect that increases the movement of water from the brain, CSF, and anterior portion of the eyes into interstitial fluid and plasma. This action reduces cerebral edema, ICP, CSF volume, and intraocular pressure. Large doses of urea inhibit the reabsorption of water and solutes in the renal tubules and induce diuresis by affecting the osmotic pressure gradient of the glomerular filtrate.

Incompatibilities
If patient is receiving blood simultaneously, don't administer urea through same administration set.

Contraindications
Active intracranial bleeding, hepatic failure, hypersensitivity to urea or its components, renal impairment, severe dehydration

Interactions
DRUGS
carbonic anhydrase inhibitors, other diuretics: Additive diuretic and intraocular pressure–reducing effects
lithium: Increased renal excretion of lithium

Adverse Reactions
CNS: Agitation, confusion, fever, headache, hyperthermia, nervousness, subarachnoid hemorrhage, subdural hematoma, syncope

---

* For diuresis; 5 to 6 hr for reduction of intraocular pressure in malignant or secondary glaucoma.

CV: Tachycardia
EENT: Dry mouth, intraocular hemorrhage
GI: Nausea, thirst, vomiting
GU: Elevated BUN level
HEME: Hemolysis
SKIN: Blemishes, extravasation with tissue necrosis and sloughing
Other: Dehydration, hypokalemia, hyponatremia, infusion site phlebitis or thrombosis

Nursing Considerations

- Expect to administer urea 60 minutes before intracranial or ocular surgery to obtain maximum reduction of ICP or intraocular pressure.
- Don't mix urea with invert sugar solution if patient has fructose intolerance from aldolase deficiency.
- Avoid infusing drug into leg veins to reduce the risk of phlebitis and thrombosis.
- Discard unused portion of drug after 24 hours.
- Be aware that rapid administration may cause hemolysis, increased capillary bleeding, and, in patients with glaucoma, intraocular hemorrhage.
- Maintain adequate hydration to minimize adverse reactions. Assess for signs of dehydration, including dry mucous membranes or tenting.
- Monitor BUN and serum electrolyte levels as well as fluid intake and output during urea therapy because prolonged use can cause diuresis.
- Store drug at 15° to 30° C (59° to 86° F); don't freeze.

PATIENT TEACHING

- Instruct patient to immediately report difficulty breathing or shortness of breath because urea can cause transient increases in circulatory volume, leading to circulatory overload, exacerbations of heart failure, or pulmonary edema.
- Advise patient to expect increased urine output.
- Encourage patient to remain on bed rest during urea therapy.

urokinase

Abbokinase, Abbokinase Open-Cath

Class and Category

Chemical: Renal enzymatic protein
Therapeutic: Thrombolytic
Pregnancy category: B

Indications and Dosages

▶ *To treat acute pulmonary thromboembolism*

I.V. INFUSION

Adults. *Initial:* 4,400 IU/kg over 10 min, followed by 4,400 IU/kg/hr for about 12 hr.

▶ *To treat acute coronary artery thrombosis*

INTRACORONARY INFUSION

Adults. 6,000 IU/min until artery is maximally opened (may take up to 2 hr). *Usual:* 500,000 IU.

▶ *To clear I.V. catheter occlusion*

INSTILLATION

Adults and children. 5,000 IU/ml instilled into occluded line.

Route	Onset	Peak	Duration
I.V.	Unknown	20 min to 2 hr	4 hr
Intracoronary	Unknown	Unknown	4 hr

Mechanism of Action

Indirectly promotes conversion of plasminogen to plasmin, an enzyme that breaks down fibrin clots, fibrinogen, and other plasma proteins, including procoagulant factors V and VIII.

Incompatibilities

Don't administer urokinase through same I.V. line as other drugs or add other drugs to urokinase solution.

Contraindications

Arteriovenous malformation, bleeding disorder, CVA during previous 2 months, hypersensitivity to urokinase or its components, internal bleeding, intracranial aneurysm, intracranial or intraspinal surgery during previous 2 months, intracranial tumor, recent cardiopulmonary resuscitation, recent trauma, severe uncontrolled hypertension (systolic blood pressure of 200 mm Hg or higher, or diastolic blood pressure of 110 mm Hg or higher)

Interactions

DRUGS

antifibrinolytics (aminocaproic acid, aprotinin): Mutual antagonism
antihypertensives: Increased risk of severe hypotension
cefamandole, cefoperazone, cefotetan, plicamycin, valproic acid: Increased risk of hypoprothrombinemia and severe hemorrhage
corticosteroids, ethacrynic acid, salicylates (nonacetylated): Increased risk of GI ulceration and bleeding

enoxaparin, heparin, NSAIDs, oral anticoagulants, platelet aggregation inhibitors: Increased risk of hemorrhage
thiotepa: Increased therapeutic effects of thiotepa

Adverse Reactions

CNS: Chills, CVA, fever, headache
CV: Arrhythmias, including tachycardia; chest pain; hypertension; hypotension
GI: Nausea, vomiting
HEME: Unusual bleeding
MS: Back pain, myalgia
RESP: Dyspnea, hypoxemia, wheezing
SKIN: Cyanosis, ecchymosis, flushing, pruritus, rash, urticaria
Other: Anaphylaxis, metabolic acidosis

Nursing Considerations

- **WARNING** Read label carefully to verify the urokinase concentration. Be aware that 250,000-IU concentration is for I.V. and intracoronary infusions only; 5,000-IU and 9,000-IU concentrations are for clearing I.V. catheter occlusions.
- Follow manufacturer's directions for reconstituting drug; mix 5,000-IU and 9,000-IU vials with supplied premeasured diluent to yield a final concentration of 5,000 IU/ml.
- Add 5 ml of sterile water for injection *without* preservatives to each 250,000-IU vial. Do *not* use bacteriostatic water for injection. Follow manufacturer's directions for further dilution for I.V. and intracoronary infusions. Discard unused portions.
- To prevent foaming, don't shake urokinase when reconstituting. Be aware that translucent filaments may form during reconstitution but won't affect drug's potency. Consult with pharmacist about giving drug through 0.45-micron or smaller cellulose membrane filter.
- Assess baseline hematocrit, platelet count, thrombin time, APTT, PT, and INR as ordered.
- Monitor heart rate and rhythm by continuous ECG during therapy, especially during rapid lysis of coronary thrombi, because arrhythmias can occur with reperfusion.
- Monitor blood pressure for hypotension. If hypotension occurs, notify prescriber and expect to reduce infusion rate.
- Check for bleeding at puncture sites and in urine and stool.
- Check for intracranial bleeding by performing frequent neurologic assessments.

- After arterial puncture is performed, apply pressure for at least 30 minutes and then apply pressure dressing. Check frequently for bleeding during therapy.
- Monitor the following patients for signs and symptoms of bleeding or hemorrhage because they're at increased risk during urokinase therapy: pregnant women; those with acute pericarditis (risk of hemopericardium, possibly leading to cardiac tamponade), cerebrovascular disease, hemorrhagic ophthalmic conditions, hypertension, mitral stenosis with atrial fibrillation (risk of embolism), septic thrombophlebitis, severe hepatic or renal disease, or subacute bacterial endocarditis; and those who have had major surgery, GI or GU bleeding, or trauma within the past 10 days.
- To prevent bleeding and associated complications, use an external blood pressure cuff to measure blood pressure; give acetaminophen (not aspirin), as prescribed, for fever; handle patient as little as possible; and avoid venipunctures and I.M. injections. If venipuncture is necessary, use a 23G or smaller needle.
- **WARNING** If serious bleeding begins and can't be controlled with local pressure, stop the infusion immediately and notify prescriber.
- Before reconstituting drug, store 250,000-IU vials at 2° to 8° C (36° to 46° F) and 5,000-IU and 9,000-IU vials at less than 25° C (77° F); don't freeze.

PATIENT TEACHING
- Instruct patient to remain on bed rest during urokinase therapy.
- Inform patient that minor bleeding may occur at wounds or puncture sites.

valproate sodium
Depacon
valproic acid
Alti-Valproic (CAN), Depakene, Deproic (CAN), Dom-Proic (CAN), Med-Valproic (CAN), Novo-Valproic (CAN), Nu-Valproic (CAN), PMS-Valproic Acid (CAN)
divalproex sodium
Depakote, Depakote Sprinkle, Epival (CAN)

Class and Category
Chemical: Carboxylic acid derivative
Therapeutic: Anticonvulsant
Pregnancy category: D

Indications and Dosages

▶ *To treat simple or complex absence seizures, complex partial seizures, myoclonic seizures, and generalized tonic-clonic seizures as monotherapy*

I.V. INFUSION, CAPSULES, DELAYED-RELEASE SPRINKLE CAPSULES, DELAYED-RELEASE TABLETS, SYRUP

Adults and adolescents. *Initial:* 10 to 15 mg/ kg/day in divided doses b.i.d. or t.i.d., increased by 5 to 10 mg/kg/day q wk, as needed and as prescribed. *Maximum:* 60 mg/kg/day.

Children. *Initial:* 15 to 45 mg/kg/day in divided doses b.i.d. or t.i.d., increased by 5 to 10 mg/kg/day q wk, as needed and as prescribed.

▶ *As adjunct to treat simple or complex absence seizures, complex partial seizures, myoclonic seizures, and generalized tonic-clonic seizures*

I.V. INFUSION, CAPSULES, DELAYED-RELEASE SPRINKLE CAPSULES, DELAYED-RELEASE TABLETS, SYRUP

Adults and adolescents. 10 to 30 mg/kg/day in divided doses, increased by 5 to 10 mg/kg/day q wk, as needed and as prescribed.

Children. 30 to 100 mg/kg/day in divided doses, as prescribed.

Mechanism of Action

Believed to decrease seizure activity by blocking the reuptake of gamma-aminobutyric acid (GABA), the most common inhibitory neurotransmitter in the brain. GABA is known to suppress the rapid firing of neurons by inhibiting voltage-sensitive sodium channels.

Contraindications

Hepatic dysfunction; hypersensitivity to valproic acid, valproate sodium, divalproex sodium, or their components

Interactions

DRUGS

aspirin, heparin, NSAIDs, oral anticoagulants, thrombolytics: Increased inhibition of platelet aggregation and risk of bleeding

barbiturates, primidone: Increased blood levels of both drugs, additive CNS effects

carbamazepine: Possibly decreased valproic acid effectiveness

cholestyramine: Decreased bioavailability of valproic acid

clonazepam: Increased risk of absence seizures

CNS depressants: Increased CNS depression

diazepam: Inhibited diazepam metabolism

ethosuximide: Unpredictable blood ethosuximide level

felbamate: Impaired valproic acid metabolism and increased blood drug level

haloperidol, loxapine, MAO inhibitors, maprotiline, phenothiazines, thioxanthenes, tricyclic antidepressants: Increased CNS depression, lowered seizure threshold

lamotrigine: Decreased lamotrigine clearance

mefloquine: Decreased blood levels of valproic acid, divalproex, and valproate sodium; increased risk of seizures

phenytoin: Increased risk of phenytoin toxicity, loss of seizure control

ACTIVITIES

alcohol use: Additive CNS depression

Adverse Reactions

CNS: Agitation, ataxia, confusion, depression, dizziness, drowsiness, euphoria, hallucinations, headache, hyperesthesia, lack of coordination, lethargy, loss of seizure control, paresthesia, psychosis, sedation, tremor, vertigo, weakness

EENT: Diplopia, nystagmus, pharyngitis, spots before eyes

ENDO: Galactorrhea, hyperglycemia

GI: Abdominal pain, anorexia, constipation, diarrhea, elevated liver function test results, hepatotoxicity, increased appetite, indigestion, nausea, pancreatitis, vomiting

GU: Menstrual irregularities

HEME: Eosinophilia, hematoma, leukopenia, prolonged bleeding time, thrombocytopenia

MS: Dysarthria

SKIN: Alopecia, diaphoresis, erythema multiforme, jaundice, petechiae, photosensitivity, pruritus, rash, Stevens-Johnson syndrome

Other: Facial edema, hyperammonemia, injection site pain, weight gain or loss

Nursing Considerations

- For I.V. infusion, dilute prescribed dose of valproate sodium with at least 50 ml of compatible diluent, such as D_5W, NS, or LR, and discard any unused portions. Use prepared solution within 24 hours if stored in glass bottles or polyvinyl chloride bags at controlled room temperature. Infuse over 60 minutes.
- Be aware that patient should be switched from I.V. to P.O. form of valproic acid as soon as possible.
- Give oral valproic acid or divalproex with food to minimize GI irritation, if necessary.

- Don't mix syrup with carbonated beverages; doing so may produce an unpleasant-tasting mixture and irritate the mouth and throat.
- Don't break or allow patient to chew delayed-release tablets.
- As needed, sprinkle contents of delayed-release sprinkle capsules on small amount of semisolid food just before administration. Instruct patient not to chew contents of delayed-release sprinkle capsules.
- Administer drug at least 2 hours before or 6 hours after cholestyramine.
- Be aware that patient with hypoalbuminemia or another protein-binding deficiency is at increased risk for valproic acid toxicity.
- Assess for signs and symptoms of decreased hepatic function, including anorexia, facial edema, jaundice, lethargy, loss of seizure control, malaise, vomiting, and weakness.
- Monitor liver function test results, as ordered. Assess for signs and symptoms of hepatotoxicity during first 6 months of treatment, especially in children under age 2. Notify prescriber immediately if you suspect hepatotoxicity.
- Be aware that hyperammonemia may occur even if patient's liver function test results are normal.
- Monitor platelet count, as ordered, for signs of thrombocytopenia, and notify prescriber if they appear.
- Store valproate sodium injection at 15° to 30° C (59° to 86° F). Consult manufacturer's instructions for storing oral forms.

PATIENT TEACHING

- Advise patient to avoid potentially hazardous activities during valproate sodium therapy because drug may affect mental and motor performance.
- Caution patient to avoid alcohol during therapy.
- Urge female patient to notify prescriber immediately about suspected or known pregnancy.
- Advise patient to notify prescriber if she develops a tremor, which may be dose-related.
- Instruct patient to swallow capsules whole to prevent irritation to mouth and throat. If she's taking delayed-release sprinkle capsules, tell her that she may open them and mix contents with soft food, such as applesauce, for easier swallowing. Emphasize that she should swallow—not chew—the contents of these capsules.

vancomycin hydrochloride
Vancocin

Class and Category
Chemical: Tricyclic glycopeptide derivative
Therapeutic: Antibiotic
Pregnancy category: C

Indications and Dosages
▶ *To treat bacterial endocarditis caused by methicillin-resistant* Staphylococcus aureus
I.V. INFUSION
Adults. 30 mg/kg/day in equally divided doses b.i.d. for 4 to 6 wk. *Maximum:* 2 g/day.
▶ *As adjunct to treat bacterial endocarditis caused by methicillin-resistant* S. *aureus in patients with prosthetic heart valve*
I.V. INFUSION
Adults. 30 mg/kg/day in equally divided doses b.i.d. to q.i.d. for 6 wk or longer in conjunction with rifampin and gentamicin. *Maximum:* 2 g/day.
▶ *To treat bacterial endocarditis caused by* Streptococcus bovis *or* Streptococcus viridans
I.V. INFUSION
Adults. 30 mg/kg/day in equally divided doses b.i.d. for 4 wk. *Maximum:* 2 g/day.
▶ *As adjunct to treat bacterial endocarditis caused by enterococci*
I.V. INFUSION
Adults. 30 mg/kg/day in equally divided doses b.i.d. for 4 to 6 wk in conjunction with gentamicin. *Maximum:* 2 g/day.
▶ *To treat bacterial septicemia, bone and joint infections, pneumonia, and skin and soft-tissue infections caused by* Staphylococcus, *including methicillin-resistant strains, and life-threatening infections*
I.V. INFUSION
Adults and children age 12 and older. 500 mg q 6 hr or 1 g q 12 hr infused over at least 60 min. *Maximum:* 4 g/day.
Children ages 1 month to 12 years. 10 mg/kg q 6 hr or 20 mg/kg q 12 hr infused over at least 60 min.
Neonates ages 1 week to 1 month. *Initial:* 15 mg/kg followed by 10 mg/kg q 8 hr infused over at least 60 min.
Neonates under age 1 week. *Initial:* 15 mg/kg followed by 10 mg/kg q 12 hr infused over at least 60 min.

Mechanism of Action
Inhibits bacterial RNA and cell wall synthesis and may alter the permeability of bacterial membranes; these actions lead to cell wall lysis and cell death.

Incompatibilities
Don't administer vancomycin through the same I.V. line as other drugs. Don't add vancomycin to albumin-containing solutions, alkaline solutions, aminophylline, amobarbital sodium, aztreonam, cefepime, ceftazidime, chloramphenicol sodium succinate, chlorothiazide sodium, dexamethasone sodium phosphate, foscarnet sodium, heparin sodium, methicillin sodium, penicillin G, pentobarbital sodium, phenobarbital sodium, piperacillin sodium and tazobactam sodium, secobarbital sodium, or sodium bicarbonate. Drug may form precipitate with heavy metals.

Contraindications
Hypersensitivity to vancomycin or its components

Interactions
DRUGS

aminoglycosides (amikacin, gentamicin, tobramycin), amphotericin B, bacitracin (parenteral), bumetanide, capreomycin, carmustine, cidofovir, cisplatin, cyclosporine, ethacrynic acid, furosemide, paromomycin, pentamidine (parenteral), polymyxins, salicylates (parenteral), streptozocin: Additive nephrotoxicity or ototoxicity

antihistamines, buclizine, cyclizine, meclizine, phenothiazines, thioxanthenes, trimethobenzamide: Masked symptoms of ototoxicity
dexamethasone: Decreased penetration of vancomycin into CSF
nephrotoxic drugs: Increased risk of nephrotoxicity

Adverse Reactions
CNS: Chills, dizziness, vertigo
CV: Hypotension
EENT: Ototoxicity
GI: Nausea
GU: Nephrotoxicity
HEME: Eosinophilia, neutropenia
RESP: Dyspnea, wheezing
SKIN: Exfoliative dermatitis; extravasation with pain, tenderness, thrombophlebitis, and tissue necrosis; pruritus; rash; toxic epidermal necrolysis; urticaria
Other: Anaphylaxis, drug-induced fever, injection site inflammation, superinfection

Nursing Considerations

- To reconstitute 500-mg vial of vancomycin for I.V. use, add 10 ml of sterile water for injection; further dilute with at least 100 ml of compatible I.V. solution, such as D₅W or NS. To reconstitute 1-g vial of dry, sterile powder, add 20 ml of sterile water for injection; further dilute with at least 200 ml of compatible I.V. solution, such as D₅W or NS.
- Be aware that a premixed form of vancomycin (500 mg/dl) is also available. Store this form at −20° to −10° C (−4° to 14° F) before use, and thaw at room temperature or in refrigerator, not in warm bath or microwave. Don't refreeze. When administering premixed form, don't use I.V. lines with series connections to prevent air embolism. Use within 72 hours if stored at room temperature or within 30 days if refrigerated. Don't use solution if it contains precipitate or is cloudy.
- **WARNING** Infuse drug over at least 1 hour. Rapid administration may cause hypotension or transient "red man syndrome," characterized by chills; fainting; fever; flushing of face, neck, upper arms, and torso; hypotension; nausea; tachycardia; and vomiting.
- Monitor blood vancomycin levels, as ordered; therapeutic trough levels are 10 to 15 mcg/ml and peak levels are 30 to 40 mcg/ml. Prescriber may adjust dosage for patients with impaired renal function based on blood drug level.
- Monitor CBC results and serum creatinine and BUN levels during therapy.
- Monitor I.V. infusion site for signs and symptoms of extravasation, including necrosis, pain, tenderness, and thrombophlebitis. If extravasation occurs, discontinue infusion immediately and notify prescriber.
- Monitor patient's hearing during therapy. Transient or permanent ototoxicity may occur if patient receives an excessive amount of drug, has an underlying hearing loss, or receives concurrent aminoglycosides.
- Monitor patient receiving prolonged therapy for signs of superinfection, such as severe diarrhea and white patches on tongue.
- Before reconstituting vancomycin, store it at 15° to 30° C (59° to 86° F).

PATIENT TEACHING
- Advise patient to report if no improvement occurs after a few days of vancomycin therapy.
- Emphasize the importance of completing the full course of vancomycin, as prescribed.

- Caution patient to consult prescriber before taking an antidiarrheal because diarrhea may signal superinfection.
- Instruct patient to keep follow-up medical appointments so that her progress can be monitored during and after treatment.

verapamil hydrochloride
Isoptin

Class and Category
Chemical: Phenylalkylamine derivative
Therapeutic: Antiarrhythmic
Pregnancy category: C

Indications and Dosages
▶ *To prevent or treat supraventricular tachycardia*
I.V. INJECTION
Adults and adolescents age 15 and older. *Initial:* 5 to 10 mg slowly over 2 min; then 10 mg, as prescribed, if response is inadequate after 30 min.
Children ages 1 to 15. *Initial:* 100 to 300 mcg/kg slowly over 2 min, up to maximum of 5 mg; then 10 mg, as prescribed, if response is inadequate after 30 min.
Infants up to age 1. *Initial:* 100 to 200 mcg/kg slowly over 2 min.
DOSAGE ADJUSTMENT Drug is administered to elderly patients over 3 minutes.

Route	Onset	Peak	Duration
I.V.	1 to 5 min	3 to 5 min	10 min to 6 hr

Mechanism of Action
Inhibits calcium movement into coronary and vascular smooth-muscle cells by blocking slow calcium channels in cell membranes. The resulting decrease in the intracellular calcium level has the following effects:
- inhibits smooth-muscle–cell contractions
- decreases myocardial oxygen demand by relaxing coronary and vascular smooth muscle, reducing peripheral vascular resistance, and decreasing systolic and diastolic pressures
- slows AV conduction time and prolongs AV nodal refractoriness
- interrupts reentry circuit in AV-nodal reentrant tachycardias.

Incompatibilities

Don't mix verapamil with albumin, amphotericin B injection, co-trimoxazole (sulfamethoxazole and trimethoprim) injection, hydralazine hydrochloride injection, or nafcillin. Solutions with pH above 6.0 cause precipitation.

Contraindications

Cardiogenic shock, concomitant use of beta blockers, hypersensitivity to verapamil or its components, hypotension, severe heart failure unless secondary to supraventricular tachycardia that responds to verapamil, severe left ventricular dysfunction, sick sinus syndrome or second- or third-degree heart block unless artificial pacemaker is in place, ventricular tachycardia

Interactions

DRUGS

alpha blockers, antihypertensives, hydrocarbon inhalation anesthetics, prazosin: Hypotensive effects

beta blockers: Increased risk of heart failure, hypotension, and severe bradycardia

calcium supplements: Decreased response to verapamil

carbamazepine, cyclosporine, theophylline, valproate: Increased risk of toxicity from these drugs

cimetidine: Decreased metabolism and increased blood level of verapamil

dantrolene: Increased risk of hyperkalemia and myocardial depression

digoxin: Increased blood digoxin level and risk of digitalis toxicity

disopyramide, flecainide: Additive negative inotropic effects

lithium: Increased risk of neurotoxicity

neuromuscular blockers: Prolonged recovery from neuromuscular blockade

NSAIDs, sympathomimetics: Decreased antihypertensive effect of verapamil

phenobarbital: Increased verapamil clearance

procainamide: Possibly further prolongation of Q-T interval, additive negative inotropic effects

protein-bound drugs (hydantoins, salicylates, sulfonamides, sulfonylureas, and warfarin and other oral anticoagulants): Altered blood levels of these drugs

quinidine: Increased risk of quinidine toxicity, possibly further prolongation of Q-T interval, additive negative inotropic effects

rifampin: Decreased bioavailability of oral verapamil
ACTIVITIES
alcohol use: Increased blood alcohol level and prolonged CNS effects

Adverse Reactions

CNS: Dizziness, fatigue, headache
CV: Angina, AV conduction disorders, bradycardia, claudication, heart failure, hypotension, peripheral edema, tachycardia
GI: Constipation, nausea
GU: Galactorrhea, menstrual irregularities
RESP: Dyspnea, pulmonary edema, wheezing
SKIN: Flushing, rash

Nursing Considerations

- Administer verapamil with compatible solutions, including Ringer's injection, D₅W, or NS.
- Maintain continuous ECG monitoring and keep emergency resuscitative equipment and drugs readily available during verapamil therapy.
- Assess patient with hypertrophic cardiomyopathy for early development of hypotension and pulmonary edema because second-degree AV block and sinus arrest can result.
- Assess for bradycardia and hypotension, and notify prescriber if heart rate or blood pressure declines significantly.
- **WARNING** Be aware that disopyramide or flecainide should not be given for 48 hours before or 24 hours after verapamil because additive negative inotropic effects can result.
- Institute measures to prevent constipation, including a high-fiber diet and a stool softener, as prescribed.
- Store drug at 15° to 30° C (59° to 86° F); protect from freezing and light.

PATIENT TEACHING

- Caution patient about possible dizziness and the need to avoid potentially hazardous activities until verapamil's CNS effects are known.
- Instruct patient to immediately report chest pain, dizziness, rash, or shortness of breath.
- Inform patient that rash and flushing may subside with continued use. Advise her to report a persistent rash.
- Encourage patient to increase dietary fiber intake to help prevent constipation. Advise her to report persistent or severe constipation.

vinblastine sulfate
Velban, Velbe (CAN)

Class and Category
Chemical: Vinca alkaloid
Therapeutic: Antimicrotubule antineoplastic
Pregnancy category: D

Indications and Dosages
▶ *To treat breast or testicular cancer, gestational trophoblastic tumors, histiocytosis X, Hodgkin's disease or non-Hodgkin's lymphoma, Kaposi's sarcoma, or mycosis fungoides*

I.V. INJECTION

Adults. *Initial:* 100 mcg (0.1mg)/kg or 3.7 mg/m² over 1 min q 7 days, increased in weekly increments of 50 mcg (0.05 mg)/kg or 1.8 to 1.9 mg/m² until leukocyte count falls to 3,000/mm³. *Maintenance:* 50 mcg (0.05 mg/kg) or 1.8 to 1.9 mg/m² less than final initial dose. *Maximum:* 500 mcg (0.5 mg)/kg or 18.5 mg/m².
Adolescents and children. *Initial:* 2.5 mg/m² over 1 min q 7 days, increased in weekly increments of 1.25 mg/m² until leukocyte count falls to 3,000/mm³. *Maintenance:* 1.25 mg/m² less than final initial dose. *Maximum:* 7.5 mg/m².
DOSAGE ADJUSTMENT Dosage decreased by 50% for patients with direct serum bilirubin concentration above 3 mg/dl.

Mechanism of Action
Binds to tubulin, a protein component of microtubules, which normally contribute to cell structure and movement, thereby inhibiting microtubule assembly and arresting cells in metaphase. Vinblastine may also interfere with amino acid metabolism. This drug is cell-cycle–phase specific for the M phase of cell division.

Incompatibilities
Prepare vinblastine solution using NS. Don't mix solution with any other drug.

Contraindications
Bacterial infection; granulocytopenia resulting from condition other than disease being treated

Interactions
DRUGS
blood-dyscrasia–causing drugs (such as cephalosporins and sulfasalazine): Increased risk of leukopenia and thrombocytopenia

bone marrow depressants (such as carboplatin and lomustine): Possibly additive bone marrow depression

hepatic enzyme inhibitors (such as allopurinol and cimetidine): Possibly earlier onset or increased severity of vinblastine adverse effects

itraconazole: Possibly earlier onset or increased severity of neuro-muscular adverse effects

phenytoin: Possibly decreased blood phenytoin level and increased risk of seizures

vaccines, killed virus: Possibly decreased antibody response to vaccine

vaccines, live virus: Possibly decreased antibody response to vaccine, increased adverse effects of vaccine, and severe infection

Adverse Reactions

CNS: Malaise, neurotoxicity, weakness
CV: Hypertension
EENT: Jaw pain, stomatitis
GI: Anorexia, constipation, nausea, vomiting
GU: Uric acid nephropathy
HEME: Anemia, leukopenia, thrombocytopenia (transient)
MS: Bone pain, tissue pain at tumor site
SKIN: Alopecia
Other: Hyperuricemia, injection site pain or redness

Nursing Considerations

- Follow facility protocols for preparation and handling of anti-neoplastic drugs and for appropriate disposal of used equipment.
- Be aware that vinblastine dosage may vary, depending on dosage schedule and regimen being used.
- Be aware that adverse reactions can vary when vinblastine is administered in combination therapy. Review information for all drugs administered as part of a specific regimen, including drug interactions and adverse effects.
- Monitor liver function test results; hematocrit, hemoglobin, and platelet count; and leukocyte count (total and differential) before and periodically during treatment, as ordered.
- Monitor blood uric acid level of patients with a history of gout or renal calculi before and periodically during therapy to detect hyperuricemia. Expect to give allopurinol, as ordered, to patients with elevated blood uric acid levels to prevent uric acid nephropathy. Be aware that patients already receiving antigout drugs, such as allopurinol, colchicine, probenecid, or sufinpyrazone, may require an adjustment in antigout drug dosage.

- Be aware that vinblastine is available in a 1-mg/ml preparation or as a powder for reconstitution. To reconstitute vinblastine, add 10 ml of 0.9% sodium chloride injection to a vial containing 10 mg/ml to yield a final concentration of 1 mg/ml. If the diluent contains a preservative, such as benzyl alcohol, use diluted solution within 28 days if stored at 2° to 8° C (36° to 46° F). If the diluent doesn't contain a preservative, use solution immediately and discard unused portion.

- **WARNING** When preparing vinblastine for administration to neonates or premature infants, don't use a diluent that contains benzyl alcohol because this preservative has been linked to a fatal toxic syndrome characterized by CNS, respiratory, circulatory, and renal impairment and metabolic acidosis.

- If vinblastine solution comes in contact with your skin or mucosa, wash if off thoroughly with warm water. If drug comes in contact with your eye, irrigate eye thoroughly with water to prevent irritation or corneal ulceration.

- **WARNING** Clearly label syringe containing prepared dose "FATAL IF GIVEN INTRATHECALLY. FOR I.V. USE ONLY" and place in overwrap. Label overwrap with the same warning and the additional statement "DO NOT REMOVE COVERING UNTIL THE MOMENT OF INJECTION." Don't administer drug intrathecally because potentially fatal paralysis may occur.

- Inspect I.V. site for signs of infiltration and leakage into surrounding tissues. If extravasation occurs, stop injection immediately and notify prescriber. Then resume injection in another vein. Apply warm heat to affected area, and expect to administer a local injection of hyaluronidase, if ordered, to help decrease discomfort and reduce the risk of cellulitis.

- Be aware that subsequent doses of vinblastine shouldn't be administered until leukocyte count after previous dose has returned to at least 4,000/mm^3, even if 7 days has passed.

- Monitor patients who have, or have recently been exposed to, chicken pox or who have herpes zoster for signs and symptoms of severe generalized disease.

- Be aware that patients who have previously received cytotoxic therapy and those who are receiving concurrent or consecutive radiation therapy are at risk for additive bone marrow depression.

- If patient develops thrombocytopenia, implement protective precautions according to facility policy.

- Assess for signs of infection, such as fever, if patient develops leukopenia. Expect to obtain appropriate specimens for culture

and sensitivity testing and implement protective precautions according to facility policy.
- Before reconstituting powder form or using diluted form, store vinblastine at 2° to 8° C (36° to 46° F).

PATIENT TEACHING
- Advise patient to have dental work completed before beginning vinblastine treatment, if possible, or to defer such work until blood counts return to normal because vinblastine can delay healing and cause gingival bleeding. Teach patient proper oral hygiene, and advise her to use a soft-bristled toothbrush.
- Advise patient to immediately report burning at injection site or other signs of extravasation.
- Instruct patient who develops bone marrow depression to avoid people with infections. Advise her to report fever, chills, cough, hoarseness, lower back or side pain, or painful or difficult urination because these signs and symptoms may indicate an infection.
- Instruct patient to avoid touching her eyes or inside of her nose unless she washes her hands immediately beforehand.
- Caution patient to avoid receiving immunizations unless approved by prescriber. Instruct her to avoid people who have recently received vaccines or to wear a protective mask over her nose and mouth if she must be around them.
- Instruct patient to immediately report unusual bleeding or bruising, black or tarry stools, blood in urine or stools, or red pinpoint spots on skin.
- Stress the importance of avoiding accidental cuts from sharp objects, such as razor blades or fingernail clippers, because excessive bleeding or infection may occur.
- Encourage patient to drink plenty of fluids to increase urine output and help excrete uric acid.
- Suggest that patient with stomatitis eat bland, soft foods served cold or at room temperature to decrease irritation.
- Caution patient to avoid contact sports or other situations that put her at risk for bruising or injury.
- Stress the importance of complying with the dosage regimen and of keeping follow-up medical appointments and appointments for laboratory tests.
- Reassure patient that her hair should grow back after vinblastine therapy has been completed.
- Urge patient to use contraception because of the risk of fetal harm from vinblastine therapy. Instruct her to notify prescriber immediately if she becomes pregnant.

vincristine sulfate

Oncovin, Vincasar PFS

Class and Category

Chemical: Vinca alkaloid
Therapeutic: Antineoplastic
Pregnancy category: D

Indications and Dosages

▶ *To treat acute lymphocytic leukemia, Hodgkin's disease or non-Hodgkin's lymphoma, neuroblastoma, or Wilms' tumor*

I.V. INJECTION

Adults. 10 to 30 mcg (0.01 to 0.03 mg)/kg or 400 mcg (0.4 mg) to 1.4 mg/m² over 1 min q wk. Dosage adjusted based on patient's clinical response and presence or severity of toxicity.

Children who weigh more than 10 kg. 1.5 to 2 mg/m² over 1 min q wk.

Children who weigh 10 kg and less. 50 mcg (0.05 mg)/kg over 1 min q wk.

DOSAGE ADJUSTMENT Dosage decreased by 50% for patients with direct serum bilirubin concentration above 3 mg/dl.

Mechanism of Action

Inhibits the formation of microtubules, which normally contribute to cell structure and movement, thus arresting cells in metaphase. Vincristine is cell-cycle–phase specific for the M phase of cell division.

Incompatibilities

Don't administer vincristine with solutions that lower or raise pH outside the range of 3.5 to 5.5. Administer only with NS or D₅W.

Contraindications

Demyelinating form of Charcot-Marie-Tooth syndrome

Interactions

DRUGS

asparaginase, itraconazole, neurotoxic drugs: Possibly additive neurotoxic effects

bleomycin: Increased susceptibility of cancer cells to bleomycin

blood-dyscrasia–causing drugs (such as cephalosporins and sulfasalazine): Increased risk of leukopenia and thrombocytopenia

bone marrow depressants (such as carboplatin and lomustine): Possibly additive bone marrow depression

doxorubicin: Increased risk of myelosuppression when used in combination with vincristine and prednisone

phenytoin: Possibly decreased blood phenytoin level and increased risk of seizures

vaccines, killed virus: Possibly decreased antibody response to vaccine

vaccines, live virus: Possibly decreased antibody response to vaccine, increased adverse effects of vaccine, and severe infection

Adverse Reactions

CNS: Fever, headache, progressive neurotoxicity (including blurred or double vision, decreased reflexes, difficulty walking, neuritic pain, and paresthesia)

CV: Hypertension, hypotension

EENT: Stomatitis

ENDO: Syndrome of inappropriate ADH secretion (SIADH)

GI: Bloating, constipation (severe), diarrhea, nausea, vomiting

GU: Dysuria, polyuria, uric acid nephropathy, urine retention

HEME: Anemia, leukopenia, thrombocytopenia

RESP: Bronchospasm, dyspnea

SKIN: Alopecia, rash

Other: Allergic reaction, hyperuricemia, injection site pain or redness, weight loss

Nursing Considerations

- Follow facility protocols for preparation and handling of antineoplastic drugs and for appropriate disposal of used equipment.
- Be aware that vincristine dosage may vary, depending on dosage schedule and regimen being used.
- Be aware that adverse reactions can vary when vincristine is administered in combination therapy. Review information for all drugs administered as part of a specific regimen, including drug interactions and adverse effects.
- Monitor liver function test results; hematocrit, hemoglobin, and platelet count; and leukocyte count (total and differential) before and periodically during treatment, as ordered.
- Monitor blood uric acid level of patients with a history of gout or renal calculi before and periodically during therapy to detect hyperuricemia. Expect to give allopurinol, as ordered, to patients with elevated blood uric acid levels to prevent uric acid nephropathy. Be aware that patients already receiving antigout drugs, such as allopurinol, colchicine, probenecid, or sufinpyrazone, may require an adjustment in antigout drug dosage.
- If vincristine solution comes in contact with your skin or mucosa, wash it off thoroughly with warm water. If drug comes in

contact with your eye, irrigated the eye thoroughly with water to prevent irritation or corneal ulceration.

- **WARNING** After withdrawing appropriate amount of drug from vial, as ordered, clearly label syringe "FATAL IF GIVEN INTRATHECALLY. FOR I.V. USE ONLY" and place in overwrap. Label overwrap with the same warning and the additional statement "DO NOT REMOVE COVERING UNTIL THE MOMENT OF INJECTION." Don't administer drug intrathecally because potentially fatal paralysis may occur.
- Administer vincristine over a 1-minute period by I.V. bolus, or inject it into a free-flowing I.V. infusion of NS or D_5W.
- Inspect I.V. site for signs of infiltration and leakage into surrounding tissues. If extravasation occurs, stop the injection immediately and notify prescriber. Then resume the injection in another vein. Apply warm heat to affected area, and expect to administer a local injection of hyaluronidase, if ordered, to help decrease discomfort and reduce the risk of cellulitis.
- Administer a prophylactic enema or laxative, if ordered, to prevent ileus.
- Monitor patient for hypotension and signs of neurotoxicity, such as paresthesia, decreased reflexes, and weakness. If such signs occur, notify prescriber and expect to decrease dosage or discontinue therapy, as ordered.
- Monitor patients who have, or have recently been exposed to, chicken pox or who have herpes zoster for signs and symptoms of severe generalized disease.
- Be aware that patients who have previously received cytotoxic therapy and those who are receiving concurrent or consecutive radiation therapy are at risk for additive bone marrow depression.
- If patient develops thrombocytopenia, implement protective precautions according to facility policy.
- Assess for signs of infection, such as fever, if patient develops leukopenia. Expect to obtain appropriate specimens for culture and sensitivity testing.
- Store vincristine at 2° to 8° C (36° to 46° F) in a light-resistant container.

PATIENT TEACHING
- Advise patient to immediately report burning at injection site or other signs of extravasation during vincristine therapy.
- Instruct patient who develops bone marrow depression to avoid people with infections. Advise her to report fever, chills, cough, hoarseness, lower back or side pain, or painful or difficult uri-

nation because these signs and symptoms may indicate an infection.

- Instruct patient to avoid touching her eyes or inside of her nose unless she washes her hands immediately beforehand.
- Caution patient to avoid receiving immunizations unless approved by prescriber. Urge her to avoid people who have recently received vaccines or to wear a protective mask over her nose and mouth if she must be around them.
- Instruct patient to immediately report unusual bleeding or bruising, black or tarry stools, blood in urine or stool, or red pinpoint spots on skin during vincristine therapy.
- Stress the importance of avoiding accidental cuts from sharp objects, such as razor blades or fingernail clippers, because excessive bleeding or infection may occur.
- Caution patient to avoid contact sports or other situations that put her at risk for bruising or injury.
- Encourage patient to drink fluids to increase urine output and help excrete uric acid; however, caution her not to drink excessive amounts because of the risk of SIADH.
- Suggest that patient with stomatitis eat bland, soft foods served cold or at room temperature to decrease irritation.
- Advise patient to consult prescriber about using a laxative if she develops constipation.
- Reassure patient that her hair should grow back after vincristine therapy has been completed.
- Urge patient to use contraception because of the risk of fetal harm from vincristine therapy. Instruct her to notify prescriber immediately if she becomes pregnant.
- Stress the importance of complying with the dosage regimen and of keeping follow-up medical appointments and appointments for laboratory tests.

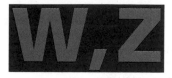

warfarin sodium
Coumadin

Class and Category
Chemical: Coumarin derivative
Therapeutic: Anticoagulant
Pregnancy category: X

Indications and Dosages
▶ *To prevent or treat pulmonary embolism; recurrent MI; thrombo-embolic complications from atrial fibrillation, heart valve replacement, or MI; and venous thrombosis (and its extension)*

I.V. INJECTION

Adults. *Initial:* 2 to 5 mg/day infused over 1 to 2 min. *Usual:* 2 to 10 mg/day infused over 1 to 2 min. *Maximum:* Determined by target PT and INR results, as prescribed.

TABLETS

Adults. *Initial:* 2 to 5 mg/day for 2 to 4 days. *Usual:* 2 to 10 mg/day based on target PT and INR results. *Maximum:* Determined by target PT and INR results, as prescribed.

DOSAGE ADJUSTMENT For patients with hepatic dysfunction, dosage reduced to 0.1 mg/kg, as prescribed. For elderly patients, dosage possibly reduced based on PT and INR results.

Route	Onset	Peak	Duration
I.V.	Unknown	3 to 4 days	2 to 5 days

Mechanism of Action
Interferes with the liver's ability to synthesize vitamin K–dependent clotting factors, depleting clotting factors II (prothrombin), VII, IX, and X. This action, in turn, interferes with the clotting cascade. By depleting vitamin K–dependent clotting factors and interfering with the clotting cascade, warfarin prevents coagulation.

Incompatibilities

Don't mix warfarin in same solution with amikacin sulfate, epinephrine hydrochloride, metaraminol tartrate, oxytocin, promazine hydrochloride, tetracycline hydrochloride, or vancomycin hydrochloride.

Contraindications

Bleeding or bleeding tendencies; blood dyscrasias; cerebral or dissecting aneurysm; cerebrovascular hemorrhage; diverticulitis; eclampsia or preeclampsia; history of warfarin-induced necrosis; hypersensitivity to warfarin or its components; malignant or severe uncontrolled hypertension; malnutrition and emaciation; mental state or condition that leads to lack of patient cooperation; pericardial effusion; pericarditis; polyarthritis; pregnancy; prostatectomy; recent or planned neurosurgery, ophthalmic surgery, or spinal puncture; severe hepatic or renal disease

Interactions

DRUGS

acetaminophen, aminoglycosides, amiodarone, androgens, beta blockers, cephalosporins, chloral hydrate, chloramphenicol, chlorpropamide, cimetidine, clofibrate, corticosteroids, cyclophosphamide, dextrothyroxine, diflunisal, disulfiram, erythromycin, fluconazole, gemfibrozil, glucagon, hydantoins, ifosfamide, influenza virus vaccine, isoniazid, ketoconazole, loop diuretics, lovastatin, metronidazole, miconazole, mineral oil, moricizine, nalidixic acid, NSAIDs, omeprazole, penicillins, phenylbutazones, propafenone, propoxyphene, quinidine, quinine, quinolones, salicylates, streptokinase, sulfamethoxazole-trimethoprim, sulfinpyrazone, sulfonamides, tamoxifen, tetracyclines, thyroid hormones, urokinase, vitamin E: Increased anticoagulant effect of warfarin, increased risk of bleeding

aminoglutethimide, barbiturates, carbamazepine, cholestyramine, dicloxacillin, estrogens, ethchlorvynol, etretinate, glutethimide, griseofulvin, nafcillin, oral contraceptives, rifampin, spironolactone, sucralfate, thiazide diuretics, trazodone, vitamin C, vitamin K: Decreased anticoagulant effect of warfarin

I.V. lipid emulsions and other medical products that contain soybean oil: Possibly decreased vitamin K absorption and increased anticoagulant effect of warfarin

nicotine patch: Altered response to warfarin

FOODS

certain multivitamins, enteral feedings, foods rich in vitamin K: Decreased effects of warfarin

ACTIVITIES

alcohol use: Increased risk of hypoprothrombinemia
smoking cessation: Altered response to warfarin

Adverse Reactions

CNS: Intracranial hemorrhage, weakness
EENT: Epistaxis, intraocular hemorrhage
GI: Abdominal cramps and pain, diarrhea, hepatitis, nausea, vomiting
GU: Hematuria, vaginal bleeding (abnormal)
HEME: Potentially fatal hemorrhage (from any tissue or organ)
SKIN: Alopecia, ecchymosis, jaundice, petechiae, pruritus, purple-toe syndrome, tissue necrosis

Nursing Considerations

- Reconstitute parenteral warfarin just before administration with 2.7 ml of sterile water for injection to yield 2 mg/ml. Administer slowly over 1 to 2 minutes through peripheral I.V. line. Use within 4 hours.
- Expect to administer another parenteral anticoagulant, such as heparin or enoxaparin, with oral warfarin for at least 3 days, or until desired response occurs, before giving warfarin only.
- Avoid I.M. injections during warfarin therapy, if possible, because they can result in bleeding, bruising, and hematoma.
- Monitor INR (daily in acute care setting) and assess for therapeutic effects, as prescribed. Therapeutic INR levels are 2.0 to 3.0 for bioprosthetic heart valve, nonvalvular atrial fibrillation, and venous thromboembolism, and 2.5 to 3.5 for mechanical heart valve and after MI.
- Expect treatment to last up to 12 weeks for bioprosthetic heart valve, 1 to 3 months for nonvalvular atrial fibrillation or venous thromboembolism, and for rest of patient's life for mechanical heart valve replacement and after MI.
- **WARNING** Be aware that patients with cerebral ischemia (for example, from recent transient ischemic attack or minor ischemic CVA) and INR of 3 to 4.5 are at increased risk for intracranial hemorrhage. If INR exceeds 4, withhold next warfarin dose and give vitamin K, as prescribed, to decrease the risk of bleeding.
- Assess for occult bleeding if patient receives I.V. lipid emulsion or other medical product that contains soybean oil. Such products can decrease vitamin K absorption and increase warfarin's anticoagulant effect.

- Store drug at 15° to 30° C (59° to 86° F); protect from freezing and light.

PATIENT TEACHING

- Explain that warfarin therapy aims to prevent thrombosis by decreasing clotting ability while avoiding the risk of spontaneous bleeding.
- Urge patient to immediately report unusual bleeding and unexplained symptoms, such as abnormal vaginal bleeding; dizziness; easy bruising; gum bleeding; headache; nosebleeds; prolonged bleeding from cuts; red, black, or tarry stools; red or dark brown urine; swelling; and weakness.
- Instruct patient who's taking oral warfarin to take drug exactly as prescribed at the same time each evening.
- Urge patient to keep weekly follow-up appointments for blood tests after discharge until PT and INR levels are stabilized.
- Advise patient to avoid alcohol during warfarin therapy.
- Urge patient to take precautions against bleeding, such as using an electric shaver and a soft-bristled toothbrush. Advise him to continue these precautions for 2 to 5 days after therapy stops, as directed, because anticoagulant effect may persist during this time.
- Caution patient to avoid activities that could cause traumatic injury and bleeding.
- Advise patient to eat consistent amounts of vitamin K–rich foods, such as dark green, leafy vegetables.
- Advise patient to consult prescriber before taking other drugs including OTC drugs—during therapy.
- Instruct female patient of childbearing age to stop taking warfarin and notify prescriber immediately about known or suspected pregnancy.
- Explain that drug may cause reversible purple-toe syndrome but that this syndrome isn't harmful.
- Urge patient to carry medical identification that reveals he's receiving warfarin therapy.

zidovudine
Retrovir

Class and Category
Chemical: Synthetic pyrimidine nucleoside analogue
Therapeutic: Antiviral
Pregnancy category: C

Indications and Dosages

▶ *To treat HIV infection*

I.V. INFUSION

Adults and children over age 12 (United States). 1 mg/kg infused over 1 hr five or six times a day. *Maximum pediatric dose:* 160 mg.

Adults and children over age 12 (Canada). 1 to 2 mg/kg infused over 1 hr q 4 hr. *Maximum pediatric dose:* 160 mg.

DOSAGE ADJUSTMENT Adult dosage reduced to 1 mg/kg q 6 to 8 hr for patients with end-stage renal disease.

▶ *To prevent maternal-fetal HIV transmission*

I.V. INFUSION

Mother. 2 mg/kg infused over 1 hr at the start of labor and delivery, followed by 1 mg/kg/hr by continuous infusion until umbilical cord is clamped.

Neonate. 1.5 mg/kg infused over 30 min q 6 hr.

Mechanism of Action

Ultimately converted by thymidine kinase and other cellular enzymes to zidovudine triphosphate. Zidovudine triphosphate is incorporated into growing chains of viral DNA polymerase, an enzyme used in the viral DNA replication process, thus inhibiting DNA viral replication of HIV.

Incompatibilities

Don't mix zidovudine with biological or colloidal solutions, such as blood products or protein-containing solutions.

Contraindications

Hypersensitivity to zidovudine or its components

Interactions

DRUGS

atovaquone: Possibly decreased zidovudine clearance and increased blood zidovudine level

blood-dyscrasia–causing drugs (such as cephalosporins and sulfasalazine), bone marrow depressants (such as carboplatin and lomustine): Increased risk of additive myelosuppressive effects

clarithromycin: Decreased blood zidovudine level and time to peak zidovudine concentration

cytotoxic drugs, ganciclovir, interferon alfa: Increased risk of hematologic toxicities

hepatic glucuronidation–metabolized drugs (such as acetaminophen, aspirin, benzodiazepines, cimetidine, indomethacin, morphine, and sulfonamides): Possibly decreased clearance and toxicity of both drugs
methadone, rifampin: Possibly altered blood zidovudine level
phenytoin: Possibly decreased blood phenytoin level and decreased zidovudine clearance
probenecid: Possibly increased blood ziduvodine level and flulike symptoms
ribovirin, stavudine: Possibly antagonized antiviral effect

Adverse Reactions

CNS: Chills, fever, headache, insomnia, tiredness, weakness
EENT: Pharyngitis
GI: Nausea
HEME: Anemia, bone marrow depression, granulocytopenia, leukopenia, neutropenia, platelet count changes
MS: Myalgia
SKIN: Altered skin pigmentation, hyperpigmentation (bluish-brown bands) of nails, pallor

Nursing Considerations

- Be aware that I.V. infusion of zidovudine is ordered only until oral drug can be administered.
- Dilute ziduvodine with D_5W to a maximum concentration of 4 mg/ml. Use within 8 hours if stored at room temperature or within 24 hours if stored at 2° to 8° C (36° to 46° F) to decrease the risk of microbial contamination. Discard solution if you observe particles or discoloration before administration.
- Administer zidovudine by I.V. infusion at a constant rate over 1 hour; don't administer drug by rapid infusion or by I.M. injection.
- Monitor CBC periodically during zidovudine therapy. Be aware that anemia most commonly occurs after 4 to 6 weeks of therapy and that patient may require dosage adjustment, discontinuation of drug, blood transfusions, or epoetin treatment if hemoglobin level is less than 7.5 g/dl or if granulocyte count is less than 750/mm^3.
- Assess patient for dyspnea, tachypnea, or decreased blood bicarbonate level; if she exhibits such findings, expect zidovudine to be discontinued until a diagnosis of lactic acidosis can be ruled out.
- Before diluting drug, store it at 15° to 25° C (59° to 77° F) and protect from light.

PATIENT TEACHING
• Advise mothers being treated for HIV infection not to breast-feed infant to prevent transmission of virus.
• Instruct patient to use a condom to decrease the risk of transmitting HIV. Also, urge patient not to share needles with anyone.
• Teach patient proper oral hygiene, and advise her to use a soft-bristled toothbrush to decrease the risk of infection or delayed healing.
• Inform patient who is also receiving cidofovir that zidovudine dosage may need to be adjusted or therapy temporarily discontinued on the day of cidofovir therapy.
• Explain to patient that zidovudine is not a cure for HIV infection. Stress the importance of complying with dosage regimen and of keeping follow-up medical appointments and appointments for laboratory tests.

zinc acetate
(contains 25 or 50 mg of elemental zinc per capsule)
Galzin
zinc chloride
(contains 1 mg of elemental zinc per ml for I.V. infusion)
zinc gluconate
(contains 1.4 mg of elemental zinc per lozenge; 1.4, 2, 4, 7, 8, 10, 11, 13, 31, 50, or 52 mg of elemental zinc per tablet)
Orazinc
zinc sulfate
(contains 1 or 5 mg of elemental zinc per ml for I.V. infusion)
Zinca-Pak

Class and Category
Chemical: Trace element, mineral
Therapeutic: Copper absorption inhibitor, nutritional supplement
Pregnancy category: C (I.V.), A (oral)

Indications and Dosages
▶ *To prevent zinc deficiency based on U.S. and Canadian recommended daily allowances*
I.V. INFUSION
Adults and children. 2.5 to 4 mg q.d. added to total parenteral nutrition (TPN) solution. *Maximum:* 12 mg/day.

Children from birth to age 5. 100 mcg/kg/day added to TPN solution.

Premature infants weighing up to 3 kg. 300 mcg/kg/day added to TPN solution.

CAPSULES, E.R. TABLETS, LOZENGES, TABLETS

Male adults and children age 11 and older. 15 mg (9 to 12 mg Canadian) of elemental zinc daily.

Female adults and children age 11 and older. 12 mg (9 mg Canadian) of elemental zinc daily.

Pregnant females. 15 mg (15 mg Canadian) of elemental zinc daily.

Breast-feeding females. 16 to 19 mg (15 mg Canadian) of elemental zinc daily.

Children ages 7 to 10. 10 mg (7 to 9 mg Canadian) of elemental zinc daily.

Children ages 4 to 6. 10 mg (5 mg Canadian) of elemental zinc daily.

Children from birth to age 3. 5 to 10 mg (2 to 4 mg Canadian) of elemental zinc daily.

▶ *To treat zinc deficiency*

I.V. INFUSION

Adults and adolescents. 2.5 to 4 mg q.d. added to TPN solution. *Maximum:* 12 mg/day.

Children from birth to age 5. 100 mcg/kg/day added to TPN solution.

Premature infants weighing up to 3 kg. 300 mcg/kg/day added to TPN solution.

CAPSULES, E.R. TABLETS, LOZENGES, TABLETS

Adults and children. Dosage individualized based on severity of deficiency.

Mechanism of Action

Necessary for proper functioning of more than 200 metalloenzymes (enzymes containing tightly bound zinc atoms as an integral part of their structures), including carbonic anhydrase, carboxypeptidase A, alcohol dehydrogenase, alkaline phosphatase, and RNA polymerase. Zinc also helps maintain nucleic acid, protein, and cell membrane structure and is essential for certain physiologic functions, including cell growth and division, sexual maturation and reproduction, night vision, wound healing, host immunity, and taste acuity. This mineral also provides cellular antioxidant protection by scavenging free radicals.

Contraindications

Hypersensitivity to zinc or its components

Interactions

DRUGS

copper supplements: Impaired copper absorption (with large doses of zinc)

oral iron supplements, oral phosphate salts, penicillamine, phosphorus-containing drugs: Decreased zinc absorption

quinolones, tetracyclines: Decreased absorption and possibly decreased effectiveness of these antibiotics

thiazide diuretics: Increased urinary excretion of zinc

zinc-containing preparations: Increased blood zinc level

FOODS

fiber- or phylate-containing foods (such as bran, whole-grain breads, cereal), phosphorus-containing foods (including milk, poultry): Decreased zinc absorption

Adverse Reactions

None with the usual dosages.

Nursing Considerations

- **WARNING** Don't administer zinc preparations that contain benzyl alcohol to neonates or premature infants because this preservative may cause a fatal toxic syndrome characterized by metabolic acidosis and CNS, respiratory, circulatory, and renal function impairment.
- Be aware that zinc is administered by I.V. infusion only to patients who are unable to take oral forms—for example, those with nausea, vomiting, or malabsorption syndrome.
- Administer oral zinc supplements 1 hour before or 2 to 3 hours after meals. Also, administer them at least 2 hours after administering oral iron supplements or phosphorus-containing drugs (to prevent decreased zinc absorption) or copper supplements (to prevent decreased copper absorption). Administer oral zinc supplements at least 6 hours before or 2 hours after administering quinolone or tetracycline antibiotics to prevent decreased absorption of these drugs.
- Monitor patient receiving long-term zinc therapy for sideroblastic anemia, which may result from zinc-induced copper deficiency and is characterized by anemia, leukopenia, neutropenia, granulocytopenia, and bone marrow problems. Be aware that these effects are reversible after zinc is discontinued.

- Monitor patient with preexisting copper deficiency for exacerbation of this condition because zinc therapy can further decrease serum copper level.
- Assess for signs and symptoms of zinc deficiency, such as growth retardation, hypogonadism, delayed sexual maturation, alopecia, impaired wound healing, skin lesions, immune deficiencies, behavioral disturbances, night blindness, and impaired sense of taste.
- Monitor blood alkaline phosphatase (ALP) level monthly, as ordered, because ALP level may increase during zinc therapy.
- Store drug at 15° to 30° C (59° to 86° F); don't freeze.

PATIENT TEACHING
- Explain to patient why she needs a zinc supplement.
- Instruct patient to take oral zinc on an empty stomach, at least 1 hour before or 2 hours after meals. Caution her not to take zinc within 2 hours of iron or copper supplements or phosphorus-containing drugs. Also advise patient to take oral zinc at least 6 hours before or 2 hours after taking quinolone or tetracycline antibiotics to prevent decreased absorption of these drugs.
- Instruct patient to allow zinc lozenge to dissolve in mouth slowly and completely, not to swallow it whole or chew it. Advise her not to take zinc lozenges more often than directed.
- Caution patient to keep lozenges out of children's reach to prevent choking.

zoledronic acid

Zometa

Class and Category

Chemical: Bisphosphonate
Therapeutic: Antihypercalcemic, bone resorption inhibitor
Pregnancy category: C

Indications and Dosages

▶ *To treat hypercalcemia caused by cancer*
I.V. INFUSION
Adults. 4 mg infused over at least 15 min. After 7 days, patient receives another 4 mg if serum calcium level doesn't return to normal or remains elevated. *Maximum:* 4 mg/dose.

Mechanism of Action

Inhibits osteoclastic bone resorption and induces osteoclastic cellular breakdown. By binding to bone, zoledronic acid blocks the osteoclastic resorption of mineralized bone and cartilage. In cancer patients with hypercalcemia, osteoclastic hyperactivity leads to excessive bone resorption. As bone is resorbed, excessive amounts of calcium are released into the blood, resulting in polyuria, GI disturbances, progressive dehydration, and decreasing glomerular filtration rate. This, in turn, leads to increased resorption of calcium by the kidneys, setting up a cycle of worsening hypercalcemia. Zoledronic acid interrupts this process.

Incompatibilities

Don't mix zoledronic acid with calcium-containing I.V. solutions such as LR because a precipitate may form.

Contraindications

Hypersensitivity to zoledronic acid, other bisphosphonates, or their components

Interactions

DRUGS

aminoglycosides: Possibly further lowering of serum calcium level
loop diuretics (such as furosemide): Possibly increased risk of hypocalcemia

Adverse Reactions

CNS: Chills, fever, somnolence
EENT: Conjunctivitis
GI: Nausea, vomiting
GU: Elevated serum creatinine level
MS: Arthralgia, myalgia
Other: Hypocalcemia, hypomagnesemia, hypophosphatemia, infusion site redness and swelling

Nursing Considerations

- Be aware that zoledronic acid is not indicated to treat hypercalcemia caused by hyperparathyroidism or other non-tumor-related conditions.
- Expect to aggressively hydrate hypercalcemic patient with I.V. NS before and throughout zoledronic acid therapy, as prescribed, to achieve and maintain urine output of about 2 L/day.

- **WARNING** During hydration, frequently monitor fluid intake and output and assess patient (especially if she has heart failure) for potentially life-threatening signs and symptoms of overhydration.
- Reconstitute zoledronic acid by adding 5 ml of sterile water for injection to drug vial to yield a solution of 4 mg of zoledronic acid. Make sure that drug is completely dissolved before you withdraw it. Further dilute drug in 100 ml of NS and infuse it over no less than 15 minutes.
- **WARNING** Be aware that a single dose of zoledronic acid should not exceed 4 mg and that drug should not be infused over less than 15 minutes to decrease the risk of significant renal function deterioration and, possibly, renal failure, which can result from rapid infusion.
- Before administering drug, inspect reconstituted and diluted solution and discard if it contains particles or is discolored.
- Refrigerate reconstituted drug at 2° to 8° C (36° to 46° F); discard after 24 hours.
- Administer drug as a single I.V. solution in a separate I.V. line.
- **WARNING** Assess patient's renal status, including renal function test results, as ordered, before and during zoledronic acid therapy to assess for deteriorating renal function. For patients with a normal serum creatinine level who develop an increase of 0.5 mg/dl within 2 weeks of receiving drug, expect to withhold the next dose until serum creatinine is within at least 10% of patient's baseline value. For patients with an abnormal serum creatinine level who develop an increase of 1 mg/dl within 2 weeks of receiving drug, expect to withhold the next dose until serum creatinine level is within at least 10% of baseline.
- Monitor serum calcium, magnesium, and phosphate levels, as ordered, throughout zoledronic acid therapy. If hypocalcemia, hypomagnesemia, or hypophosphatemia occurs, expect to administer appropriate short-term supplemental therapy, as prescribed.
- Assess aspirin-sensitive asthma patients for worsening of respiratory symptoms during zoledronic acid therapy because other bisphosphonates have caused bronchoconstriction in these patients.
- Store drug at 25° C (77° F).

PATIENT TEACHING

• Teach patient receiving zoledronic acid the importance of maintaining a nutritious diet that includes adequate amounts of calcium and vitamin D.

• Advise patient to report muscle or bone pain.

• Stress the importance of keeping follow-up medical appointments and undergoing prescribed diagnostic tests to evaluate effectiveness of treatment.

EQUIANALGESIC DOSES FOR OPIOID AGONISTS

An equianalgesic dose of a synthetic opioid agonist is the dose that produces the same level of analgesia as 10 mg of I.M. or S.C. morphine, the principal opioid obtained from opium poppies. If your patient is switched from one opioid to another, expect to use the equianalgesic dose to decrease the risk of adverse reactions while increasing the likelihood of adequate pain relief. The chart below compares equianalgesic doses (oral and parenteral) for adults and children who weigh 50 kg (110 lb) or more.

Opioid agonist	Oral dose	Parenteral dose
codeine	200 mg (Not recommended dose)	120 to 130 mg
hydrocodone	30 mg	Not applicable
hydromorphone	7.5 mg	1.5 mg
levorphanol	4 mg	2 mg
meperidine	300 mg	75 to 100 mg
morphine (around-the-clock dosing)	30 mg	10 mg
morphine (single or intermittent dosing)	60 mg	10 mg
oxycodone	30 mg	Not applicable

CALCULATING THE STRENGTH OF A SOLUTION

Most solutions come prepared in the required strength by the pharmacy or medical supply source. But sometimes only the concentrated form is available, and you'll need to dilute the solution or solid to administer the prescribed strength.

When a solid form of a drug is used to prepare a solution, the drug must be completely dissolved. Solid drug forms, such as tablets, crystals, and powders, are considered 100% strength. (An exception to this is boric acid, which is only 5% at full strength.) The final diluted solution is stated in terms of liquid measurement. To prepare a solution, you'll need to add the prescribed solid or liquid form of the drug (the solute) to the prescribed amount of diluent (the solvent). Two of the most common diluents used in the clinical setting are normal saline solution and sterile water.

You can use either of two formulas to calculate the strength of a solution, as shown in the examples below.

Method 1: Calculating percentage and volume
Use the following formula:

$$\frac{\text{Weaker solution}}{\text{Stronger solution}} = \frac{\text{Solute}}{\text{Solvent}}$$

Example: You need to dilute a stock solution of 100% strength to a 5% solution. How much solute will you need to add to obtain 500 ml of the 5% solution?

Calculate as follows:

$$\frac{5\ (\%)\ (\text{Weaker solution})}{100\ (\%)\ (\text{Stronger solution})} = \frac{X\ (g)\ (\text{Solute})}{500\ ml\ (\text{Solvent})}$$

$$100\ X = (500)(5)\ \text{or}\ 2,500$$

$$X = 25\ g$$

Answer: You'll need to add 25 g of solute to each 500 ml of solvent to prepare a 5% solution.

(continued)

CALCULATING THE STRENGTH OF A SOLUTION *(continued)*

Method 2: Calculating percentage and volume

Use the following formula:

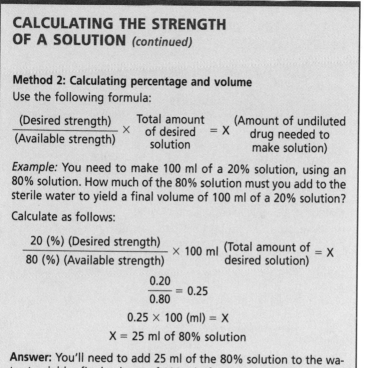

$$\frac{\text{(Desired strength)}}{\text{(Available strength)}} \times \frac{\text{Total amount of desired solution}}{} = X \quad \frac{\text{(Amount of undiluted drug needed to make solution)}}{}$$

Example: You need to make 100 ml of a 20% solution, using an 80% solution. How much of the 80% solution must you add to the sterile water to yield a final volume of 100 ml of a 20% solution?

Calculate as follows:

$$\frac{20\ (\%)\ \text{(Desired strength)}}{80\ (\%)\ \text{(Available strength)}} \times 100\ \text{ml} \quad \frac{\text{(Total amount of desired solution)}}{} = X$$

$$\frac{0.20}{0.80} = 0.25$$

$$0.25 \times 100\ \text{(ml)} = X$$

$$X = 25\ \text{ml of 80\% solution}$$

Answer: You'll need to add 25 ml of the 80% solution to the water to yield a final volume of 100 ml of a 20% solution.

CALCULATING PARENTERAL DRUG DOSAGES

You may need to calculate drug dosages when you're asked to administer a drug that is available in one measure, but prescribed in another. To make such calculations, you can use any of the three common methods of ratio and proportion shown in the examples below.

Example: You need to administer a prescribed dose of 1 mg morphine sulfate from a unit-dose cartridge that contains 4 mg per 2 ml. How many milliliters will you need to give to equal the prescribed dose of 1 mg?

Method 1: Using labeled amount of drug

In this method, the proportions between the drug label and the prescribed dose are used to determine ratio and proportion. The drug label, which states the amount of drug in one unit of measure (in this case, 4 mg in 2 ml), is the first ratio and is expressed as follows:

milligrams : milliliter = milligrams : milliliter
4 mg (amount of drug) : 2 ml (unit of measure)

The prescribed dose—in this case, 1 mg—is the second ratio; it must be expressed in the same order and units of measure as the first, as follows:

$$4 \text{ mg} : 2 \text{ ml} = 1 \text{ mg} : X \text{ ml}$$

Calculate as follows:

$$4X = 2$$

$$X = \frac{2}{4}$$

$$X = 0.5 \text{ ml}$$

Answer: You'll need to give 0.5 ml of morphine sulfate to equal the prescribed dose of 1 mg.

CALCULATING PARENTERAL DRUG DOSAGES *(continued)*

Method 2: Using an established formula
Use this formula:

$$\frac{\text{Prescribed dose}}{\text{Dose available}} \times \text{Quantity (unit of measure)} = X \text{ (unknown quantity to be given)}$$

Calculate as follows:

$$\frac{1 \text{ mg}}{4 \text{ mg}} \times 2 \text{ ml} = X \text{ (number of ml)}$$

$$\frac{4}{2} = 0.5$$

Answer: You'll need to give 0.5 ml of morphine sulfate to equal the prescribed dose of 1 mg.

Method 3: Calculating according to proportion size
To determine the correct amount of morphine sulfate to give using this method, use the following formula:

smaller : greater = smaller : greater
milligrams : milligrams = milliliters : milliliters

Critical thinking leads us to believe that 1 mg is less than 4 mg and that you'll need less than 2 ml to give 1 mg of the drug; therefore, 1 mg goes into the smaller part of the first ratio, and X goes into the smaller part of the second ratio. Set up the proportion as follows:

$$1 \text{ mg} : 4 \text{ mg} = X \text{ (ml)} : 2 \text{ ml}$$

$$4X = 2$$

$$X = \frac{2}{4}$$

$$X = 0.5$$

Answer: You'll need to give 0.5 ml of morphine sulfate to equal the prescribed dose of 1 mg.

CALCULATING I.V. FLOW RATES

When an I.V. solution is delivered by gravity, you must calculate the number of drops needed per minute for proper infusion. To calculate I.V. flow rates, you need to know three things:
- the drip factor—or the number of drops contained in 1 ml for the type of I.V. set you'll be using—which is provided on the individual package label
- the amount and type of fluid that you'll infuse, as prescribed on the physician's order sheet
- the infusion duration time in minutes.

Once you've gathered this information, you can calculate the I.V. flow rate using the following equation:

$$\frac{\text{Total number of ml}}{\text{Total number of min}} \times \text{drip factor (gtt/ml)} = \text{flow rate (gtt/min)}$$

Example 1: If the physician prescribes 1,000 ml of D_5W to infuse over 10 hours, and the drip rate for your administration set is 15 drops (gtt)/ml, calculate as follows:

$$\frac{1,000 \text{ ml}}{10 \text{ hr} \times 60 \text{ min}} \times 15 \text{ gtt/ml} = X \text{ gtt/min}$$

$$\frac{1,000 \text{ ml}}{600 \text{ min}} \times 15 \text{ gtt/ml} = X \text{ gtt/min}$$

$$1.67 \text{ ml/min} \times 15 \text{ gtt/ml} = X \text{ gtt/min}$$

$$25.05 \text{ gtt/min} = X$$

Answer: To infuse, round off 25.05 to 25 gtt/min or according to your institution's policy.

CALCULATING I.V. FLOW RATES (continued)

Example 2: If the physician prescribes 500 ml of 0.45NS to infuse over 2 hours, and the drip rate for your administration set is 10 gtt/ml, calculate as follows:

$$\frac{500 \text{ ml}}{2 \text{ hr} \times 60 \text{ min}} \times 10 \text{ gtt/ml} = X \text{ gtt/min}$$

$$\frac{500 \text{ ml}}{120 \text{ min}} \times 10 \text{ gtt/ml} = X \text{ gtt/min}$$

$$4.17 \text{ ml/min} \times 10 \text{ gtt/ml} = X \text{ gtt/min}$$

$$41.7 \text{ gtt/min} = X$$

Answer: To infuse, round off 41.7 to 42 gtt/min or according to your institution's policy.

Note: When a controlled infusion device is being used for I.V. administration, the electronic flow-regulator will either count drops using an electronic eye or use a controlled pumping action to deliver the fluid in milliliters. Your final calculation will be based on the unit of measure used by the device: drops per minute, or milliliters per hour.

SELECTED COMMON TOXICITY CRITERIA

The National Cancer Institute developed the Common Toxicity Criteria (CTC) in 1982 to provide standard language for reporting adverse events occurring in cancer trials that it sponsored. Since then, the list has expanded from 49 adverse events grouped in 18 categories to more than 200 adverse events in 24 categories. The following chart

Adverse Event	Grade 0	Grade 1	
Acute respiratory distress syndrome	Absent	N/A	
Allergic reaction, hypersensitivity (including drug fever)	None	Transient rash, drug fever <38° C (<100.4° F)	
Arthralgia (joint pain)	None	Mild pain that doesn't interfere with function	
Ataxia (incoordination)	Normal	Asymptomatic but abnormal on physical exam; doesn't interfere with function	
Bilirubin	WNL	>ULN to 1.5 × ULN	
Bone pain	None	Mild pain that doesn't interfere with function	
Cardiac ischemia, infarction	None	Nonspecific T-wave flattening or changes	
Cardiac left ventricular function	Normal	Asymptomatic decline of resting ejection fraction of ≥10% but <20% of baseline value; shortening fraction of ≥24% but <30%	

KEY: N/A = not applicable; LLN = lower limits of normal; ULN = upper limits of normal; WNL = within normal limits.

is a condensed version of selected criteria from the expanded list. Be sure to have the entire CTC, Version 2.0, available when grading adverse events. You can access the current CTC and other supporting information at http://ctep.info.nih.gov/CTC3/default.htm.

Grade 2	Grade 3	Grade 4
N/A	N/A	Present
Transient rash, drug fever ≥38° C (≥100.4° F), and/or asymptomatic bronchospasm	Symptomatic bronchospasm requiring parenteral medications, with or without urticaria; allergy-related edema or angioedema	Anaphylaxis
Moderate pain: pain or analgesics that interfere with function, but not with activities of daily living (ADLs)	Severe pain: pain or analgesics that severely interfere with ADLs	Disabling
Mild symptoms that interfere with function, but not with ADLs	Moderate symptoms that interfere with ADLs	Bedridden or disabling
>1.5 to 3 × ULN	>3 to 10 × ULN	>10 × ULN
Moderate pain: pain or analgesics that interfere with function, but not with ADLs	Severe pain: pain or analgesics that severely interfere with ADLs	Disabling
Asymptomatic ST- and T-wave changes suggesting ischemia	Angina without evidence of infarction	Acute MI
Asymptomatic, but resting ejection fraction below LLN for laboratory, or decline of resting ejection fraction of ≥20% of baseline value; shortening fraction of <24%	Congestive heart failure (CHF) that is responsive to treatment	Severe or refractory CHF or need for intubation

(continued)

SELECTED COMMON TOXICITY CRITERIA *(continued)*

Adverse Event	Grade 0	Grade 1	
Colitis	None	N/A	
Conduction abnormality, AV heart block	None	Asymptomatic, not requiring treatment (such as Mobitz type I [Wenckebach] second-degree AV block)	
Cough	Absent	Mild; relieved by OTC medication	
Diarrhea (patients without colostomy)	None	Increase of <4 stools/day over pretreatment period	
Dizziness, light-headedness	None	Not interfering with function	
Dyspnea (shortness of breath)	Normal	N/A	
Edema	None	Asymptomatic, not requiring therapy	
Erythema multiforme (such as Stevens-Johnson syndrome or toxic epidermal necrolysis)	Absent	N/A	
Extrapyramidal or involuntary movements, restlessness	None	Mild involuntary movements that don't interfere with function	
Fever (without neutropenia, where neutropenia is defined as absolute granulocyte count of $<1 \times 10^9$/L)	None	38° to 39° C (100.4° to 102.2° F)	
Fibrinogen	WNL	$\geq$0.75 to $<1 \times$ LLN	

Grade 2	Grade 3	Grade 4
Abdominal pain with mucus or blood (or both) in stools	Abdominal pain, fever, change in bowel habits with ileus or peritoneal signs, and documentation by radiography or biopsy	Perforation, toxic mega-colon, or need for surgery
Symptoms that don't require therapy	Symptoms that require treatment (such as Mobitz type II second-degree AV block, third-degree AV block)	Life-threatening (such as arrhythmia associated with CHF, hypotension, syncope, or shock)
Requiring narcotic antitussive	Severe cough or coughing spasms poorly controlled or unresponsive to treatment	N/A
Increase of 4 to 6 stools/day or nocturnal stools	Increase of ≥7 stools/day, incontinence, or need for parenteral support for dehydration	Hemodynamic collapse; physiologic consequences requiring intensive care
Interfering with function, but not with ADLs	Interfering with ADLs	Bedridden or disabling
Dyspnea on exertion	Dyspnea at normal level of activity	Dyspnea at rest or requiring ventilator support
Symptoms that require therapy	Symptomatic edema that limits function and is un-responsive to therapy or that requires drug discontin-uation	Anasarca (severe generalized edema)
Scattered, but not generalized, eruption	Severe or requiring I.V. fluids (such as generalized rash or painful stomatitis)	Life-threatening (such as exfoliative or ulcerating dermatitis or type that requires enteral or parenteral nutritional support)
Moderate involuntary move-ments that interfere with function, but not with ADLs	Severe, involuntary move-ments or torticollis that interferes with ADLs	Bedridden or disabling
39.1° to 40° C (102.3° to 104° F)	>40° C (>104° F) for <24 hr	>40° C (>104° F) for >24 hr
≥0.5 to <0.75 × LLN	≥0.25 to <0.5 × LLN	<0.25 × LLN

(continued)

SELECTED COMMON TOXICITY CRITERIA *(continued)*

Adverse Event	Grade 0	Grade 1	
Hand-foot skin reaction	None	Skin changes or dermatitis without pain (such as erythema and peeling)	
Hemoglobin	WNL	<LLN to 10 g/dl <LLN to 100 g/L <LLN to 6.2 mmol/L	
Hypertension	None	Asymptomatic, transient increase of >20 mm Hg diastolic or to >150/100 mm Hg if previously WNL; not requiring treatment	
Hypotension	None	Changes that don't require treatment (including transient orthostatic hypotension)	
Infection without neutropenia	None	Mild, with no active treatment	
Injection site reaction	None	Pain, itching, or erythema	
Hearing—inner ear	Normal	Hearing loss on audiometry only	
Hearing—middle ear	Normal	Serous otitis without subjective decrease in hearing	
Keratitis (corneal inflammation or ulceration)	None	Abnormal ophthalmologic changes with or without symptoms (such as pain and irritation) and without visual impairment	
Leukocytes (total WBC)	WNL	<LLN to 3×10^9/L <LLN to 3,000/mm^3	
Muscle weakness (not due to neuropathy)	Normal	Asymptomatic with weakness on physical exam	

Grade 2	Grade 3	Grade 4
Skin changes with pain that doesn't interfere with function	Skin changes with pain that interferes with function	N/A
8 to <10 g/dl 80 to <100 g/L 4.9 to <6.2 mmol/L	6.5 to <8 g/dl 65 to <80 g/L 4 to <4.9 mmol/L	<6.5 g/dl <65 g/L <4 mmol/L
Recurrent, persistent, or symptomatic increase of >20 mm Hg diastolic or to 150/100 mm Hg if previously WNL; not requiring treatment	Need for treatment or more intensive treatment than previously	Hypertensive crisis
Need for brief fluid replacement or other treatment, but not hospitalization; no physiologic consequences	Need for treatment and sustained medical attention, but resolves with no persistent physiologic consequences	Shock (associated with acidemia and impairing vital organ function because of tissue hypoperfusion)
Moderate, localized infection requiring local or oral treatment	Severe systemic infection requiring IV antibiotic or antifungal treatment or hospitalization	Life-threatening sepsis (such as septic shock)
Pain or swelling with inflammation or phlebitis	Ulceration or necrosis that is severe or prolonged or that requires surgery	N/A
Tinnitus or hearing loss that doesn't require hearing aid or treatment	Tinnitus or hearing loss that is correctable with hearing aid or treatment	Severe unilateral or bilateral hearing loss (deafness) that is not correctable
Serous otitis or infection requiring medical intervention, subjective decrease in hearing, rupture of tympanic membrane with discharge	Otitis with discharge, mastoiditis, or conductive hearing loss	Necrosis of soft tissue or bone in the canal
Symptoms that interfere with function, but not with ADLs	Symptoms that interfere with ADLs	Unilateral or bilateral loss of vision (blindness)
≥2 to <3 × 10⁹/L ≥2,000 to <3,000/mm³	≥1 to <2 × 10⁹/L ≥1,000 to <2,000/mm³	<1 × 10⁹/L <1,000/mm³
Symptoms that interfere with function, but not with ADLs	Symptoms that interfere with ADLs	Bedridden or disabling *(continued)*

SELECTED COMMON TOXICITY CRITERIA (continued)

Adverse Event	Grade 0	Grade 1	
Nausea	None	Able to eat	
Neuropathy—cranial	Absent	N/A	
Neuropathy—motor	Normal	Subjective weakness but no objective findings	
Neuropathy—sensory	Normal	Loss of deep tendon reflexes or paresthesia (including tingling) that doesn't interfere with function	
Nodal or junctional arrhythmia	None	Asymptomatic, not requiring treatment	
Pericardial effusion or pericarditis	None	Asymptomatic effusion, not requiring treatment	
Petechiae, purpura (hemorrhage, bleeding into skin or mucosa)	None	Rare petechiae of skin	
Platelets	WNL	$<$LLN to 75×10^9/L $<$LLN to 75,000/mm^3	
Pleural effusion (nonmalignant)	None	Asymptomatic, not requiring treatment	
Pneumonitis or pulmonary infiltrates	None	Radiographic changes but no symptoms or symptoms that don't require steroids	
Pruritus	None	Mild or localized; relieved spontaneously or by local measures	
Rash or desquamation	None	Macular or papular eruption or erythema without associated symptoms	

Grade 2	Grade 3	Grade 4
Oral intake significantly decreased	No significant intake; requires I.V. fluids	N/A
Present but doesn't interfere with ADLs	Present and interferes with ADLs	Life-threatening or disabling
Mild objective weakness that interferes with function, but not with ADLs	Objective weakness that interferes with ADLs	Paralysis
Objective sensory loss or paresthesia (including tingling) that interferes with function, but not with ADLs	Sensory loss or paresthesia that interferes with ADLs	Permanent sensory loss that interferes with function
Symptoms that don't require therapy	Symptoms that require treatment	Life-threatening (such as arrhythmia associated with CHF, hypotension, syncope, or shock)
Pericarditis (rub, ECG changes, or chest pain)	Having physiologic consequences	Tamponade (requiring drainage or pericardial window)
Petechiae or purpura in dependent areas of skin	Generalized petechiae or purpura of skin or petechiae of any mucosal site	N/A
$\geq$50 to <75 $\times$ 10^9/L $\geq$50,000 to <75,000/mm^3	$\geq$10 to <50 $\times$ 10^9/L $\geq$10,000 to <50,000/mm^3	<10 $\times$ 10^9/L <10,000/mm^3
Symptomatic and requiring diuretics	Symptomatic and requiring oxygen or therapeutic thoracentesis	Life-threatening (such as requiring intubation)
Radiographic changes and need for steroids or diuretics	Radiographic changes and need for oxygen	Radiographic changes and need for assisted ventilation
Intense or widespread; relieved spontaneously or by systemic measures	Intense or widespread and poorly controlled despite treatment	N/A
Macular or papular eruption or erythema with pruritus or other associated symptoms covering <50% of body surface area, or localized desquamation or other lesions covering <50% of body surface area	Symptomatic generalized erythroderma or macular, papular, or vesicular eruption or desquamation covering $\geq$50% of body surface area	Generalized exfoliative dermatitis or ulcerative dermatitis

(continued)

SELECTED COMMON TOXICITY CRITERIA *(continued)*

Adverse Event	Grade 0	Grade 1	
Renal failure	None	N/A	
SGPT (serum glutamic pyruvic transaminase); also known as ALT	WNL	>ULN to 2.5 × ULN	
Stomatitis, pharyngitis (oral, pharyngeal mucositis)	None	Painless ulcers, erythema, or mild soreness without lesions	
Thrombosis or embolism	None	N/A	
Urticaria (hives, welts, wheals)	None	Requiring no medication	
Vasculitis	None	Mild, not requiring treatment	
Vertigo	None	Not interfering with function	
Vomiting	None	1 episode in 24 hours over pretreatment	

Grade 2	Grade 3	Grade 4
N/A	Requiring dialysis but reversible	Requiring dialysis and irreversible
>2.5 to 5 × ULN	>5 to 20 × ULN	>20 × ULN
Painful erythema, edema, or ulcers, but able to eat or swallow	Painful erythema, edema, or ulcers requiring I.V. hydration	Severe ulceration or need for parenteral or enteral nutritional support or prophylactic intubation
Deep vein thrombosis that doesn't require anti-coagulant therapy	Deep vein thrombosis that requires anticoagulant therapy	Embolic event, including pulmonary embolism
Requiring oral or topical treatment or I.V. medication or steroids for <24 hours	Requiring I.V. medication or steroids for ≥24 hours	N/A
Symptoms that require medication	Need for steroids	Ischemic changes or need for amputation
Interfering with function, but not with ADLs	Interfering with ADLs	Bedridden or disabling
2 to 5 episodes in 24 hours over pretreatment	≥6 episodes in 24 hours over pretreatment or need for I.V. fluids	Hemodynamic collapse, need for parenteral nutrition, or physiologic consequences requiring intensive care

I.V. ANTINEOPLASTIC DRUGS

Antineoplastic drugs have become the standard of treatment for most types of cancer today. Most of these drugs work by inhibiting cell proliferation, thereby leading to cell death. They're most effective at killing cells that are actively dividing. Cell-specific antineoplastics exert their actions during one or more phases of the cell cycle. S-phase antineoplastics interfere with DNA synthesis; M-phase drugs interfere with the formation of microtubules and disrupt mitosis. Most antineoplastics impair DNA in one of the following four ways:

- preventing separation of DNA strands
- inhibiting DNA repair
- mimicking DNA bases
- disrupting the triplicate codons or producing oxygen free radicals that damage the DNA.

Antineoplastic drugs are cytotoxic, which means that they affect both neoplastic cells and normal cells. As a result, they may cause serious and sometimes life-threatening adverse reactions. Antineoplastics are most harmful to normal cells that exhibit rapid activity and growth, such as bone marrow tissue, the epithelium of the GI mucosa, and hair follicles. When they suppress bone marrow activity, the patient may develop leukopenia, thrombocytopenia, or anemia. When the drugs affect the GI mucosa, the patient may experience nausea, vomiting, anorexia, bowel dysfunction, and mucosal ulcerations. When they affect the hair follicles, the result is hair loss (alopecia), one of the most common adverse reactions; although not life-threatening, hair loss can be emotionally traumatic for patients, especially women.

Drug Classification
Antineoplastics are classified according to their mechanism of action.

Alkylating drugs, the first drugs developed to fight cancer, are most effective against slow-growing tumors. These agents can damage tissue at the injection site and produce systemic toxicity. They can damage cells during all stages of growth, causing mitotic arrest. Because their actions are not limited to neoplastic cells, they also cause myelosuppression, a predictable adverse reaction. They can also result in secondary tumor development, even years after the initial therapy.

I.V. ANTINEOPLASTIC DRUGS *(continued)*

Antibiotic antineoplastics originated from a genus of fungus-like bacteria called *Streptomyces*. Their classification is based on their origin, not on mechanism of action, toxicity, pharmacokinetics, or varying clinical indications. Many of these drugs bind to specific bases and block DNA synthesis, thus interfering with cell replication.

Antimetabolites are cell-cycle-phase–specific drugs that act by preventing synthesis of nucleotides or inhibiting enzymes by mimicking nucleotides. These drugs tend to be more effective when used in combination.

Antimitotic antineoplastics disrupt the formation of microtubule structures within the cell during mitosis. This breakdown of microtubule production stops the formation of the mitotic spindle, inhibiting cellular reproduction.

Biological response modifiers alter tumor-host metabolic and immunologic relationships.

Antineoplastic enzymes interfere with the breakdown of extracellular asparagine, an endogenous enzyme that leukemic cells depend on for their survival. The rapid depletion of asparagine eventually kills leukemic cells by fragmenting them into membrane-bound particles that are eliminated by phagocytosis.

Hormonal antineoplastics act as agonists to inhibit tumor cell growth or as antagonists to compete with endogenous growth-promoting hormones. Steroid hormones form specific receptor complexes that bind to certain nuclear proteins necessary for DNA transcription.

Miscellaneous antineoplastics act in a variety of ways, such as by destroying microtubules that are essential for tumor cell structure before mitosis and by inhibiting topoisomerase, the enzyme that affects the degree of supercoiling in DNA by cutting one or both strands. This inhibition causes DNA strands to break and synthesizes toxic compounds that inhibit DNA strand repair.

You'll find complete entries for some of the most common I.V. antineoplastics in this book. The following chart lists the generic and common trade names of additional I.V. antineoplastics, which are grouped according to mechanism of action. It also includes FDA-approved indications and the usual adult I.V. dosage for each drug.

(continued)

I.V. ANTINEOPLASTIC DRUGS *(continued)*

Generic and Trade Names	Indications	Usual Adult Dosages
Alkylating drugs		
busulfan Busulfex, Myleran	To provide palliative treatment of chronic myelocytic leukemia	0.8 mg/kg I.V. over 2 hr q 6 hr for 4 days for a total of 16 doses as an adjunct with cyclophosphamide
carmustine (BCNU) BiCNU, Gliadel Wafer	To treat primary brain tumors, Hodgkin's disease, non-Hodgkin's lymphoma, and multiple myeloma	150 to 200 mg/m^2 by slow I.V. infusion as a single dose q 6 to 8 wk; or 75 to 100 mg/m^2 by slow I.V. infusion q.d. for 2 days q 6 wk; or 40 mg/m^2 by slow I.V. infusion q.d. for 5 days q 6 wk
ifosfamide IFEX	To treat germ cell testicular tumors	1.2 g/m^2/day by I.V. infusion for 5 days q 3 wk
mechlorethamine hydrochloride (nitrogen mustard) Mustargen	To treat Hodgkin's disease, non-Hodgkin's lymphoma, and mycosis fungoides	0.4 mg/kg I.V. as a single dose or in divided doses over 2 to 4 days
streptozocin Zanosar	To treat islet cell or pancreatic carcinoma	500 mg/m^2 I.V. for 5 days q 6 wk, or 1,000 mg/m^2 I.V. q wk for 2 wk
thiotepa (TESPA, triethylenethiophosphoramide, TSPA) Thioplex	To treat breast cancer, epithelial ovarian cancer, and Hodgkin's disease	0.3 to 0.4 mg/kg I.V. q 1 to 4 wk, or 0.2 mg/kg for 4 to 5 days q 2 to 3 wk
Antibiotic antineoplastics		
bleomycin sulfate Blenoxane	To treat non-Hodgkin's lymphoma, squamous cell carcinoma, and testicular cancer	0.25 to 0.5 unit/kg or 10 to 20 units/m^2 1 or 2 times/wk I.V., or 0.25 unit/kg or 15 units/m^2 q.d. by I.V. infusion over 24 hr
	To treat Hodgkin's disease	0.25 to 0.5 unit/kg I.V. or 10 to 20 units/m^2 1 or 2 times/wk

I.V. ANTINEOPLASTIC DRUGS (continued)

Generic and Trade Names	Indications	Usual Adult Dosages
Antibiotic antineoplastics (continued)		
dactinomycin (actinomycin-D) Cosmegen	To treat Ewing's sarcoma, gestational trophoblastic or Wilms' tumor, rhabdomyo-sarcoma, sarcoma botryoides, and testicular cancer or tumors	0.5 mg I.V. q.d. for 5 days; may repeat after 3 wk
daunorubicin hydrochloride Cerubidine	To treat acute lymphocytic leukemia	45 mg/m^2 I.V. q.d. for first 3 days of a 32-day course of combination therapy with vincristine, predni-sone, and asparaginase
	To treat acute nonlymphocytic leukemia	45 mg/m^2 I.V. q.d. for first 3 days of first course of combination therapy with cytarabine and first 2 days of second course of combination therapy with cytarabine
daunorubicin, liposomal DaunoXome	To treat AIDS-related Kaposi's sarcoma	40 mg/m^2 I.V. over 60 min q 2 wk
epirubicin hydrochloride Ellence	To treat breast cancer	100 to 120 mg/m^2 by I.V. infusion over 3 to 5 min by a free-flowing I.V. solution as a single dose on day 1 or in divided doses on days 1 and 8; repeated q 3 to 4 wk for 6 cycles in combination with other chemothera-peutic drugs
idarubicin hydrochloride Idamycin	To treat acute nonlymphocytic leukemia	12 mg/m^2/day I.V. over 10 to 15 min for 3 days in combination with cytarabine

(continued)

I.V. ANTINEOPLASTIC DRUGS (continued)

Generic and Trade Names	Indications	Usual Adult Dosages
Antibiotic antineoplastics (continued)		
mitomycin (mitomycin-C) Mutamycin	To treat gastric or pancreatic cancer	20 mg/m^2 I.V. as a single dose q 6 to 8 wk
pentostatin (2'-deoxycoformycin) Nipent	To treat hairy cell leukemia	4 mg/m^2 by rapid I.V. injection or diluted for infusion over 20 to 30 min as a single dose q other wk
plicamycin (mithramycin) Mithracin	To treat testicular cancer	0.025 to 0.03 mg/kg I.V. q.d. over 4 to 6 hr for 8 to 10 days
	To treat hypercalcemia and hypercalciuria	0.015 to 0.025 mg/kg I.V. q.d. over 4 to 6 hr for 3 to 4 days; may repeat dose q wk as needed
Antimetabolites		
cladribine (2-CdA, 2-chloro-deoxyadenosine) Leustatin	To treat hairy cell leukemia	0.1 mg/kg/day by continuous I.V. infusion for 7 days
cytarabine (ARA-C, cytosine arabinoside) Cytosar, Cytosar-U	To treat acute nonlymphocytic leukemia	Initially, 100 mg/m^2/day by continuous I.V. infusion for 7 days, alone or in combination with other drugs; or 100 mg/m^2 I.V. q 12 hr on days 1 to 7, then consult manufacturer's literature for specific dosage; or high-dose therapy of 2 to 3 g/m^2 I.V over 1 to 3 hr for 2 to 6 days, then consult manufacturer's literature for specific dosage.
	To prevent or treat acute lymphocytic leukemia and chronic myelocytic leukemia	Consult manufacturer's literature for specific dosage.

I.V. ANTINEOPLASTIC DRUGS *(continued)*

Generic and Trade Names	Indications	Usual Adult Dosages
Antimetabolites *(continued)*		
fludarabine phosphate Fludara	To treat chronic lymphocytic leukemia	25 mg/m^2 I.V. infused over 30 min for 5 days; cycle repeated q 28 days
Antimitotic antineoplastics		
docetaxel Taxotere	To treat breast cancer	60 to 100 mg/m^2 by I.V. infusion over 1 hr q 3 wk
	To treat non-small-cell lung carcinoma	75 mg/m^2 by I.V. infusion over 1 hr q 3 wk
vinorelbine tartrate Navelbine	To treat non-small-cell lung carcinoma	30 mg/m^2 I.V. over 6 to 10 min q wk, alone or in combination with cisplatin 120 mg/m^2 on days 1 and 29, and thereafter q 6 wk
Biological response modifiers		
aldesleukin (IL-2, interleukin-2) Proleukin	To treat renal cancer and metastatic melanoma	600,000 IU/kg by I.V. infusion over 15 min q 8 hr for 14 doses, followed by 9 days of no drug; then course of 14 doses repeated for total of 28 doses
denileukin diftitox Ontak	To treat cutaneous or T-cell lymphomas, including mycosis fungoides	9 or 18 mcg/kg/day by I.V. infusion over at least 15 min for 5 days; repeated q 21 days
Antineoplastic enzymes		
asparaginase Colaspase, Elspar, Kidrolase (CAN)	To treat acute lymphocytic leukemia	200 IU/kg I.V. q.d. for 28 days
pegaspargase (PEG-L-asparaginase) Oncaspar	To treat acute lymphoblastic leukemia in adults up to age 21	2,500 IU/m^2 I.V. q 14 days

(continued)

I.V. ANTINEOPLASTIC DRUGS *(continued)*

Generic and Trade Names	Indications	Usual Adult Dosages
Miscellaneous antineoplastics		
dacarbazine DTIC (CAN), DTIC-Dome	To treat Hodgkin's disease	150 mg/m^2 I.V. q.d. for 5 days in combination with other drugs, possibly repeated q 28 days; or 375 mg/m^2 q 15 days in combination with other drugs
	To treat malignant melanoma	2 to 4.5 mg/kg I.V. q.d. for 10 days and q 28 days thereafter; or 250 mg/m^2 I.V. q.d. for 5 days and q 21 days thereafter
gemcitabine hydrochloride Gemzar	To treat non-small-cell lung carcinoma	1,000 mg/m^2 by I.V. infusion over 30 min q.d. on days 1, 8, and 15 q 28 days in combination with cisplatin 100 mg/m^2 on day 28; or 1,250 mg/m^2 I.V. q.d. on days 1 and 8 q 21 days in combination with cisplatin 100 mg/m^2 I.V. on day 21
	To treat pancreatic cancer	1,000 mg/m^2 by I.V. infusion over 30 min q wk for 7 wk, followed by 1 wk of no drug; then q wk for 3 wk, followed by 1 wk of no drug; then 4-wk cycle repeated

I.V. ANTINEOPLASTIC DRUGS (continued)

Generic and Trade Names	Indications	Usual Adult Dosages
Miscellaneous antineoplastics (continued)		
mitoxantrone hydrochloride Novantrone	To treat hormone-refractory prostate cancer	12 to 14 mg/m^2 I.V. q 21 days
	To treat acute nonlymphocytic leukemia	12 mg/m^2 by I.V. infusion through free-flowing NS or D$_5$W solution over 3 min q.d. on days 1 and 3 in combination with cytarabine 100 mg/m^2/day by continuous I.V. infusion on days 1 to 7; if response is inadequate, second course of same dosage may be given
porfimer sodium Photofrin	To treat esophageal cancer and non-small-cell lung carcinoma	2 mg/kg I.V. over 3 to 5 min, followed by laser light illumination and debridement of tumor; course may be repeated q 30 days three times
topotecan hydrochloride Hycamtin	To treat ovarian cancer and small-cell lung carcinoma	1.5 mg/m^2 I.V. over 30 min q.d. for 5 days; repeated q 21 days
trastuzumab Herceptin	To treat breast cancer	4 mg/kg I.V. over 90 min, followed by 2 mg/kg I.V. over 30 min q 7 days

BODY MASS INDEX CALCULATION

Body mass index (BMI) is a formula used to determine obesity; it's calculated by dividing a person's weight in kilograms by his height in meters squared (kg/m^2). A BMI of 25 or higher increases your patient's risk of developing hypertension, cardiovascular disease, type 2 diabetes mellitus, and stroke. It also increases the risk that he won't respond effectively to the usual drug dosages. If your patient has an abnormal BMI, be prepared to make dosage adjustments that are individualized based on body weight, as prescribed.

WEIGHT (POUNDS)

HEIGHT (INCHES)																		
58	91	96	100	105	110	115	119	124	129	134	138	143	148	153	158	162	167	17⋯
59	94	99	104	109	114	119	124	128	133	138	143	148	153	158	163	168	173	17⋯
60	97	102	107	112	118	123	128	133	138	143	148	153	158	163	168	174	179	18⋯
61	100	106	111	116	122	127	132	137	143	148	153	158	164	169	174	180	185	19⋯
62	104	109	115	120	126	131	136	142	147	153	158	164	169	175	180	186	191	19⋯
63	107	113	118	124	130	135	141	146	152	158	163	169	175	180	186	191	197	20⋯
64	110	116	122	128	134	140	145	151	157	163	169	174	180	186	192	197	204	20⋯
65	114	120	126	132	138	144	150	156	162	168	174	180	186	192	198	204	210	21⋯
66	118	124	130	136	142	148	155	161	167	173	179	186	192	198	204	210	216	22⋯
67	121	127	134	140	146	153	159	166	172	178	185	191	198	204	211	217	223	23⋯
68	125	131	138	144	151	158	164	171	177	184	190	197	203	210	216	223	230	23⋯
69	128	135	142	149	155	162	169	176	182	189	196	203	209	216	223	230	236	24⋯
70	132	139	146	153	160	167	174	181	188	195	202	209	216	222	229	236	243	25⋯
71	136	143	150	157	165	172	179	186	193	200	208	215	222	229	236	243	250	25⋯
72	140	147	154	162	169	177	184	191	199	206	213	221	228	235	242	250	258	26⋯
73	144	151	159	166	174	182	189	197	204	212	219	227	235	242	250	257	265	27⋯
74	148	155	163	171	179	186	194	202	210	218	225	233	241	249	256	264	272	28⋯
75	152	160	168	176	184	192	200	208	216	224	232	240	248	256	264	272	279	28⋯
76	156	164	172	180	189	197	205	213	221	230	238	246	254	263	271	279	287	29⋯
	19	20	21	22	23	24	25	26	27	28	29	30	31	32	33	34	35	3⋯

BODY MASS INDEX

The table below will help you find your patient's BMI easily. It converts pounds to kilograms and inches to meters, and then it shows the BMI. To use it, simply find the patient's height on either side of the table; then move across the row to the weight that most closely matches your patient's. At the bottom of the column containing the weight, you'll find the BMI for that patient. For example, the BMI for a patient who is 70" tall and weighs 208 lb is 30.

WEIGHT (POUNDS)

																		HEIGHT (INCHES)
77	181	186	191	196	201	205	210	215	220	224	229	234	239	244	248	253	258	58
83	188	193	198	203	208	212	217	222	227	232	237	242	247	252	257	262	267	59
89	194	199	204	209	215	220	225	230	235	240	245	250	255	261	266	271	276	60
95	201	206	211	217	222	227	232	238	243	248	254	259	264	269	275	280	285	61
02	207	213	218	224	229	235	240	246	251	256	262	267	273	278	284	289	295	62
08	214	220	226	231	237	242	248	254	259	265	270	278	282	287	293	299	304	63
15	221	227	232	238	244	250	256	262	267	273	279	285	291	296	302	308	314	64
22	228	234	240	246	252	258	264	270	276	282	288	294	300	300	312	318	324	65
29	235	241	247	253	260	266	272	278	284	291	297	303	309	315	322	328	334	66
36	242	249	255	261	268	274	280	287	293	299	306	312	319	325	331	338	344	67
43	249	256	262	269	276	282	289	295	302	308	315	322	328	335	341	348	354	68
50	257	263	270	277	284	291	297	304	311	318	324	331	338	345	351	358	365	69
57	264	271	278	285	292	299	306	313	320	327	334	341	348	355	362	369	376	70
65	272	279	286	293	301	308	315	322	329	338	343	351	358	365	372	379	386	71
72	279	287	294	302	309	316	324	331	338	346	353	361	368	375	383	390	397	72
80	288	295	302	310	318	325	333	340	348	355	360	371	378	386	393	401	408	73
87	295	303	311	319	326	334	342	350	358	365	373	381	389	396	404	412	420	74
95	303	311	319	327	335	343	351	359	367	375	383	391	399	407	415	423	431	75
04	312	320	328	336	344	353	361	369	377	385	394	402	410	418	426	435	443	76
37	38	39	40	41	42	43	44	45	46	47	48	49	50	51	52	53	54	

BODY MASS INDEX

ABBREVIATIONS

The following abbreviations, which are common to nursing practice, are used throughout the book.

ABG	arterial blood gas
a.c.	before meals
ACE	angiotensin-converting enzyme
ADH	antidiuretic hormone
AIDS	acquired immunodeficiency syndrome
ALT	alanine aminotransferase
ANA	antinuclear antibodies
APTT	activated partial thromboplastin time
AST	aspartate aminotransferase
ATP	adenosine triphosphate
AV	atrioventricular
b.i.d.	twice a day
BUN	blood urea nitrogen
°C	degrees Celsius
cAMP	cyclic adenosine monophosphate
(CAN)	Canadian drug trade name
cap	capsule
CBC	complete blood count
cGMP	cyclic guanosine monophosphate
CK	creatine kinase
Cl	chloride
cm	centimeter
CMV	cytomegalovirus
CNS	central nervous system
COPD	chronic obstructive pulmonary disease
C.R.	controlled-release
CSF	cerebrospinal fluid
CV	cardiovascular
CVA	cerebrovascular accident
D_5LR	dextrose 5% in lactated Ringer's solution
D_5NS	dextrose 5% in normal saline solution
$D_5/0.2NS$	dextrose 5% in quarter-normal saline solution
$D_5/0.45NS$	dextrose 5% in half-normal saline solution
D_5W	dextrose 5% in water
$D_{10}W$	dextrose 10% in water
$D_{50}W$	dextrose 50% in water
dl	deciliter
DNA	deoxyribonucleic acid
DS	double-strength

ABBREVIATIONS (continued)

EC	enteric-coated
ECG	electrocardiogram
EEG	electroencephalogram
EENT	eyes, ears, nose, and throat
ENDO	endocrine
E.R.	extended-release
°F	degrees Fahrenheit
FDA	Food and Drug Administration
g	gram
GFR	glomerular filtration rate
GI	gastrointestinal
GU	genitourinary
H_1	histamine$_1$
H_2	histamine$_2$
HDL	high-density lipoprotein
HEME	hematologic
HIV	human immunodeficiency virus
HPV	human papilloma virus
hr	hour
h.s.	at bedtime
HSV	herpes simplex virus
HZV	herpes zoster virus
ICP	intracranial pressure
I.D.	intradermal
IgA	immunoglobulin A
IgE	immunoglobulin E
I.M.	intramuscular
INR	international normalized ratio
IU	international unit
I.V.	intravenous
IVPB	intravenous piggyback
kg	kilogram
KIU	kallikrein inactivator unit
L	liter
LA	long-acting
LD	lactate dehydrogenase
LDL	low-density lipoprotein
LOC	level of consciousness
LR	lactated Ringer's solution
M	molar
m^2	square meter
MAO	monoamine oxidase

(continued)

ABBREVIATIONS *(continued)*

mcg	microgram
mEq	milliequivalent
mg	milligram
MI	myocardial infarction
min	minute
ml	milliliter
mm	millimeter
mm^3	cubic millimeter
mmol	millimole
mo	month
MS	musculoskeletal
Na	sodium
NaCl	sodium chloride
NG	nasogastric
NPH	human isophane insulin
NPO	nothing by mouth
NS	normal saline solution
0.225NS	quarter-normal saline (0.225%) solution
0.45NS	half-normal saline (0.45%) solution
NSAID	nonsteroidal anti-inflammatory drug
OTC	over the counter
p.c.	after meals
PCA	patient-controlled analgesia
P.O.	by mouth
P.R.	by rectum
p.r.n.	as needed
PSVT	paroxysmal supraventricular tachycardia
PT	prothrombin time
PTCA	percutaneous transluminal coronary angioplasty
PVC	premature ventricular contraction
q	every
q.d.	every day
q.i.d.	four times a day
q.o.d.	every other day
RBC	red blood cell
REM	rapid eye movement
RESP	respiratory
RNA	ribonucleic acid
RSV	respiratory syncytial virus
SA	sinoatrial
S.C.	subcutaneous
sec	second

ABBREVIATIONS (continued)

S.L.	sublingual
S.R.	sustained-release
stat	immediately
supp	suppository
tab	tablet
T_3	triiodothyronine
T_4	thyroxine
t.i.d.	three times a day
U	units
USP	United States Pharmacopeia
UTI	urinary tract infection
VLDL	very low-density lipoprotein
WBC	white blood cell
wk	week

INDEX

- **Generic and alternate names:** lowercase initial letter
- **Trade names:** uppercase initial letter
- **Illustrations:** *i* after page number
- **Tables:** *t* after page number

A

Abbokinase, 691
Abbokinase Open-Cath, 691
abciximab, 1–3
Abelcet, 39
Acetazolam, 3
acetazolamide, 3–6
acetazolamide sodium, 3–6
Acova, 58
actinomycin-D, 745t
Activase, 21
Activase rt-PA, 21
acyclovir sodium, 6–10
Adenocard, 10
adenosine, 10–12
Adrenalin, 277
adrenaline, 277–280
Adriamycin PFS, 257
Adriamycin RDF, 257
Adrucil, 322
Adverse reaction, xx
Aerosporin, 598
Aggrastat, 673
Agonists, xix
A-hydroCort, 364
Akineton Lactate, 86
Ak-Zol, 3
alatrofloxacin mesylate, 12–14
aldesleukin, 747t
Aldomet, 467
alglucerase, 15–16
Alkylating drugs, 742, 744t
Allergic reaction, xx
allopurinol sodium, 16–19
Aloprim, 16
alpha₁–antitrypsin, 19–20

alpha-difluoromethylornithine, 272–273
alpha₁–proteinase inhibitor (human), 19–20
alteplase, recombinant, 21–24
Alti-Doxycycline, 265
Alti-Valproic, 694
AmBisome, 39
A-methaPred, 469
Amicar, 26
amikacin sulfate, 24–26
Amikin, 24
aminocaproic acid, 26–28
aminophylline, 28–31
amiodarone hydrochloride, 31–34
ammonium chloride, 34–36
amobarbital sodium, 36–39
Amphocin, 39
Amphotec, 39
amphotericin B, 39–44
amphotericin B cholesteryl sulfate complex, 39–44
amphotericin B liposomal complex, 39–44
amphotericin lipid complex, 39–44
ampicillin sodium, 44–47
ampicillin sodium and sulbactam sodium, 48–51
Ampicin, 44
amrinone lactate, 381–383
Amytal, 36
Ana-Guard, 277
Anaphylactic reaction, xx–xxi
Ancef, 120
Anergan 25, 615
Anergan 50, 615

Anexate, 319
Angiomax, 88
Aniflex, 542
anisoylated plasminogen-
    streptokinase activator
    complex, 51–53
anistreplase, 51–53
Antagonists, xix–xx
Antibiotic antineoplastics, 743,
    744–746t
Antilirium, 590
Antimetabolites, 743, 746–747t
Antimitotic antineoplastics, 743,
    747t
Antinaus 50, 615
Antineoplastic drugs, 742–743,
    744–749t
Antineoplastic enzymes, 743,
    747t
antithrombin III, human, 54–55
Anzemet, 249
Apo-Acetazolamide, 3
Apo-Atenol, 60
Apo-Benztropine, 80
Apo-Doxy, 265
Apo-Metoprolol (Type L), 476
Apo-Perphenazine, 572
Apresoline, 361
aprotinin, 55–57
ARA-C, 746t
Aramine, 455
Aranesp, 208
Aredia, 554
argatroban, 58–60
asparaginase, 747t
Astramorph PF, 497
AT-III, 54–55
atenolol, 60–63
Ativan, 439
ATnativ, 54
atracurium besylate, 63–65
atropine sulfate, 65–67
Azactam, 73
azathioprine, 67–70
azathioprine sodium, 67–70
azithromycin, 70–73
aztreonam, 73–76

B

Bactocill, 544
Bactrim, 193
Banflex, 542
basiliximab, 77–79
BCNU, 742t
Beesix, 627
Benadryl, 243
benzquinamide hydrochloride,
    79–80
benztropine mesylate, 80–83
Betaloc, 476
betamethasone sodium
    phosphate, 83–86
Betaxin, 665
Biamine, 665
BiCNU, 742t
Biological response modifiers,
    743, 747t
biperiden lactate, 86–88
bivalirudin, 88–91
Blenoxane, 91, 744t
bleomycin sulfate, 91–94, 744t
Blood products, administering,
    xxxi
Blood types, xxxii
Body mass index calculation,
    750–751t
Bretylate, 95
bretylium tosylate, 95–97, 96i
Bretylol, 95
Brevibloc, 294
bumetanide, 97–99
Bumex, 97
Buprenex, 99
buprenorphine hydrochloride,
    99–102
busulfan, 744t
Busulfex, 744t
butorphanol tartrate, 102–105

C

Caelyx, 261
Calciject, 107

Calcijex, 106
Calcilean, 357
Calciparine, 357
calcitriol, 106–107
calcium chloride, 107–111
calcium gluceptate, 107–111
calcium gluconate, 107–111
Calcium Stanley, 107
Camptosar, 394
Cancidas, 113
Capastat, 111
capreomycin sulfate, 111–113
Carbacot, 461
carbamide, 689–691
Cardene, 522
Cardene I.V., 522
Cardene SR, 522
Cardizem, 238
carmustine, 742t
caspofungin acetate, 113–116, 114i
2–CdA, 746t
Cefadyl, 158
cefamandole nafate, 116–119
cefazolin sodium, 120–123
cefepime hydrochloride, 123–126
Cefizox, 149
cefmetazole sodium, 126–129
Cefobid, 131
cefonicid sodium, 129–131
cefoperazone sodium, 131–134
Cefotan, 138
cefotaxime sodium, 135–138, 139i
cefotetan disodium, 138–142
cefoxitin sodium, 142–145
ceftazidime, 145–149
ceftizoxime sodium, 149–152
ceftriaxone sodium, 152–155
cefuroxime sodium, 155–158
Celestone Phosphate, 83
cephapirin sodium, 158–160
Ceptaz, 145
Cerebyx, 331
Ceredase, 15
Cerubidine, 745t

chloramphenicol sodium succinate, 161–163
chlordiazepoxide hydrochloride, 163–165
2–chlorodeoxyadenosine, 746t
Chloromag, 442
Chloromycetin, 161
chlorothiazide sodium, 166–169, 167i
chlorpromazine hydrochloride, 169–172
cidofovir, 172–175
Cidomycin, 347
cimetidine hydrochloride, 175–177
ciprofloxacin, 178–180
Cipro I.V., 178
cisplatin, 181–185
cladribine, 746t
Claforan, 135
Cleocin, 185
clindamycin phosphate, 185–187
codeine phosphate, 187–190
Cogentin, 80
Colaspase, 747t
colchicine, 190–193, 191i
Common Toxicity Criteria of NCI, 732–741t
Compazine, 610
Controlled substance schedules, viii
Cordarone, 31
Corlopam, 310
Cortastat, 213
Corvert, 373
Cosmegen, 745t
co-trimoxazole, 193–195
Coumadin, 712
Culture, drug dosage and, xxi
cyclophosphamide, 195–200
cyclosporin A, 200–203
cyclosporine, 200–203
cytarabine, 746t
Cytosar, 746t
Cytosar-U, 746t
cytosine arabinoside, 746t
Cytovene, 341

Cytovene-IV, 341
Cytoxan, 195

D

dacarbazine, 748*t*
dacliximab, 204–205
daclizumab, 204–205
dactinomycin, 745*t*
Dalacin C Phosphate, 185
Dalalone, 213
Dalgan, 221
Dantrium, 205
Dantrium Intravenous, 205
dantrolene sodium, 205–208
darbepoetin alfa, 208–211
daunorubicin, liposomal, 745*t*
daunorubicin hydrochloride, 745*t*
DaunoXome, 745*t*
Dazamide, 3
DDAVP Injection, 211
Decadrol, 213
Decadron Phosphate, 213
Decaject, 213
Demadex, 678
Demerol, 447
denileukin diftitox, 747*t*
2'-deoxycoformycin, 746*t*
Depacon, 694
Depakene, 694
Depakote, 694
Depakote Sprinkle, 694
Deproic, 694
Desired effect, xx
desmopressin acetate, 211–213
Dexacorten, 213
dexamethasone sodium
    phosphate, 213–217
Dexasone, 213
DexFerrum, 399
DexIron, 399
Dexone, 213
dexrazoxane, 217–219
dextrose, 219–221
2.5% Dextrose Injection, 219
5% Dextrose Injection, 219

10% Dextrose Injection, 219
20% Dextrose Injection, 219
25% Dextrose Injection, 219
30% Dextrose Injection, 219
40% Dextrose Injection, 219
50% Dextrose Injection, 219
60% Dextrose Injection, 219
70% Dextrose Injection, 219
dezocine, 221–223
DFMO, 272–273
D.H.E. 45, 235
Diamox, 3
Diamox Sequels, 3
Diazemuls, 224
diazepam, 224–227
diazoxide, 227–229
Didronel, 302
Diflucan, 317
Digibind, 233
digoxin, 230–233
digoxin immune Fab (ovine),
    233–235
dihydroergotamine mesylate,
    235–237
Dihydroergotamine-Sandoz, 235
dihydromorphinone, 367–370
1,25–dihydroxycholecalciferol,
    106–107
Dilantin, 584
Dilaudid, 367
Dilaudid-HP, 367
diltiazem hydrochloride, 238–240,
    238*i*
dimenhydrinate, 241–243
Dinate, 241
diphenhydramine hydrochloride,
    243–245
Diprivan, 618
dipyridamole, 245–246
disoprofol, 618–620
Diuril, 166
divalproex sodium, 694–697
Dizac, 224
dobutamine hydrochloride,
    246–249
Dobutrex, 246
docetaxel, 747*t*

dolasetron mesylate, 249–251
Dom-Proic, 694
dopamine hydrochloride, 251–255
Dopram, 255
Doryx, 265
doxapram hydrochloride, 255–257
Doxil, 261
Doxine, 627
doxorubicin hydrochloride, 257–261
doxorubicin hydrochloride liposome, 261–265
Doxycin, 265
doxycycline calcium, 265–269
doxycycline hyclate, 265–269
Dramanate, 241
droperidol, 269–271
Drug absorption, xvi–xvii
Drug classification, xv
Drug distribution, xvii–xviii
Drug excretion, xviii
Drug interaction, xxi
Drug metabolism, xviii
Drug nomenclature, xv–xvi
DTIC, 748t
DTIC-Dome, 748t
Duramorph, 497

E

Edecrin, 299
eflornithine hydrochloride, 272–273
Elderly patients, special considerations and, xxi–xxii
Ellence, 745t
Elspar, 747t
Emete-Con, 79
Eminase, 51
enalaprilat, 274–277
Epimorph, 497
epinephrine, 277–280
epinephrine hydrochloride, 277–280
epirubicin hydrochloride, 745t

Epival, 694
EPO, 280–283
epoetin alfa, 280–283
Epogen, 280
epoprostenol sodium, 283–286
Eprex, 280
eptifibatide, 286–289
Erythrocin, 289
erythromycin gluceptate, 289–293
erythromycin lactobionate, 289–293
erythropoietin alfa, 280–283
esmolol hydrochloride, 294–296
estrogens (conjugated), 297–299
ethacrynate sodium, 299–302
Ethnicity, drug dosage and, xxi
etidronate disodium, 302–303
Etopophos, 303
etoposide, 303–307
etoposide phosphate, 303–307

F

famotidine, 307–309, 308i
fenoldopam mesylate, 310–311
fentanyl citrate, 312–314
Ferrlecit, 652
filgrastim, 314–317
Flagyl, 479
Flagyl I.V., 479
Flagyl I.V. RTU, 479
Flexoject, 542
Flolan, 283
Floxin, 536
fluconazole, 317–319
Fludara, 747t
fludarabine phosphate, 747t
flumazenil, 319–321
fluorouracil, 322–326
Folex, 463
Folex PFS, 463
folic acid, 326–327
Folvite, 326
Fortaz, 145
foscarnet sodium, 327–331
Foscavir, 327

fosphenytoin sodium, 331–336
5-FU, 322–326
Fungizone Intravenous, 39
furosemide, 337–340

G

Galzin, 718
Gamimune N 5%, 378
Gamimune N 10%, 378
Gamimune N 5% S/D, 378
Gamimune N 10% S/D, 378
Gammagard S/D, 378
Gammagard S/D 0.5 g, 378
Gammar-P IV, 378
ganciclovir sodium, 341–344
Garamycin, 347
gatifloxacin, 344–347
gemcitabine hydrochloride, 748*t*
Gemzar, 748*t*
gentamicin sulfate, 347–350
Gliadel Wafer, 744*t*
glucagon, 350–352
Glucagon Diagnostic Kit, 350
Glucagon Emergency Kit, 350
glucose, 219–221
glyceryl trinitrate, 526–529
glycopyrrolate, 352–356
G-Mycin, 347
granisetron hydrochloride,
    356–357
granulocyte colony-stimulating
    factor, 314–317
Gravol, 241

H

Hepalean, 357
heparin calcium, 357–361
heparin co-factor I, 54–55
Heparin Leo, 357
Heparin Lock Flush, 357
heparin sodium, 357–361
Herceptin, 681, 749*t*
Hexadrol Phosphate, 213

Histanil, 615
Hormonal antineoplastics, 743
Humulin R, 388
Hycamtin, 749*t*
hydralazine hydrochloride,
    361–363
Hydrate, 241
hydrocortisone sodium
    phosphate, 364–367
hydrocortisone sodium succinate,
    364–367
Hydrocortone Phosphate, 364
hydromorphone hydrochloride,
    367–370
hyoscyamine sulfate, 370–372
Hyperstat, 227
Hyrexin, 243

I

ibutilide fumarate, 373–375
Idamycin, 745*t*
idarubicin hydrochloride, 745*t*
Idiosyncratic response, xx
IFEX, 744*t*
ifosfamide, 744*t*
IGIV, 378–381
Ilotycin, 289
IL-2, 747*t*
imipenem and cilastatin sodium,
    375–378
immune globulin intravenous
    (human), 378–381
immune serum globulin, 378–381
Imuran, 67
inamrinone lactate, 381–383
Inapsine, 269
Inderal, 620
Indocid PDA, 383
Indocin I.V., 383
indomethacin sodium trihydrate,
    383–385
InFeD, 399
infliximab, 386–388
Infusion devices, xxvii–xxviii
Inocor, 381

insulin human injection, buffered regular, 388–391
insulin human injection, regular, 388–391
insulin injection, regular, 388–391
Integrilin, 286
interferon alfa-2b, recombinant, 391–394
interleukin-2, 747*t*
Intron A, 391
Intropin, 251
irinotecan hydrochloride, 394–398
iron dextran, 399–401
iron sucrose, 401–403
ISG, 378–381
isoproterenol hydrochloride, 403–406
Isoptin, 701
Isuprel, 403
itraconazole, 406–409
I.V. drug administration, principles of, xxiii–xxxii
Iveegam, 378
I.V. flow rates, calculating, 730–731
IVIG, 378–381
I.V. therapy, complications of, xxviii–xxix
I.V. therapy, nursing process and, xxxiii–xxxviii
I.V. therapy, teaching patient about, x–xi

J

Jenamicin, 347

K

Kabikinase, 657
kanamycin sulfate, 410–411
Kantrex, 410
Kefurox, 155
Kefzol, 120
ketorolac tromethamine, 412–414

Kidrolase, 747*t*
Kytril, 356

L

labetalol hydrochloride, 414–417
Lanoxin Injection, 230
Lanoxin Injection Pediatric, 230
Largactil, 169
Lasix, 337
Lasix Special, 337
lepirudin, 417–419
Leustatin, 746*t*
Levaquin, 420
levarterenol bitartrate, 531–533
Levo-Dromoran, 423
levofloxacin, 420–423
Levophed, 531
levorphanol tartrate, 423–426
Levothroid, 426
levothyroxine sodium, 426–428
Levsin, 370
Librium, 163
lidocaine hydrochloride, 428–430
lignocaine hydrochloride, 428–430
Lincocin, 431
lincomycin hydrochloride, 431–433
linezolid, 433–436, 434*i*
liothyronine sodium, 436–439
Liquaemin, 357
Lopresor, 476
Lopressor, 476
lorazepam, 439–441
L-thyroxine sodium, 426–428
L-triiodothyronine, 436–439
Luminal, 576

M

magnesium chloride, 442–444
magnesium sulfate, 442–444
Mandol, 116
mannitol, 445–447
Maxipime, 123

mechlorethamine hydrochloride,
744*t*
Med-Valproic, 694
Mefoxin, 142
Megacillin, 561
meperidine hydrochloride,
447–450
mephentermine sulfate, 450–453
meropenem, 453–455
Merrem I.V., 453
Mestinon, 624
Mestinon-SR, 624
Mestinon Timespans, 624
metaraminol bitartrate, 455–459
methicillin sodium, 459–461
methocarbamol, 461–463
methotrexate sodium, 463–467
methyldopate hydrochloride,
467–469
methylprednisolone sodium
succinate, 469–473
metoclopramide hydrochloride,
473–476
metoprolol tartrate, 476–479
Metro I.V., 479
metronidazole, 479–482
metronidazole hydrochloride,
479–482
Mexate, 463
Mexate-AQ, 463
Mezlin, 482
mezlocillin sodium, 482–485
midazolam hydrochloride,
485–488
milrinone lactate, 488–490, 489*i*
Minocin, 491
minocycline hydrochloride,
491–493
Miolin, 542
Mio-Rel, 542
Mithracin, 746*t*
mithramycin, 746*t*
mitomycin, 746*t*
mitomycin-C, 746*t*
mitoxantrone, 493–497

mitoxantrone hydrochloride, 749*t*
Monocid, 129
Morphine Extra-Forte, 497
Morphine Forte, 497
Morphine H.P., 497
morphine sulfate, 497–502
Mustargen, 744*t*
Mutamycin, 746*t*
Myleran, 744*t*
Myotrol, 542

N

Nafcil, 503
nafcillin sodium, 503–505
nalbuphine hydrochloride,
505–508
Nallpen, 503
nalmefene hydrochloride, 508–510
naloxone hydrochloride, 510–512
Naming drugs, xv
Narcan, 510
Natrecor, 515
Navelbine, 747*t*
Nebcin, 675
Needlestick injuries, preventing,
xxix
Nembutal, 569
Neoral, 200
Neosar, 195
neostigmine methylsulfate, 513–514
Neo-Synephrine, 582
nesiritide, 515–517
Nestrex, 627
netilmicin sulfate, 517–520
Netromycin, 517
Neupogen, 314
niacin, 520–522
niacinamide, 520–522
nicardipine hydrochloride,
522–526
nicotinamide, 520–522
nicotinic acid, 520–522
Nipent, 746*t*

Nipride, 529
Nitro-Bid I.V., 526
nitrogen mustard, 742*t*
nitroglycerin, 526–529, 527*i*
Nitroject, 526
Nitropress, 529
nitroprusside sodium, 529–531
norepinephrine bitartrate, 531–533
Norflex, 542
Normodyne, 414
Novantrone, 493, 749*t*
Novo-Atenol, 60
Novo-Cimetine, 175
Novolin ge Toronto, 388
Novolin R, 388
Novometoprol, 476
Novo-Valproic, 694
Nubain, 505
Nu-Metop, 476
Numorphan, 547
Nursing process, I.V. drug therapy and, xxxiii–xxxviii
Nu-Valproic, 694

O

Octostim, 211
octreotide acetate, 534–536
ofloxacin, 536 540, 538*i*
Omnipen-N, 44
Oncaspar, 747*t*
Oncovin, 708
ondansetron hydrochloride, 540–542
Ontak, 747*t*
Opioid agonists, equianalgesic doses for, 725*t*
Orazinc, 718
Orfro, 542
Ornidyl, 272
orphenadrine citrate, 542–544
Orphenate, 542
Osmitrol, 445

oxacillin sodium, 544–546
oxymorphone hydrochloride, 547–549

P

paclitaxel, 550–554
2–PAM chloride, 606–608
pamidronate disodium, 554–557
Pantoloc, 557
pantoprazole sodium, 557–558
Parenteral drug dosages, calculating, 728–729
Parenteral fluids, administering, xxix
paricalcitol, 559–561
Patient-controlled analgesia, xxviii
Pediatric patients, special considerations and, xxii
pegaspargase, 747*t*
PEG-L-asparaginase, 747*t*
Penbritin, 44
penicillin G potassium, 561–563
Pentacarinat, 563
Pentam 300, 563
pentamidine isethionate, 563–565
Pentazine, 615
pentazocine lactate, 565–568
Pentids, 561
pentobarbital sodium, 569–572
pentostatin, 746*t*
Pepcid, 307
perphenazine, 572–575
Persantine, 245
pethidine hydrochloride, 447–450
Pfizerpen, 561
PGI$_2$, 283–286
PGX, 283–286
Pharmacodynamics, xviii–xx
Pharmacokinetics, xvi–xviii
Pharmacotherapeutics, xx–xxi
Phenazine 25, 615
Phenazine 50, 615

Phencen-50, 615
Phenergan, 615
Phenerzine, 615
phenobarbital sodium, 576–580
Phenoject-50, 615
phentolamine mesylate, 580–581
phenylephrine hydrochloride,
    582–584
phenytoin sodium, 584–590
Photofrin, 749*t*
physostigmine salicylate, 590–591
piperacillin sodium, 592–595
piperacillin sodium and
    tazobactam sodium, 595–598
Pipracil, 592
Platinol, 181
Platinol-AQ, 181
plicamycin, 746*t*
PMS Benztropine, 80
PMS Perphenazine, 572
PMS-Valproic Acid, 694
Polycillin-N, 44
Polygam S/D, 378
polymyxin B sulfate, 598–601
porfimer sodium, 749*t*
potassium acetate, 601–603
potassium chloride, 601–603
potassium phosphates, 604–606
pralidoxime chloride, 606–608
Pregnancy, special considerations
    and, xxii
Pregnancy risk categories, vii
Premarin, 297
Primacor, 488
Primaxin, 375
Primaxin ADD-Vantage, 375
Primaxin IV, 375
Primethasone, 213
Pro-50, 615
procainamide hydrochloride,
    608–610
prochlorperazine edisylate,
    610–614
Procrit, 280
Procytox, 195
Prolastin, 19

Proleukin, 747*t*
Promacot, 615
Pro-Med 50, 615
Promet, 615
promethazine hydrochloride,
    615–618
Pronestyl, 608
propofol, 618–620
propranolol hydrochloride,
    620–622
Prorex-25, 615
Prorex-50, 615
prostacyclin, 283–286
Prostaphlin, 544
Prostigmin, 513
protamine sulfate, 623–624
Prothazine, 615
Protonix, 557
Protonix I.V., 557
Protopam Chloride, 606
Pyri, 627
2-pyridine aldoxime
    methochloride, 606–608
pyridostigmine bromide, 624–626
pyridoxine hydrochloride,
    627–628

Q

quinidine gluconate, 629–631
quinupristin and dalfopristin,
    631–634

R

ranitidine hydrochloride,
    634–636
recombinant erythropoietin,
    280–283
Refludan, 417
Regitine, 580
Reglan, 473
Regonol, 624
Regular Iletin II, 388
Regular Insulin, 388

Remicade, 386
remifentanil hydrochloride, 636–639, 638*i*
ReoPro, 1
Resectisol, 445
Retavase, 640
reteplase, 640–642
Retrovir, 715
Revex, 508
Revimine, 251
Rexolate, 654
rG-CSF, 314–317
Rh factor, xxxii
r-HuEPO, 280–283
Rifadin, 642
Rifadin IV, 642
rifampicin, 642–645
rifampin, 642–645
"Rights" of drug administration, xxiv–xxvi
Rimactane, 642
Rituxan, 645
rituximab, 645–647
Robaxin, 461
Robinul, 352
Robinul Forte, 352
Rocephin, 152
Rodex, 627
Rofact, 642
Rogitine, 580
Romazicon, 319
Rubex, 257

S

Sandimmune, 200
Sandoglobulin, 378
Sandostatin, 534
SangCya, 200
scopolamine hydrobromide, 647–650
Selestoject, 83
Septra, 193
Shogan, 615
Simulect, 77

Skelex, 461
sodium bicarbonate, 650–652
sodium ferric gluconate, 652–654
sodium L-triiodothyronine, 436–439
sodium phosphates, 604–606
sodium thiosalicylate, 654–656
Solu-Cortef, 364
Solu-Medrol, 469
Solurex, 213
Solution, calculating strength of, 726–727
Sporanox, 406
Stadol, 102
Staphcillin, 459
Storzolamide, 3
Streptase, 657
streptokinase, 657–659
streptozocin, 744*t*
Sublimaze, 312
sulfamethoxazole and trimethoprim, 193–195
Synercid, 631–634
Synthroid, 426

T

T_3, 436–439
T_4, 426–428
Tagamet, 175
Talwin, 565
Taxol, 550
Taxotere, 747*t*
Tazicef, 145
Tazidime, 145
Tazocin, 595
tenecteplase, 660–662
Tenormin, 60
Tequin, 344
TESPA, 744*t*
Tham, 687
theophylline ethylenediamine, 28–31
theophylline in dextrose injection, 662–665

thiamine hydrochloride, 665–667
Thioplex, 744*t*
thiotepa, 744*t*
Thorazine, 169
Thrombate III, 54
thyronine sodium, 436–439
thyroxine sodium, 426–428
Ticar, 667
ticarcillin disodium, 667–670
ticarcillin disodium and
    clavulanate potassium,
    670–673
Timentin, 670
tirofiban hydrochloride, 673–675
tissue plasminogen activator,
    recombinant, 21–24
TNKase, 660
Tobi, 675
tobramycin sulfate, 675–678
Toposar, 303
topotecan hydrochloride, 749*t*
Toradol, 412
torsemide, 678–681
Totacillin-N, 44
Total parenteral nutrition,
    administering, xxxi
Toxic agents, safe handling of,
    xxix
Tracrium, 63
Trandate, 414
trastuzumab, 681–684, 749*t*
Trasylol, 55
Tridil, 526
triethylenethiophosphoramide,
    744*t*
triflupromazine hydrochloride,
    684–687
Trilafon, 572
Trilafon Concentrate, 572
Triostat, 436
tromethamine, 687–689
trovafloxacin mesylate, 12–14
Trovan, 12
Trovan I.V., 12
TSPA, 744*t*
Tusal, 654

U

Ultiva, 636
Unasyn, 48
Unipen, 503
urea, 689–691
Ureaphil, 689
Uritol, 337
urokinase, 691–694

V

Valium, 224
valproate sodium, 694–697
valproic acid, 694–697
Vancocin, 698
vancomycin hydrochloride,
    698–701
Vasotec I.V., 274
Velban, 704
Velbe, 704
Velosulin BR, 388
Venofer, 401
Venoglobulin-I, 378
Venoglobulin-S 5%, 378
Venoglobulin-S 10%, 378
Venous access, types of, xxvi–xxvii
VePesid, 303
verapamil hydrochloride, 701–703
Versed, 485
Vesprin, 684
V-Gan-25, 615
V-Gan-50, 615
Vibramycin, 265
Vibra-Tabs, 265
vinblastine sulfate, 704–707
Vincasar PFS, 708
vincristine sulfate, 708–711
vinorelbine tartrate, 747*t*
Vistide, 172
Vitabee 6, 627
vitamin B$_1$, 665–667
vitamin B$_3$, 520–522
vitamin B$_6$, 627–628
vitamin B$_9$, 326–327

W

warfarin sodium, 712–715
Water and electrolyte solutions,
    xxx*t*
Wyamine, 450

X

Xylocaine, 428
Xylocard, 428

Z

Zanosar, 744*t*
Zantac, 634

Zefazone, 126
Zemplar, 559
Zcnapax, 204
zidovudine, 715–718
Zinacef, 155
zinc acetate, 718–721
Zinca-Pak, 718
zinc chloride, 718–721
zinc gluconate, 718–721
zinc sulfate, 718–721
Zinecard, 217
Zithromax, 70
Zofran, 540
zoledronic acid, 721–724
Zometa, 721
Zosyn, 595
Zovirax, 6
Zyvox, 433

COMPATIBLE DRUGS IN A SYRINGE

The chart below lets you know at a glance whether particular drugs are compatible for at least 15 minutes when mixed together in a syringe for immediate administration. However, keep in mind that drugs listed as compatible when mixed in a syringe may not be compatible when prepared for other routes of administration. Drug combinations

	atropine	chlorpromazine	dexamethasone	diazepam	diphenhydramine	droperidol	furosemide	glycopyrrolate	haloperidol	heparin	hydromorphone
atropine		C	n/a	n/a	C	C	n/a	C	I	n/a	C
chlorpromazine	C		n/a	n/a	C	C	n/a	C	n/a	I	C
dexamethasone	n/a	n/a		n/a	I	n/a	n/a	n/a	n/a	n/a	C
diazepam	n/a	n/a	n/a		n/a	n/a	n/a	I	n/a	I	n/a
diphenhydramine	C	C	I	n/a		C	n/a	C	I	n/a	C
droperidol	C	C	n/a	n/a	C		I	C	n/a	I	n/a
furosemide	n/a	n/a	n/a	n/a	n/a	I		n/a	n/a	C	n/a
glycopyrrolate	C	C	I	C	C	C	n/a		C	n/a	C
haloperidol	n/a	n/a	n/a	n/a	C	n/a	n/a	n/a		I	C
heparin	C	I	n/a	I	n/a	I	C	n/a	I		n/a
hydromorphone	C	C	n/a	n/a	C	n/a	n/a	C	C	n/a	
hydroxyzine	C	C	n/a	n/a	C	C	n/a	C	I	n/a	C
ketorolac	n/a	n/a	n/a	I	n/a	n/a	n/a	n/a	I	n/a	I
lidocaine	n/a	n/a	n/a	n/a	n/a	n/a	n/a	C	n/a	C	n/a
lorazepam	n/a	n/a	n/a	n/a	n/a	n/a	n/a	n/a	n/a	n/a	C
meperidine	C	C	n/a	C	C	C	n/a	C	n/a	I	n/a
metoclopramide	C	C	n/a	n/a	C	C	I	n/a	n/a	C	C
midazolam	C	C	n/a	n/a	C	n/a	n/a	C	C	n/a	C
morphine	C	C	n/a	n/a	C	C	n/a	C	I	C*	n/a
pentobarbital	C	I	n/a	n/a	I	I	n/a	I	n/a	n/a	C
prochlorperazine	C	n/a	n/a	n/a	C	C	n/a	C	n/a	n/a	I
ranitidine	C	I	C	n/a	C	n/a	n/a	C	n/a	n/a	C
scopolamine	C	C	n/a	n/a	C	C	n/a	C	n/a	n/a	C

* Compatible only with morphine doses of 1 mg, 2 mg, and 5 mg.